THE ROYAL COLLEGE OF NURSING
MANUAL OF FAMILY HEALTH

ROYAL COLLEGE OF NURSING
Manual of Family Health

Everyday care in the home

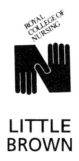

LITTLE
BROWN

A *Little, Brown* Book

First published in Great Britain in 1992 by Little, Brown and
Company

Copyright © Little, Brown and Company (UK) Limited and
Scutari Press 1992

The right of the Royal College of Nursing to be identified as
author of this work has been asserted in accordance with the
Copyright, Designs and Patents Act 1988.

A CIP catalogue record for this book is available from the
British Library.

ISBN 0 356 20051 5

Little, Brown and Company (UK) Limited
165 Great Dover Street
London SE1 4YA

Conceived and produced by
Martin Marix Evans MA, Book Packaging and Marketing,
3 Murswell Lane, Silverstone, Towcester,
Northants NN12 8UT

Designed, typeset and illustrated by
Oxprint Ltd, Aristotle Lane, Oxford OX2 6TR

Printed and bound in Great Britain by
BPCC Hazells Ltd
Member of BPCC Ltd

CONTENTS

CONTENTS

PART III

APPENDICES

Editorial Direction

The Manual of Family Health was produced under the direction of Scutari Press, a division of Scutari Projects, the publishing company of the Royal College of Nursing, with the help and support of the members of the Department of Nursing Policy and Practice of the Royal College of Nursing

Senior Editorial Adviser

Mark Jones BSc(Hons), RGN, RHV (Higher Dip),
Community Health Adviser to the Royal College of Nursing

Additional Editorial Advisers

June Andrews MA(Hons), MA(Nott), RGN, RMN;
Dr St.J. Dowling MB FRCGP;
Rosemary Morris RGN, RM, RSCN, Dip.N, RNT

Consultant Editorial Advisers
Jo Alexander RGN, RM, MTD, JBCNS Course 900;
Anne Betts MSc, BSc(Hons), RGN, RNT; Chris Corfield MRPharmS;
Paul Lloyd RGN, OHN Cert; Vicki Nix RGN, RM, FETC, DMS;
Christine Norton MA, RGN; Linda Thomas RGN;
Barbara Weller MSc, RGN, RSCN, RNT; Pauline Weston RGN, RM, ADM;
WING (Work Injured Nurses Group)

Editor

Richenda Milton-Thompson BA(Hons), M.Litt

Additional editorial help from
Jessica Anderson; Linda Bailey RGN; Anne Blandford (Citizens' Advice Bureau Worker); Jim McCarthy RMN; Carrie Walker MA, MB, BS; Sarah Windsor BA(Hons)

Contributors

Jo Alexander RGN, RM, MTD, JBCNS Course 900;

Susan C Bailey RGN, NDN, Cert.ICN;

Pamela A Barnes Cert.Ed, SKTC Dip, Counselling Dip;

Anne V Betts MSc, BSc(Hons), RGN, RNT;

Jenifer A Booth RGN, ONC, RCNT, Dip.N, FETC;

Christine G Brooker BSc, SRN, SCM, RNT;

Sue Cluroe SRN, RSCN, RCNT;

Greta Curtis SRN, RM, ONC;

Liz Day MA, BA, RGN, NDN, HV, PGCEA;

Brendan Egan RMN, FETC, Cert.Counselling;

Scilla Erskine BA(Hons), RGN;

Laura Ferguson RGN, Dip.N, Onc.Nursing Cert;

Dinah Gould BSc, M.Phil, RGN, Dip.N, Cert.Ed;

Jill Gregson MSc, RGN, RSCN;

Peter E Hodgkinson BA, MPhil, AFBPSS, C.Psychol;

Angela Huggett RGN, NDN, PWT, PGCEA, DNT;

Chris Jackson PhD, BA(Hons);

Mark Jones BSc(Hons), RGN, RHV(Hgr Dip.);

Caroline R Lamming RGN,NDN, RHV, Dip.N;

Jenny Langford RGN, RM, ADM, MTD, PGCEA;

Sandra Lask BA(Hons), MSc, PGCEA, RGN, RNT;

Valerie Levy RGN, RM, MTD;

Paul V Lloyd RGN, OHN Cert;

Paul Mangan RGN, EN(G);

Alison McCormick RMN;

Donna Mead MSc, RGN, RNT, RCNT, Dip.N, DANS;

Julia Mingay MSc, RGN, RMN, Dip.N, Dip.N.Ed., RCNT, RNT, Cert.Counselling;

John Morgan RMN, Dip.N, Cert.Ed, RNT;

Elizabeth Morris BSc, SRN, RMN, RNT;

Rosemary Morris RGN, RM, RSCN, Dip.N, RNT;

David Mossman PhD, BSc;

Linda Nazarko RGN;

Sarah Peters Dip.COT, SROT;

Moira Plant PhD, RGN, RMN;

Brenda Poulton MSc, BA(Hons), RGN, RHV, FWT, Cert.Ed;

Marion Richardson BD(Hons), RGN, RCNT, Dip.N;

Ruth Sander RGN, RCNT, Dip.N;

Ruth Scudamore RGN, RSCN, SCM, RHV, PGCEA;

David Sines PhD, BSc(Hons), RMN, RMNH, FRCN;

Carol Smith RGN, RM;

Linda Thomas RGN;

Stephen Thomas RGN;

Verena Tschudin BSc(Hons), RGN, RM, Dip.Counselling Skills;

Jackie Tyler MSc, SRN, ONC, NDN, PWT, Cert.Ed(FE), RNT;

Carolyn M Walker MA, MB, BS;

Jan Ward RMN;

Jane Warner RGN, Dip.N, Cert.Clin. Teaching;

Mary Watkins MN, RGN, RMN;

Valerie Watson RGN, RMN, RM, Dip.Prof. Studies;

Pat Webb RGN, RNT, Dip.Soc.Res;

Barbara F Weller MSc, RGN, RSCN, RNT;

Pauline Weston RGN, RM, ADM;

Marion Wood RGN, RCNT;

Kay Wright RGN, RCNT, Dip.N;

Ann P Young BA, RGN, RNT;

Lynn Young RGN, Dip.N, PWT;

Pat Young BA(Hons)

FOREWORD

I am delighted to have been asked to introduce *The Royal College of Nursing Manual of Family Health*.

This is the first time that such a guide to family health has been produced by nurses. Written by nurses and allied professionals, it is a particularly timely publication, for more and more people are recognising the invaluable contribution made by good nursing practice to the well-being of the nation's population.

By looking at issues like job loss, being bullied at school and the death of a loved one, the *Manual* promotes health by looking at the whole person. Nurses know that the stresses and strains of everyday living take their toll on the health of the individual. There is little point treating the middle-aged man's insomnia without recognising that redundancy and the consequent fears of failure and financial problems are the prime cause.

Illustrated, easy to read and highly informative, the manual provides indispensable information for all sections of the community, whatever their particular health needs are at the different stages of their lives. While giving guidance on caring for sick people, the manual also concentrates on how to stay healthy.

Using this innovative format, the guide begins with the basics. General information is given on fitness and health, caring for sick people at home and coping with normal life events like adolescence, marriage and having children.

Subsequent chapters are divided by age, starting with birth and ending with the over 60s. A series of Appendices include information on how the body works, first aid, further reading and useful addresses.

I am convinced that every family in the United Kingdom will gain vital health information from this manual. I am especially proud that the Royal College of Nursing has seized the initiative and produced such a worthwhile guide. I am sure that its style will ensure its appeal to all.

Christine Hancock
General Secretary
Royal College of Nursing

HEALTH AND CARING

1 KEEPING FIT AND HEALTHY

1.1 DIET

The link between what we eat and the state of our health has been well established for a long time, and most people now accept that their eating habits can affect them in one way or another.

Eating well and enjoying your food is a very important part of keeping fit and healthy. Many of us, however, develop eating habits which can easily undermine our health rather than contribute to promoting it.

- What is your diet like?

- Do you think that you are eating properly?

Good nutrition plays a central role in managing stress, preventing illness and in promoting health and feelings of well-being.

Some people will need to take particular care of their nutritional needs as their requirements for nutrients and vitamins will be increased. These groups of people include:

- Those recovering from an illness or surgery;

- People with a long term chronic illness;

- Individuals experiencing considerable amounts of stress, over work or worry;

- Individuals who smoke cigarettes and who drink alcohol;

- Mothers of small children;

- Pregnant women and nursing mothers;

- City dwellers – exposed to pollution;

- Those taking prescribed drugs, e.g. the Pill, antidepressants.

Many Western countries do not have a very good reputation for healthy eating. On the whole we tend to eat too much of some things, like foods containing a lot of fat, sugar and salt. This causes problems. In the United Kingdom, for example, 36 per cent of the population are overweight. Being too fat is more of a problem for men than it is for women, who are more likely to have lower blood levels of vitamin C and iron than may be desirable.

1.1(a) GETTING THE BEST FROM YOUR FOOD

Modern diets – bad for your health?

Unfortunately, food today is just not what it used to be! Since the Second World War modern intensive farming methods have been developed which use millions of gallons of pesticides, nitrogen, potash and phosphate fertilisers. These chemicals not only deplete the soil of nutrients but may also contaminate the food itself. Maximum crop yields depend upon massive use of these substances which, in their turn, create ideal conditions for pests and diseases. Fungi thrive and aphids, often carrying viral disease, reproduce faster on nitrogen rich soils.

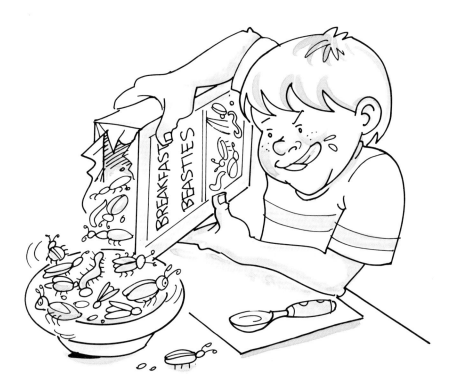

We have all heard about the grain and butter mountains and wine lakes in Europe – we produce far more than we need. So, not only may the food not be as tasty as it could be, it may also have been in storage for years, going stale and losing its vitamins.

All in all it is far better for your health to eat freshly produced organic foods, to eat them slowly and to take pleasure in your meals. If you are concerned about your diet in any way, it may be useful to complete a food diary for a week or so. Just write down everything that you eat and drink for a whole week, as indicated on the opposite page, and then examine your eating patterns. From this basis you can explore how gradual improvements can be made.

MEAL	DAY 1	DAY 2	DAY 3	DAY 4
Breakfast	1 cup of coffee with milk. Bowl of cereal. 2 slices of toast and butter.			
Snacks and drinks	1 cup of coffee with milk. 1 plain biscuit			
Lunch	One round of cheese & pickle sandwiches. One apple One can of diet cola One bar of chocolate			
Etc. ↓				
COMMENTS:				

Food diary

1.1(b) HEALTHY EATING – A FEW HINTS

There are a few basic principles to bear in mind when thinking about eating well, aiming for fitness and health.

The first, and most important, principle is to take your time over your food. There is so much emphasis on fast and instant foods these days, and arguably most people do not have the time to spend hours over preparation. However it is really worth while taking time to eat, to relax over a meal. A calm attitude whilst you are eating helps you to absorb the nutrients more efficiently. Give yourself time to eat slowly, peacefully and with concentration. You will be more aware when you have eaten enough and will be less likely to overeat. Digestion is aided by a peaceful mind and body.

Another important principle is to make sure that you actually absorb all the nutrients that you eat. There are some foods which when eaten together will inhibit the absorption of other nutrients.

Top ten foods	Other good foods
• Apricots, peaches and nectarines	• Blackcurrants
• Broccoli, brussels sprouts and cabbage	• Mangoes, pawpaw
• Carrots	• Polyunsaturated margarine
• Citrus fruits	• Offal (but not liver for pregnant women)
• Fish, particularly oily varieties such as herring, mackerel, salmon	• Parsley
• Garlic	• Peas
• Oats	• Peppers
• Olive oil	• Prunes
• Lentils	• Wholemeal bread, flour, pasta etc.
• Nuts	

Compiled from information produced by the World Health Organisation in the book Diet, Nutrition and Chronic Diseases *(see Appendix VIII) and an article by J. Marshall in* The Independent, *2nd February 1991*

Tea, coffee and fizzy canned drinks have powerful inhibiting effects upon the absorption of iron and zinc. It is better not to have these drinks with a meal, but to wait for a while and have them afterwards or to find alternatives. Keep alcohol consumption to a minimum, no more than 2–3 units 2–3 times a week for women and 3–4 units 3–4 times a week for men (units of alcohol are defined in the figure below).

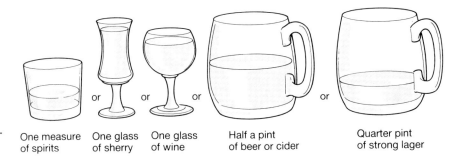

Units of alcohol

One measure of spirits • One glass of sherry • One glass of wine • Half a pint of beer or cider • Quarter pint of strong lager

Bran and unleavened wheat, particularly wholegrain wheat, when used in pastry, biscuits, chappatis and sauces thickened with wholemeal flour can block the absorption of minerals including calcium, magnesium and zinc.

Further principles for healthy eating include the following:

- Don't smoke;

- Keep sugar and refined carbohydrates to a minimum;

- Reduce both animal and vegetable fats – to about 75 per cent of your usual amount – avoid fried foods, pies, sausages, preserved and tinned meats;

- Ensure a good intake of fibre – this may help with conditions like constipation, as well as having long term health benefits (high fibre foods include beans, pulses, fruits, vegetables and cereals such as wheat, oats, barley, rye);

- Try to eat a varied and interesting diet;

- Ensure a good but not excessive intake of protein rich foods. These include lean meats, fish, eggs, poultry without the skin, nuts, seeds, peas, beans, lentils, sprouted beans and whole grains.

How much nourishment do you need? Look at the diagram below and check the chart overleaf to see if you need to make any changes.

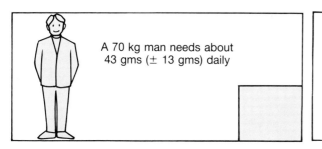
A 70 kg man needs about 43 gms (± 13 gms) daily

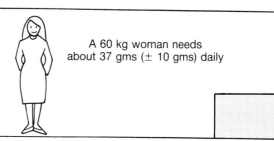
A 60 kg woman needs about 37 gms (± 10 gms) daily

Average protein requirements

One kg is equivalent to (approximately) 2lb 3oz. 100 gms is equivalent to (approximately) 3½ oz

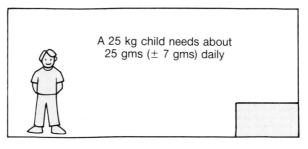
A 25 kg child needs about 25 gms (± 7 gms) daily

1.2 EXERCISE

We are not designed to live slow, inactive or sedentary lifestyles and those people who do engage in recreational exercise regularly may feel better and fitter than those who do not. They tend to enjoy more positive health and are more likely to remain within their normal weight range, which reduces their chances of illness.

Are you eating well?

Sign or symptom	Can be caused by deficiency of
Cracking at the corners of the mouth	Iron, vitamins B_2, B_6, folic acid
Recurrent mouth ulcers	Iron, folic acid, vitamin B_{12}
Dry, cracked lips	Vitamin B_2
Enlargement of taste buds of the tip of the tongue	Vitamin B_2, B_6
Bruising or enlargement of veins at the tip of the tongue	Vitamin C
Red, greasy skin on face especially sides of nose	Vitamin B_2, B_6, zinc or essential fatty acids
Skin conditions such as eczema, dry, rough, cracked or peeling skin	Zinc, essential fatty acids
Poor hair growth	Iron or zinc
Bloodshot, gritty, sensitive eyes	Vitamin A or B_2
Brittle or split nails	Iron, zinc or essential fatty acids
White spots on nails	Zinc

Many people use up a lot of energy in the course of their normal daily activities; however these physical and repetitive movements may not help you to feel fitter and may cause stresses and strains in one particular area. Physical work does not usually contribute to an increase in all round physical fitness or mental exhilaration.

Physical fitness usually contributes to a long and fulfilling life, while inactivity and obesity increase the possibility of early death. It is possible to engage in some enjoyable exercise, even when you have a limited amount of time, whatever your age.

How active are you? When there is a choice do you take the stairs, walk instead of driving or take some physical exercise?

1.2(a)　GUIDELINES FOR EXERCISE

Exercise is meant to be enjoyable and it may be helpful to turn your sporting activity into a social event, so that there is outside support to encourage you. However it can also be convenient to design a routine for yourself, to do at home to music for example.

A good variety of exercise is important. Your programme should include exercises for flexibility and for strength, like yoga or keep fit, and for increasing your heart and lung capacity, like swimming, cycling, netball, or squash. In addition, women who have reached the menopause should continue with exercises, such as brisk walking or cycling, which strengthen their bones.

The exercise that you choose will be influenced by your age, general level of health, interest and past experience.

1.2(b) SAFETY

Many people believe that the way to get the most out of exercising is to stretch and strain until they are sore. It is vital to avoid injury however. Exercise is supposed to make you feel better, not worse.

Physical activity should not pose any problems or hazards for most people, but there may be some who should seek medical advice about the type of activity most suitable for them. Such people include those with heart trouble, frequent pains in the heart or chest, dizzy spells, or high blood pressure.

Find out as much as you can about the activity you would like to get involved in. Talk to others about the type of injuries that commonly occur and ask about ways to avoid them.

Make sure you do strengthening exercises before beginning a new sport, and always warm up prior to any sporting activity.

Go slowly. The older you are, the more slowly you should start, and improve gradually.

Minimise competition. If you do want to compete, find someone your own level. The sport you may have done at school would probably have been competitive, and may have put you off. There is no need at all for sport to involve competing against others.

Finally take a few minutes to cool down slowly after any activity.

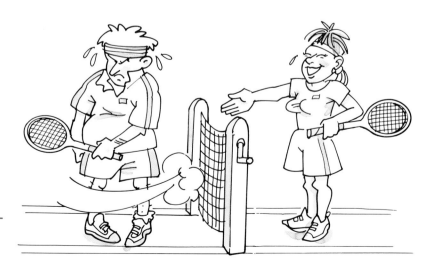

It doesn't matter whether you win or lose – unless you lose

1.2(c) PREPARATION

Mental preparation

Ask yourself 'Why do I want to exercise?' It might be because you feel you ought to, or because you want to get fit. Sometimes you feel like exercise for the enjoyment of the sport itself, or maybe because you feel stressed and tense and want to let off some steam, or release tension.

For some the joy of competition and winning is the drive behind the wish to exercise. Sometimes this competitive drive interferes with the enjoyment or the stress releasing aspects of the exercise. So develop an awareness of your motives. Sorting out in your mind exactly what you want from the physical activity can help.

STRETCHING EXERCISES

Wear comfortable and loose clothing. Remove your shoes and socks.

Hamstring stretch

Bend at the waist clasping the backs of the calves with your hands. Feet 6 inches apart. Hold for up to 10 seconds and repeat five times. You should feel the stretch at the back of your legs.

Thigh muscle stretch

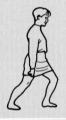

Bend the left knee and stretch the right leg out behind you, as far as you can go. Balance body over the left knee and hold for 3–5 seconds. Keep right foot flat on the floor. Repeat the other side.

Ankle stretch

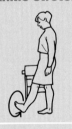

You may need to hold on to something for this one. Lift the right leg off the floor and stretch the leg in front of you with the foot a few inches off the ground. Start rotating your ankle in one direction making small circles with your foot. Repeat three times in one direction then three times in the other. Place the foot back on the ground and repeat with the other ankle.

Arm circling

Lift arms to the side and make 3–5 vigorous circles with both arms. Repeat in both directions.

Body preparation

A warm-up period of five minutes stretching before the more intensive forms of exercise is necessary to prevent injury, prepare the body, and improve performance.

Well developed flexibility prevents damage to the body from sudden exertion. It requires the stretching of certain muscle groups and, in order to stretch adequately, it is important to learn to relax the muscles too.

Stretching is a very important part of the warm up period so remember to concentrate on the stretch, don't think about other things but give it your full attention, and focus on the feelings of relaxation afterwards.

Shoulder circles

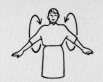

Raise your arms sideways again, parallel to the floor. With your fingers outstretched begin to make small circles with your fingers rotating your arms at the shoulder joint. Gradually increase the circles then decrease them. Repeat three times in one direction and three times in the other bringing your arms to rest by your side between each time.

Neck roll

Let your head fall down to your chest with your chin tucked in. Slowly rotate your head to the left bringing your ear as close to your left shoulder as you can. Take your head back and round over the right shoulder and finally bring your chin round to the front. Repeat three times – with your eyes closed – breathing in as you take your head back and breathing out as you bring your head forward. Repeat in the opposite direction three times.

Stair climbing

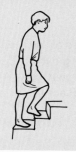

If you have stairs at home spend 5 minutes climbing up and down. Start slowly and gradually increase the pace and time spent. Remember to co-ordinate your movement and to breathe regularly.

Back posture

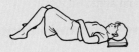

Lie on the floor on your back. Use a few books to support your head (books are better than a pillow for this exercise). Have your knees bent up and your feet about 12–18 inches apart. Your arms should be lying symmetrically on your tummy. Close your eyes and concentrate on breathing rhythmically and evenly. Stay in this position for as long as you have time for. When you get up, roll slowly to one side and sit up first before standing.

Always stretch within your limits. Be aware of your breathing, allow it to become slow and rhythmical – don't hold your breath during the stretch.

Exercise should be self rewarding: the more you do the better you feel both physically and mentally.

Have a go at the programme outlined in the chart on the previous page, and enjoy yourself!

1.3 SLEEP

For most people, the purpose of sleep is to recuperate and to rest the body and mind. After a good night's sleep you wake refreshed and invigorated ready to meet the challenges of the day with enthusiasm.

It is important to sleep well when attempting to keep fit and healthy, although we probably need much less sleep than we would like. If you do suffer from a sleep problem, take heart, you are not alone. Many adults have some problem or another.

1.3(a) SLEEP PATTERNS

During sleep the body has the opportunity for repair and growth. Psychologists have been fascinated by sleep and have set up sleep laboratories where their subjects will be (painlessly) wired up to monitoring machines which can record the brain wave patterns that occur. They have found that there are various stages of sleep, which progress from light to deep sleep followed by a dreaming period called REM (Rapid Eye Movement) sleep. The sleep cycle lasts about 90 minutes and then begins again. At the beginning of the night the REM stage is very short, only a few minutes, but gets longer throughout the night.

The research that has been done on sleep deprivation has usually used young, fit, healthy men, who have been kept awake for a few

The stages of sleep

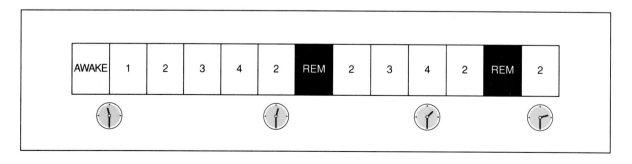

days at a time. It was found that after a few days the men became irritable, unable to concentrate and forgetful. Eventually they also became suspicious and suffered hallucinations.

Most people who suffer from sleep deprivation will not be fit, healthy young men but will be older people or women caring for young children or dependent relatives.

Sleep difficulties tend to fall into the following categories:

- Difficulty in falling asleep;

- Waking up frequently during the night;

- Waking up too early in the morning, say at about 4 am, and not being able to go back to sleep again.

In a survey taken amongst the middle aged population in Switzerland, more than half of the people polled responded that they suffered from insomnia at least occasionally, and an alarming 7 per cent of men and 12 per cent of women answered that they slept badly every night.

In general it has been found that sleep disorders are more common among women and that they tend to increase with age.

Many people experience mild and occasional sleep disorders, which should give them no grounds for concern, and which are caused by one or more of the following:

- Strong emotions – anger, fear, joy or ideas and problems occupying the mind;

- New surroundings;

- Mild illnesses – colds, 'flu, pain.

1.3(b)   SLEEP PROBLEMS: POSSIBLE RESPONSES

Many people resort to medication to help them sleep; this may be valuable in the short term, but should never be considered for long.

See also Appendix III on Drugs and medicines

In 1983 family practitioners in England issued over 23 million prescriptions for tranquillisers, and about 80 per cent of these were for sleeping problems. It seems as if nearly half the population were in such a state that they required help to relax and sleep. Fortunately, however, the situation has now become more sensible; doctors have taken stock and reduced the amount of drugs they prescribe. About one in seven British adults now take tranquillisers.

Barbiturates, which act as a very strong type of sleeping pill, were commonly prescribed in the 1960s – about 16 million per year in Britain at this time. Now they are not used at all for sleeping problems, due to the introduction of safer medications.

There are many positive things that you can do to ensure a better night's sleep before you resort to medication.

Sleeping pills do not bring about natural sleep. They change the normal progression of sleep stages, and reduce the amount of essential dreaming sleep you have. They often continue to work during the day, which may result in fatigue, 'hangover' and impaired performance, and they can become habit forming and lead to dependency and addiction after long use.

1.3(c)   GOOD SLEEP PROGRAMME

Preparation

Analyse your sleep problem. Try and identify what it is that is causing the problem. Is it to do with you? are you worried, angry, sad, fearful? too many thoughts buzzing around your mind?

An exercise called 'left luggage' can be very useful. Organise your worries and thoughts into a manageable order, say into four or five different categories, and then imagine yourself putting all of these worries into a suitcase, and taking the suitcase to a 'left luggage' at a railway station.

Remember it is important for you to get some good sleep and at the moment your life's luggage is a bit too heavy for you to carry around with you all the time. So you need to put it somewhere for safekeeping.

Say to yourself that you will come back and collect it again when you wake up refreshed, when you will feel stronger and more able to carry it around. You can always leave it there again in the day

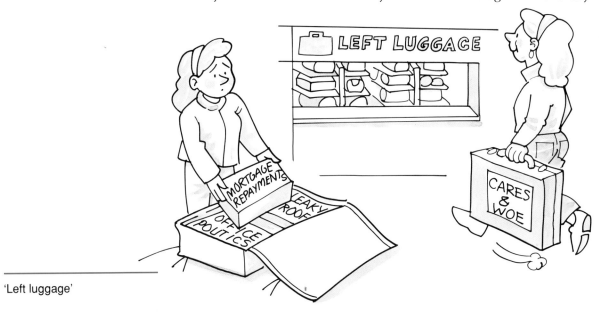

'Left luggage'

sometimes, when you are feeling a bit weary, and hopefully you will find that gradually it becomes a bit lighter.

If your sleep problem is due to waking to take care of someone else, then every so often try and get someone else to do a shift for you so that you get the break you deserve.

Practical approaches

See also section 1.5 below for more advice on coping with stress

- Develop a regular bedtime ritual – a hot drink often helps, but avoid coffee, nicotine and other stimulants.

- Exercise in the day can make your body relax better and relaxation for your mind can help too.

- If you cannot sleep, get up and find something to do – reading, knitting, or another manual activity – until you are tired.

Remember it is perfectly all right not to sleep well, provided it is not upsetting you. You can probably cope with a limited amount of sleep, so there is no need to expend energy on worrying about it.

1.4 WORK AND RECREATION

The work that you do has a very important influence on your health. Your attitude to your occupation is crucial – a positive approach to a difficult and challenging job can make all the difference.

See also Chapter 7, section 10(d) on Occupational disorders

There are many occupations which can cause health risks and hazards. One of the first work hazards documented was mercury poisoning from the felt of those making hats (hence the expression 'mad as hatters'). Nowadays we are familiar with hazards such as asbestos-related illness, backache in nurses (accounting for 764,000 working days lost to the NHS in Britain) and occupational skin disorders (accounting for 630,000 working days lost in the United Kingdom). Furthermore, the UK alone sees a staggering 274,000 non-fatal accidents per year occurring at work.

American scientists estimate that as many as 30 per cent of all diseases in that country could have occupationally related causes.

Other signs of poor working practices can be seen in unsatisfactory working relationships and confusing communications resulting in general malaise, stress, unhappiness and lack of satisfaction with work.

Being unemployed can make you ill too. More unemployed people are likely to suffer depression, anxiety, and poor self-esteem in addition to an increased likelihood of physical illness. Those in employment work too hard and they get ill; those without get ill too. So how do you strike the right balance?

1.4(a) TIME-SPENDING CIRCLES

How you actually spend your time each day can be crucial to your health. One way of deciding whether your habits are health enhancing or not is to complete this time-spending exercise.

Take the previous 24 hours, say from 8.00 am to 8.00 am and work out how much time you spent in the following activities:

- Work outside the home (including travel to and fro);
- Housework (cooking, cleaning, child care, shopping, looking after others in the family);
- Body maintenance (eating, bathing, etc.);
- Sleep;
- 'Time off' (everything that you regard as free time).

Look at the examples given and then complete circles for yourself and your family members. Next write down your attitude to each category.

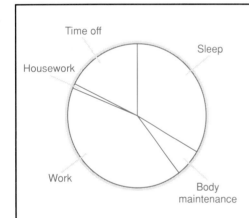

Time-spending circle: Fiona

Fiona is a 22 year old chemistry student in her final year. Her time-spending circle worked out as shown.

Sleep	8 hours – loves it, but feels she would like some more
Body maintenance	1½ hours – quite enjoys it, bathing and putting on her make-up
Work	10 hours – mixed feelings, generally positive although the time spent travelling to and from college can be a bit stressful
Housework	15 minutes – loathes it; spent the time washing her underwear and coffee mug
Time off	4¼ hours – adores it; spent the time chatting to friends and drinking in the college bar

So what is the relationship between our work, our free time and our attitudes?

Your 'time off' or leisure can only really be enjoyed if it is perceived as either a reward or a respite from work.

Many people do not have a structured day with a prescribed amount of time allotted for leisure. Housewives, mothers, carers, the retired, ill patients and the unemployed and those who work from home do not usually have a structured working day, and so might consequently not enjoy their leisure time as much as those who can easily define what is work and what is not.

A healthy time-spending circle would have a balanced amount of each of the five activities, and a positive attitude to all areas. It can be seen from the examples given that one's relationship to work and leisure are very closely linked. What makes people healthy is a good balance so that their leisure can actually be enjoyed – we only really enjoy it if it is a rest or a reward from work.

Think about how you can develop a healthier balance between the activities that you do. Plan your leisure so that it invigorates you, enabling you to perform better in your work.

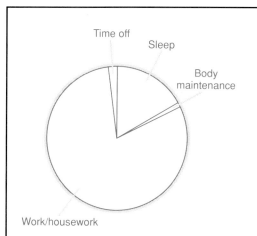

Time-spending circle: Alison

Alison is Fiona's 29 year old sister. She has given up teaching to look after her two small children. Her time chart is markedly different.

Sleep 4 hours, in two lots of 2 hours; she feels very much in need of more and is totally exhausted most of the time

Body maintenance 15 minutes – no time for any longer

Work/housework 19¼ hours; she has very mixed feelings about this – she loves her children but experiences resentment as well as happiness at her lot

Time off ½ an hour; too tired to enjoy it really, watches the news on TV

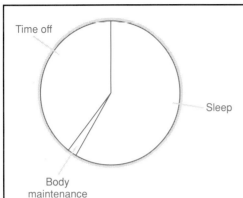

Time-spending circle: Simon

Simon, the father of these two women, is 61 and was made redundant some months ago. His chart looks like this.

Sleep 14 hours – he goes to bed at midnight and gets up at 2 pm the next day; he feels sleepy a lot of the time

Housework Nil

Body maintenance ½ an hour – washes and shaves – finds it a chore

Work Nil – he misses it

Time off 9½ hours – he watches TV and finds it boring

Time-spending circle: Nigel

Nigel, Simon's brother, is 56. He is still working as a printer, and his chart is different again.

Sleep 6 hours – this is plenty; he enjoys it and wakes refreshed

Housework 1½ hours – he is happy to do his share; washes up and cleans the kitchen floor each evening, shops for groceries and does more on his day off

Work 8 hours – Nigel loves his work

Body maintenance 1 hour – he enjoys his shower

Time off 7½ hours – he loves his leisure time and spends it playing squash, watching TV, socialising with his family and pursuing his hobbies

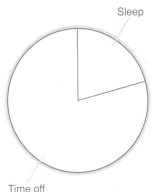

Time-spending circle: Sylvia

Sylvia, grandmother to Fiona and Alison, is 82. She is bed-bound with rheumatoid arthritis. Sylvia lives with her son Simon and is looked after by Fiona's mother.

Sleep 5 hours; she really can't sleep for longer but would like to

Body maintenance None – it is all done for her; she feels very resentful about this

Housework None; she regrets that she is unable to do things her way and feels bitter that she is so handicapped

Work None – she misses her work in the factory and all the friends she made there

Time off 19 hours – she is bored and depressed for most of the time

---

1.5 STRESS

We will all experience stress to a greater or lesser degree at some time as it is an inevitable part of life. It comes in two varieties – good and bad. Good stress, we experience as arousal or excitement. A first date, a rousing concert, Christmas Eve for small children are all stressful occasions, but they do contribute to the quality of life and life would be very dull without them.

Bad stress (*dis*-stress) is the other side of the coin. Stress can be seen as the general wear and tear of the body, as high levels of mental unease accompanied by bodily tension, which can exceed an individual's ability to cope, sometimes resulting in disease.

Stressors are factors in our lives which induce stress. They can be internal, that is coming from within ourselves like a sad memory or a fear, or external, coming from outside ourselves like other people, noise, or work.

1.5(a) PEOPLE AS STRESSORS

Other people are often the most stressful stressors that we have to deal with. Occasionally, these people are mere strangers, like the aggressive bus conductor or the surly shop assistant, but, more often than not, the people who are able to distress us the most are our family and friends, or our work colleagues – the people we have to communicate with every day of our lives.

Some relatives seem to be able to send us into fits of depression, guilt or anger by the tone of their voice, or a few carefully chosen words. Most people will have agonised over something they have said, the way they said it, or issues left unspoken.

It can be very important to have a few communication rules to abide by, so that things do not get out of hand too often.

Good communication

This is an approach to communicating with people which, if you stick to the rules, will guarantee that you have communicated in a positive manner. Using this approach will mean that you have done the best you could and can leave each encounter feeling proud and worth while.

The rules are fairly simple to understand, but rather more difficult to integrate into our everyday patterns of behaviour.

The diagram shown below illustrates the communication approach, representing four types of behaviour. When talking to people the rules are:

- Always keep above the line;

- Attempt to balance your communication behaviour evenly between assertive and responsive behaviour;

- Never use the aggressive or passive response – there are no situations or individuals which deserve them.

In this approach people's characteristics are divided up into two types: 'A' behaviour and 'R' behaviour.

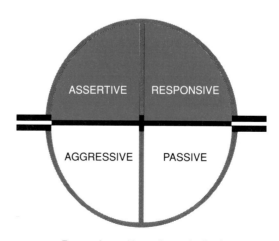

Person to person: good communication

Remember – Keep above the line!

The 'A' behaviour is made up of all the energy and drives which go into the creative aspects of our nature, the emotions and energy needed to shape and influence events, to make and create things, and to defend our rights and principles. It has a positive communication behaviour called *assertion* and a negative communication behaviour called *aggression*.

The 'R' or responsive characteristics are our energy and drives which can be used to respond to others, to fit in well with them, to accommodate people and to be responsive, nurturing, caring and supportive. The positive behaviour is *responsive* and the negative behaviour is *passive*.

The quiz given overleaf will help you to determine which type of communication behaviour you habitually use. In it, you will find a series of paired statements. All you have to do is to distribute 10 points between the two statements. Give more points to the statement which comes closest to describing your behaviour or feelings. You may find that you give all 10 points to the 'A' type, or you give 5 each to both if both statements fit your behaviour about equally. Any combination is possible as long as for each question 'A' plus 'R' equals 10.

Communication styles

Assertive communication   When using this style you are standing up for yourself and presenting your views and ideas in such a way that the other person's rights or views are respected. Both parties in the conversation are being treated with respect and consideration – yourself and the other person.

Your intention is to influence the other, to use your ideas and talents in order to gain self-respect without diminishing the other person. Your aim is to find out *what* is right not who is right.

You hold a belief of 'I win/You win' and 'I'm OK – You're OK'.

When using this style the effect on other people is that they feel informed and enhanced by you.

Aggressive communication   The person using an aggressive style is concerned about standing up for his views and ideas but has no regard for the rights or views of the other person. His intention is to be 'on top', to put others down. He may be patronising or sarcastic; he may show contempt or be insulting. Aggressive behaviour is used to get your own way without regard for the consequences. The effect on others is that they may feel hurt, they may become defensive, and feel humiliated, fearful, resentful and dependent.

The belief held is 'I win/you lose' or 'I'm OK – You're *not* OK'. This behaviour is dominating, overpowering and self-enhancing at the expense of others. It is seen as attacking and accusatory.

'A' statements	'R' statements
1. I enjoy making decisions and following them through forcefully Points _____	I enjoy thinking about problems and solving them Points _____
2. I am quick and incisive Points _____	I am reflective and thoughtful Points _____
3. When I am with other people I spend more time talking than listening Points _____	When I am with other people I spend more time listening than talking Points _____
4. My ability to be a strong competitor has paid off for me Points _____	My ability to be co-operative and to build collaborative relationships has paid off for me Points _____
5. In most groups I am one of the people who initiates ideas and makes suggestions Points _____	In most groups I am one of the people who provides stability and balance Points _____
6. I get things done by shaping events, and having a direct impact on people Points _____	I get things done by 'tuning in' on and responding to the people and situations around me Points _____
7. When I am dissatisfied with someone's behaviour I become more demanding and make suggestions for improvement Points _____	When I am dissatisfied with someone's behaviour I observe, listen and try to understand Points _____
8. If I err it is on the side of being too tough Points _____	If I err it is on the side of being too tolerant Points _____
9. If I err it is on the side of being impulsive Points _____	If I err it is on the side of being cautious Points _____
10. Under pressure my strength lies in my ability to get 'fired up' while retaining a clear picture Points _____	Under pressure my strength lies in my ability to stay calm while remaining involved Points _____
11. When people disagree with me I tend to 'speed up' and try to convince them Points _____	When people disagree with me I tend to 'slow down' and consider their reservations Points _____
Total 'A' _____	**Total 'R'** _____

How did you do? If your scores were about even then you are probably using your emotions and skills appropriately. If there is a large difference you may be overusing one at the expense of the other.

Aggressive behaviour is a poor method of communicating and in the long term unsuccessful. It is likely to lead to more aggressive behaviour or the other negative type, passive behaviour.

Passive communication   In this style you are failing to stand up for yourself, your views or your ideas. It is like aggressive behaviour turned in on yourself. The belief you hold is 'I lose/You win and 'I'm *not* OK – You're OK'.

Your intention is to be 'safe', to appease, to let others take responsibility for you. You rely on the resources of others in order to get help and sympathy. You find that you deny your own abilities, needs, interests and resources.

When using this style your behaviour comes over as whining, apologetic and passive with 'lots of hurt feelings'. Often, you may put yourself down whilst placing the blame on others (e.g. 'I'm not very good at this but I might have succeeded if only you had given me more help'). The effect on others is that they often feel guilty or angry. They may feel like joining you in your attack on yourself, or pity and regret that they mentioned something. They feel they can't disagree with you without hurting or being seen as hostile. They feel frustrated.

If someone asks you whether you have had a good weekend and you reply in this style you might say: 'Me? No, not really. I never have much to do as I'm on my own you see. Nobody ever asks me to spend time with them'.

Responsive communication   When using this style you are aware of, and responsive to, the rights and resources of others without denying or limiting your own rights and abilities.

Your intention is to try and understand the other person, to show respect for others without diminishing yourself. You want to find out what is right, not who is right.

The beliefs you hold are the same as in the assertive mode of 'I win/You win' and 'I'm OK – You're OK'. Your behaviour is seen as responsive, seeking, sharing, understanding, showing willingness to change – taking on new ideas enthusiastically and learning. The effect on others is that they feel valued and warm towards you.

The aim of using this approach is to encourage you to use only the two styles above the line – to develop an assertive/responsive communication style. It may take some practice. However the two negative styles – aggressive and passive – always leave someone with a bad feeling, and an overload of stress and unhappiness, which is very unhelpful. Everybody deserves to be treated with the skills above the line – be they children, elderly, people with a handicap, even those behaving in an irrational or deluded way or people who are displaying stupid and offensive behaviour.

1.5(b) RESPONDING TO STRESS

The way we respond to stress is vitally important. There are a variety of ways in which we habitually respond to stress, responses that form our personality and character. There are two major types of responses:

• Fighting;

• Fleeing (flight).

Problems arise when stress responses become automatic – we respond from habit and overuse one response. When this occurs it can lead to further stress and ill-health.

However, this stress response need not be automatic. By considering alternative responses, we can begin to choose how we will react. We need to learn to use an appropriate stress response, one that will enhance our health and not harm it.

The quiz given in the box aims to give you some idea of how you respond to stress. If most of the ticks are for the statements in the right hand column, you exhibit what has become known as 'Type A behaviour'. You are probably fairly impulsive, time conscious, achievement orientated and hard driving. Because of these traits you are at a greater risk of suffering from a heart attack and should think about slowing down. You are most likely using the 'fight' response mentioned above.

Instant stress detector

Reproduced with kind permission of Thames Methuen from *All in the Mind* by Professor Cary Cooper, page 109

This short quiz has been devised by a professor from the University of Manchester Institute of Science and Technology. For each of the questions below, tick whichever phrase applies to you.

Are you casual about appointments? ☑	Or never late? ☐
Are you not competitive? ☐	Or very competitive? ☐
Are you a good listener? ☐	Or do you often interrupt? ☐
Are you never rushed? ☐	Or always rushed? ☐
Can you wait patiently? ☐	Or are you impatient? ☐
Do you usually express your feelings? ☐	Or do you tend to hide your feelings? ☐
Do you take one thing at a time? ☐	Or do you do lots of things at once? ☐
Are you easy going? ☐	Or are you hard driving? ☐

The 'fight' response In fact there are two main types of fight response, the first of which is that displayed by the hot ambitious individuals mentioned above, who are likely to be very successful and leaders. At their worst, such individuals can be aggressive, irritable and overbearing. When they become very stressed their pattern

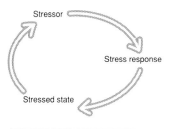

Vicious stress cycle

of behaviour tends to overstimulate the heart and circulation, and is associated with heart disease.

The other type of fight response is called the *internal fight response*. In this case, the individual turns all the aggression in on himself. Such people like to be 'in control' and tend to be orderly, tidy, precise and consistent. They can appear unemotional and, at their worst, can become obsessional and repetitive in thoughts and actions. There can be difficulties in coping with unforeseen events which challenge their need to be in control.

When they become stressed they may develop gastrointestinal disease, like peptic ulcers or irritable bowel syndrome.

The 'flight' response   The individuals who use this response always attempt to avoid the stressor. They don't like to discuss difficult issues, and may not pay their bills, for example. This response can lead to cautious and conservative behaviour, and can develop into a manner that appears vulnerable, dependent and non-assertive. They can feel themselves to be at 'the mercy of the world', withdrawing into their own private self where they remain aloof, isolated and suspicious. The consistent use of the flight response is associated with the 'phobic' personality or the despair syndrome, which has recently been linked to the development of certain types of cancer.

Warning signs

Each one of us has our own individual way of responding to the stressors in our lives; however there are many common warning signs which we can be on the lookout for.

Physical warning signs   These include flushing, sweating, dry mouth, tightness in the chest, heart palpitations and pounding pulse, headaches, general aches and pains, feelings of weakness, vomiting and diarrhoea, fatigue, loss of appetite, insomnia, breathlessness and dizziness. Warning signs witnessed as muscular symptoms include general tightness in muscles, tremors, tics, spasms, an increased startle reaction (overreaction to sudden noise or unexpected movement), lots of deep sighing and clumsiness.

Psychological and social warning signs   Emotional states which can warn us of too much stress include agitation, shakiness, increased tiredness, panicky feelings, depression, irritability and frequent bouts of anger.

Mental states can warn us too: too much worrying, feelings of dread, difficulty maintaining attention, forgetfulness, nightmares, fear of death, loss of self-confidence and difficulty in making decisions can alert us to make changes.

Stress can change our behaviour and this can be seen by increases in drinking alcohol, smoking and taking other drugs, and in becoming accident prone.

1.5(c) BREATHING AS A RESPONSE TO STRESS

So, what can be done about all this stress? One excellent strategy for breaking into the cycle of responding habitually, without thought, to stressors is by *diaphragmatic breathing.*

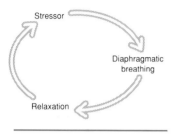

Benign stress cycle

Breathing is one the few bodily processes that can be either voluntary or involuntary. Breathing can take place automatically without us thinking about it, or we can alter it consciously and at will. Breathing is one of the most sensitive indicators or warning signs of stress that we possess because of this link between mind and body. By using our mind, we can influence our bodily reaction, through the link with breathing.

There are two main types of breathing, chest breathing and diaphragmatic breathing.

Chest breathing   If we chest breathe, there is an upward and outward movement of the chest. We chest breathe during vigorous exercise and in emergency situations. If we use this method all the time, it keeps the body in a state of constant tension and arousal; the body acts as if it is experiencing stress, even if it is not.

Diaphragmatic breathing   The diaphragm is a dome shaped muscle which separates the chest and abdominal cavities. When we breathe this way our abdominal wall or tummy is pushed out when we breathe in and flattens when we breathe out. Try the following exercise to see which way you breathe. Sit comfortably in a chair with your eyes closed and place one hand on your upper chest and the other hand on your abdomen. Get someone to time you and count your breaths for one minute. Also note which hand moves the most. If it is the hand on your abdomen, then you habitually use diaphragmatic breathing. Don't try to alter your breathing at this stage, just see which one you use.

Diaphragmatic breathing is by far the healthier way to breathe as the lungs are able to fill completely, thus providing the body with sufficient oxygen. It also forces the waste product, carbon dioxide, from the lungs.

The movement of the diaphragm gently massages the abdominal contents which increases their blood circulation and function.

Learning to relax

Many chest breathers can learn how to change their breathing quite easily, and thereby reduce their stress levels. When confronted by a stressful situation everybody can consciously breathe diaphragmatically. We all breathed that way once: watch a young baby or even a cat breathe and you will see the belly moving up and down while the chest stays completely still.

Carry out the instructions for diaphragmatic breathing until you begin to feel tension gradually slipping away. Some people need considerable practice to make diaphragmatic breathing their usual method, so don't worry if it does not come very easily. Practice makes perfect.

Whenever you feel under stress or unable to cope, if you ever have something important to do or say, just take a few seconds to check your breathing and away you go.

DIAPHRAGMATIC BREATHING

Where	Find a quiet room where you will be undisturbed for about 10–15 minutes (you may have to plan this in advance). Lie down on the bed or the floor. The floor is better if you have a soft bed. Undo tight clothing and take off your shoes. Spend a few minutes just settling yourself down and clearing your mind of thoughts and worries. Support your head with a few books or a slim pillow, spread your feet 12–18 inches apart and check that your head, neck and spine are in a straight line.
Check your breathing	Close your eyes and focus your attention on your breathing. Do not try to change anything, just become aware of your breathing. Is it fast or slow? Is it regular and rhythmical or jerky and uneven with gaps, pauses, and sighs? Notice whether you are breathing with your chest or with your diaphragm.
Hand on diaphragm	Now put one hand on your chest and the other on your abdomen, just below your rib cage, and relax. After a while as you breathe out, press the lower hand to flatten your abdomen. As you breathe in (inhale), allow the abdomen to rise, and as you breathe out again (exhale) allow the abdomen to flatten. When you get into a pattern, reduce the amount of movement in the chest.
Rhythm	Take time to get into a rhythm, and allow your breath to become smooth, easy and regular. Don't worry about any gaps or pauses, just continue to think about making the rhythm smooth and even.
Slow it down	When you feel confident about the lower hand rising when you inhale *slow down your exhalation* and allow the inhalation to follow smoothly and easily. If any distractions, thoughts or worries come into your mind, allow them to come and then allow them to go, and bring your attention back to breathing. Gradually make the exhalation longer and the rhythm smooth.
Finish	When you are ready to finish this exercise, take a few deep breaths in, and get up slowly by rolling over onto your side first.

CARING AT HOME

2

2.1 ## INTRODUCTION

Nursing someone at home can be a worrying responsibility for the carer. Most people will be called upon at some time to care for someone with a brief illness when the sufferer can feel dreadful for a few days or more. Some will find themselves in the position of looking after a person with a longer, more disabling illness. With the emphasis on early mobilisation and early discharge from hospital, the period of acute illness may merge with a period of convalescence. Patients may be discharged home from hospital needing help not only with everyday needs but also with managing pain, a surgical wound, a course of medication or learning to live with a plaster of Paris or crutches. They may still feel quite unwell and exhausted by their experience.

For more serious and long term illness or disability there is help available in the community although it may not always be offered if you appear to be managing well. The doctor will explain the nature of the illness to the patient and family. If this is not explained in terms that can be readily understood, ask for clarification and he will go over it again. Appendix I describes the basic working of the human body and there are also many sources of reference available which explain specific illnesses. This manual describes common problems in sections covering various age groups (see also the Index).

Further sources of help are specialist nurses working in the community. The doctor will put you in touch with them but sometimes it may be necessary to ask for help or advice. Nurses in the community include district nurses who undertake home nursing, health visitors who advise on health problems, psychiatric nurses who have special skills to treat the mentally ill and their families, and specialist nurses who are available in many areas. They include nurses with skills to help people who have a stoma (where part of the bowel is temporarily or permanently brought through the abdomen), those who help diabetics and those who care for the dying. These services will depend on the geographical location of the family. People living in isolated areas fare less well. The carer may well feel alone and housebound but help is often available for the asking. It is worth remembering that the family, friends and neighbours are usually willing to provide a break. This may take a

See Appendix I for a brief description of How the body works

See Appendices V and VII for more details of how to get help

bit of organisation. Be specific in your request – e.g. 'Could you look after Bill to give me a break to go to my evening class on Tuesday? I would like to be out between 7 and 10 pm.' When friends come to help, give a list of specific guidelines and advice to enable them to feel competent to help; such a list might include, for example, the fact that the patient can manage to go to the bathroom if he has a stick and a supporting arm. Leave the telephone number of the doctor and a neighbour and where you may be contacted.

Every family has its own routine, values and customs. These will be moulded by tradition, circumstances, religious beliefs and cultural background. The helper may well have different routines, values and ideas. It is courteous therefore to avoid conflict both for the patient and the helper. A willing helper may be less willing to return if rebuffed when attempting to provide companionship and conversation at a time when the patient always listens to a favourite radio programme for example. Similarly, a helper who has given up chocolates for Lent may be embarrassed if pressed upon to accept one by someone from a different religious tradition. Those helpers who find the role satisfying, and who do not find themselves in a position of fear or uncertainty, are likely to return gladly another day.

2.1(a) THE SICK ROOM

Sick people should not be in bed if they feel well enough to move around or sit in a chair for a while. They are usually the best judge of how they feel but may need some encouragement to be up and about to keep the circulation flowing and to prevent the complications of not getting any exercise.

It may not be practical to create an ideal sick room. Adaptability is the secret of home nursing, making use of the facilities available. Where it is possible, however, the bedroom should be:

- Warm but well ventilated – this can be achieved by opening a window when the patient is up and about but remember to close it before the room is reoccupied;

- Pleasant and not full of clutter – it is easy for both patient and carer to trip over things;

- A room with a view of the outside world;

- Equipped with essentials such as books, a radio, stationery and pens, a mirror and nursing equipment such as a bed table which can be improvised, a urinal, medicines etc.;

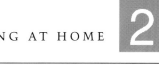

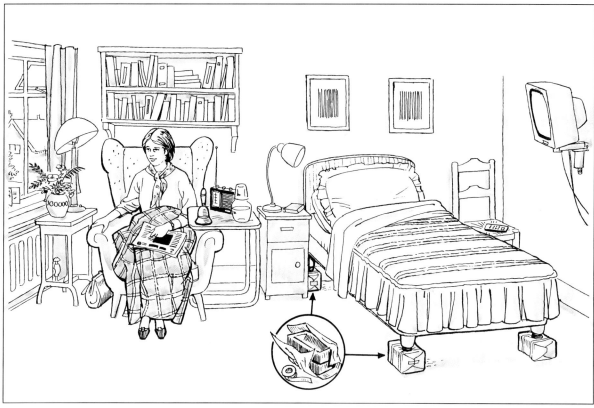

The sick room

An imaginative carer can achieve much

See section 2.4(a) below which summarises the principles of safe lifting

- Equipped with some means of calling others such as a bell or an intercom (an intercom used for a baby is ideal); be careful in the choice of bell – a harsh sound can be irritating to everyone;

- Equipped with a suitable bed at the right height for the carer; a few bricks can raise the height of the bed enough to enable the carer to avoid backache without making it difficult for the patient to get in and out; ideally, access should be possible from both sides of the bed.

2.1(b) RESPONDING TO ILLNESS

Coming to terms with temporary or permanent illness is as individual an experience as people's personalities and background. Most people who are normally healthy and independent kick against being deprived of their freedom to do what they want to do and earn their living when they become obliged to rely on others to meet their personal and economic needs. Young people will worry about falling behind at school or college. It is unusual for people to exploit their illness to gain attention or manipulate others but it can happen.

2

The best way to find out how people feel about being ill is to ask them. The response, which may not necessarily be immediately forthcoming, may be surprising. Professional nurses make an assessment of their patients based on what the patient cannot do for himself, asking what help is needed. A plan of care will be devised together so that everyone is agreed about the goals of care on a daily basis. This can also be done informally at home.

It is all too easy to waste time and effort on nursing care that is quite unacceptable to the sick person. It is easy either to over nurse or to neglect. For example, breakfast could be offered on a tray but the patient may prefer to be helped downstairs to the kitchen for half an hour, where he would be able to check his tomatoes on the window sill, have a chat and feel normal. This would help to make a tidied bed or a comfortable armchair more welcome later.

Illness does not necessarily draw people closer together as resentment and misunderstanding can build up on both sides. The carer may unconsciously expect gratitude while possibly becoming the butt of the sick person's anger at being dependent. It is vital, therefore, both to communicate and to be sympathetic. It is not too difficult to say something like 'You must feel rotten with that high temperature. Are you feeling well enough for a quick bath or shower?' With a bit of luck the patient might respond with, 'That would be lovely but I want you to put your feet up for a bit afterwards'. Don't bank on it though. Sick people are usually self-absorbed as their world shrinks rapidly to the four walls of their prison and they can be consumed with anxieties about their daily lives and the outcome of their illness. An indication of the fact that they are recovering is that they will begin to be concerned about their normal lives and the outside world.

2.1 (c)   THE ART OF HOME NURSING

Caring is a natural art for both men and women. It is directly connected to looking after the young. Some skills are innate while others can be learned.

The following pages will provide a step by step guide to helping people with things they are temporarily or permanently unable to do for themselves. All the normal activities of daily living will be considered individually. Taken one by one, the carer can ask the question 'What can't he manage to do that he would usually do automatically, without thought?' If a verbal or a written plan is made it not only makes life easier, but it can be very satisfying to help someone get better or enable them to use all their own resources in adapting to, perhaps, a permanent disability or progressive illness.

HELPING THE SICK PERSON AT HOME WITH THE ACTIVITIES OF LIVING

2.2(a) WHAT ARE ACTIVITIES OF LIVING?

In order to live from day to day, an individual carries out certain activities known as 'activities of living'. All of these activities – which are listed below – are necessary for the health and welfare of each of us. The activities of living are:

- Breathing;

- Eating and drinking;

- Eliminating;

- Sleeping and resting;

- Dressing and undressing;

- Keeping warm (or cool);

- Keeping clean and well groomed;

- Avoiding danger;

- Communicating and expressing needs;

- Practising religious beliefs;

- Working;

- Recreation.

You will probably have noticed that all of these activities involve the individual in 'doing' something. This is important for two reasons. Firstly, it encourages the individual to take an interest in himself and, secondly, it encourages independence. Both of these factors are important.

Individuals should be encouraged to take an interest in themselves as a means of retaining some control over events which might otherwise seem overwhelming. A person who feels 'in control' will be able to participate in making decisions about his own care. This activity and interest helps to alleviate the boredom and frustration often experienced by someone who is ill or handicapped – an important factor since prolonged boredom and frustration can affect the physical and mental well-being of the individual.

Encouraging independence also gives control back to the individual. Another important point is that an independent person means a reduced caring role for you. It may be quicker for you to wash and dress the person you are caring for, even if she is able to perform some activities for herself. In the long term, however, you will be making her dependent on you for all of her needs. It is much better, for example, to allow an hour in the evening when you might have more time to supervise the individual washing parts of her body for herself than to 'take over' because you are in a hurry.

Time to relax or be unhurried with regard to an activity such as washing or dressing also helps to remove some of the stress of caring. Often it also provides opportunities for you both to talk about how you might be feeling and to express your needs.

Activities of living are carried out by each individual but to different levels or degrees. The degree to which an activity is performed is unique to each person. There are degrees or levels which are recognised as being 'normal', for example walking without a limp or without pain. However, for an individual born with a defect to the hip, walking with a limp may be quite normal. If the limp became more pronounced or suddenly painful, then that would need investigation. Since you are involved in caring for the individual, you will need (or you may be asked) to watch out for changes which you know are not normal for that person.

In the following sections relating to activities of living, some of the changes have been described. Information is also provided to help you in your role as carer.

2.2(b)   BREATHING

Everyone needs to take in a sufficient amount of air in order for the body cells to grow and remain healthy. Breathing, or respiration, consists of a process of inspiration (breathing in) and expiration (breathing out) which is prompted by movements of the chest and the diaphragm.

See Appendix I, section vii for more information about the respiratory system

Outward movement of the chest wall allows the lungs to expand, drawing air into the tiny sacs or alveoli within the lung tissue. It is in these sacs that oxygen from the air passes into the blood stream and carbon dioxide passes out of the blood. Relaxation of the muscles of the chest wall forces air, containing carbon dioxide, out through the air passages. The process of respiration

Possible causes of breathlessness

• Anaemia	• Endocarditis
• Asthma	• Hypertension
• Bronchiectasis	• Left ventricular failure
• Bronchitis	• Obstructive airways disease
• Carcinoma of bronchus	• Pleurisy
• Carcinoma of lung	• Pneumonia
• Congenital heart disease	• Pulmonary oedema
• Coronary heart disease	• Rheumatic heart disease
• Emphysema	

ensures that oxygen is transported by the blood to all parts of the body.

Unfortunately, some individuals may experience difficulties with breathing during the course of an illness. These difficulties may be caused directly by the illness, for example in the case of a chest infection, or they may be caused indirectly by reduced mobility, for example following an accident. Difficulties with breathing may occur when the lungs are not able to expand sufficiently. They may also occur if an individual remains in the same position for long periods at a time.

Posture

It is important to be aware of the importance of alternating an upright or semi-upright posture with other positions. It is also important to ensure that an open posture is used. (An open posture means that the shoulders are back and the spine is supported.) This position allows the lungs to expand as fully as possible even if the patient is lying on his side.

Using a selection of firm and soft pillows, it is possible to support a frail or sick patient either in bed or in a chair in the correct position. The objective should always be to support the spine so that the shoulders fall back. The lungs are then able to expand to maximum capacity.

If the patient smokes regularly then it is even more important to encourage him to breathe deeply because his lung capacity may be already reduced by inhaling cigarette or pipe smoke.

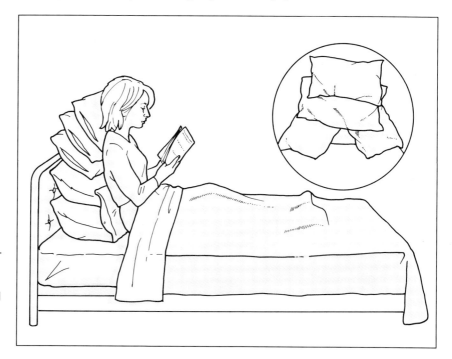

A variety of firm and soft pillows, arranged in one of the ways shown, can be used to support the individual in an upright or semi-upright position

Character of breathing

Under normal circumstances, breathing is recognised as being quiet and regular. The rate of breathing varies with age. Normal breathing rate for an infant will be 30–35 breaths per minute and this decreases to 16–21 for an adult. The rate of breathing can be counted by watching the rise and fall of the patient's chest, each rise and fall counting as one breath. However some people, who may have lived with a chronic chest condition for many years, may consider their breathing pattern to be normal even though it may sound harsh to you. Other individuals, for example those suffering from asthma, may always have had a cough. It is important to recognise these differences as being normal for that individual. This is because you may be asked to look out for changes in breathing. As the person most closely working with the patient, you will probably be the first person to notice a change or difficulty.

Things to look out for   Any alteration which may occur to the pattern of breathing may be a sign of a developing chest infection or a deterioration in the patient's condition. Such alteration could be indicated by a number of symptoms, as outlined in the boxed feature below.

BREATHING: SIGNS THAT SHOULD CONCERN YOU	
Changes in the noise, depth or frequency of intake of air	Breathing may become harsh or rasping. Alternatively, it may become very quiet. The depth of breathing may also change so that it becomes either deep and pronounced or shallow and faint. Along with the changes already described, breathing may also become rapid or it may become intermittent. This intermittent type of breathing (Cheyne-Stokes respiration) may occur in the late stages of very severe illness. The patient is observed to take a deep breath which may be held for several seconds before exhaling and the sequence being repeated. This type of breathing may last for 2–3 hours or longer and can be frightening if you are not prepared.
A cough which may develop with or without changes in breathing	Although it is also important to be aware of the patient who already has a persistent cough, you should observe any changes which may take place. The cough may be described as dry, when no sputum is produced, or wet, when the cough will be accompanied by varying quantities of sputum. The cough may be infrequent or totally overwhelming and exhausting.
A pain developing in the chest region	Each individual will have his own way of describing pain and it should never be ignored. Pain in the chest should always be reported to the doctor or nurse at the earliest opportunity. There are many reasons for chest pain which would need to be investigated. Pain which may be associated with a chest infection is usually described as being at the side of the rib cage. Patients often describe the pain as being worse when they breathe in.

What can be done

See section 2.4 on Lifting and transfers

You can do a great deal to help the patient to prevent either a chest infection or further deterioration of an existing illness. Where possible, the patient should be encouraged to move around the room every 2–3 hours during the day. If this is not possible then she should be helped and encouraged to sit out of bed, preferably in a high backed chair.

If the patient is unable to get out of bed then deep breathing exercises, every hour or so, should be encouraged. Whether the patient is in or out of bed, it is important to maintain good posture (as described above). It is also beneficial to encourage gentle exercises of the arms and legs which will help to improve the circulation. Improving the circulation will also help the supply of oxygen to all parts of the body.

If the patient complains of chest pain, a well protected hot water bottle applied to the area can be very comforting. Tissues and a waste paper receptacle will be needed to contain any sputum which may be coughed up.

See section 2.2(g) below, for details of simple exercises

Exercises   Simple mobilising exercises will also help to exercise the lungs. This is because the heart and lungs will have to work harder to keep the body supplied with oxygen.

Deep breathing exercises may be taught by a physiotherapist but it is also possible to carry out simple breathing exercises which will be of benefit.

- The individual should sit or lie, well supported with pillows, so that the shoulders fall back naturally.

- Place the palms of the hands, fingertips touching, across the front of the chest along the lower edge of the rib cage. (The individual may do this for himself.)

- Ask the individual to breathe in slowly and deeply through the nose, so that the rib cage moves upwards and outwards. This movement allows the lungs to inflate as fully as possible.

If the exercise is being performed correctly, it should be possible to see or feel the fingertips move apart.

- Ask the individual to breathe out slowly through the mouth.

- The fingertips should move back towards one another as the rib cage moves back to its resting position as the lungs deflate.

- Repeat the sequence six times every hour during the day.

It is important to remember that deep breathing should be a gentle exercise. If it is carried out excessively, it may cause giddiness. It must also be remembered that all exercise should be balanced with periods of rest, otherwise the individual will become exhausted.

FATING AND DRINKING

Each individual needs sufficient food for all of the mechanisms of the body to function satisfactorily. The requirement is necessary whether the person is well or ill. The dietary needs of each individual will vary according to other influences such as the degree of mobility.

Often the term 'diet' is used in relation to weight loss but this is really an inappropriate use of the term. 'Diet' means the total amount of food and drink required by an individual. The word is often used in conjunction with the term 'balanced' to describe the amount of each food constituent required by an individual in order to meet his particular needs.

In some instances, additional information is required in order to meet special needs. For example, in cases where a person may be suffering from diabetes, a dietitian or other health professional will be able to give advice.

The amount and type of food which individuals are able to consume will vary according to a number of factors. Some of these are described below:

- Personal taste – which may limit the choice available to you in terms of providing a balanced diet.

- The presence or absence of teeth. The poor state of an individual's teeth will affect his ability to chew some foods. In addition, ill-fitting or broken dentures will also cause problems with chewing.

- Reduced sense of taste or smell which may be caused by poor mouth hygiene or may be a result of the illness. Sometimes medicines affect the taste of food making meal times an unpleasant experience.

- Difficulty in swallowing – which may be caused by the disease but can also be caused by infections of the mouth or throat.

- Nausea and vomiting which may be caused by reaction to medicines being taken. However, the problem may also be associated with the illness.

It is important to remember that an individual who is unable to manage solids can still receive adequate nourishment in liquid form. The difficulty in this case will be associated with trying to provide sufficient variety in flavour, colour and consistency.

A balanced diet

The constituents of a balanced diet which are necessary for maintaining health in a well person are even more important for one

See Chapter 1, section 1 on Diet for a description of a balanced diet

See section 2.2(d) below on Eliminating and vomiting

whose health needs restoring. This can be difficult if the sick person does not feel much like eating, but some measures can be taken to help tempt an ailing appetite.

The importance of an adequate fluid intake should not be overlooked either. Water is required throughout the body systems. It provides a means to transport products through the body and to excrete waste products. Water in its natural form, or in the form of other liquids, is just as important as the other nutrients.

An individual needs between 1.5 and 2 litres of fluid each day unless medical advice has been given to the contrary.

It is a fallacy that incontinence can be 'cured' by reducing the intake of fluid.

Food preparation

The method of preparing food is important. The nutritional value of some foods may be decreased during this process; for example potatoes cooked in their skins provide more roughage than if the skin is removed. Equally, some foods benefit from long cooking times – for example meat may be tenderised by a long, slow cooking process to aid digestion. Steaming vegetables helps to retain the vitamin content.

If the individual has difficulty chewing, a food liquidiser may be invaluable. Nourishing soups may be made very simply or foods may be puréed prior to serving.

It is also important to remember when preparing foods that cooked and uncooked foods should not be allowed to come into contact with one another.

The use of a food thermometer when you are reheating pre-cooked food will ensure that it is thoroughly heated. Such measures will help to reduce the risk of food poisoning.

Presentation

However small the amount of food being taken, presentation is important. Food which is arranged attractively on a plate is much more appealing to the eye and therefore aids the appetite. Even food which is minced or sieved should be carefully arranged on the plate.

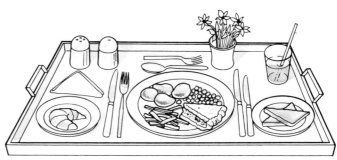

Food that is attractively presented is more likely to tempt a failing appetite

The use of colour and the texture of the food also helps to improve the appetite. For example, small portions of carrot, mashed potato and meat will look more attractive than mashed potato, steamed white fish and parsley sauce.

Dietary supplements

It is possible to obtain dietary supplements in liquid form. These can be obtained either in cans ready for use or in powder form, the latter requiring the addition of milk or water before serving.

These products are available in a variety of flavours. Some brands may be purchased, while others will be available on prescription. They contain all of the nutrients required by the body in varying amounts.

Aids

See Chapter 7, section 12 for more information about specialised crockery and cutlery. See also Appendix VII for Addresses of useful organisations

It is possible to hire or buy a wide variety of items which will aid the activity of eating and drinking. Such equipment may be obtained from a variety of sources including your occupational therapist, Social Services Department or an organisation such as the Disabled Living Foundation. Items include plate guards which clip onto the side of the plate, non-slip mats to place under dishes or plates, cutlery with extended or angled handles and cutlery fitted with increased handgrips.

2.2(d)   ELIMINATING AND VOMITING

See also Chapter 8, section 4(b) on Physical care of the elderly

The manner in which individuals eliminate waste material from the body varies according to each person. It is important to be able to recognise changes to the normal pattern for that person. It is also important to recognise that some changes, for example incontinence, are not always an inevitable consequence either of the disease or of the ageing process.

Faeces

• **Toxins**
  Poisonous substances

Waste material in the form of faeces needs to be eliminated from the bowel regularly. If this does not happen then toxins may be absorbed into the body from the faeces. This may cause nausea and even vomiting. However, the frequency of elimination varies considerably from one person to another. Some individuals may have daily bowel actions while others may only empty their bowel every two or three days. As long as the motion is formed and soft, there is no need for concern. Faeces are usually brown in colour.

Constipation If the length of time between bowel actions becomes much longer than usual for that individual, or if the faeces become hard and painful to pass, then a little help may be required.

The first thing to consider is the diet. The individual needs to eat plenty of fresh fruit and vegetables which will help to provide roughage. The amount of fluid taken should also be increased to at least two litres each day.

The amount of exercise taken is also a contributing factor which may or may not be easy to rectify. Also some medicines, for example analgesics, can cause constipation.

- Analgesics
  Pain killing medicines

Frequent use of laxatives is not usually recommended; however it may be necessary to ask the doctor to prescribe something which will help in the short term.

Diarrhoea The individual who complains of persistent diarrhoea needs to be seen by the doctor. Sometimes diarrhoea may be a sign of severe constipation, strange though that may seem. However, it may also be caused by medicines taken. If the cause proves to be neither of these, then the doctor will arrange for further tests to be carried out. You should save a sample of the diarrhoea for the doctor (see the box below). You should also make a note of any changes in the colour of the faeces. The doctor will need this information in order to make a diagnosis.

Saving a specimen of faeces

- If a specimen of faeces has been requested then the individual will need to pass the faeces into a bedpan or commode so that it can be saved.

- If the doctor has asked for the specimen but has not provided a container, the faeces should be left in a covered bedpan or commode for the doctor to observe.

- If the doctor has provided a specimen container, it will contain a small spoon attached to the lid. After the individual has passed faeces, a specimen should be spooned into the container using the special spoon. The container should be labelled with the individual's name, the date and the time that the specimen was collected.

- Depending on the arrangements that have been made, the container may then be taken to the doctor's surgery or kept at home for the doctor to collect.

- The bedpan or commode can then be emptied and cleaned in the usual way. You should then wash and dry your hands very carefully.

- Haemorrhoids
  Piles

- Anus
  The lower opening of the
  bowel

Discomfort   Pain or discomfort when emptying the bowel may be the result of trying to pass very hard faeces. In this case, when the constipation is eased, the discomfort will disappear.

Discomfort may also be caused by haemorrhoids around or just inside the anus. These are caused by straining too hard to empty the bowel and will require treatment.

There are creams available from the chemist which may help. Sometimes an ice cube wrapped in an old piece of linen and held over the area will ease the discomfort. (Care must be taken to avoid burning the skin as a result of using unprotected ice.) In the long term haemorrhoids may need to be removed by surgery. Persistent instances of pain should always be reported to the doctor or district nurse.

Stoma   Some individuals empty their faeces through an opening on the abdominal wall. This opening is called a stoma. The faeces are collected in a specially designed bag (a colostomy or ileostomy bag) which is attached to the skin by adhesive. This is not normally painful for the individual and the bags are not difficult to change. Fresh supplies of bags are available on prescription from the chemist. Some drug companies also operate a delivery service to the home. In cases of difficulty, a specialist nurse will visit in order to advise you.

Some individuals need to pass their faeces through an opening in the abdomen into a specially designed bag

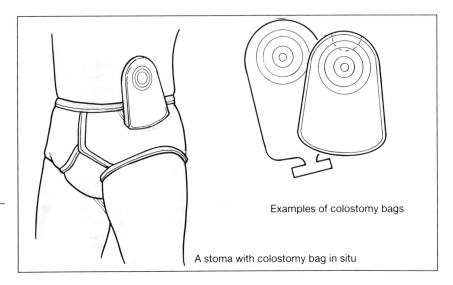

Examples of colostomy bags

A stoma with colostomy bag in situ

Facilities

Sometimes pain, discomfort and constipation may be caused by a lack of appropriate toilet facilities. Difficulties may be due to any of the following:

- A toilet seat which is either too high or too low;

- A toilet seat which is too hard;

- The toilet being inaccessible due to steps or stairs;

- The bathroom being too small to accommodate a wheelchair or walking frame;

- The toilet being too cold;

- Lack of privacy;

- Lack of security – for example, the toilet may be outside;

- Unsafe facilities – for example, the commode may need servicing.

It is possible to obtain raised toilet seats for the toilet which is too low and blocks to put at the foot of the toilet to ease access to the toilet seat which may be too high.

A piece of 5 cm (2 inch) thick foam cut to shape will make the toilet seat more comfortable.

If the toilet is inaccessible a commode may be obtained from various sources (talk to your district nurse or occupational therapist). A chemical type which needs emptying only every few days, or a conventional type of commode, is usually available.

Once the individual is seated safely, she should be left alone if possible for several minutes.

Provision of suitable facilities will help the individual to achieve maximum independence.

Urine

The bladder normally stores urine which the individual is able to pass several times during a 24 hour period. Passing of urine is not normally painful or uncomfortable. Fresh urine usually has no smell and is a clear, straw coloured liquid.

Disorders   Since urine is stored in a dark, warm 'container' (the bladder) within the body, it provides an ideal breeding ground for bacteria. Urinary infections are therefore quite common, particularly in women. One reason for the high incidence of infection is the close proximity of the openings of the urinary passage and the bowel. Bacteria which normally live in the bowel may easily be transmitted into the urinary passage. For this reason, it is important always to wipe, wash or dry the genital area from front to back.

The first signs of a urinary infection may be:

- Dark urine;

- An offensive smell (often fishy);

- Pain or a burning sensation on passing urine;

- The urge or need to pass urine more often.

If the person shows signs of having a urinary tract infection, the doctor may ask for a specimen of urine. The box below tells you how to collect this.

Collecting a specimen of urine

- If you have a bedpan, urinal or commode then the urine can be passed directly into it providing that the receptacle is clean and free of disinfectant.

- You can then transfer a small amount of urine into a clean jam jar or other small container, cover it with cling film or replace the lid.

- Keep the urine, in its container, in a cool place away from other items.

- If the patient passes faeces at the same time as voiding urine then the specimen cannot be saved for testing.

- If the individual is able to use the toilet then he should be provided with a small container and asked to pass some urine directly into it.

- Incontinence
  An inability to control the passage of urine or faeces

Another disorder which may occur is incontinence of urine. This may be caused by:

- Poor muscle control or tone;

- Urinary tract infections;

- Some illnesses or major trauma.

The cause of incontinence will need to be established before it can be treated. Often simple exercises which strengthen the muscles around the urinary tract can be practised with good effect.

See also Chapter 4, section 6 for pelvic floor exercises specific to women after childbirth

The pelvic floor, like any other muscle, gets stronger with 'regular use and exercise'. You cannot see the pelvic floor muscles so it is often quite difficult, at first, to know which muscle to exercise.

In order to identify the muscles which need exercising, firstly sit, stand or lie and without tensing the muscles of your legs, abdomen or buttocks imagine that you are trying to control diarrhoea by consciously tightening the ring of muscle around the back passage. This will help you to identify the back part of the pelvic floor.

Secondly, when you are passing urine, try to stop the flow, then restart it. Do this every time you empty your bladder. Gradually you will then become aware of the muscles at the front of the pelvic floor.

These two groups of muscles are the ones to be exercised in order to regain strength and tone in the pelvic floor as a means of increasing urinary control.

You will not notice any difference at first so do try to be patient. Improvement will be gradual over a period of three months. A large number of people, male and female, can help to maintain or improve urinary control, some with complete success. However, in order to maintain the improvement gained, the following exercises should be carried out every day.

- Tighten the muscles around the back passage. Slowly count to four, then release them.

- Tighten the muscles around the front passage. Slowly count to four, then release them.

- Repeat the sequence four times.

- Repeat the sequence four times morning and evening and whenever possible in between.

You can perform the exercises anywhere, while watching television, while waiting for a bus or driving the car, while washing up or cleaning your teeth. There is no need to hide or to feel ashamed because no one will know that you are doing the exercises unless you tell them.

If the incontinence results from an infection, then it should resolve once the infection is cleared.

Catheters and catheter care   Some illnesses or major accidents can result in a lack of control in the muscles surrounding and acting upon the urinary tract. In these cases, the flow of urine may be controlled by inserting a catheter (tube) along the urinary tract into the bladder. Urine then passes into a bag and can be emptied into the toilet or a suitable container. The catheter is usually inserted by a doctor or nurse but some individuals may be taught to do this for themselves.

Catheters will usually be connected to what is known as a 'closed drainage system'. The system means that the catheter will not normally be disconnected from the drainage bag unless the catheter or the bag needs to be changed. This will be done by the doctor or nurse. It is important that the catheter remains connected to the system in order to prevent the passage of bacteria along the catheter and into the bladder.

If a leg bag is used during the day this should not be disconnected from the catheter at night. Instead the overnight bag can be connected directly onto the leg bag outlet. This enables the closed system to be maintained and helps to prevent infections.

The position of the tubing and bag should be such as to allow the urine to flow downhill continuously. It is important to avoid kinking in the tubing so that urine is able to flow freely.

Hands must be washed and dried thoroughly before and after handling the catheter or any part of the system. A clean jug or container should always be used to collect urine for disposal. The drainage bag should either be attached to the patient's leg or to a free standing holder. This ensures that the drainage outlet does not come into contact with the floor.

In both male and female patients care must be taken to wash the genital area. This should be performed, using soap and water, every day and after every bowel action. Washing and drying of the catheter site should always be carried out separately from the perineal area and should always be from front to back.

It is not necessary to add disinfectant to the water although specially prepared, disposable wipes can be purchased and used if the individual prefers.

The patient should be encouraged to carry out this procedure for himself whenever possible.

Incontinence aids   It is possible to obtain pads and special pants which can be worn to control incontinence. This method is more acceptable to some people. There is a large variety of both pads and pants available. Each individual will be assessed and, after discussion, advice will be given on the most appropriate type. The assessment is usually made by a district nurse.

Providing that the pads are changed as recommended and the skin washed and dried carefully, there is usually no problem with this method. Sometimes the use of a barrier cream on the genital and buttock area will be advised. Special water-proofed sheets are also available which can be used on the bed or to protect upholstered chairs.

- **Perineal area**
  The area between the genitals and the anus

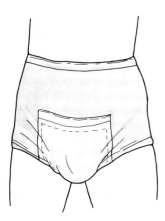

Incontinence pants

With this type, an incontinence pad can be slipped into a pocket as shown, and changed easily

Vomiting

Vomiting can be very distressing not only for the individual but for the carer. A feeling of nausea may persist for several hours before the individual actually vomits. However, vomiting may also occur without warning.

Persistent vomiting may result in:

- Loss of weight, leading to general weakness;

- Disturbances to the level of mineral salts in the body, leading to giddiness or confusion;

- Cramp caused by imbalance in the body fluids;

- Anxiety and depression.

Causes   Vomiting may be caused by any of the following:

- Contaminated food;
- The illness or disease;
- Allergic reaction to some medicines.

The individual should be provided with a bowl or bucket to collect the vomit. This should be covered and emptied as soon as possible, after each episode of vomiting. The container should then be cleaned thoroughly.

Some people like to put a small amount of disinfectant into the bottom of the container but this is not necessary. Indeed the smell of disinfectant may actually precipitate an episode of vomiting.

You may be asked to save a specimen of vomit for the doctor to examine. In such cases, a small amount of vomit should be transferred to a covered container and kept, preferably in a cool place, until it can be examined.

Changes in the frequency, type and colour of the vomit should also be noted and reported to the doctor or nurse.

Treatment   Offer the person a warm flannel and towel with which to refresh his hands and face after each episode of vomiting. Clothing and bedlinen should be changed as necessary.

A mouthwash, which may be obtained from the chemist, should be offered after each episode of vomiting. Some people also like to clean their teeth.

If the individual has dentures, these should be removed prior to the spell of vomiting if possible. Obviously, this is not always easy since there may be no time. In such cases, dentures should be removed after the episode, cleaned thoroughly and returned after the individual has used a mouthwash.

Sips of water should be offered frequently to help prevent dehydration. Proprietary drugs such as Dioralyte are available from chemists and these can help to replace body salts lost through persistent vomiting. However, there is a danger associated with consuming too much in the way of mineral supplements. The advice of the doctor should always be sought.

Food should not be withheld for more than 24 hours unless on the advice of the doctor.

2.2(e)   SLEEPING AND RESTING

Each individual needs to be able to spend periods of time both resting and sleeping. It is important that this time is balanced with other activities so that the individual becomes neither bored nor exhausted. The amount of sleep needed by different individuals varies considerably. As with other activities, it is changes to the normal pattern for that person which need to be recognised.

An individual whose activity levels are reduced may find that resting periods are increased, whereas sleeping hours may be reduced. As long as the period of time spent asleep is of good quality then the individual will be refreshed. The fact that the period of time is reduced may not cause difficulties. However, if the sleep pattern is disturbed then difficulties may occur. Anxiety or worry about the lack of sleep increases the disturbance to the sleep pattern. The individual may then enter a downward spiral of sleep disturbance and increased anxiety which needs to be broken.

Sleep disturbances may have a variety of causes, including the following:

- Inappropriate bedclothes resulting in the individual being too hot or too cold;

- Cramp;

- Joint pains;

- Difficulty in breathing;

- Persistent cough;

- Frequent urge to pass urine;

- Anxiety or depression;

- Hunger;

- Use of stimulants (e.g. tea, coffee or cigarettes) particularly in the evening.

There are several simple measures which can be tried in order to promote sleep and adequate rest.

See also section 2.2(g) below on Keeping warm/cool

Warmth Warmth is usually beneficial in promoting a relaxed state which aids sleep. A hot water bottle or an electric blanket may prove useful. Bedclothes should be lightweight but warm. Alternatively, a bedcradle or some other means of alleviating the weight of the bedclothes should be used. Loose fitting nightwear is more comfortable, avoiding tight necks or waistbands, and bed-socks may be helpful. A warm, milky drink may be enjoyed by some individuals and will help to alleviate pangs of hunger.

Position The use of a selection of firm and soft pillows will help to provide adequate support in a comfortable position. Breathing difficulties may be alleviated by sleeping in an upright or semi-upright position. This position may also help to relieve a persistent cough. It may also be necessary to provide a bed table. The person may find it beneficial to rest forwards over pillows placed on the bed table as shown below.

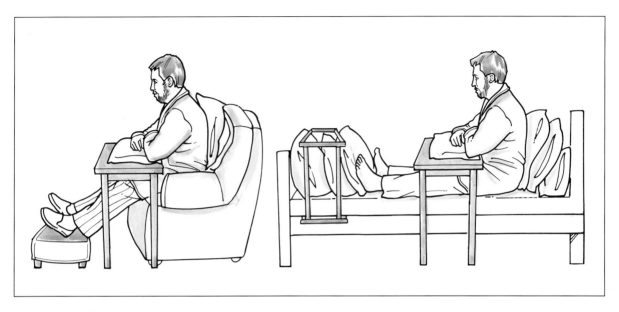

Some individuals may be more comfortable if enabled to lean forwards over a bed table

Relieving discomfort Cramp may be caused by long periods spent in uncomfortable positions. It may also be caused by dietary imbalance. Cramp may be relieved by changes of position every three or four hours. It may also be necessary to take mineral supplements – should this be the case the supplements will be prescribed by the doctor.

Joint pains may be caused by lack of mobility or by long periods spent in the same position. Locally applied warmth in the form of gel packs or suitably protected hot water bottles may help. Medication may be prescribed and this should be taken regularly. It may be useful to take the evening dose at least 30 minutes before settling down to sleep.

If discomfort is caused by a persistent cough, then a glass of water or a supply of lozenges placed within reach may be of benefit. If relief is not obtained, ask the doctor to prescribe a suitable linctus.

Other remedies It is possible to obtain herbal drinks which have a calming or soothing effect. When taken at night, these can be beneficial. Herbal remedies may be obtained from some chemists and all health food shops.

Relaxation techniques in the form of deep breathing or relaxation exercises are easy to learn and are beneficial when practised regularly. Tapes and books are available which aid the learning of such techniques.

See the instructions for Diaphragmatic breathing in Chapter 1, section 5(c)

DRESSING AND UNDRESSING

As with other activities of living, the aim should be to encourage maximum independence. An individual can be helped to achieve this goal in many ways. Working towards maximum independence will also help to reduce the work of caring.

Increased motivation also stems from increased independence. It has been shown that changes of clothing help the individual to feel better about herself. Spending long periods of the day in night-wear may emphasise the sick role which can be depressing.

Whenever possible, once the person has recovered from the severe effects of fever or from the immediate after-effects of an operation, he should be encouraged to change into a different set of clothing for daytime. The individual may not feel well enough, at first, to dress fully in day clothes since the whole procedure may be too exhausting, but he should be encouraged to try a little more each day.

Fastenings and designs

Front fastenings for dresses are much easier to manage than side or back openings. Zips or medium sized buttons along a centre front seam aid independence. There is no need to spend large sums of money on clothes with front openings since adaptations to existing clothes are fairly simple. In such cases, a piece of velcro at the neck edge to replace the original buttons, or a zip, will facilitate dressing and undressing.

Velcro strips or elasticated waistbands make skirts manageable. Often if the individual is confined to a wheelchair, a skirt which fastens only at the waist will make using the toilet easier. Velcro fly and waistband fastenings for trousers also help with toileting as well as with dressing and undressing.

Trousers with wide legs make emptying drainage bags easy. Alternatively, the inside leg seam could be unstitched. Fastening with velcro or tapes will facilitate access.

Nightdresses set on a yoke are useful. Dresses, pyjama jackets and blouses with raglan or dropped sleeves can also aid dressing and undressing.

Hold-up stockings are easier to manage than tights; however tights are preferable to ordinary stockings with homemade garters. Garters can be dangerous since they may impede the circulation to the legs.

Materials

Nightwear and underwear made of cotton is most appropriate during a period of ill-health since it is more absorbent. Loose fitting nightwear together with a cardigan, jumper or bedjacket is practical and also means that the person will be better prepared to deal with the swings in temperature often associated with some illnesses. Layers of clothing may then be added or removed according to the level of fever or the temperature of the day.

Cotton mixed with polyester makes washing and drying easier and also helps to reduce the amount of ironing necessary.

Crimpelene or other man made fibres tend to give and therefore make dressing and undressing easier. These materials will stretch over fixed shoulder or elbow joints and so cause less discomfort.

All of these materials are easy to wash.

Dressing aids

Stocking and sock aids and long handled shoes horns may be obtained from occupational therapy departments or from the Disabled Living Foundation shops. These aids are very useful in helping the person to put on stockings, socks and shoes. Elasticated shoe laces may also be obtained. These enable a lace up shoe, which provides greater support, to be worn without the worry of tying shoe laces.

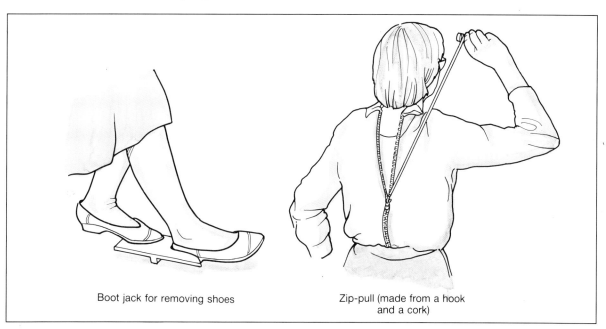

Boot jack for removing shoes

Zip-pull (made from a hook and a cork)

There are a number of aids to dressing and undressing which can be purchased, borrowed or improvised

If a back zip fastening is unavoidable, a piece of fine cord or string attached to the catch facilitates opening and closing the zip and will help to maximise independence.

Putting clothes on

It is easier when dressing someone to insert the weaker arm or leg into the garment first. This is particularly useful if movements are severely restricted. When undressing the individual, the reverse applies. If the person is very frail or partially paralysed it is often helpful to dress her in stages.

The first stage involves putting on underpants, socks or stockings, trousers to thigh level and also shoes.

The second stage consists of putting on the upper garments. This can be achieved either while the person is lying down or while she sits on the edge of the bed.

The third stage involves the person standing, if possible, so that the lower and upper garments can be adjusted. The adjustment can be achieved just as successfully by rolling the person from side to side while she lies in bed.

This method of dressing reduces movement to a minimum and is less tiring for the individual concerned. By reversing the process she can be helped to undress with minimum effort.

It is advisable for the person to wear shoes rather than slippers because of the degree of support shoes offer. They should be checked regularly for signs of wear and tear so that they remain in a safe condition.

2.2(g) KEEPING WARM/COOL

Under normal circumstances the majority of people are able to keep themselves warm. However, reduced mobility and some illnesses affect the body's ability to regulate body temperature. This may apply to persons of any age.

Normal body temperature is usually acknowledged to be around 37°C (98.4°F). However, it is important to remember that for some individuals, 'normal' body temperature may be slightly higher or several degrees lower than this.

When caring for an individual, you may wish to record her temperature and pulse as a guide to monitoring progress.

Taking a temperature

You may need to measure a temperature orally (that is under the tongue) or in the axilla (or armpit). The temperature recorded in the axilla will be 1–2° lower than that obtained from an oral reading. The oral reading is generally considered to be the most reliable. However, if the individual is either too ill to understand or comply with instructions, or is confused, then the temperature should not be taken orally.

A temperature is taken using a glass thermometer which is self-registering. The thermometer is approximately 10 cm (4 inches) long and contains a fine tube along which mercury travels. The mercury is contained in a bulb at the base of the thermometer.

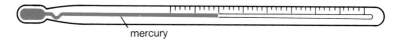

Glass clinical thermometer
with a mercury-filled bulb

Care must be taken to check the thermometer for cracks before it is used. The individual must also be warned not to clamp her mouth and teeth onto the thermometer otherwise it might break.

The temperature should not be taken immediately after activity, food or fluid intake as this may alter the result, but should be delayed for at least 15 minutes. Situations where taking a temperature should be delayed include the following:

- Following a hot or cold drink;

- Following hot or cold food;

- Following exercise;

- Following a steam inhalation, bath or shower;

- Following a cigar, cigarette or pipe.

Taking a temperature orally

- Shake the thermometer so that the mercury falls to below 35°C.

- Insert the bulb in the patient's mouth, under the tongue.

- Ask the patient to close her mouth gently and not to suck or bite the thermometer. She should be encouraged not to talk.

- Leave the thermometer in position for at least two minutes.

- Remove the thermometer and read the result.

The heat of the patient's body will have caused the mercury to travel along the central cavity. The point at which the mercury stops indicates the temperature of the individual.

- Rinse the thermometer, wipe it dry with a clean tissue, shake the mercury down and return it to its container.

- Record the result in a notebook or on a pad.

Taking a temperature in the axilla

- Wipe but do not wash the axilla so that it is dry (perspiration may give an inaccurate reading).

- Shake the thermometer so that the mercury falls to below 35°C.

- Place the thermometer in the axilla and hold the arm firmly against the body so that the bulb of the thermometer is in direct contact with the skin.

- Hold the thermometer in position for four minutes.

- Remove the thermometer and read the result.

- Rinse the thermometer, wipe it dry, shake the mercury down and return it to its container.

- Rearrange the patient's clothing.

- Record the result in a notebook or on a pad.

Taking a pulse rate

The pulse can be most easily felt and counted at places on the body where an artery (blood vessel) passes over a bone, near to the surface of the skin. The pulse is most frequently counted at the wrist but may also be felt at the side of the temple or on the neck, just below the angle of the jaw.

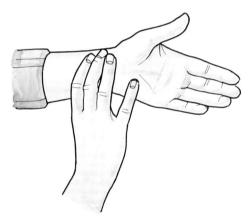

Taking a pulse

By placing two fingers gently but firmly over the pulse sites it is possible to count the pulse rate. Each beat which you will be able to feel against your fingers is counted as one. The pulse rate should be counted for one minute and the number of beats recorded. As with the temperature, individual pulse rates vary considerably and can also be affected by disease or by drugs which the individual may be prescribed. The 'normal' range may vary from 60–72 beats per minute.

During the course of a fever, the pulse rate may rise up to 100 beats per minute and be quite difficult to count.

Some patients may be prescribed drugs which act to slow the pulse rate down in the case of certain heart conditions.

Dealing with a fever

As mentioned above, a fever can cause a rise in the pulse rate. It also causes rises in temperature which may sometimes be quite dramatic. Such rises in temperature and pulse rate can make the individual feel very uncomfortable.

When an individual's temperature rises the skin becomes flushed, the amount of perspiration produced increases and the individual complains of feeling hot. In severe cases there may be reduced output of urine, loss of appetite and sometimes the person may become confused.

During the course of a fever, the patient may prefer to lie in bed and should be allowed to rest quietly. She will be most comfortable wearing loose fitting cotton nightwear which will absorb excessive perspiration.

You may also find it necessary to remove some of the bedclothes, perhaps leaving only a sheet and a light blanket on the bed. However, it is advisable to keep other bedlinen and blankets available since, firstly, an individual with a fever may suffer from extreme swings of temperature and additional blankets may be required from time to time, and secondly, bedlinen may need to be changed more often.

If an electric fan is available, this may be helpful in reducing body temperature.

Frequent drinks should be offered to replace fluid lost from the body in perspiration. Sachets of Dioralyte may be purchased from chemists and are a useful means of replacing body salts especially if perspiration is excessive and prolonged. Mouthwashes are also refreshing if offered regularly.

Tepid sponging   An alternative measure for helping to reduce body temperature, which is not only effective but also comforting, is a procedure known as 'tepid sponging'.

The requirements for tepid sponging are:

- A bowl (e.g. a clean washing-up bowl);

- Six flannels/pieces of linen/towelling squares;

- Warm (tepid) water;

- A bucket for soiled water;

- Two large towels or bath sheets.

The procedure is as follows:

- Close all windows and the bedroom door.

- Remove nightclothes and spread a large towel over the bottom sheet for the patient to lie on. Place the other towel over him.

- Wring out the flannels in tepid water and place one on the forehead, one in each armpit and one in each groin.

- As the flannels become warm, wring out again in tepid water and replace them as before.

- At the same time, gently sponge the individual's body and pat it dry. Do not rub the skin as this encourages blood flow and will therefore increase feelings of discomfort.

- On completion of the sponging, replace the individual's nightclothes and leave him to rest.

Dealing with exceptionally hot weather

Many of the above suggestions will also benefit an individual who is confined either to bed or to a chair during a period of excessively hot weather. Frequent cool drinks, loose clothing, and the use of a fan will all be helpful.

It may not be appropriate to carry out tepid sponging but the individual will probably appreciate the opportunity to wash himself at each end of the day. The use of cologne or a cold flannel placed across the forehead may also be beneficial.

If the individual is unfortunate enough to be wearing a plaster cast, it is vital that he appreciates the importance of not scratching inside the cast in order to relieve the itching caused by the heat. Reducing the body temperature will help to alleviate the irritation; in the meantime the individual should be encouraged to participate in activities which help to pass the time and therefore divert attention from the irritation.

Keeping warm

Reduced mobility, some illnesses, poverty and mental confusion may all affect individuals' ability to keep themselves warm. The elderly and the very young are likely to be at particular risk of becoming chilled but anyone may find difficulty keeping warm in the wrong set of circumstances. Some practical suggestions to carers, to help them enable their sick or frail relative to keep warm, are given below.

Clothing   Clothing should be comfortable and loose fitting. Tight clothing may cause skin soreness or may interfere with the circulation. For example, tight socks or garters may result in chilblains or other circulatory problems.

It is better to provide several layers of clothing rather than one heavy jumper or cardigan. Air trapped between the layers is an excellent form of insulation.

Cotton underwear or nightwear (if it is available) is preferable to nylon or other synthetic materials. Perspiration will be absorbed more easily by cotton material, and this will help to alleviate skin soreness.

In particularly cold weather hats are beneficial even if the individual is confined to the house or to bed. This is because a great deal of body heat is lost through the head.

Bedclothes Flannelette or brushed cotton sheets are useful because of their softness and warmth. Several cellular blankets will provide greater warmth than solid blankets with less weight. Many people prefer to feel the weight of several blankets as well as a quilt rather than a duvet. Unfortunately, the weight of the bedclothes may restrict the movements of some frail individuals. Greater attention therefore will need to be paid to the condition of the skin.

Sheepskin underblankets will help to provide additional warmth. Electric blankets which are thermostatically controlled can be beneficial, but should not be used if the patient is incontinent. Hot water bottles may also be used as an additional form of heating. These should not be filled with boiling water and must be well wrapped to protect the patient from burns. Hot water bottles should not be placed directly against the skin and should never be used for people who are confused, immobile or very frail, nor for babies.

Heating system The room which is to be used by the sick or handicapped person should be maintained at a suitable temperature. The room temperature should be kept between 18°C and 21°C (65°F and 70°F) depending on whether the individual is sitting in or out of bed. If the room temperature is allowed to fall below 18°C for long periods then the patient may be at risk of hypothermia, a condition discussed in more detail overleaf and later in the book.

During the winter months, fuel bills may be reduced by moving the bed into the living room. This may allow one room to be kept at an acceptable and safe temperature. The bed should also be placed against an internal wall and away from the window if possible.

See also Appendix VI on Benefits

Grants may be available for loft insulation in some situations. The Social Security department or your local Citizens' Advice Bureau will advise on benefits which may be available to assist in meeting fuel bills etc.

Exercise Individuals who have restricted mobility are also likely to be at risk from the cold.

It is important to remember that it is possible for a person to exercise even if confined to bed. Simple arm, hand, leg and foot exercises performed for five minutes every hour will help to improve the circulation. These exercises will also help to keep the individual warm.

If an exercise hurts then stop and try again, less strenuously, an hour later. Performing the exercises to music occasionally will provide variety and will help to make them fun.

Hand and arm exercises

- Clench the hand slowly to make a fist, relax and straighten the fingers. Repeat five times for both hands.

- Keeping the arms still, gently circle each hand five times to the left and then five times to the right.

- Holding the arms out in front of the body, move the back of the hands up towards the arm for a count of five and then relax them. Do this five times with both hands.

- Raise both arms out to the side, keeping the elbows straight. Lift the arms to shoulder height to a count of five and then lower to the sides. Repeat this five times.

- Raise the arms as high as possible, trying to clap hands over the top of the head. Don't worry if you can't get your hands together, just raise them as high as possible. Do this five times.

Leg and foot exercises

- While sitting in a chair, shoes or slippers off, place your feet together on the floor. Lift your thigh and knee up towards your chest and keep it there for a count of two. As you get stronger, which may take several weeks, lift your knee for a count of five.

- Again, while sitting in a chair, stamp feet alternately ten times, lifting your knees as high as possible.

- Circle each foot, first round to the left and then to the right. Do this five times in each direction.

- Finally, move your foot up so that the top of the foot and the toes move towards your knee, keeping the heels on the ground. Hold your foot in this position for a count of five. Do this exercise five times with each foot.

There is no reason why carer and patient shouldn't exercise together sometimes. However, it is important to remember that exercise should always be balanced with periods of rest.

Hypothermia

This is the name given to a condition which occurs if the body temperature falls below 35°C (or 95°F). Regulation of body temperature is a function of the brain aided by the nervous system. As stated above, this function may be affected by internal factors (such as a disease process) or external circumstances (such as inadequate clothing or heating).

See Chapter 8, section 6(f) for more information on Hypothermia and how to prevent and treat it

Hypothermia is preventable. Adequate heating and appropriate clothing will reduce the risk.

2.2(h)   KEEPING CLEAN AND WELL GROOMED

During the periods of time when we are well, a great deal of time and energy may be spent on caring for the skin, hair and nails. The care and time that each of us spends on such activities is part of our self-image. It helps to make us feel good about ourselves.

During periods of ill-health, however, individuals will need varying amounts of help in order to meet such needs. Whenever possible the patient should be encouraged to care for herself to the standard she held prior to her illness. This is important since it helps to maintain the individual's feelings of self-worth.

The skin

During a lifetime the skin undergoes numerous changes. The firm, smooth skin of childhood becomes wrinkled and lax. In later years, the skin may become so thin as to be transparent. Hormonal changes may result in the appearance of facial hair or patches of brown pigmentation may appear on the skin.

Keeping skin healthy   The skin secretes varying amounts of sebum and sweat which mix with dust from the atmosphere and with dead skin cells. If this combination is allowed to remain on the surface of the skin it can become very unpleasant. Some areas, which are warm and moist, may give rise to skin soreness and odour. Examples of such areas are under the breasts, underarms and groins. Daily washing with soap and water is necessary. Special care should be taken to wash and dry skin folds and creases. A light dusting of talcum powder may help, particularly in the skin creases and between the toes, but too much may clog the pores.

While washing the patient, it is important to examine the skin for signs of redness or soreness. Skin soreness, particularly under the breasts and in the groins, may give rise to infection if it is not treated. Skin redness may be the first sign of pressure over a particular area.

Pressure sores   Pressure sores occur when the blood supply to an area of skin is interrupted by continuous pressure. Patients who are unable to move freely are likely to suffer damage to the skin. Pressure sores are NOT inevitable and a great deal can be done to minimise or prevent them. The figure overleaf shows the areas of the body which are most likely to be affected.

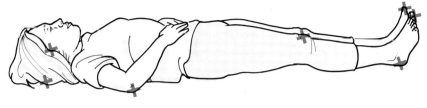

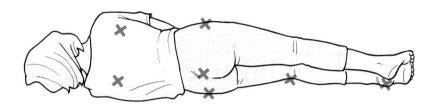

Parts of the body most likely to be affected by prolonged pressure

Other causes of pressure sores include the following:

- Soiled or wet bedlinen;

- Soiled or wet clothing;

- Starched sheets;

- Patched or seamed sheets;

- Crumbs in the bed;

- Long periods spent on a hard chair;

- Incorrect lifting or moving in bed;

- Impaired sensation as a result of an injury or illness;

- Inadequate diet;

- Failure to rinse excess soap from the skin.

Preventing pressure sores   Until quite recently it was considered appropriate to massage areas of skin considered to be at risk from pressure. However, research has shown massage to be ineffective and possibly even damaging to the skin.

The individual should be helped to wash and dry himself as often as is necessary to keep the skin surfaces clean. Barrier cream should be applied after careful washing if the individual is incontinent.

The patient's position should be changed at least every four hours and pressure areas examined at each change of position.

Taking the necessary steps to avoid the causes of pressure will help to avoid unnecessary discomfort. It the patient is very ill or if his mobility is severely restricted, special equipment may be obtained through the district nurse. Special mattresses and sheepskins will help to alleviate pressure.

See section 2.4 below on Lifting and transfers

Washing and bathing

If the person you are looking after needs help with bathing, you may find some of the numerous bath aids helpful. These include:

- Non-slip bath mats;

- Bath seats;

- Wall bars;

- Bath handles;

- Hoists.

Many of these can be obtained on loan through your local family doctor or from organisations such as the Red Cross – ask your community nurse for details of what help may be available for you.

You may find it easier to help your relative to have a shower rather than a bath by placing a special seat in the shower cubicle for him to sit on.

People who are unwell should never lock the bathroom door, in case they should fall or become faint while in the bathroom. You may need to consider some alternative way of letting other members of the household know that someone is in the bathroom, for example by hanging 'vacant' and 'engaged' cards on the outside handle of the door.

People who are very frail or feverish should not be left in the bathroom alone at all if it can possibly be helped. They could slip or the heat could make them dizzy or faint. Support such a person in and out of the bath and help him to sit down. A bath mat placed in the centre of the bath before the water starts running will prevent slipping in the bath itself. As you take the person out of the bath, cover him with a large, warm towel.

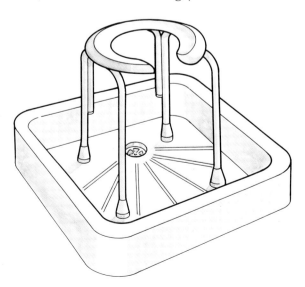

A special stool in the shower can make washing much easier for people who find standing difficult

Lifting a person from the bath is probably easier if done from the back. Make sure the person's armpits arc dry so he isn't slippery, and get him to hold his own wrists across his chest. Put your hands under his armpits and grasp his wrists firmly. Tell him to press on his heels to help you lift. You should be able to get a normal sized patient onto the back ledge of the bath in this way, and from there onto a stool or chair which has been covered previously with a clean, dry towel.

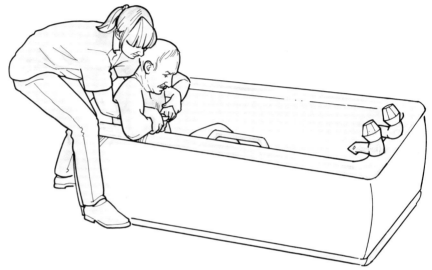

Helping a person out of the bath

You may find it easier to stand behind the person, and put your hands under his armpits to grasp his wrists

It is important to ensure that the person is properly dried after a bath or shower – especially in any areas where folds of skin meet such as the groins, under the breasts for a woman, under the arms and between fingers and toes.

Make sure that the bath is cleaned, the bathroom tidied and the room well ventilated after completion of the bath.

If the person is unable to be bathed in the bathroom, there are plenty of ways to improvise, always remembering to preserve the person's modesty by keeping that part of the body not being washed covered with towels and redressing the person as soon as possible. The box opposite gives advice on carrying out a bed bath.

If there are real difficulties associated with bathing your elderly, sick, or disabled relative at home, it may be possible to arrange for her to have a weekly bath in a local Day Hospital. Talk to your doctor or district nurse about whether this might be a suitable option for you.

Hair

Psychologically many people feel much better if their hair is clean and tidy. Dry shampoos can be obtained from the chemist if it is not possible to wash the hair in the conventional manner.

Giving a bed bath

You will need:

- Jugs of hot and cool water.
- A large bowl (such as a clean washing-up bowl) from which to wash the person.
- A bucket into which you can empty used water.
- Clean face cloths and soap.
- Teeth cleaning equipment and glass of fresh water.
- Two clean towels, one of which should be placed underneath the part of the patient's body that is being washed.

Make sure you have everything to hand before you start.

Strip the bedclothes, leaving the patient covered only by a light warm blanket.

Begin by washing the person's face in clean water. Dry his face and allow him to clean his teeth.

Now wash all other parts of the body, uncovering only a small area at a time (e.g. an arm or leg) to be washed and dried. Change the water regularly. When you have washed an area, cover it up again, before moving on to the next part.

Once the bed bath is over, the patient will probably appreciate a change of clothing and the opportunity to shave or to brush his hair.

However, with a little manoeuvring it is possible to wash a patient's hair while she remains in bed. This can be achieved by removing the headboard (of a single bed) and positioning a bowl on a chair at the head of the bed (as shown below). Alternatively, if the patient is able to move freely, a bowl could be placed either on a chair at the side of the bed or on a bed table.

Many hairdressers offer a full hairdressing service in the home.

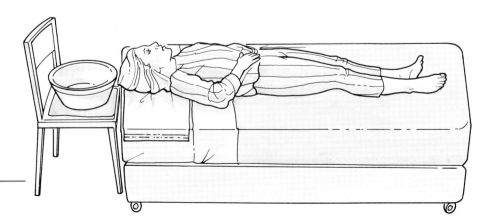

Positioning a bowl for hairwashing

Nails

It is important for hygiene purposes to keep nails short and clean. Fingernails should be cut or filed to follow the shape of each finger. Toenails, unless cared for by a chiropodist, should not be cut down at each side but rather straight across. It is easier to cut toenails if the feet are soaked for five minutes before cutting with special nail clippers.

Often toenails become thickened as a result of the ageing process. Such nails may need to be treated by a chiropodist.

2.2(i) AVOIDING DANGER

See also Chapter 7, section 7 on Safety at home and outside

Within the home environment there are numerous potential hazards to well-being. It is generally recognised that the old and the very young are most at risk of accidents in the home. However, accidents may involve any age group.

Accidents may be the result of human factors or factors associated with the environment.

Human factors include the following:

- Frailty and lack of co-ordination;

- Impaired vision or hearing;

- Reduced mobility;

- Confusion;

- Loneliness which may result in apathy or carelessness.

Material factors include the following:

- Dangerous improvisation;

- Lack of space to mobilise safely;

- Poorly maintained equipment;

- Faulty equipment.

Common types of accidents include falls, burns and scalds, and poisoning (which may be related to medication).

Falls

Falls may be caused by any of the following:

- Slipping on wet or highly polished floors;

- Tripping over obstacles, loose rugs or flexes;

- Lack of hand rails on stairways or baths;

- Poor lighting;

- Moving from bed to chair or onto a toilet or commode;

- Underlying illness;

- Side-effects of medication.

The risk of falls may be increased by poor eyesight which results in an inability to see hazards clearly, or by hearing loss which may result in failure to hear instructions. Delays in using the toilet or commode may result in hurried actions in order to avoid accidents. Rushing, together with reduced mobility or giddiness, may also result in falls.

Prevention of falls   The risk of falls can be reduced quite easily by taking several precautions:

- Use of non-slip polish;

- Removal of loose rugs;

- Ensuring that toys etc. are not left lying around;

- Wiping up spillages immediately;

- Removing excess furniture whenever possible to allow safe passage around the room or across to the bathroom;

- Use of non-slip mat and safety rails on the bath;

- Extra hand rails on the staircase;

- Hand rails by the toilet;

- Beds and chairs of the correct height.

These items may be obtained from your local Social Services department or from the occupational therapy department at your local hospital. (If you are unsure, your doctor or community nurse will be able to advise you.)

It is important to ensure that flexes or cables from electrical appliances do not trail across the floor. Flexes should be hidden behind furniture or placed along skirting boards.

Another important safety aspect relates to footwear. If the individual is able to walk around the room, he should be encouraged to wear shoes rather than slippers as they give more support. Shoes need to be kept in good repair.

For peace of mind, it is also possible to obtain an alarm call device which can be worn around either the neck or the wrist. The call system is linked to a monitoring service which will alert identified carers in an emergency. This may be particularly useful if your relative lives in a self-contained part of the house.

Burns and scalds

Burns may result from falling onto or coming too close to a fire or some other type of heater. Clothing may catch fire as a result of a fall or may be set alight by sparks from a coal fire. Burns may also result from careless use of smoking materials. Faulty or over-full hot water bottles can cause serious scalds. Scalds may also be caused by hot drinks – the risk may be increased if the individual has reduced mobility.

Faulty electric blankets can also be a hazard.

Prevention of burns and scalds All fires should be contained within a full size fireguard, preferably a fixed, box type. Ideally, portable heaters should be placed well away from other pieces of furniture and bedlinen.

Cigarettes, matches and other smoking items should not be left unattended on upholstered furniture. Individuals should not smoke in bed unless it is really necessary and then they should, ideally, be supervised.

Electric blankets should be kept dry and should be serviced regularly by a recommended agent. These items should always be stored flat.

Poisoning

Poisoning may occur as a result of inhalation of poisonous fumes or from unintentional overdose of medicines.

Accidents involving gas heaters are quite common. These may result from poor ventilation, inappropriate installation or failure to have the appliance serviced regularly. Accidental poisoning may also occur through absent minded behaviour or confusion.

Prevention of gas poisoning Suspected gas leaks should be reported to the Gas Board who will always investigate such reports. Gas appliances should be serviced regularly either by the Gas Board or by a recommended dealer. It is important to ensure adequate ventilation of the room if a gas heater is being used. It is also a good idea to check that pilot lights are lit especially in stormy weather conditions.

Medicines Unintentional overdose of medicines may occur through confusion and/or mistakes.

Confusion can result from misunderstanding instructions relating to timing and amounts of medicine to be taken.

Prevention of poisoning by medication Medicines should be kept in a separate cupboard away from bleaches, lotions and disinfectants. Ideally the cupboard should be kept locked and the key stored in a safe place.

See also Chapter 8, section 7(a) on Poly-medication and getting it right

Medicines should always be kept in their original containers. The containers and their contents must be returned to the chemist if the labels become difficult to read. Clear adhesive tape placed over new labels will help to keep them clean and therefore legible.

Large print labels are available for the individual whose vision is impaired.

Medicines which are no longer required should be returned to the chemist who will destroy them.

If the patient is taking several different types of tablets, it is a good idea to make a tick chart for the times when tablets should be taken. This will help to avoid unintentional second doses being taken.

Answering the door

Unfortunately there are cases of bogus callers who may be allowed access to the home. It is important that the credentials of callers are confirmed (unless you know them) before they are allowed access. A bona fide caller will not mind proving his identity before gaining entry. If the patient is alone in the house, it may be appropriate to ask the caller to come back at another time.

2.2(j) COMMUNICATING AND EXPRESSING NEEDS

Individuals vary in the degree to which they need to socialise, although the majority need 'to belong'. Some people enjoy spending long periods of time alone without feeling lonely, whereas others, who may always appear in a crowd or want to be with others continuously, still experience loneliness. The individuality of each person should always be considered and respected.

The issue of visitors when someone is ill is one which may cause distress to the visitor as well as to the person being visited. Often, people who are ill cannot face the prospect of making conversation or worse, the prospect of visitors talking amongst themselves, while the invalid is trying to rest. Individuals should always be asked whether or not they would like visitors and their wishes acknowledged.

Unfortunately, unless handled sensitively, the individual who feels too ill or uncomfortable to see visitors may unwittingly spark arguments or distress. As the main carer, you may need to be very strict about ensuring that the individual has sufficient time during the day for rest. You may also need to ensure privacy for some visits, which might be requested for personal, religious or business reasons.

If the individual feels unable to cope with visitors, she may prefer to make contact by telephone. Letters are also a useful form of contact and the person may like to write or dictate letters to friends or relatives. Advances in technology have produced other aids to communication in the form of videos and cassette tapes; such devices bring the messages 'alive' and may be very much appreciated.

Illness, whether long or short term, can place an enormous strain on relationships. This may be particularly so if the person is being 'protected' from bad news. In many cases, the individual will have deduced the nature of the illness and its possible outcome. Thus the attempt to 'protect' becomes part of a conspiracy of silence. An illness can be a time for sharing and for drawing closer together for partners and families, but only if you all feel able to express your needs. Some people find it difficult to express their feelings and needs in relation to the situation they find themselves in.

Carers too have needs of their own and require time and space in which to meet those needs. Caring for someone at home is an enormous responsibility and it may seem as if you are all alone. Indeed, for many hours of the day and night you may well be alone. Many people will find themselves isolated within their own homes because of the responsibility of caring.

It may be that you feel that you have a duty to provide the care required by a sick relative or close friend. Often people feel very guilty if they do not take on the role of carer; however, carers may also work full or part time, have a growing family each with individual needs, or they may already be caring for a sick or disabled relative. It is important that you feel able to express your needs to agencies who may be able to help you. In cases of brief or prolonged illness or disability, your local Social Services or family doctor should be able to arrange various types of help or support.

See section 2.6 below on Help for the carers

You should not feel guilty, nor a failure, if you ask for help. Nursing someone at home can be exhausting even if the period of time is short.

In addition to communicating with other people, relatives or professionals, you need to be able to communicate effectively with your patient. It is also important for the patient to be able communicate with you. Difficulties in communicating may arise through hearing loss, poor or absent vision or speech impairment. Unfortunately for some people, more than one of these difficulties may be present at the same time. The frustration of not being able to communicate effectively will add to the anxieties already felt as a result of the illness or disability. The frustration may be experienced by the carer as well as by the patient.

Hearing

See also Appendix I, How the body works, section xii on The eye and ear

Sound is collected by the external area of the ear and travels along the hearing canal to the ear drum. Vibrations of this membrane are transmitted by a series of tiny bones to a complicated system of canals which allow the sounds to be interpreted by sensory and auditory nerves.

Hearing loss may be caused by damage to either the sensory or the auditory nerves. Damage may be the result of incomplete development or it may result from some childhood diseases. It may also result from pressure or other damage to the hearing centre of the brain.

Hearing loss may also occur as a result of wax in the ear canal. Wax or cerumen is a normal secretion of the ear but sometimes it accumulates and may cause dizziness as well as deafness.

What can be done If the patient normally wears a hearing aid then it is important to ensure that he continues to do so. You will need to ensure that the ear piece is clean and that the batteries are working. Changing the batteries is a simple procedure, but if you are at all unsure then the doctor or nurse will advise you.

If, however, the patient suddenly becomes hard of hearing, it may be that the problem has been caused by an accumulation of wax. You should not attempt to remove the wax yourself. If you contact your doctor, a quick examination should reveal the nature of the problem.

If wax is present then you may be asked to insert drops into the patient's ear two or three times each day for a few days. The drops help to soften the wax. A safe way to remove the softened wax is by flushing it gently out with warm water using a special syringe. The doctor or district nurse will carry out this procedure.

If wax is not the cause of the hearing loss then the doctor may arrange for further tests to be carried out. In the mean time, a pad and pencil can be used to convey messages.

Sight

The sense of sight is just as important as hearing in communicating or expressing needs. People are able to show how they are feeling by making or avoiding eye contact or by facial expressions. A frown or a smile will often convey more than words.

Equally important is the ability to participate in family activities and decision making. Individuals will also be able to participate more effectively in day to day events if they are able to watch television or read newspapers. Reading books may also help to alleviate boredom.

What to do During the course of a chronic illness the need for an eye test may be overlooked for various reasons. Many opticians will visit patients in their own homes in order to provide eye care. An eye test should be carried out once each year unless the patient is already receiving eye treatment.

It is important for the patient's spectacles to be within easy reach so that he may read or carry out other activities. A magnifying glass may be obtained from the optician if necessary.

It is also possible to obtain books written in large print from local libraries. Tape recordings of a large variety of books are also available and tape recorders may be borrowed on free loan. Books and other items such as clocks and watches are available in Braille.

Speech

Some illnesses (for example, stroke) may affect the patient's ability to speak. The individual may know what she wishes to say but may be unable to form the words. Alternatively, she may be able to communicate in single words but unable to form sentences. This is a devastating blow because speech is very important to all of us. The individual may become frustrated and angry or withdrawn, particularly if she feels ignored.

What to do   You can help the person by being very patient. It is important to give her every opportunity to construct the words for herself. You must try hard not to complete half sentences for her, however much you may be tempted to do so.

If the patient is unable to construct words then you can use a pad and pencil for messages. Another method is to make picture cards of everyday items which can then be used to express needs.

The doctor may also arrange for the person to be assessed by a speech therapist.

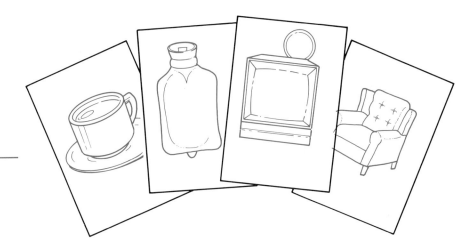

Cards with pictures of everyday objects on them may help a person with speech problems to communicate her wishes

Touch

Whether or not you are able to communicate by sight or sound, touch is important to all of us. A touch or a hug can be very comforting to someone who is ill, particularly if that person is by nature demonstrative.

2.2(k)   PRACTISING RELIGIOUS BELIEFS

Despite ill-health or confinement to the home as a result of reduced mobility, many people need to be able to continue to practise their faith. Some individuals find themselves turning back to religious practices which may have lain dormant for some years, while others look to spiritual beliefs as a means of support and comfort in times of physical or emotional distress. Whatever the reason, the individual should be helped to meet this need with as much energy as any of the other activities of living.

It is important that time and privacy are provided in order for the individual to meet her spiritual needs. It may also be necessary for you to get in touch with a member of the appropriate group as a first point of contact.

Most religious groups offer a visiting or counselling service for those in need of this type of support. They will also give advice on preferred types of food or special requirements.

If the person you are caring for is not of the same religion, elders or religious leaders will be pleased to help you.

2.2(l)   WORKING

In consideration of this activity of living, a fairly general view has been taken – that is to say, general in terms of allowing and encouraging all individuals, as far as they are able, to spend part of each day in activities which are productive for them. These activities may involve the individual in spending time away from the home as part of the general work force. This may be in a voluntary capacity, in sheltered workshops or in mainstream employment. Alternatively, the individual may be able to work from home.

The development of computers and other devices has meant that many individuals at one time denied fulfilment with regard to occupation are now able to meet this need. The emphasis should be on encouraging ability rather than on being over concerned with disability.

Loss of productivity can be devastating but the effect may be much worse when considered in addition to long term restricted activity and poor health. Chronic ill-health need not necessarily mean that work opportunities will be denied to the individual; however it may well mean considerable change in the ability of the person to remain the provider or wage earner.

A great deal of emotional support and practical help will be required in order to help the individual to come to terms with this change in role as a wage earner. In addition, the person may need help to adjust to what he may perceive as a detrimental change in status.

Access

Although there remain many buildings where access is difficult, particularly for wheelchairs, much has been done. Ramps, automatic doors, lifts and access to toilet facilities are improving in many areas. These arrangements enable many individuals to follow careers or occupations of their choice despite reduced mobility or other limitations.

Disablement Resettlement Officers

These professionals are available to assist in assessing and training – or retraining – individuals, particularly following major accidents. Individuals are helped to develop skills which they may use either in sheltered workshops, in the general workplace or in the home.

Voluntary groups

See Appendix VII for Addresses of useful organisations and support groups

Many self-help and other voluntary groups are organised and run by individuals who are themselves affected by the illness. This involvement may include organising events or speakers. Some may be involved in producing a newsletter.

These groups provide a vital service, often meeting an otherwise unmet need. They also provide opportunities for individuals to socialise and to feel like useful members of society.

Information is available in libraries and Citizens' Advice Bureaux, both on the groups available and also on the setting up of new groups.

2.2(m) RECREATION

Most individuals have a need to undertake some form of recreational activity. These activities not only help to sustain an interest in life but also help to provide the necessary balance between activity and rest.

The individual who is forced into early retirement as a result of ill-health may find a hobby related activity fulfilling. It may also provide opportunities for social outings and interaction which will help to alleviate feelings of boredom or isolation.

Recreational activities cannot make up for loss of income but they are a means of maintaining feelings of self-worth.

Education

Some individuals are able to pursue postal courses in vocational or academic subjects. Unfortunately, however, these courses may prove to be expensive in terms of course and assessment fees. Open University degrees are also possible although some courses require the individual to attend summer school which may prove difficult but not impossible. Many people who are confined to the home through reduced mobility are able to pursue these options.

Hobbies

Many people use the period of enforced relative inactivity to pursue new or existing hobbies or activities. If manual dexterity is not a problem, then embroidery, painting or writing may be enjoyed.

For individuals who are able to attend Day Centres, basket work or pottery, amongst other activities, may be possible. For those who prefer less creative pastimes, card games provide opportunities to socialise.

Leisure

Individuals who enjoy listening to music may take advantage of the music section in most libraries. Music, like reading, may allow the individual to escape from the realities of ill-health or restricted mobility. Most libraries now have a vast repertoire of tapes and records to suit most tastes.

As for reading, all libraries have a varied selection of books in large print for those with reduced vision. A large selection of 'talking books' can also be obtained.

2.2(n) IMPROVISING EQUIPMENT

By using simple, everyday items, it is possible to:

- Improve the level of independence;

- Add to the comfort of the individual;

- Simplify the caring role;

- Reduce the stress and strain of caring.

It may be necessary to improvise if you are unable to obtain items of equipment for a few days, for example at a weekend or over a bank holiday when many departments are closed. It may also be necessary to improvise for a short time if items are unobtainable due to shortages.

Some innovations make moving an individual from wheelchair to toilet or wheelchair onto a bath seat easier. Other items help by easing the weight of bedclothes or by helping to prevent the individual from constantly slipping down in bed.

Whatever the innovation, the aim is always to improve the quality of life for the individual. The indirect results of the innovation will also help the carer.

Moving in bed

Items of equipment which help the individual while in bed can not only help to prevent breathing difficulties but may also help to prevent pressure sores.

A loop of rope, knotted at intervals and attached to the foot of the bed, can enable the individual to sit herself up or forwards.

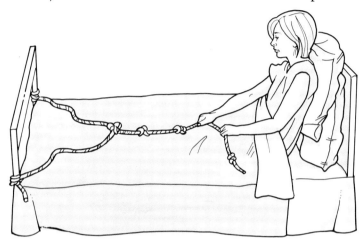

A knotted rope attached to the foot of the bed can be used to help the individual to pull herself into a sitting position

A single or double width sheet containing a bolster or several pillows in the shape of a cracker can be used to help keep the individual sitting up in bed. The filled 'cracker' should be placed across the bed at the level of the feet. The ends of the sheet are then tucked firmly under the mattress. This device will also help to keep the weight of the bedclothes off the legs and feet.

Alternatively, a medium sized carboard box, stuffed with cushions or a pillow, and placed under the top bedclothes at the foot of the bed will help to relieve pressure on lower limbs.

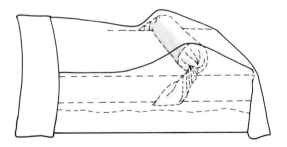

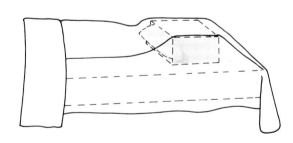

Improvising a footrest

Either a pillow wrapped in a sheet like a 'cracker' or a cardboard box filled with cushions will make a comfortable soft footrest for the patient in bed

Both of these measures will help in the prevention of pressure sores on heels and knees.

Moving from or to a wheelchair

If the individual has a good sense of balance and strong upper limbs then he may be able to help himself actively in moving in and out of the wheelchair.

See also section 2.4 below on Lifting and transfers

A suitably prepared wooden board can be used by the individual to move across between the wheelchair and other suitable pieces of furniture. The board needs to be smooth, strong (at least 1 cm thick) and at least 25 cm (or 10 inches) wide. It also needs to be long enough to span the gap safely. Such boards may be obtained from Social Services departments, and will help to reduce the amount of lifting performed by the carer. It is crucial, however, that the individual is physically active in the upper part of the body and confident in his ability.

Comfort

The individual who has lost a lot of weight or who is frail may suffer a great deal of discomfort from toilet or commode seats. A piece of 5 cm (or 2 inch) thick foam rubber cut to fit the shape of the seat will help to relieve the discomfort. Such foam is easy to wash and dry should it become soiled accidentally.

Dexterity

It is possible to adapt cutlery for the person who has limited manual dexterity by making tubes of 2.5 cm (or 1 inch) thick foam rubber. The handles of knives, forks and spoons can then be inserted into the tubes.

The foam is easily removed for washing and will help with difficulties in gripping some objects. Of course, the foam will not be as useful in cases where arm and wrist movements are also restricted. In such instances, specially adapted cutlery is required.

Very thin pieces of foam or a damp J-cloth placed under a dish or plate will help to stop the item of crockery from sliding across the table. This is helpful in maintaining independence if the person has the use of only one arm or hand.

Drinking straws, particularly the 'bendy' variety, are often preferable to invalid cups. They help to improve the quality of life and level of independence which are important in maintaining feelings of self-worth.

2.3 COPING WITH PAIN

The word pain covers an enormous variety of sensations. It can vary from slight tenderness caused by a splinter to crushing chest pain during a heart attack, from the dull throbbing ache of a sprained ankle to the intense pain of a burnt hand. Whatever the type of pain only the person who has it knows what it feels like. No two people have identical pains; it is an individual sensation. The effectiveness of pain relief is therefore also individual.

Pain is usually considered to be a warning that something is amiss in the body. It may be present to prevent injury or further injury, or to enforce rest. The exception to this is the pain felt during childbirth when the body is carrying out a normal function.

The interpretation of pain depends on the person's previous experience and knowledge. For example, someone with a chronic pain may see no end to it. Because pain is so individual it is important to listen to the description of the pain given by the person feeling it.

2.3(a) PAIN THEORY

Several theories as to the causes of pain have been developed over the centuries. Great strides have been made in the last three decades in understanding the mechanism of pain and the body's reaction to it.

It is now thought that the sensation of pain is transported to the brain by nerve fibres and that there is a gate-like mechanism in the pathway. Other messages, such as touch or heat, passing up to the brain, can shut the gate and reduce the level of pain. The gate can also be shut by endorphins which are morphine-like substances released by the body. When someone is tense the release of endorphins can be inhibited.

The amount of pain is affected by the person's psychological state. His previous experience, beliefs and attitudes are important in this respect. Pain will often improve when the person is told that the cause is something minor and the worry of a major illness and the corresponding upset to his life is removed. The feeling of pain is very complex and its workings are still to be fully comprehended.

2.3(b) PAIN ASSESSMENT

One of the most difficult parts of pain control is the assessment of the pain. The assessment needs to be objective and there are now several recognised methods. At home it may be helpful if a diary is kept to record the pain and the effectiveness of any drugs or pain relieving methods used. Try drawing an outline of the body and shading in the area where pain is felt, as shown opposite. This will not always correspond with the area where the pain originates as pain can be superficial, deep or referred to another area of the body. The amount of pain can be recorded by using a number according to the scale. It may be useful to record the amount of pain before

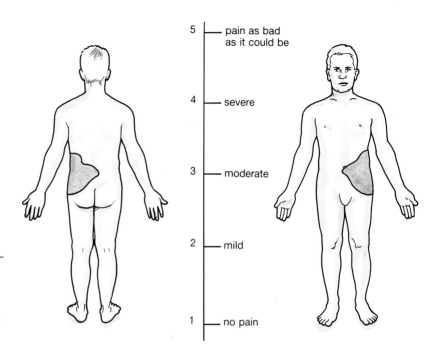

5 — pain as bad
as it could be

4 — severe

3 — moderate

2 — mild

1 — no pain

Pain assessment: shade in
the area on the body outline
where the pain is felt. Record
the amount of pain by using a
number from the scale

any pain-relieving drugs and also half way between doses. This will
indicate the effectiveness of the drugs or other methods used and
will provide valuable information to the carer, doctor or district
nurse. Noting down when pain-relieving drugs are used also helps
to give an objective assessment of their need. Drugs and complementary therapies can then be used constructively and
improvements in the levels of pain can be seen.

2.3(c) DRUGS

*See also Appendix III
for more information
about Drugs and
medicines*

Many of the stronger pain-relieving drugs are only given by prescription. These should be taken according to the instructions
given by the doctor or pharmacist. Both of these professionals are
able to answer queries about dosages, timing and side-effects. If the
pain is long term and drugs are prescribed to be taken regularly
then do follow the prescription. It is easier to keep pain away than
to remove it once it is already being felt. Any side-effects of the
drugs (such as sickness) should be mentioned to the doctor so that
either the prescription can be changed or the side-effects controlled
by further drugs or other methods.

There are many other drugs for pain relief which can be bought
over the counter. Asking for the drug by the approved name rather
than by trade name will often give you a cheaper bottle of the same
thing. If other drugs are already being taken your doctor or
pharmacist should be consulted.

2.3(d) ALTERNATIVE METHODS

Pain relief can be achieved using many methods other than drugs. Pain felt can be much worse if someone is tired, cold, hungry or thirsty. Basic physical needs should be provided for in combination with pain relief methods. If one has a very full bladder, or is desperate for a drink, the discomfort felt will often increase.

One of the simplest ways of relieving pain, or of enhancing a drug's effectiveness, is by a change of position. This may involve adding extra pillows for support or turning onto the other side if in bed. Stretching out limbs, tensing them then allowing them to relax may help. If the person has been in bed for a long time get her to stand up or sit in a chair. Similarly, if someone is normally up and about it may be worth getting her to lie down for an hour or so. These measures carried out after the taking of drugs may help the drugs' effectiveness or may postpone the need to take drugs.

It is now recognised that stimulation of nerve fibres can interfere with the sensation of pain. This can be done by using a small electric current, warmth or touch. TENS (transcutaneous electrical nerve stimulation) is sometimes effective in pain relief. A TENS machine consists of a small box with two or four electrodes. These send a minute electric current to the skin which causes a tingling sensation. If this method has been advised the machines can be hired from the manufacturers or supplied by pain clinics.

Often warmth applied to a painful area will be extremely effective. A hot water bottle is the simplest method although care

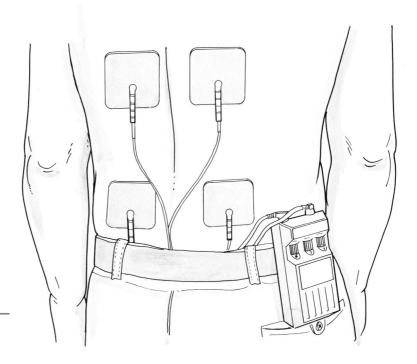

Transcutaneous electrical
nerve stimulation

must be taken to ensure that the bottle is not hot enough to burn. It should not be used if the sufferer is unable to remove it himself or if he has reduced sensation in that area. Massage has long been used to relieve pain. It works mainly by releasing tense muscles. Simple stroking of a hand or head may help to block pain, releasing the body's own pain killers and promoting relaxation.

Several techniques involving the mind can be useful by themselves or as a complement to drugs. Some of these are described in the boxed feature below.

2.3(e) ACUTE PAIN

In an emergency it is these non-drug methods of pain relief which can be used to help someone suffering from acute pain while waiting for the doctor. Drugs used to stop the pain may interfere with the signs and symptoms that the doctor needs to observe while making a diagnosis. If you can keep the person comfortable, talk to him, touch him and try to reassure him that help is on the way, then the pain may be more bearable.

2.3(f) CHILDREN

Children are very difficult to help when in pain. They do not have the knowledge or ability to describe accurately the pain or where it is. More information is often gained by observation of their behaviour.

All the pain-relieving methods described above can be used with children. Distraction, in the form of books, television or friends, can work wonders but there may be a relapse as soon as the distraction ends. Children may be easier to reassure and comfort than adults as they do not have past experience of or knowledge of what pain may mean. However the blind faith that they put in you, the

ALTERNATIVE METHODS OF COPING WITH PAIN	
Relaxation	This can be learnt from a professional, by attending yoga classes or from a tape.
Visualisation	The person imagines herself in a more comfortable situation. She can also concentrate on the area where the pain is, imagining it as a warm point or visualising the healing process taking place.
Distraction	This can encourage the person to think about something other than the pain. Watching television or immersing herself in music can help. This again may promote relaxation and the release of the body's own pain controlling substances.

2

carer, may place an extra strain on you. As far as drugs are concerned, aspirin should not be given to children under the age of 12 so a liquid form of paracetamol is usually the drug of choice. You should be careful however not to exceed the stated dose.

2.3(g)   PAIN – A SUMMARY

Pain is distressing for the person feeling it but it is also distressing for the carer. Often you feel helpless and hate to see someone near to you suffer. Several ways you can help have been described above. A combination of methods is often more effective than one alone, and trying different approaches at different times may have different effects. Most of all listen to the sufferer and respond to what she says works for her.

2.4   **LIFTING AND TRANSFERS**

If you are caring for someone who is bedridden, disabled or very frail you are likely to have to provide a considerable amount of heavy physical help on a regular basis. It is particularly important in such a situation that you take care of your own health as unnecessary lifting and overstraining could result in your becoming badly injured yourself. This section aims to give you some advice on how to move a patient without endangering yourself but it must be stressed that reading a book is no substitute for adequate help and correct demonstration by a trained person. It is very important that you talk to your district nurse or community physiotherapist about what help is available to you and ask her to show you the best way of moving your patient. You can further help to avoid injury by remembering the following important principles:

• Lifting a person who cannot give you considerable help should never be attempted unless the person is reasonably light and you have an able helper;

• Keep your back as straight as possible when lifting or performing any other nursing task (see the figure opposite);

• Never attempt to lift or handle at arm's length;

• Know your own limitations and never try to overstretch yourself;

• Make sure that your general practitioner and district nurse know if you are finding the situation difficult. There are other sources

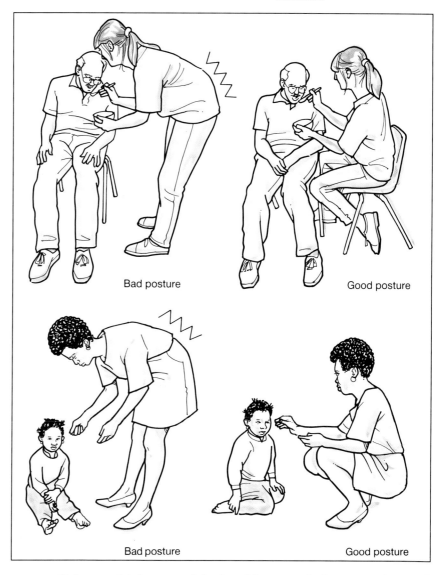

Bad posture

Good posture

Bad posture

Good posture

Good and bad posture

It is important to keep your back straight whenever possible

as well from which you might be able to get help. A mechanical lifting device may be obtained for heavy dependent patients and you should not hesitate to ask for one.

The lifting and moving procedures that you are most likely to have to perform will now be described.

2.4(a) MAKING A BED WITH A PATIENT IN IT

• You will need a second person to help you with this task.

Make sure that the room is warm – your patient will have fewer covers on him for a while. If he uses a duvet, have a blanket to hand to cover him with while you change the bottom sheet. Put a chair at the end of the bed to put the bedclothes on, remove all but one pillow and loosen the bedclothes all around the bed.

Now take off all the blankets except for one which you should leave over the patient. Remove the top sheet from under the blanket. The bedclothes should be put neatly over the chair in order so that the first to go back on the bed will be on top of the pile. If the patient has a duvet, one person should roll it back slowly while the other replaces it with the blanket so that the patient does not get cold.

The two carers should stand one on each side of the bed. The patient should be rolled onto his side and towards one of you. Talk to him as you are doing this and let him know what to expect at every stage. Then while one carer supports him, facing her on his side, the other should roll the bottom sheet up towards his back – as shown in the figure. A clean sheet should be put over the un-covered side of the bed with its rolled up edge against that of the old sheet. Between them, the carers now turn the patient onto his back and roll him over onto his other side towards the second carer

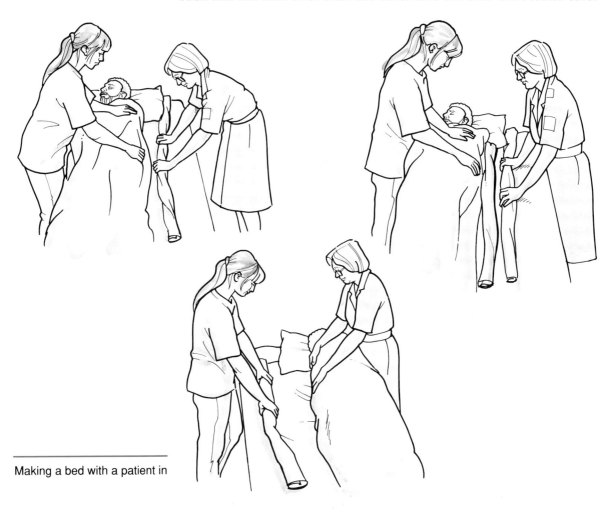

Making a bed with a patient in

so that he is now lying on the clean sheet. The second carer supports him while the first one removes the old sheet and tucks the clean one in. After this, the person's position can be adjusted for comfort as the rest of his pillows are returned (with clean covers as appropriate) and a clean top sheet and blankets or a duvet can be put back over him, smoothed down and tucked in (but not too tightly). The chair can now be replaced in its original position and the dirty linen removed.

2.4(b) MOVING SOMEONE UP THE BED

See the introduction to this section for a summary of the principles of safe lifting

• You will need a second person to help you with this task.

The first step in moving a patient up the bed is to raise her into a sitting position. The two carers should position themselves one on each side of the bed, facing towards the headboard (as shown in the figure). If the bed is low, as most beds in private houses are these days, each carer should put one knee up on the bed and the other foot flat on the floor.

Be careful to keep your back straight while lifting.

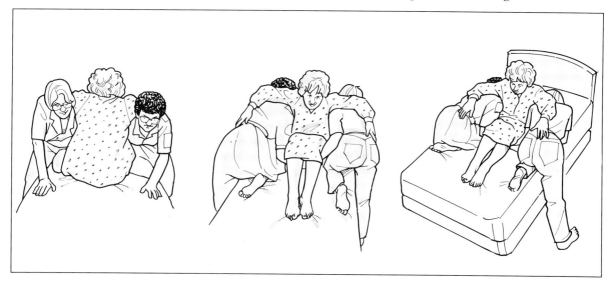

Moving the patient up the bed

Both carers should place their inner shoulder under the patient's armpit and grasp each other's wrists under her knees, as shown in the figure. They will need to synchronise their movements as they lift the patient up the bed on the inner arm and shoulder by pressing on the floor with the outer foot and against the mattress with the outer hand.

If the patient is in a double bed, one of the carers will have to kneel actually on the bed beside her, while the other adopts the position described above.

2 CARING AT HOME

2.4(c) MOVING A BARELY MOBILE PATIENT FROM BED TO CHAIR

See the introduction to this section for a summary of the principles of safe lifting

• You will need a second person to help you with this task.

The chair should be positioned close to the patient's bed and you should ensure that there is no clutter (or ridges of carpet, etc.) to complicate the journey.

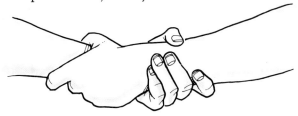

Grasping each other's wrists prior to lifting the patient

The first step is to raise the patient into a sitting position. Then you should ease his feet gently over the side of the bed and help him to put on slippers (and socks if necessary) and a dressing gown or cardigan.

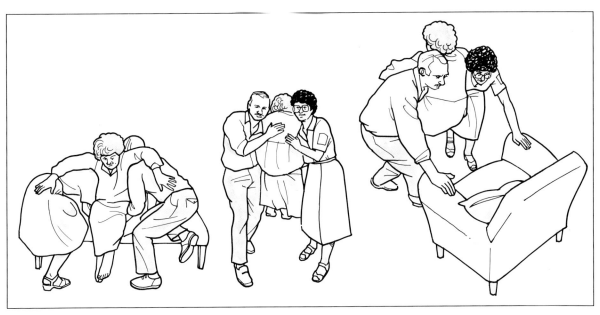

Transferring a patient from bed to chair

You will then need to lift him, supporting him with your inner shoulder against his armpit and your inner hand grasping the other carer's wrist under the patient's knees in the same way as if you were preparing to lift him up the bed (see above). Synchronising your movements, you and the other carer should straighten your knees to stand up, lifting the patient as shown in the figure. You can then move slowly towards the chair and lower him gently into it.

The patient will probably need a rug or blanket over his knees while sitting the chair unless the weather is very warm.

2.4(d) HELPING THE MORE MOBILE PATIENT FROM BED TO CHAIR

See the introduction to this section for a summary of the principles of safe lifting

The more mobile patient, able to bear some of her own weight, will probably be able to move herself to a sitting position on the edge of the bed with just a moderate amount of help from one person. Now you can help her to put on her dressing gown and slippers, or she may be well enough to wear comfortable daytime clothes. When she is ready to be moved, ask her to put her arms around your shoulders or waist. Put your hands under her armpits and bend your knees. Straighten your legs to help her to her feet. Wait until she is steady before you attempt to move, then support her as you both walk with small steps towards the chair. She should continue to bear much of her own weight until she is sitting down again.

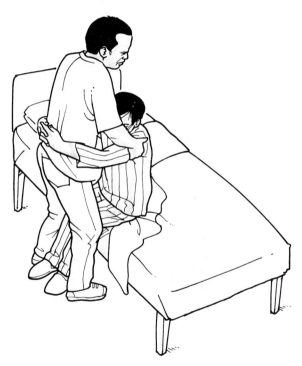

Helping the patient with some mobility to stand up

2.4(e) TURNING THE PATIENT WHO CANNOT MOVE HIMSELF

See section 2.2(h) above for more information about pressure sores

If a person is too ill or disabled to move himself, you will need to move him regularly so that he does not develop pressure sores. This procedure should be performed every two hours if at all possible and every four hours at least. If sore areas appear to be developing show them to your district nurse. It may be that your patient is not being moved often enough.

As with any other procedure, it is important that while you are moving the patient you tell him what is going on and what you will be doing to him next. You should do this even if the person is unconscious as there is some evidence that he may still be able to hear. You will need to remove the bedcovers before you start turning a patient, so you should first ensure that the room is sufficiently warm.

If at all possible, turning a patient should be done by two people, and the following instructions are for the carer who is accompanied by a helper.

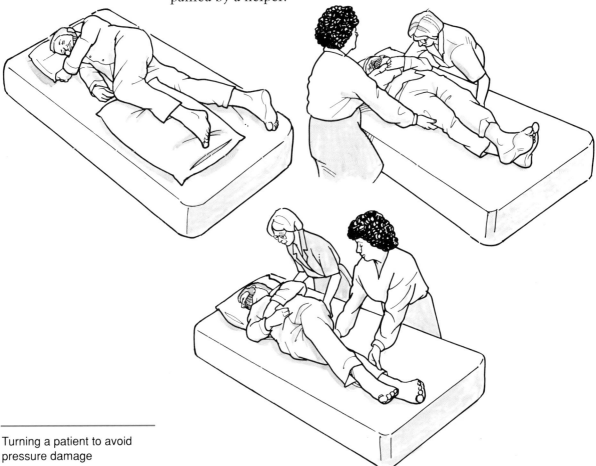

Turning a patient to avoid pressure damage

Assuming that the person is lying on his right side, with a pillow between his knees as shown in the top left hand figure, the following steps describe how to move him into the same position on his left side.

The two carers should stand one each side of the bed. The carer on the right should gently remove the pillow and straighten the left leg so that the foot rests just in front of the right foot. The carer on the left should roll the patient carefully towards her so that he is lying flat on his back.

Now the carers must turn the patient's head to the left, fold his arms across his chest and lift his right leg over his left one.

Both carers should now stand with their feet apart, on the side of the bed opposite to the one the patient will be facing when he has been turned to his new position. Both must insert their hands and arms under the patient's shoulders, buttocks and upper thighs. They should slide the patient, who will still be lying on his back, towards them, using their forearms as skids.

• No lifting is necessary, nor should it be attempted.

The patient can now be turned onto his left side, into a comfortable lying position in the middle of the bed. A pillow under the slightly bent, right knee will protect the bony part of the knee from becoming too sore.

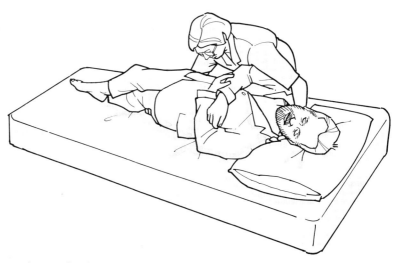

Turning the patient without a helper

If you find yourself alone with the patient when it is time to turn him, you will have to perform the task yourself. The mechanics are similar to the two-person turn. You should first remove the pillow from between the patient's legs and roll him onto his back as described above. Folding his arms across his chest and turning his head to the left should not be too difficult, neither should arranging his right leg over his left one, as shown above.

Position yourself on the right hand side of the bed and slide one hand under the patient's shoulders and the other under his hips. Straighten your back and bend your knees. With one smooth movement, slide the patient, still lying on his back, to the side of the bed on which you are standing. Cross his outer leg over his inner leg on the side to which he is to be turned. Now go round to the opposite side of the bed. Cross the patient's arms over his chest, take hold of his furthest hip and pull him over towards you.

He will now be lying on his side in the centre of the bed. Rearrange his limbs and clothing to make him comfortable.

2.5   PEOPLE WITH SPECIAL NEEDS

2.5(a)   CHILDREN

As any parent knows, children are not small adults. What they are, however, is unique and complex individuals whose needs may change rapidly as they grow and develop.

Caring for a child, whether your own or somebody else's, can be very demanding. It can also be a source of anxiety, frustration, and most of all of great joy.

The United Nations Declaration of the Rights of the Child recognises the precious (and dependent) nature of childhood, as well as the responsibilities of those who have children in their care. Some of these rights may be granted or withheld by governments or political bodies world wide but the first, 'The right to affection, love and understanding' is one that every parent can aspire to fulfil.

The United Nations Declaration of the Rights of the Child

> - The Right to affection, love and understanding
> - The Right to adequate nutrition and medical care
> - The Right to free education
> - The Right to full opportunity for play and recreation
> - The Right to special care if handicapped
> - The Right to be among the first to receive relief in time of disaster
> - The Right to be a useful member of society and to develop individual abilities
> - The Right to be brought up in a spirit of peace and universal brotherhood
> - The Right to enjoy these rights regardless of race, colour, sex, religion, national or social origin

All children may go through phases when they may cause their parents more anxiety than delight and specific problems that can arise (be they physical or behavioural) are explored in more detail in Chapters 5 and 6 of this book. It is hoped too that these chapters will give some helpful advice to parents wishing to promote their children's health, happiness and well-being.

The sick child

Most children from time to time have episodes of sickness at home. In many instances it is sufficient to take a common sense approach to providing care for simple problems such as the

*See also Chapter 5,
section 11 and
Chapter 6, section 3 on
Caring for a sick child
at home*

common cold or a 'tummy' upset. But for the new parent or one faced with a new illness or change in the child's condition it is sometimes difficult to know when to seek advice. However, nobody knows the child as well as the parent who, better than anyone else, will recognise when the child is not progressing as well as she should be.

Caring for a sick child can be quite taxing and worrying for parents. Try to eat and rest sensibly, recognising that there are times when you will feel the need for a break even if only for an hour or so. Enlist the help of friends or family members to take over, or consider a timetable of 'shared care' with your partner.

Does the child need to go to bed? Few children feel ill enough to want to be quiet all the time. Be guided by your child, who may be happier sitting in a cosy chair with the rest of the family rather than being bored and alone in a bedroom. Try to introduce some change of position during the day to provide a change of scene, perhaps by moving the chair or bed to be nearer a window.

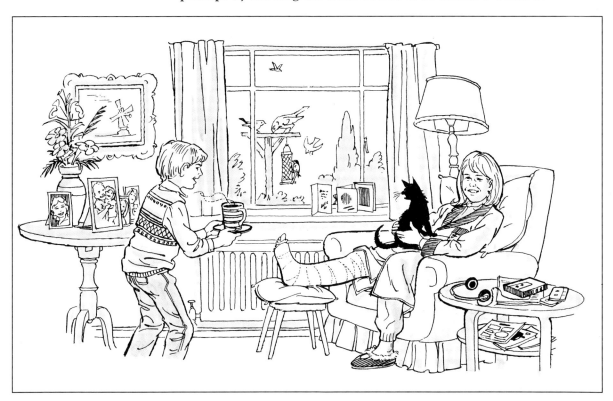

Moving the child to another room, near the rest of the family, during the day will prevent feelings of boredom and isolation

While it is important for the sick child to be kept warm, avoid overheating. A comfortable room temperature with the appropriate amount of fresh air for the family will usually suit the child.

If the child is breathless or has a cough, sitting up well supported with pillows and cushions will enable her to be more comfortable.

At night time it may be necessary to add more pillows – particularly for the older child. If a limb is in a plaster cast or the child has a pain in a particular place, instinctively the position of least discomfort will be adopted. The gentle placing of pillows for support and protection of the affected part will often help the child to feel more comfortable and secure.

Food and drink   The sick child will eat normally again when he feels ready to do so and should never be 'force fed'. (This applies to well children too.) Once he has recovered, lost weight will be regained rapidly. Special diets are seldom needed; if they are the doctor will advise you. Children who are feverish will need extra fluids to replace that which is lost in sweating. Small amounts given frequently are usually well tolerated although some encouragement may be needed. Use a wine glass, different bendy straws or offer ice chips or homemade ice lollies to provide variety with fluid intake.

When to call the doctor   Advice should always be sought for:

- The baby who starts to refuse feeds and is generally off colour;
- The drowsy irritable child with a headache or earache;
- The child who is vomiting, in pain or has diarrhoea;
- The child with breathing difficulties;
- The child with unexplained bruises and bleeding;
- The child with a high fever;
- The child who has become confused or loses normal skills.

It is a good idea to make a note of your own observations to tell the doctor as it is very easy to forget them if you are worried. Some parents also find it helpful to list the questions that they wish to ask the doctor.

Pain management   Measures to relieve pain and discomfort may include an ice pack held over a bruise or swelling, a cold wet flannel applied to the forehead for a headache, or a covered hot water bottle or heat pad which may be very comforting for the older child with a stomach ache.

See also section 2.3 above on Coping with pain

There is no reason why your child should be in continuous pain. Painkillers such as paracetamol are readily available and usually most effective especially if given before the pain becomes too severe. Always follow the manufacturer's instructions carefully. All medicines should be kept in a safe and secure place.

- It is important to remember that aspirin should never be given to children under the age of 12 as it may occasionally cause complications.

Anxiety and fear can often make the child's pain more difficult to bear. Answer all questions about the pain or the child's illness simply and truthfully – knowing what is happening makes acceptance and co-operation much easier.

Play and occupation A bored child is likely to be a miserable child, so it is in both of your interests to keep the child occupied. To help you, here are a few play pointers.

- Provide a good steady surface e.g. a tray for the child to play on while in bed or sitting in a chair.

- Some form of covering to protect bedding may be needed, especially for the younger child.

- Sick children tire quickly; toys and activities will need frequent changing.

- It is a good idea to have in reserve an assortment of oddments of wool, material, cards, magazines for 'cutting up', pencils, paper, paints and pens etc., for when suddenly faced with the task of amusing a sick child.

PLAY/OCCUPATION IDEAS	
For babies	Mobiles hung above cot and pram (need to be changed from time to time) Varied rattles . . . hand hold size, sealed tins with a piece of wood inside Squeaky soft toys Musical toys/boxes
For toddlers	Old Christmas/birthday cards Crayons/felt tip pens (washable) and paper A bag or box to unpack, filled with a variety of surprises Play dough/plasticine Bubbles to blow Building bricks Glove/sock puppets
For older children	Organised projects e.g. making a scrap book, writing a diary, starting a stamp collection Construction kits Make-up and mirror Sewing, knitting, patchwork, embroidery Origami, modelling Jigsaws Video/computer games

The child who has been in hospital   It is not unusual for a child who has been in hospital to appear difficult and demanding on return home. Younger children often regress to more childish behaviour – for example a child who had stopped using a bottle may refuse to drink from a cup. This is quite normal and usually settles quickly once the family routine has been re-established.

See also Chapter 5, section 9 on The child who needs to visit hospital

2.5(b)   PEOPLE WITH A LEARNING DISABILITY

The majority of people with a learning disability (mental handicap) live at home with their families or in homes which they share with friends and colleagues of their choice. In the past parents were faced with the difficult dilemma of coping 'alone' or 'sending' their child into residential care or hospital. Nowadays circumstances have changed and improvements in home care services (through Community Mental Handicap teams) provide parents and carers with practical assistance and advice. Increases in financial allowances and benefits have also enhanced the quality of life for people and their carers, helping to promote opportunities and lifestyles in the community.

See Chapter 7, section 13 on The adult with a learning disability for more information about the work of Community Mental Handicap teams

Caring for someone at home can present particular difficulties from time to time and this will largely depend on presenting needs at different stages of the person's life. This is further complicated by the fact that learning disability does not often follow a particular course and the actual extent of a person's handicap or needs will determine the amount of care and supervision required.

There are many variations within the learning disability speciality which range from mild learning difficulties (requiring minimal support and care) to more intensive needs of a degree that respond only to intensive supervision and home based nursing care. This section will consider the needs of those persons who present particular challenges and needs.

It may be assumed that between four and five people in every thousand fall into this category. They may acquire their condition in one of the following ways:

- By congenital deformity (e.g. Down's syndrome);

- Because of a birth injury;

- As a result of a variety of other factors ranging from nutritional deficiency to metabolic disorders (disturbances in the body's chemistry).

Of this group it is estimated that just under half may have additional needs such as epilepsy (seizures), respiratory or cardiac complications and in some cases, spasticity of the limbs.

Despite the rather apparent worrying combination of some of these conditions, the majority of people can expect to live as long as other members of the general population and to enjoy their lives within the context of their families or with friends in their local communities.

One myth should be dispelled at an early stage. The majority of people do *not* need to live in specialist hospitals and do *not* require skilled nursing care. In fact many nurses are now of the opinion that the very best approach to meeting the needs of some of our more disabled people is to support parents in delivering care directly in their own home. In other words, there is no substitute (in most cases) for a caring family who are supported in their task by trained and accessible professionals.

People with learning disabilities are people first and any approach adopted in meeting their needs should always acknowledge this fact. It may, in fact, be all too easy to respond to the needs of some individuals with a learning disability in a condescending or patronising manner, and while this may be understandable, particularly during childhood, it is not so acceptable in later life. A personal and dignified approach is required which respects the actual needs and wishes of each individual. After all people with learning disabilities have feelings and emotions just like any other member of the family of the same age and as such require life experiences that enrich learning opportunities.

All people (no matter how severe their disabilities may appear) can develop and respond to education and positive stimulation. One way of understanding this is to recognise that some people may take a little longer to acquire or consolidate some of the learning experiences that we take for granted in our everyday lives. In many cases the way in which we provide these experiences may be different to the way in which we respond to other members of the family whose senses and communication skills may be more advanced or developed. However, while some of the more obvious forms of communication (such as speech) may not be so well developed, other senses such as smell, touch and hearing may develop normally to compensate. Consequently one of the most important rules in providing care is to identify a specific communication system (advice will be available from your speech therapist or community mental handicap nurse) and to implement it consistently. Non-verbal communication systems (examples of which are 'Makaton' or the 'British Sign Language') have been used successfully with people with severe learning disabilities.

Thus communication is one of the most important areas to master before appropriate care and stimulation can be given. Similarly it is important that parents and professionals reach agreement about their expectations of the person's potential, and this is best achieved by open and frank discussion. Setting one's sights too high can result in disappointment for both parents and clients, while setting them too low may encourage underachievement and overprotection. Once this delicate balance has been accepted and negotiated it may then be possible to consider how to reduce the effects of any presenting handicap and to encourage the maximisation of learning potential for clients.

The majority of home based techniques fall into two categories:

- Those which reduce the effects of 'handicap' and ill health;

- Those which encourage the acquisition of new skills (and the reduction of inappropriate ones!).

The first category may involve the introduction of passive exercises to manipulate limbs (under the supervision of a physiotherapist) when cerebral palsy (spasticity) presents, or the introduction of muscle exercises to improve 'floppy' muscles and tone. Other needs may demand the use of specific feeding techniques which may range from the preparation of special diets and soft food to 'tube feeding' in a very few instances. The monitoring of epilepsy is a rather more common requirement and some 40 per cent of people who fall into the 'severe' category of learning disability may require medicines to control the frequency of seizures. Parents will also need to exercise vigilance whenever seizures occur in order to administer appropriate care and first aid.

See also Appendix II on First aid

The second group of interventions usually demands the use of specific and consistent routines based on the design of 'training programmes'. These may vary from toilet training and feeding programmes to those that encourage literacy and numeracy. Others may be designed to change inappropriate behaviours which may disrupt patterns of family living – e.g. sleep disturbance, self-inflicted injury and temper tantrums. Clinical psychologists, consultant psychiatrists in mental handicap and community mental handicap nurses may be particularly useful in advising on the use of these programmes which are based on the principles of learning theory and 'behaviour modification'.

See Chapter 7, section 13 for more information about the work of the various health professionals

2.5(c)   THE EMOTIONALLY ILL

It has been estimated that approximately one in every five women and one in every seven men will receive treatment for emotional problems at some point in their lives. Today, emphasis is placed largely on treatment being given at home or day centres rather than in a hospital setting.

See also Chapter 7, section 10(b) on Depression and anxiety

Emotional illness can take many forms. It may be an acute reaction to an incident which has occurred in a person's life such as bereavement or redundancy, or an illness which requires longer term care such as schizophrenia or dementia.

Acute episodes

Following acute life events, people often respond to the emotional pain they are feeling by crying, feeling depressed or sometimes becoming angry. These are healthy reactions to emotional distress and you should encourage a person responding in this way to talk freely without feeling pressured or guilty. Initially, you may find that he seems to be suffering from a form of emotional shock, and is unable to carry out day to day tasks like caring for himself, children or the home. If this is the case, you may find as a carer that your first role will be to enlist practical support from other friends or family to help out (other people are usually very supportive in times like this so don't be afraid to ask).

Making sure that the person has adequate food, drink and rest will probably be your next priority. Remember that a person's appetite is often greatly reduced at times of extreme stress but light, appetising meals should be offered regularly. Fresh fruit juice or milky drinks are a welcome change from lots of tea and coffee which, because they contain caffeine, will hinder sleep and can make individuals feel more on edge if taken in large quantities.

See also Chapter 1, section 3 on Sleep

Many people find it difficult to sleep when they are feeling stressed or ill, usually because they are unable to relax fully and stop thoughts from going around in their mind. 'Catnapping' during the day should be avoided, unless the person is extremely tired, as it prevents good rest at night. A warm bath and a milky drink before bed work well for some people, while during the day, it may be helpful to suggest deep breathing and relaxation exercises. These exercises are very easy to learn, but concentration is needed to gain maximum benefit. Suggest that the person:

• Lies down in a darkened, warm room away from noise;

• Then, he should concentrate on breathing slowly and deeply (it sometimes helps to count slowly to five on each breath in and out);

• When the breathing has become restful, he should imagine the tension in his toes slowly being released on each breath out;

• Next he should imagine the tension being released in his ankles, calves, and so on until he reaches the top of his head.

See also Chapter 1, section 1.5(c) on Breathing as a response to stress

Concentrating all the time on the breathing is the key to this type of relaxation, and you may find that your local library or health centre can lend you a pre-recorded tape which will include similar exercises.

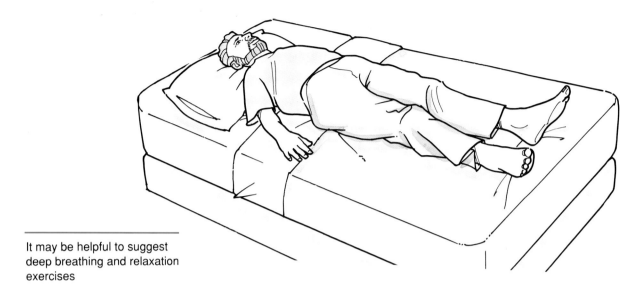

It may be helpful to suggest deep breathing and relaxation exercises

Explain that the aim of this type of relaxation exercise is not to sleep, but to make the person feel calmer, as this may help the person who is anxious about sleeping.

Following an acute episode like this, it is important to allow the person gradually to build up his confidence again and begin to carry out normal activities. Giving appropriate praise and showing warmth and affection are very powerful tools in helping someone regain his self-esteem.

Perhaps the most helpful thing that you can do for anyone who is going through an emotionally stressful period is to spend time listening to her and being with her. If, however, someone is suffering from a more serious form of illness her behaviour may be very different from that described earlier. You may be caring for someone whose thoughts appear to become confused, or who thinks that she can hear voices, and this can make her behave in a different way to usual – for example, by making her more withdrawn or angry with no obvious cause. If this starts to happen suddenly, or without any apparent reason, it is important to seek help as soon as you can. Many undiagnosed physical illnesses can cause behaviour like this, but it may be the beginning of a longer term emotional problem.

Longer term illness

People with a long term mental illness are no longer automatically placed in hospitals or institutions as they can lead normal lives in their own homes or hostels with different levels of support. People with this type of illness usually have times when symptoms are very acute as well as periods of relative wellness. Many support

See Appendix V for more information about People and resources available to help you, and Appendix VII for Addresses of useful organisations and support groups

groups and charities now offer practical help and support to carers who have a relative or friend with long term mental illness, and your library, health centre or telephone directory will have a local contact number to put you in touch with people in a similar situation to your own.

Sometimes, it is the less obvious symptoms of the illness which are the most difficult to deal with at home. You may find that your relative or friend has great difficulty getting up in the morning, begins to neglect his appearance, withdraws from other people or spends a lot of time alone. Occasionally he may begin to talk about or act on strange ideas or thoughts. Encouraging him to find non-stressful but worthwhile activities may help, but it is important to keep a balance between activity and rest as concentration and tolerance may be more limited than usual.

You may find that medication in the form of injections or tablets is prescribed by your doctor to help with symptoms of the illness. If these are prescribed, it is very important they are taken regularly to give maximum benefit, but it is worth asking if there are also other forms of treatment or support available such as visits from a community psychiatric nurse, or a Day Centre or workshop that the person could attend. This not only provides some structure and interest for the person, but will also give you and other members of the family an opportunity to spend some time together.

See also section 2.6 below on Help for the carers

You should not forget your own needs when caring for someone with a long term emotional illness as it can be very stressful for you and other members of the household. Give yourself some time to be alone, continue with hobbies or interests, and look after yourself physically. If you feel you are becoming increasingly under stress or your relative or friend appears to be becoming unwell again you should seek help from the support services immediately.

2.5(d) VICTIMS OF VIOLENCE AND DISASTER

See Chapter 3, section 10 for a discussion of Bereavement and loss

Every day, people suffer personal disasters such as assaults or accidents, in which they may feel their lives or health have been at risk. Personal disasters may involve bereavement but this section deals solely with the experience of trauma. You should also be aware that those who lose loved ones in a sudden, unexpected and violent way will suffer many of the feelings described below in addition to grief.

The experience of trauma

Immediately after some sort of trauma, there is often a reaction of numbness and detached calm. Alternatively, some people may show a brief but strong emotional reaction, seeming to recover from this quickly. Being reunited with loved ones hours later may be the trigger for a stronger reaction, or reactions may develop slowly over the following days or weeks, after a superficial return to normality.

In the longer term, the following reactions may develop.

Re-experiencing This involves the person having intrusive thoughts or mental images about the event. These may also come in the form of nightmares. Flashbacks may be triggered by reminders of the event.

Avoidance and emotional numbing Emotional numbing prevents the person from experiencing too much pain at any one time. It thus serves as a protection and, as such, should be respected. Most people move in and out of numb under-reaction and strong painful memories of the event. You will need to be sensitive to when the person is more open to talking about his experiences.

Other people may avoid actual reminders of the trauma, such as the place it happened, other parties involved etc. This can cause difficulties if it handicaps an individual's life. People who have experienced trauma may seem changed in a number of ways: they may lose interest in activities they used to find enjoyable, they may feel and appear cut off or detached from loved ones, they may seem to have a restricted range of feelings, for example appearing to be less 'loving' than before. They may also seem pessimistic about the future. These reactions are often misinterpreted as depression rather than the reaction to trauma. When coupled with the irritability referred to below, these changes may lead to problems in relationships.

Increased physical arousal People may be very physically aroused – literally, their 'adrenaline is flowing'. They may have difficulty in sleeping, may be irritable or have outbursts of anger, have difficulty concentrating, be very jumpy or vigilant for dangers around them, and they may have physical symptoms such as a racing heart (palpitations), sick stomach, excessive sweating etc.

Guilt Guilt is an important emotion. The person may question why she survived when others did not. Guilt may also be focused on actual actions or their absence: 'Did I do enough, could I have saved someone?' This sort of guilt may be very difficult to discuss.

Helping those who have experienced trauma

The first two things that anyone who has been involved in a traumatic event needs are *information* about what has happened and will now happen (e.g. at hospital or in legal proceedings), and simple *comfort*. It is a mistake to assume automatically that people need counselling, but they do need the space and opportunity to talk about what has happened in the hours that follow. You need simply to allow this to happen, to be a witness to the person's thoughts, feelings and questions which have no answers, without feeling that you yourself have to do anything or say anything that 'makes things better'. Your task will be to listen, and this may not be easy as it will involve blocking off a natural reaction to make sympathetic remarks, which are experienced as platitudes, the reaction of wanting not to hear any more, or not to hear the same things repeated again and again.

Experiencing intense feelings after trauma may lead individuals to question profoundly their understanding of the person they thought they were ('I thought I was strong, could handle things'), or life itself ('What is the meaning of a life in which these awful things can happen?'). You can help someone who has suffered trauma in the days that follow by reviewing what happened, what he thought and felt at the time and what he has been feeling since. He will need to understand that his reactions are *understandable reactions to abnormal events*, rather than the signs of any 'illness'.

The details listed above should be used to enable people to see that their reactions are not unique. It is important that you should not expect a traumatised individual's reactions to go away quickly. Also, it is easy to forget the needs of children, who may be less articulate or may be bewildered by how the adults are reacting and frightened of upsetting them further. Do include them in discussion about what has happened.

Seeking further help

Some people will need further help in resolving their reactions. You should seek further help:

- If you feel you cannot handle intense feelings or bodily sensations, or that your emotions are not falling into place with time;

- If you continue to feel numb, rather than experience the normal reactions described, perhaps keeping active so as not to feel;

- If you continue to have nightmares or poor sleep, or feel chronic tension, confusion, or exhaustion;

- If you have no one to share your feelings with or your relationships suffer, or sexual difficulties develop;

- If you take to using tobacco, alcohol or drugs to excess;

- If your work performance suffers;

- If you have accidents.

2

CARING AT HOME

Many people are reluctant to seek help, because they feel, and believe others think, that they 'should be over it by now'; there is embarrassment attached to asking for help. There is also the feeling that talking may 'make things worse', although this is rarely the case. Help may be sought through your general practitioner or local Victim Support Scheme, whose number will be found in the local telephone directory. Your local branch of the Red Cross will have a leaflet 'Coping with a Personal Crisis'.

See Appendix VII for Addresses of useful organisations and support groups

2.5(e) PEOPLE WITH LONG TERM DISABILITY

Difficulties facing the adult with a physical disability vary from those confronting the severely handicapped to those of people whose disability and handicap are not always so obvious and whose difficulties are not always appreciated.

Problems encountered are probably more noticeable by people in their adult life than when they were younger. Gone are the days when society saw 'the disabled' as dependent on the state to be cared for at all levels. Aside from those with a more severe disability, independence and a worthwhile role within our society is what the majority of those with disability expect of themselves.

The accepted definition of disablement is given in box below.

ACCEPTED DEFINITION OF DISABLEMENT	
Impairment	Any loss or abnormality of physical, psychological or anatomical structure or functions (i.e. parts of the body that do not work).
Disability	Any restriction or lack (resulting from impairment) of ability to perform an activity in the manner or within the range considered normal for a human being (i.e. things people cannot do).
Handicap	A disadvantage to an individual resulting from impairment or disability that limits or prevents the fulfilment of a role, taking into account age, sex, social and cultural factors for that individual. This is seen in relation to a particular environment or relationship with other people.

Social attitudes and disability

Many people with physical disability are extremely innovative and resourceful in finding ways to cope with any problems encountered. However there are, even today, individuals who find it difficult to face and deal with other people's disability. Attitudes swing across society from non-acceptance – if you don't look it's not there – practically ignoring those with a physical disability, to the other extreme of a patronising attitude. It must at all times be remembered that a 'mechanical malfunction' of limb does not automatically equate with the intellect being impaired. Motor neurone disease is a classic example of a progressive disability where the sufferer's intellect remains unchanged.

Time and again we hear those with a disability, especially if they use a wheelchair, complain 'I wish others wouldn't treat me as though I were an idiot.' This still occurs. It shouldn't.

It must also be borne in mind that physical disability, especially when resulting from trauma, does not necessarily equate with illness. Allowing for limitations, the person with a physical disability can indeed be quite 'fit'.

Society is largely responsible for the environment in which we live. Accessibility to public buildings, shops, etc. is still not as good as it should be. The invention and introduction of the automatic swing door is a boon to those in a wheelchair or on crutches. The same cannot be said of the revolving door. Most government buildings are now equipped with lifts that have the operating panel at a level that can be used by all. (Many government buildings also have the addition of Braille operating instructions.) Local authorities are responsible for civic buildings and the installation of ramps where appropriate. After working hard to achieve any degree of independence, not being obliged to have to ask all the time should be an automatic right, just as it is for the able bodied.

Adjustment

Physical disability in the adult can be due to a congenital abnormality, trauma or disease. Where impairment is due to a congenital condition (e.g. cerebral palsy) the cause would have been established before adulthood was reached. Physical disability that arises in adulthood can create radical changes within the family who may have been totally unprepared for such a turn of events, whereas the adult with a congenital impairment/disability may cause increasing pressures on a family who were able to cope during the childhood years. Physical growth itself can cause many problems. No longer is it relatively easy to lift the disabled person. Parents who are getting older may no longer have the physical ability to care for their offspring. They will also become increasingly concerned about the long term welfare of their child, for when the time inevitably comes that they are no longer around to be involved in her care.

The family of anyone facing a new disability needs to adjust to the situation, just as much as does the person herself. This adjustment may take time. No longer will the person who is disabled be able to fulfil her role and participate in family life in the manner in which she did formerly. However it is important that, with support, any person faced with disability is encouraged and made to feel that she is no less valuable than before.

Leisure and social life

Activities in which the handicapped person participates should as far as possible be encouraged, although recently disabled people may feel very self-conscious about meeting others who previously saw them as fit and active. Once the hurdle of meeting those friends and contacts has been crossed, the self-consciousness should begin to disappear.

Physical disability can lead to the person participating in new activities; for example, disco dancing may be out, but swimming may take its place.

Handicapped people may find they need to have driving tuition to enable them to achieve independence through mobility. Cars may need to be adapted or changed. A wheelchair can mean the difference between being confined indoors, or taking part in activities outside the home.

The question of whether or not to join a group of people with similar handicaps is one of personal choice. The advantages of joining a group catering for disabled people, however, can be educational as well as social. One can learn from other members how they cope with their disability. Through joining a group, the handicapped person may learn of benefits which are available that he did not know about, or did not think he would be eligible to claim. He may learn more about provisions for the disabled, such as suitable equipment which would provide an aid to daily living.

Generally speaking it is advantageous for a person with a long term disability to be enabled to engage in as many normal social activities as possible, if he so wishes. For example, a visit to a pub or restaurant can be an enjoyable way to relax for many people. One point that should be remembered, however, is that the consumption of alcohol may need to be avoided or reduced if the person is taking certain medications. It would be wise to discuss this possibility with your doctor.

2.5(f) PEOPLE LIVING ALONE

Being ill is never a nice experience, but when you live alone it is even worse. You feel lonely and isolated, wishing there was someone to comfort and look after you. Even if you are feeling really bad, there are some important things you must do for yourself.

Good ventilation is imperative when you are ill because a hot and humid room is the ideal place for micro-organisms to multiply, and stale unpleasant odours linger. An open window or an ioniser reduces pollution in a room, providing clearer, sweeter-smelling air to breathe. If you are experiencing difficulty in breathing, you should sit upright, as this opens the airway, allowing more oxygen to enter the lungs. It can be frightening when you can't breathe properly; this makes you panic and find breathing even harder. Try to relax and take slow, deep breaths. If your breathing is very distressed, you may be prescribed oxygen. Remember never to smoke or use a naked flame in its presence. If you are having difficulty breathing, you shouldn't be smoking anyway, especially not in bed, as this is a fire risk.

Normal body temperature is between 36 and 37.5°C. When you are unwell, your temperature may rise or fall. Usually if you are feeling ill, you are less active and this lowers body temperature. There are some simple tasks you can do to increase it. A little physical activity, wearing extra clothing and blankets, the use of hot water bottles and electric blankets, remembering not to fall asleep when they are on, can all help. So too can simple exercises. Heating is expensive, but if you can keep the room you are in warm, you will feel better, as being in a cold, damp room not only makes you feel cold and miserable, but also slows down the rate of recovery. If your temperature is high, do the reverse of the above. Antibiotics and aspirin can also lower temperatures.

See Chapter 2, section 2(g) above on Keeping warm/cool

Although you may not feel like eating, it is important, as the water and nutrients from food are required to assist in fighting infection and aid recovery. With a reduction in activity, you won't need as many calories, so a light diet is ideal. Fluid is also important when you are ill; the daily requirement is at least 1½ litres (3 pints). If you are in bed, a jug of squash or a flask of tea beside you will save you getting up every time you want a drink.

With a reduction in mobility and dietary intake when you are feeling ill, you are more prone to constipation. If you eat high fibre food and increase your fluid intake, this can help prevent it. You may have vomiting, diarrhoea or even both at the same time. It is important to replace that lost fluid with extra drinks. If your mobility is poor and you may not reach the bathroom in time, a commode beside the bed may help you. It is important to remember to wash your hands properly after using the toilet and before preparing food, because, when you are ill, your natural defence mechanisms are already under stress and less able to fight infection, and this is an easy way of re-infecting yourself.

As a result of being ill, your level of activity has probably been reduced. It is important to have a small amount of exercise, however. A walk to the kitchen or bathrooom every few hours may be all that is needed. If you spend a lot of time immobile, you are at risk of suffering from constipation, blood clots as the circulation system slows down and, most important, pressure sores. These are usually caused by pressure on the skin because of immobility, as well as lack of oxygen to the site, and wet skin. Changing positions, with a little exercise, ensuring skin is clean and dry, and a varied diet can help to prevent pressure sores developing.

See section 2.2(h) above for more information on pressure sores

When you live alone and don't expect any visitors, you may not bother taking pride in your appearance, especially when you are unwell. By washing, brushing your hair, cleaning your teeth, shaving, wearing some make-up, even using after-shave or perfume, you will improve your self-esteem. Changing your bed linen and clothes will also increase your feelings of cleanliness and comfort.

When you are ill, you may well sleep for longer than the average requirement of 7–8 hours a day, although your sleep pattern may have been altered. You may not spend eight hours asleep in one period, as it has been disturbed by your feeling too hot or too cold, by coughing or being in pain, or wanting to use the toilet, but throughout the day in broken periods you will probably gain enough sleep. It is important to remember that you may not even need your usual number of hours sleep because you have been less active and resting throughout the day.

If you are usually an active person, being confined indoors or in bed can be frustrating and boring. If your hobbies include sporting activities or country walks, you won't be able to do these, but there are alternatives.

If you are confined inside while ill, a telephone is probably the most important line of communication you have. If you are in bed, it is ideal to have a telephone and important numbers beside you. This enables you to get in touch with the doctor, family and friends, to ask for help and visitors. It also provides companionship, so you don't feel alone all the time.

If you are confined to bed, it is a good idea to have a telephone, and any important phone numbers, within easy reach

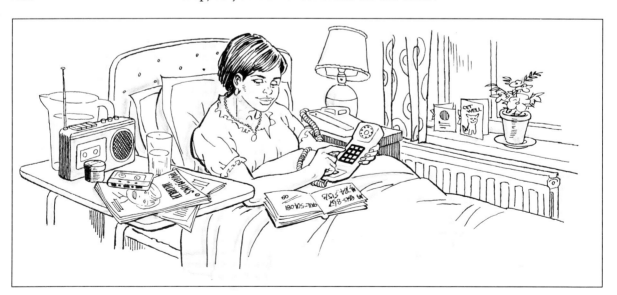

Friends and neighbours can be asked to help with the activities you can't do for yourself whilst ill. They may include collecting shopping and prescriptions, feeding and exercising pets, even keeping the car running if you are going to be ill for a long time.

Before taking any medication, it is important you remember to check that it can be taken in conjunction with others prescribed by the doctor and whether you should continue to take any medicines prescribed before this particular bout of illness.

2.5(g) THE ELDERLY

It is important not to assume that age is always accompanied by sickness or that if a person who happens to be elderly finds her health deteriorating she is necessarily on a path of irreversible decline. Some people, even some health professionals, assume that any ailment suffered by a person who happens to be elderly should be dismissed as being 'a sign of age'. Such an attitude can be very damaging for all concerned. It may mean that measures to improve the person's quality of life are simply not explored, while the sick person herself gives up hope and allows low morale to speed up the process of physical and intellectual decline.

See also Chapter 8, especially section 4 on Caring for an elderly person at home

More detailed advice on caring for a sick elderly person at home is given in Chapter 8, and it should also be stressed here that much of the information about helping sick individuals to maintain their activities of daily living in as normal a way as possible is just as relevant for a person in her seventies or beyond as for someone in early adulthood. There are, however, some specific points of which all carers should be aware.

- The elderly tend to have more than one thing wrong with them at a time.
- They tend to recover more slowly than younger people.
- Physical illness may send an elderly person into a temporary state of confusion with more ease than a younger person.

Three principles are particularly important.

- It should be remembered that many elderly people enjoy good health and lead full, useful lives. Ageist stereotypes can not only prevent many simple health problems from being taken seriously, they can also lead to younger people missing out on enriching relationships with older members of society.
- Elderly people must maintain their mobility as far as possible. An immobile person is much more vulnerable to chest infections, constipation, circulatory problems, boredom and depression. She is also likely to develop pressure sores quickly.
- Elderly people must be enabled to keep their dignity and independence – including independence of choice – for as long as they possibly can.

The complex nature of elderly people's needs

As mentioned above, elderly people are more likely than their younger counterparts to suffer from several problems at a time. This is partly because one problem often gives rise to another and then another. Awareness of potential problems before they arise may help to prevent at least some of them from occurring.

Consider, for example, the case of an 82 year old man who suffers from bronchitis. During the winter, he might contract a bad chest infection and take to his bed. Because of his age, his skin will be more fragile and he will be more likely to become sore where his body presses on the bed. Extra care will be needed to keep him moving, to ensure he is clean and dry, and to alleviate pressure on various parts of his body. He will need a good diet to keep his skin healthy and to restore his strength.

He may be stiff (and will become more so if immobile for any length of time); his sight and hearing may not be too good, especially at night. His bladder will have altered in shape and he may suffer from prostate trouble. If he tries to get out of bed in a hurry, he is more likely than a younger man to fall – and if he does fall his thinned bones are more likely to break. So, a man whose original problem was a chest infection aggravated by a chronic chest complaint could end up in hospital with a fractured femur, possibly never regaining his mobility or even returning home.

While other people cannot make absolutely certain that such an unfortunate chain of events does not occur (particularly if they are concerned with that most important principle of respecting the elderly person's independence and autonomy), steps can be taken to prevent one relatively straightforward problem from leading to a string of more complicated ones. If an elderly person takes to his bed with an infection, it is important to encourage him to change his position often (so as not to put too great a pressure on any one area of his skin) and to sit up in a chair for a while. He will probably also benefit from a little gentle exercise – ask your district nurse or community physiotherapist for advice about this. When preparing food, try to take his normal habits and likes and dislikes into account. It is better to produce a meal which is not quite as nutritious but will be eaten than one which is perfectly balanced but which will be quietly tipped into the bin while you are not looking. Be aware that immobility can lead to constipation and try to tempt your patient with fluids and foods containing fibre to counter this.

Many elderly people have increased difficulty seeing (and orienting themselves) in the dark so make sure that adequate lighting is left on to enable someone to get to the bathroom safely at night. Be careful to ensure that floors are not slippery, that there are no loose rugs or invisible steps on the way and that other family members

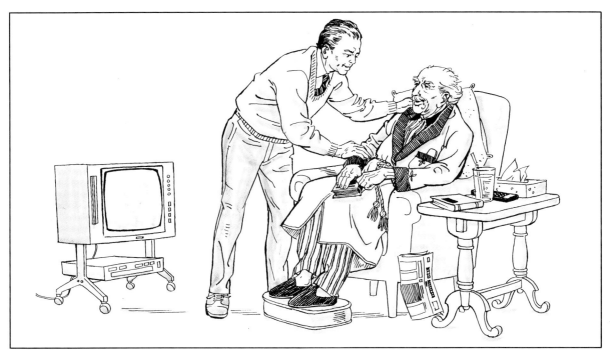

If at all possible encourage the sick elderly person to sit up in a chair for a while

do not leave clutter lying around to be tripped over. It is also a good idea to discuss with the patient whether a commode, chamber pot or urine bottle in the bedroom is acceptable as this may make many hazardous journeys unnecessary.

Confusion

A number of physical problems (including breathing difficulties, hypothermia and diabetes) can lead to an elderly person becoming confused. Confusion can also be a side effect of some drugs or can occur when an elderly person has been bereaved, has recently moved house or is depressed. So, if your elderly relative or neighbour becomes confused, don't automatically assume that something irreversible has happened and that she is becoming 'senile': talk first to your community nurse or general practitioner.

See also Chapter 8, sections 4(c), 7(b) and 7(g) for more information about confusion

Individual differences

It is only too easy to make generalisations about categories of people but really good care is sensitive to the special characteristics of each individual. Elderly people are no more alike than people in any other age group. Some may be inward looking and seemingly uninterested in the world outside their own front door. Some may appear very set in their ways. Others will be adventurous, outgoing and in every way 'young at heart'.

Even our bodily organs don't all age at the same rate. The elderly man with the chest infection considered above may have the lungs of a man in his mid-eighties, but his heart may be that of a 70 year old, his eyesight that of an average 50 year old, and his mental alertness younger again.

Each elderly person, then, is an individual with his unique likes and dislikes, character and personality. He just happens to have been born at a certain time and his habits and lifestyle will have been formed to a certain extent by the era and society which helped to mould him. He is a whole person – body, mind and spirit – and you are caring for this whole person, not just that part of him which happens to be ill.

2.5(h) THE DYING

See also Chapter 8, section 5 on Dying and death

See section 2.6 below on Help for the carers

Caring for someone close to you who is dying will make great demands upon you. It is normal to fear the unknown or unfamiliar but the person you are caring for is the same one that you have always known; that will not change. Most individuals prefer to die at home if at all possible. Having the people they love around them and being in familiar surroundings lessens their own feelings of fear and uncertainty. Even if you, the carer, are not told you are appreciated, you are. There are many practical ways you can gain help and support during this time, some of which apply equally to other situations.

Understanding how people feel

People often behave differently when they are sick or know that they are dying. It is helpful to understand why this is, so that you do not feel rejected or hurt. You have enough to cope with already.

Most people do not fear death so much as the process of dying. In particular, they may fear pain and loss of independence. These are normal human reactions but may lead to mood swings not previously seen in the individual.

Talking about it   Talking helps. If you have always talked openly about issues in life, do so now. It does not mean that you have to know the answers to life's difficult questions. It only means you care enough to share another's doubts and fears.

Some people are not used to sharing life's issues in this way. If this is the case, you may want to enlist the help of someone outside the family circle – a clergyman, solicitor, or someone else who knows the family well. There are others who give particular support to help the dying and their carers. Your general practitioner or one of his team may be the person. Specialist nurses (often funded by charities but very much a part of that team) may be called upon to help. Your general practitioner, Citizens' Advice

See Appendix VII for Addresses of useful organisations and support groups

Bureau or a helpline called 'Help for Health' will be able to give you details. There are also many voluntary organisations who run telephone helplines, support groups or counselling services. These vary depending upon the cause of your relative's illness. Details can be obtained from the sources mentioned above, or from information given elsewhere in this book.

Time for reflection It is understandable that the dying person wants to sort out his affairs and tie up the ends of his life. Old age or chronic illness may have presented physical problems which, to date, have preoccupied the person. However, when the possibility of being active has ceased or diminished, this allows time for reflection on life's past joys, satisfactions, disappointments and regrets. Your relative may feel useless and a burden to you and may regret the loss of role – as mother, father, daughter or whoever.

Feeling a burden One of the most common feelings a dying person has is that of being dependent upon another. This is of course true and there is no point denying it. However, it is very important to enable as much independence as possible for as long as possible. Self-esteem will then remain high and feelings of value and worth will be retained. Enable the dying person to contribute to family decisions and activities as much as possible. Do not exclude her. Ask her for her opinion; check with her whether or not she wants to be involved in a given activity. Avoid assuming that she is too tired or weak. The human spirit is very resilient and people want to live until they die, not be preoccupied with dying.

Physical needs of the dying

Great emphasis has, purposely, been put on the way dying people feel and react. Many of the practical issues involved in caring have been dealt with elsewhere in this book. There are, however, a few specific issues worth mentioning or emphasising.

Appetite Although eating and drinking are seen by most people as pleasant social activities, the dying person may have very little appetite and may even feel sick at the thought or smell of some foods. This can be difficult for you when you have taken considerable trouble to prepare something good and nourishing for him. However, it is best to check with him each time what he feels like eating or drinking. Tastes fluctuate and what may be acceptable one day may not be the next. Tempt him with small amounts of moist food that are easy to eat and digest. The sight of too much food will certainly take away any appetite that may have been there. The body is well able to determine what food is needed. If excess is forced, it will rebel.

Dry mouth If food and drink are not taken regularly, the mouth can become very dry and teeth or dentures encrusted and uncomfortable. Provide regular opportunities for rinsing the mouth with plain water and for cleaning teeth or dentures. This may be helpful four or more times a day – when food or drinks may normally be consumed – even if no food is taken. It is also important first thing in the morning and last thing at night.

See section 2.2 above for a detailed description of Helping the sick person at home with the activities of living

Comfortable position/general hygiene Many points have been addressed elsewhere in this manual. For the dying person these would be the same. Most people prefer to be dressed in their usual day clothes and join in with the family activities for most of the time – until they decide to do otherwise. Unless there are obvious reasons for doing so, there is no need for them to be in bed all the while, though once profound weakness overtakes them there may be no choice. The more active they can remain, the less burden on you and the greater will be their own self-esteem.

See section 2.2(h) above for more advice about Keeping clean and well groomed

General hygiene may be continued with help from the carer. A shower may be easier and safer than a bath for some. Using a stool in the bath with a detachable shower unit will meet the need of those who do not have a fixed shower unit. Hair washing and hairdressing is important for self-esteem for both men and women. This can be achieved with enterprise despite the debility of the dying person. Moving a chair to the bathroom or a bowl to the bedside is all that is required.

See section 2.2(d) above for more advice on coping with problems related to elimination

Constipation and diarrhoea Like other parts of the body, the gut may be affected by illness, treatment, effects of ageing or change in mobility and diet. These changes may result in either constipation or diarrhoea. Simple ways of trying to resolve constipation include:

- The introduction of as much roughage as can be tolerated into the diet;

- Increasing fluids of any kind but particularly clear fluids and water;

- Encouraging as much mobility as possible.

If walking with help is possible, then it is good to do a little each day as it will help not only the gut but all body systems.

Diarrhoea is more difficult to manage but may be reduced by omitting roughage, highly spiced or fatty foods from the diet. Fluids should not be discouraged though. Fluid is lost in diarrhoea and must be replaced. Water will not cause diarrhoea.

If these simple measures do not work, you should ask for help from your doctor.

See section 2.2(d) above on Eliminating and Chapter 8, section 6(b) on Urinary and bowel related problems

Incontinence This can be a problem for people at the end stages of life. Refer to the relevant sections in this manual for practical hints to help you cope with this.

Odour Infections, either from a surgical wound that has not healed or from internal disease, may cause an unpleasant odour. The person who is dying may be very aware of this which may cause further problems with self-esteem. You as a carer will certainly be aware of it and may find it so offensive that it is almost intolerable. Simple remedies are:

• Keeping the room well ventilated with fresh air;

• Changing clothes as soon as they become soiled;

• Keeping genital areas clean if these are the cause of the odour;

• Using commercial air fresheners or joss sticks to counteract odour – but do use such remedies carefully as they may make the situation worse and cause nausea in the individual.

If all of these fail, spray deodorisers or local applications are available from the chemist or by prescription from your doctor.

See also section 2.3 above for more information on Coping with pain

Pain If pain is not under control, speak to your doctor about it. There are many excellent ways to relieve pain, some of which do not require drugs, although they of course play a major part in the treatment. Pain may fluctuate and should not be allowed to return and preoccupy the person's mind.

Sleep Sleep patterns are frequently disturbed due to either physical or emotional reasons. Sleeping at night may be difficult if naps are taken during the day. Position in bed may be uncomfortable. Look at some simple remedies first. For example, it may be easier for your relative to sleep sitting up in a chair rather than in bed. It may be more helpful to accept that there are some nights when sleep will not come. Boredom at this time needs to be replaced by adequate reading, music, or other activity.

Fighting insomnia rarely works. If your relative has long periods awake, be sure there is everything nearby to occupy the time. If insomnia becomes a real problem, talk it over with your doctor.

Coping as a carer

This can be a difficult and stressful time for you, the carer. Share your feelings with others close to you and try to take some time out if you possibly can. Nothing bad will happen to your relative if you allow someone else to be with him for a while and you will return refreshed and with more resource to go on. You have to look after yourself as well. If there is no one else in the family to help you, ask for help from one of the agencies concerned. Your general practitioner or one of his team will be able to put you in touch with the appropriate people. The health professionals are there to support you as much as the dying person; be sure you use them.

2.6 HELP FOR THE CARERS

The majority of the time, carers cope with those they look after at home with help from relatives and friends and in some instances the community nursing and social services. People continue to care for as long as they are able for many reasons, the most important being that they want to do so and it gives them satisfaction. This role can become very stressful when the satisfaction from caring reduces and/or the carer begins to become tired or ill herself. Carers must not feel guilty if they begin to find their task increasingly difficult, but rather seek ways of making their job easier.

This section examines ways in which the responsibilities of caring can be best organised to reduce the load on carers, without in any way disadvantaging the person whom they are looking after.

2.6(a) LOOKING AFTER YOURSELF

This is Rule Number One, because if the carer becomes ill, the quality of care given is very likely to be reduced. All carers should check that they are getting the following:

- An adequate diet;

- Some time to themselves – involving a break from caring;

- Some time with other people;

- Sufficient sleep – this will vary from person to person;

- Support from the voluntary or statutory (social or health) services to ensure that the above items are achievable.

2.6(b) HELP AVAILABLE

General practitioner

The first port of call when seeking help is often the general practitioner (or family doctor) who will inform you of the services available locally and if appropriate, he will ask the social services or community nursing service to assist you or to make an assessment of your needs. It is now well recognised, however, that the general practitioner is not always in the best position to direct you to all the resources available. This is partly because of the growth in voluntary agencies which could help but of which he may be unaware, and also due to increasing demands made on the community health care systems resulting in some families being given a higher priority than others in terms of receiving assistance.

Voluntary and charitable organisations

See Appendix VII for Addresses of useful organisations and support groups

The following two (United Kingdom based) agencies will be able to give you information, advice and practical support regardless of the problems either you, or the person for whom you care, may have.

The Carers' National Association This national charity was founded in 1988 with the following aims:

• To encourage carers to recognise their own needs;

• To develop appropriate support for carers;

• To provide information and advice for carers;

• To bring the needs of carers to the attention of government and other policy makers.

If you become a member of the association, no one expects you to become actively involved unless that is what you want. The association's headquarters will put you in touch with your local branch and carers' support groups. Local branches hold regular meetings in order for carers to keep up with what is available to help them locally, for example if a new Day Centre opens, the branch will know. Each branch has a system to ensure that there is someone for you to talk to who will lend a sympathetic ear at those moments when you feel at the end of your tether. Remember all carers feel like this at times and it can be immensely reassuring to share your feelings with others in the same situation.

Some branches of the association arrange outings to which you can go alone, or take the person for whom you care. There is no need to be embarrassed in the event of your relative being disruptive or incontinent on an outing, because the other people would understand. Sometimes carers choose to take it in turns to go on an outing while one stays behind and looks after the other's dependent relative or friend, and vice versa.

Crossroads Care This is a voluntary agency which now has over 200 branches throughout Britain. Its purpose is to provide practical support for carers and those for whom they care in their own homes. It will, for example, provide a sitter to stay with the dependent person while the carer goes out to shop, have her hair done, visit friends, go to bingo, play bridge or follow any particular interest. In this way, carers get some time to themselves, to socialise or to be alone, depending on which suits them best. In most instances, if the carer wants to go out regularly once or twice a week to keep up with friends or family, then Crossroads will find the same regular volunteer to cover her absence. Most volunteers are well able to give the person with whom they sit a drink, take someone to the toilet and, perhaps most importantly, provide a fresh face and companionship.

Some branches of Crossroads can offer more diverse services such as taking you out for a drive or giving your relative meals and assistance during the day while you work or attend a vital appointment.

Disease or problem-specific agencies

See Appendix VII for Addresses of useful organisations and support groups

There are some societies that have developed specifically to help people who suffer from one particular disease or problem. These include, for example, the Alzheimer's Disease Society, Mencap (which works with people who have a learning difficulty and their families), the Schizophrenia Association, the British Diabetic Society, the Cystic Fibrosis Research Trust – to name but a few. If you feel that contacting one of these societies may be helpful in terms of giving you advice and support about a particular illness, then contact your local general practitioner's surgery for information or see Appendix VII in this book. If you have difficulty in obtaining information this way, it may be worth contacting the local hospital you attend. Because these societies concentrate on one particular disease or problem, they are often able to give you more help, support and advice about that condition than anyone else.

2.6(c) YOUR OWN NEEDS

Benefits and allowances

See Appendix VI for more information about Benefits

It has already been suggested that you need to look after yourself in order to look after the person for whom you are caring. There are several ways of ensuring you are getting all the benefits and assistance to which you are entitled and it is suggested that you look at Appendix VI in this manual, and pay a visit to your local Citizens' Advice Bureau.

It is very important that you claim for all benefits to which you are entitled as they will have a considerable impact on your quality of life and income. For example, the Invalid Care Allowance, added to an Attendance Allowance, can make a tremendous difference to the lifestyle of both the carer and the person for whom he cares.

Remember, nobody will come knocking on your door offering you these allowances, so you may well discover that a little bit of 'finding out' is well worth while.

Assistance from professionals

You may decide that you ought to be getting more assistance from professionals such as the district nurse, the community psychiatric nurse, social worker, home help or the general practitioner than you actually are. It may be useful to sit down and list the areas in which you would most like help before contacting any of these professional people. You may, for example, find it extremely difficult to bath the person for whom you care, to cope with her dirtying her underpants and being incontinent, or giving her her insulin. It is only if you identify the problems that you find most difficult to deal with that the professionals will be able to give you assistance in those areas. Try to be assertive and if necessary, get somebody from one of the voluntary organisations such as the Carers' National Association to back you up. Do try to remember that the professionals are meant to be there to serve and help you and the person for whom you care. This may make asking a little bit easier.

IF YOU ARE AT THE END OF YOUR TETHER	
If you suddenly feel at crisis point	Make the person you are caring for safe and get out of the room – express your anger in private, go for a walk, scream into a pillow, throw something. Do anything that helps you release tension. Ring the Samaritans, your family doctor or a social worker.
When you are calmer	Ask yourself whether you want to go on caring and if so, what help do you need to make it easier. If you feel unable to go on caring, consider how your relative or friend may best be looked after.
Later – perhaps the next day	Share the answers to the above with someone you are close to, then ask her to accompany you to see your doctor or to go to the Social Services Department. Ask for the assistance you need.
If you are driven to desperation	If, for example, you want to hit the elderly person – DON'T. It is an offence. Tell your doctor and social worker that you are being driven to this and that they must help you.
Remember	Social Services/social work departments have a responsibility under Acts of Parliament to care for disabled, elderly people. If all else fails, contact a Councillor, or write to your Member of Parliament at the House of Commons, Westminster, London SW1.

This section draws heavily on advice given in a leaflet produced by Age Concern and other societies. It can be obtained from The Distribution Dept, Age Concern, 1268 London Road, London SW16 4EJ.

2

If you are able to claim benefits and increase your income, together with getting the support that you require from the professional agencies and assistance from the voluntary agencies outlined, you are likely to be well able to look after yourself in terms of an adequate diet, having time for yourself, some periods of sleep and very importantly, some time to socialise with others. However, it is well recognised that the caring role can be difficult and, even if you do look after yourself in this way, there may be times when you feel desperately low or frustrated with the person for whom you care. These indicators are important to watch out for because if they are 'nipped in the bud', you are more likely to be able to go on caring than if they are not.

The box on the previous page gives you some advice about dealing with acute frustration.

If you get to the point where the caring role is merely a problem to you, and the rewards you receive from it very little, then it may be time to discuss with your family, or any professionals, whether the time has come to review all the options. It may be that the situation has reached the point where long stay care is now more appropriate for the person you have been looking after. If careful thought and discussion suggest that this is the case, you must not feel that you have failed. In recognising your own limits, you are in some ways ensuring that the person concerned will continue to receive an appropriate quality of care.

NORMAL LIFE
CRISES

3

3.1 ### INTRODUCTION

It is suggested that you read this chapter in conjunction with Chapter 7, section 4 (Mental health) and section 6 (Counselling skills) as well as the references cited by specific sections. You should also refer to Appendix VII for Addresses of useful organisations and support groups

Every individual can either recall an event which could be described as a crisis, or is in a position to identify periods with the potential for being a 'crisis time'. Such events may be the experience of, or anticipation of, starting a new job, moving house, children leaving home, a change in lifestyle due to relationship problems such as separation or divorce, a change in the health of a family member, or the loss, through death, of someone close.

It is the intention of this chapter to identify what normal life crises are, to describe some of the life crises encountered by individuals and to consider ways in which they may be understood. In each of the separate sections support systems will be highlighted so that readers can consider the possible choices for support.

The use of the word 'normal' indicates that there are crises which may be anticipated to occur in our lives and in the lives of others and which will have an effect upon us. A 'crisis' is often described as an event which radically alters or disturbs the normal order of a person's life. However normal it may be, the event catches the person unawares and often unprepared to manage the situation. Crisis situations are often totally new, unpredictable and have an acute emotional effect upon individuals leaving them with the feeling of not being able to cope with the situation at all. The sense of confusion that results from the crisis disrupts all previously held beliefs, values and ideas about the world around. Everything feels out of control and untrustworthy. The need to question everything that is happening becomes overpowering.

What may be a life crisis to one person may not be so to another. Previous experiences of challenging life events may have helped an individual to learn how to cope with or manage the crisis, for it is true that these skills are learnt through the experiences of life. However, even with past experiences or with anticipation of a crisis event, its occurrence may still spin the individual into a feeling of disorder and confusion. In addition, previously unresolved crises may come into sharp focus again due to the recent disruptive experience contributing further upset and distress.

An easy way of understanding the process of a crisis would be to view it as a series of steps or stages through which a person travels with a final outcome of resolution or understanding of the crisis and its impact upon the person's life. A diagrammatic representation of this process is given in the figure.

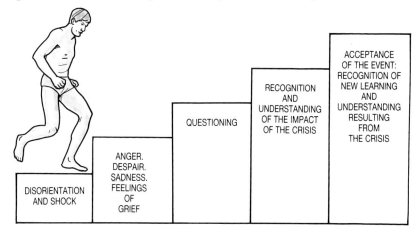

Reacting to crisis

The person must pass through a series of steps or stages before his feelings are resolved

DISORIENTATION AND SHOCK

ANGER. DESPAIR. SADNESS. FEELINGS OF GRIEF

QUESTIONING

RECOGNITION AND UNDERSTANDING OF THE IMPACT OF THE CRISIS

ACCEPTANCE OF THE EVENT: RECOGNITION OF NEW LEARNING AND UNDERSTANDING RESULTING FROM THE CRISIS

There are two key factors which may facilitate the passage through the steps or stages:

- Information;

- Support.

People experiencing a crisis often feel as though all their control over the situation, and the choices that could be made, have been taken away. Having information about the crisis event enables them to understand what is happening and then perhaps, when they are ready, to make an informed choice. Also it is possible that individuals may find themselves feeling very alone in a crisis. This is not at all unusual, indeed it may be they are alone as a result of the crisis. Alternatively, they may have isolated themselves from others in an attempt to deal with the crisis.

The steps or stages may be travelled alone but they are perhaps more easily managed and understood when the individual is supported by others. The process of talking to another helps one to keep a perspective upon the experience, reducing the repetitive thoughts going round and round, perhaps finding an understanding not previously recognised.

In some circumstances, life crises may be anticipated. For example, knowing that children will be leaving home to go to school, college or to set up their own home for some time prior to the event occurring, may not minimise the emotional upset of the actual experience. The knowledge that a loved one is going to die does not make managing the loss any easier. This therefore reinforces the fact that it is the experience of life crises, and the understanding of such events by individuals, that equips them for both the inevitable and the unexpected life crises they will meet.

See also Chapter 6, especially section 6.7

3.2 **ADOLESCENCE**

The age range of adolescence is not clearly specified, and appears to vary according to which book you read. An all encompassing view would be from the age of 12 to the late teens.

Adolescence is a time during which the individual is confronted with a range of life crises or transitions. Each of the crises makes the person reflect on her understanding of herself, her self-concept. It is during adolescence that the individual engages in a wider and expanding social arena, moving from the family group to develop relationships in school, clubs, sports and hobbies groups. The process of leaving and joining new groups is potentially hazardous, yet an essential part of adolescent development. Adolescent experiences are likely to focus around the peer group, as opposed to the experiences of childhood when the family was the key reference group. The experiences adolescents have are more likely to be their own, rather than shared family experiences, and they are not protected, therefore, by the family coping or decision making systems. The individual is confronted with making decisions for herself. This may be stressful, for often the decisions are important ones which will influence the whole of her life.

3.2(a) ROLES, MODELS AND SELFHOOD

The influence of the peer group and the media encourages adolescents to experiment with new ideas and new roles. Often the audience exposed to the experiments is the family group, and challenges are made to force an overt response. The many experiences of roles they have observed from their teachers, parents or their peer groups, and notable or notorious roles from the media world are experimented with to enable the individual to identify himself. This testing out of love, care and boundaries is essential for the adolescent, as an exploration of his significant family group which acts as a touchstone of safety and security. It may be that the response the young person wished for, a response of shock and horror as he challenges the family values, is the one he will get. It is only then, feeling more sure of his projected appearance, that he can face the world with confidence.

3.2(b) BODY IMAGE AND SEXUALITY

How they see themselves physically is a major issue for all adolescents. During puberty the child's body develops, through a series of stages, to take on the characteristics of an adult form. The individual is very sensitive to these physical changes and innocent comment may easily be interpreted as a personal assault. With the increasingly wider social group the individual engages in making comparisons between himself and others, and searching for an image which he feels portrays his image of himself.

Again the influence of media, through television, video, magazines and music, is important.

Society today is increasingly complex, with the traditional roles of men and women becoming blurred and shared. This reinforces the need for adolescents to be sure of their identity, to know and understand what sexuality means to them. Developing intimate relationships is often an area fraught with difficulty, embarrassment and experimentation.

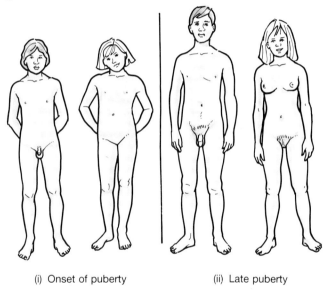

Physical changes of adolescence

(i) Onset of puberty   (ii) Late puberty

3.2(c) LOOKING AHEAD

Economic realities contribute more pressure as the adolescent makes plans for career and employment prospects. With fewer employment opportunities, a competitive climate is created amongst the peer group. This has the potential to create stress and conflict with the people to whom the adolescent feels emotionally close, and about whom she cares.

Adolescents are exposed to complex pressure from society to fulfil adult roles independently. Most adolescents manage the crises they encounter, one by one, as they arise. In so doing, they draw upon their relationship with parents and other significant family members in order to try or test out adult behaviour in a safe environment of care and respect. It could be said that the myth of the generation gap is only perpetuated by parental figures and members of society who are not prepared to listen to, or give permission to, the adolescent as she struggles to travel the path from childhood to adulthood. Taking the opportunity to listen to the young person and her peer group may pay dividends in gaining insight into this struggle. Many adolescents feel they have to manage on their own, all the while longing to talk through the issues with someone they feel really wants to listen.

3.3 THE WORLD OF WORK

3.3(a) STARTING WORK

See also Chapter 7, section 3 on Work and occupational health

Starting work is often seen by society as the legitimate mark of moving from adolescence into the adult world. Exciting and often an achievement, this is also a crisis time as it generates concerns, stresses, fears and anxieties due to the changes it brings to the individual's world.

Work is a very important part of Western lifestyle, providing individuals with colleagues, and perhaps friendship, a sense of community with fellow workers, purpose and structure for the day, a role which contributes to identity and self-esteem, and a sense of satisfaction from personal achievements. It is often the starting point of any conversation with an unfamiliar person to ask, 'What do you do for a job?'

The economic climate of the 1990s does not always permit immediate choice of occupation, due either to lack of opportunity or to competition. This may create a high level of stress and despondency with the need to take interim employment as a stepping stone to the ultimate goal. Seeking career and employment advice is wise especially if the individual has a family to consider. Taking the opportunity to talk through the implications with all concerned enables everyone to cope with changes and to support the individual in his choices.

Starting work may raise many questions about performance, achievement and interpersonal relationships. How to carry out the role of an adult at work, trying to retain personal identity but also being part of the social group, may be a constant battle until a point of balance is found. Achieving this may be very testing to those at home who see the distress such conflict can create.

An opportunity to talk experiences through with a non-judgemental listener is valuable, contributing to the ability to stand by values and beliefs that are being threatened by the new occupational environment. This will help the individual to integrate his new role into his self-image.

3.3(b) SUCCESS AT WORK

Success at work may also present as a crisis. Promotion may generate feelings of a lack of confidence in one's ability to perform as expected in the new role. There may also be the loss of familiar colleagues and a recognised support network which leaves the individual feeling bewildered, anxious or depressed. People may feel embarrassed to admit to such feelings, especially when (on the surface) promotion is seen as success. However those close to individuals in this situation will detect the stress which is being experienced. Again, it is invaluable if time can be taken to talk through the implications of such changes for all of those concerned. In this way, positive coping strategies can be used to cope with the crisis which should then soon resolve itself.

3.3(c) LOSS OF A JOB

The occupation that an individual finds himself in may not necessarily be rewarding. Many jobs are based on routine, are monotonous and offer limited opportunity for promotion. Such a scenario may precipitate a crisis.

The current economic climate means that most occupations carry the risk of redundancy and, sadly perhaps, the loss of a job may almost be considered normal. In spite of the more frequent occurrence of job loss, standards of personal success are still associated with, and measured by, work. Thus the crisis of job loss should not be underestimated.

Loss of self-esteem and a feeling of no longer being able to determine the future may be generated by unemployment. The loss of financial income has the result of restricting opportunity, creating frustration and inevitably affecting the whole family unit. The most helpful course of action is to talk, not only to those immediately involved, but also to employment and financial advisers. Often the most overwhelming desire is to play ostrich and hide one's head in the sand. But the benefits of confronting the crisis greatly outweigh the initial feelings of embarrassment.

3.4 MARRIAGE

Our society continues to be structured with a primary focus of the family. The family structure varies according to the cultural origins and values held by the family and modified by successive generations. Some cultures perpetuate an extended family network and others a nuclear approach, depending upon the lifestyle and choices of the family members. Within the majority of cultures marriage is a feature of tradition and is greeted with delight, pleasure, happiness and anticipation for the future.

For the couple getting married, however, the experience may feel like one of crisis. Many couples now take the step of cohabiting before marriage. Some see this as a trial period, others see it as preferable to a legal statement of commitment. Either way, the experience of two people coming together to live 24 hours a day may be fraught with potential problems. To the situation each person brings their culture, modes of behaviour and expectations of what the relationship will be like. So too, they bring the understanding of what roles are played, and by whom, within the family. It is within these areas that conflict may occur, when expectations or previously unquestioned roles need to be confronted.

In spite of previously held beliefs there is an essential process of negotiation to facilitate a balance and harmony within the relationship. Inevitably there may be an element of compromise on both parts. Through the process of negotiation the couple begin to develop their own set of standards, their own codes of behaviour, their interpretation of roles within the household and coping strategies to deal with the crises that will inevitably come their way in the future. A note of caution is worth while here: that having talked issues through once does not mean that future opportunities will not be needed. Nothing could be further from the truth. As a relationship develops, so too will the issues that the couple need to confront. A relationship rarely takes place in isolation from the world, and outside pressures may create conflict between the partners. Some such pressures may include:

- A demanding job;

- Money worries;

- Studying for further qualifications;

- The minor hassles of life such as parking tickets, travel difficulties and office politics.

In today's society, dual career families are increasingly common. Men are no longer the only, or even the chief, breadwinners, and there is ample potential for conflict – over child care arrangements for example.

Inevitably the most effective strategy for dealing with crises in marriage – indeed in any long term relationship – is the making of time to talk through issues and obtain an accurate understanding and appreciation of each other's point of view. Honesty is essential to generate trust. Listening will facilitate a balance of priorities and a shared compromise.

3.5   HAVING CHILDREN

See also Chapter 4 on Pregnancy and parenthood

The experience of having a child is a watershed; the mother's life, in particular, will be radically altered by the experience itself and the consequent responsibility of raising a child. There is no doubt that the process of managing the situation will be very much easier if the pregnancy is planned and seen as positive, especially if the woman feels supported by those around her.

3.5(a)   SINGLE PARENTHOOD

See Appendix VII for Addresses of useful organisations and support groups

Today, there is an increasing number of women who find themselves facing motherhood alone. The dramatic life changes that being pregnant and raising a child bring to the life of a parent should not be underestimated. Therefore opportunity to explore what these changes mean is essential. If you do not have a partner with whom you can share experiences, thoughts and feelings, it is important to take time to talk not only to professional carers, but also to members of local, voluntary or self-help groups.

3.5(b)   MIXED FEELINGS

Publicly the news of pregnancy generates excitement and anticipation of a new life being brought into the world. However the mother may not only experience the physical symptoms of pregnancy as distressing, but may also feel emotionally sensitive, find her moods labile and her emotions in a state of turmoil as she begins to come to terms with her changing role. Almost feeling guilty at not mirroring the delight of those around her the expectant mother may be distressed by such ambivalent feelings. These may be pertinent for a woman who has pursued her career and is concerned about changes that will occur. Equally, where finances may be limited, anxieties of how to manage best for the future may need to be discussed and options explored.

During pregnancy, the woman has the opportunity to talk to health professionals who can help her to adapt to the physical, psychological and social changes she is experiencing. This support can be invaluable to the mother; the father, however, does not have such an easy access to opportunities for discussing the issues and adapting to new roles and responsibilities. This imbalance, where the father adapts to the pregnancy almost by chance and third hand through his partner telling him what the health professionals say, is a potential arena for crisis.

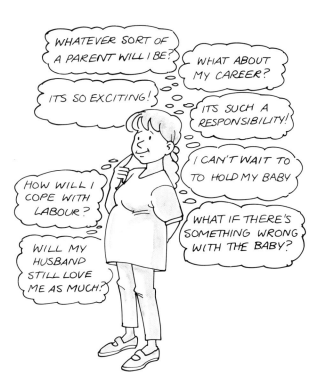

Many women have mixed feelings about their pregnancy

The couple need to make time to develop their relationship through sharing hopes and fears they have about the forthcoming pregnancy and to explore the need for compromise, flexibility and renegotiation of roles which will help them to adapt to the demands of a baby in the home.

In addition to talking with others, reading may raise questions that can be clarified with health professionals. There are many publications that make information available to couples so that they can face this watershed in an informed way.

See Appendix VIII for Suggested further reading

3.5(c) OTHER CHILDREN

See also Chapter 4 section 6(d) for advice on coping with Sibling rivalry

Additional problems may arise if the couple has a child already. The new baby may appear to usurp the elder child's position, thus creating difficulties in the formation of the new family group. Preparation for the arrival of a new baby is essential, but it should be remembered that a child's response may be very different when confronted with reality. Providing the older child continues to feel she is as important as before in the family unit and the new baby has not taken her place, adaptation will take place gradually.

The need to feel as valued and loved and cared for after the birth of the baby as before is crucial for all family members. This can only be achieved by sharing, talking and the demonstration of affection.

See also Chapter 7 section 8 for more information about Mid-life

3.6 MID-LIFE

The 'mid-life crisis' is a popular term used in an attempt to understand unexpected behaviour of individuals between the ages of 45 and 64.

This is often the time of life when the results of the hard work involved in establishing a family, financial and social security are seen and a sense of achievement may be experienced. It may also be an important time for reflection, for reviewing the present situation and perhaps choosing to address some of the missed opportunities of life to date.

3.6(a) CHANGING RESPONSIBILITIES

The constitution of the family may also change with children, now adults, leaving home or becoming increasingly independent and no longer requiring the degree of parenting needed earlier. This is often cited as 'the empty nest syndrome'.

See also Chapter 8, section 4 on Caring for an elderly person at home

With increases in life expectancy, however, it may be that there are elderly relatives to be cared for. Such demands may not have been considered previously, constituting a potential crisis point and requiring a redefinition of roles and responsibilities. This may be particularly important for the female partner as the role of carer, more often than not, is still perceived as 'women's work'. If such care arrangements need to be organised it would be wise to make formal contact with the local organisations and support groups involved with care of the elderly. It is essential that the provision of such care is not underestimated in terms of the physical and emotional stress it may create.

See also Chapter 2, section 6 on Help for the carers and Appendix VII for Addresses of useful organisations and support groups

REDEFINING ROLES

Within relationships the wish to renegotiate or redefine roles is anxiety provoking, perhaps threatening, disorientating and crisis provoking. Recognition and open acknowledgement of these feelings provides an opportunity to explore the implications of change.

Society today is open to enabling people to redefine roles, to start new careers and to take up educational opportunities that previous circumstances may have made difficult. With support from partners, acknowledging the risks that may be taken, not being put off by the reticence of others, it may open up opportunities that were felt to be lost. Just as with the feelings of the adolescent, the crisis of self-esteem and self-identity comes into focus, requiring sensitive support and understanding from family and friends.

3.6(b)

See also section 3.3(b) above on Success at work

The opportunities for promotion may also present during the mid-life years.

During these years, both men and women have to face the realities of the ageing process. It is possibly the women who experience the more dramatic effects of this through the post-menopausal symptoms of mood changes. The crisis of menopause may be traumatic for some, representing as it may, a loss of femininity. These are important issues to confront, not to be ignored, with partners and health professionals.

The mid-life years are a time to consider new opportunities and new experiences. However they are also a time when these changes will have implications for those who live within the family unit and, as such, should be discussed by all who will be affected.

3.7 RETIREMENT

See also Chapter 8, section 2 on Life after retirement and section 3.3 above on The world of work

Retirement is defined as the giving up of an occupation in order to enjoy more leisure or freedom, a positive move for some but not so, perhaps, for others. Crisis arises if an individual has invested a great deal of his energies and himself into his working role and has omitted to develop a lifestyle or social activities outside. An individual's self-concept is enhanced through his role at work. If this is taken away, he may feel that there is little or no value in taking up a positive attitude to retirement. Others look forward to having time to pursue interests which have had to take a back seat while they were in full time employment.

Retirement may also occur earlier than had been anticipated due to economic or health reasons.

Whatever the reason for retiring at a particular point, the individual needs time to adapt to the enforced change in the structure of his day and the amount of time spent in the company of other family members. Those who have had the opportunity to attend a pre-retirement course are at an advantage, as they have had access to information and may have been warned about potential hazards. This may include forewarning that the feelings of loss associated with not going to work and no longer being part of the social network may feel like the experience of grieving. If such opportunities have not been made available, it is worth enquiring whether such a course is available through your local education authority.

See section 3.10 below on Bereavement and loss

Despite the best preparation, some individuals still experience retirement as a crisis. Such people will find it valuable to talk through their feelings with family and friends. Gradually, they will find alternative ways of enhancing their self-esteem, recognising their self-worth without work. They may also find avenues whereby they can offer their knowledge and skills to society through local enterprise initiatives. Alternatively the available time and energy may be spent in developing new skills and hobbies, either independently or with their partner.

These strategies may also be relevant for those who have had to retire through ill-health. The crisis of coping not only with retirement but also with health problems means that the process of coming to terms with the change requires time, opportunity to reflect and to talk through feelings. The aim is to come to terms with personal physical limitations, all the while exploring ways of achieving satisfaction, enhanced self-esteem and new roles within a family and social support system. The stress of this should not be underestimated and support from the local social or voluntary services may be needed.

3.8   RELOCATION

Residential changes are occasions creating crises by their ambivalent nature. Most moves are seen in a positive light, yet are tinged with anxiety that the new situation may not turn out to be all that was hoped for.

3.8(a)   PRACTICAL ASPECTS

The process of planning and organising the move may act as a buffer to the crisis itself. Equally, past experiences such as leaving home, going to boarding school or previous moves equip the individual with knowledge and skills to manage the situation. The loss of a familiar social context is often counterbalanced by the new opportunities provided by the residential change. However the situation may be more complex if the move requires a number of family members to adapt to a new place to live as simultaneously a number of major changes for each member are likely to be necessary, for example new schools, new friends, new travel routines, new social networks, new cultures. Inevitably, compromise within the crisis of moving may be needed by everybody. This requires listening to and acknowledgement of, each person's feelings. Children and young adults form very close ties to their peer groups and the feelings associated with relocation should not be underestimated. Children are likely to grieve over the loss of close companions and their behaviour may provoke crisis in the household.

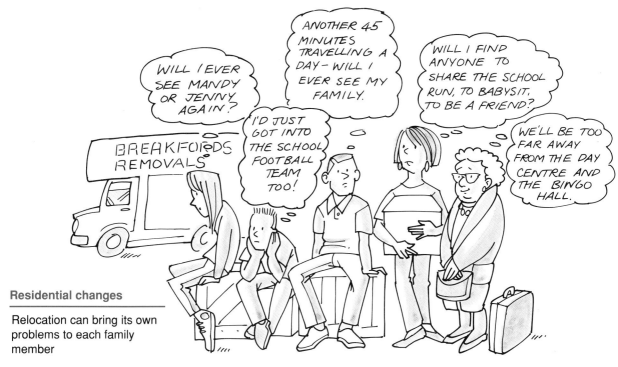

Residential changes

Relocation can bring its own problems to each family member

3.8(b) UNANTICIPATED MOVES

Unanticipated moves catch individuals unprepared spinning them into crisis. This may be the result of job transfer and if frequent in occurrence the individual or family unit develops effective coping strategies to deal with unanticipated events. Alternatively relocation may be the consequence of changes in financial status. Again the impact of the crisis lies with the accumulation of stresses, limited finances, little economic security and the environmental changes discussed previously. Taking the opportunity to talk things through is often easier said than done in such circumstances, and it may be valuable to include someone who is professionally experienced in helping people in these situations. Information helps people to make appropriate choices and often, when one is involved in a situation, it is difficult to view the options in a realistic light.

See Appendix VII for Addresses of useful organisations and support groups

3.8(c) RELOCATION FOR THE ELDERLY

Similar crises may be experienced by elderly people moving into residential accommodation. The move away from familiar social and environmental settings may require adaptation skills that an elderly person feels she simply does not possess. This can precipitate intense feelings of sorrow; therefore pre-planning in which the elderly person herself participates fully is vital.

3.9 SICKNESS AND BODY CHANGES

Modern technology has led people to assume that medicine today can diagnose, treat and cure illness. In most incidences this is likely to be the case. It is not surprising, therefore, that illness which is destined to be more long lasting often precipitates some sort of crisis. The experience of crisis may be more poignant if the illness is going to result in changes to appearance or body function, or to the person's lifestyle.

3.9(a) EMOTIONAL AND SOCIAL ASPECTS

Often the emotional experience of illness is fuelled by the fear of not knowing or understanding what is happening to the body as a result of the disease process, or what will happen in the future. One way of allaying some of the anxiety is to ask the health professionals what is happening. Sometimes it may feel as though it is 'better not to know as what you don't know you cannot worry about'. However this only adds to the fears and fantasies about what is happening.

The experience of illness may interrupt the individual's ability to fulfil the roles she normally performs. This can create the need for others in the family to take on her responsibilities, or her role will not be filled. Consequently all aspects of family life are likely to be influenced and affected by long term ill-health. The most critical is likely to be the financial aspect, and support and advice should be sought in order to minimise potential difficulties.

3.9(b) PHYSICAL ASPECTS

The physical experience of treatments to counteract the illness may be distressing, for example the side-effects of drugs. It is important in these situations that carers are informed what these symptoms and side-effects are, so that they are able to help minimise them and be understanding about what is happening to the individual.

3.9(c) INFORMATION AND SUPPORT

Individuals who are in possession of the relevant information may then be in a position to begin adapting their lifestyle to achieve goals within the limitations dictated by their illness. The focus needs to be on how to manage life, rather than on how to manage the illness.

See Appendix VII for Addresses of useful organisations and support groups

Voluntary and self-help groups, as well as statutory services, may be available to contact for support, not only for the person who has the illness, but also for the carers as it is well recognised that caring in the home can be stressful.

3.10 BEREAVEMENT AND LOSS

See also Chapter 2, section 5(h) on The dying and Chapter 4, section 3(e) on Loss and grief at or around the time of birth

Bereavement can be defined as the emotional experience that follows an actual or perceived loss. The loss of a person through death, the loss of a limb, the loss of a relationship as in divorce, the loss of a loved family pet and the loss of a home all generate similar emotional experiences of sadness and loss.

Bereavement is as natural a part of life as being born and, until recently, death was a familiar visitor to families claiming not only the old but the young too. As a result of developments in health care many people may reach middle age without having to confront the death of someone close to them. How to deal with grief and mourning is learnt through social and cultural experiences but today the majority of deaths occur in the clinical environment of a hospice or hospital reinforcing the taboo of death and minimising the rituals and customs which enable the person to begin to grieve.

An additional consequence of today's technological society is that death may come as an unexpected visitor through violent and unexpected death, such as road traffic accidents.

3.10(a)   THE STAGES OF GRIEF

Within the emotional trauma of grief there are distinct phases which each person goes through in their grief. It is suggested that it is essential for all of the stages to have been gone through before the person can be said to have fully come to terms with the loss. Stages of grief are described in the box below.

STAGES OF GRIEF	
Stage 1 Numbness	characterised by shock and disbelief
Stage 2 Rage	anger and horror
Stage 3 Realisation	of what has happened, experiencing the pain of grief
Stage 4 Acceptance	and adjustment to the changed world
Stage 5 Resolution	investment of energy into new role and relationships

*See Appendix VII for
Addresses of useful
organisations and
support groups*

These stages are helpful in providing an understandable framework to the experience which is disruptive, distressing and even incomprehensible. Each person is likely to travel through each phase in a different way, and over a different period of time. Some may even go back to a previous stage, especially when significant events or anniversaries occur. People who find they are unable to complete the stages are advised to ask for help from health professionals or one of the many relevant organisations (this can be a self referral). It is not a sign of weakness to ask for help in time of crisis, but a sign of strength to recognise a need.

3.10(b)   THE NEEDS OF CHILDREN

It is also important to remember that everyone of any age has the need to grieve for a loss, and this includes children. Children need to be included in the grieving which takes place in the home, school or for something very special to them. They should be respected and not excluded. Above all, they should not be lied to.

3.10(c)   GRIEF ON APPROACHING DEATH

The hospice, a very special place providing care and comfort for those who are terminally ill, gives a permissive atmosphere to enable people to grieve and prepare for death. The steps or phases that people who are approaching death go through are similar to those described above. They are identified as:

- Denial;
- Anger/rage;
- Bargaining;
- Depression;
- Acceptance.

Some individuals choose to spend their last days in their own homes. This can be stressful but rewarding for those who are providing the care and comfort. There are special resources and support services available to individuals and families at such times which are accessible through the local health care services.

STAGES OF LIFE

PREGNANCY AND PARENTHOOD

4.1 PREPARING FOR PREGNANCY

4.1(a) FAMILY PLANNING

To find out more about the different forms of contraception, contact your family doctor or local family planning clinic. See also Appendices VII and VIII

Any couple requiring family planning advice and supplies may go either to the family doctor or to the community or hospital family planning clinic run by the Health Authority. For selected clients, who for some reason do not attend the clinic, a domiciliary service may be available. In the United Kingdom the service is free under the National Health Service, but a charge will be made for services provided by the Family Planning Association.

Anyone is welcome, be they married or single, male or female, young or old. Partners are all invited to discuss different methods of birth control to discover the method most acceptable to them on social, religious and aesthetic grounds.

People attend family planning clinics for a variety of reasons. Different methods suit different people at different times. A couple may seek family planning advice from the beginning of their relationship to obtain information about contraception. A couple having already tried a method of birth control may return to the clinic if the method is no longer acceptable to them. By making sure that the method chosen is effective and suitable, the couple will be more relaxed and better able to enjoy intercourse. A couple may seek advice about stopping contraception to plan for a baby. This will ensure that they are aware of the optimum time to conceive. Preconception advice is often referred to at this time.

See *section 4.1(b) below for more about Preconception advice*

Female methods of contraception

The natural method (safe method or rhythm method)   This is the only method acceptable to some people. The safe period refers to the time in the menstrual cycle when conception cannot take place. The safe period will be easier for women whose menstrual cycles are regular to identify.

A women's menstrual cycle is influenced by her reproductive hormones, and divided into three phases:

- Pre-ovulatory;

- Ovulation;

- Post-ovulatory.

Effectiveness of the various
methods of contraception

Method	Percentage effectiveness
Natural methods	83–95%
Diaphragm/cap	97%
IUCD/coil	96–98%
Combined pill	Almost 100%
Mini pill	98%
Injectable contraceptives	98%
Condom	97%
Spermicides	Not effective alone
Withdrawal	Unreliable

Ovulation is the release of an ovum from the ovary to pass along the fallopian tube in preparation for fertilisation. It usually occurs around the 14th day of the cycle which is therefore the time when the woman is most fertile. Fertilisation is possible up to five days before and two days after ovulation.

The natural method involves being able to recognise the physical changes that take place around ovulation. These are:

• Variation in body temperature;

• Changes in cervical mucus.

Body temperature rises by about 0.3°C (1°F) at the time of ovulation, and this raised level continues until the end of the cycle. If you are using the 'temperature method', you should take your temperature, and chart the result, immediately on waking. For the most accuracy at least three cycles should be completed to identify this rise and fall in temperature.

The character of the cervical mucus changes throughout the menstrual cycle. For the cervical mucus (or Billings) method, you will be taught to examine the mucus each day. Following a menstrual period, there is little or no mucus for several days, after which it becomes thick, white and sticky. Three or four days before ovulation occurs the mucus becomes thinner, allowing survival and transport of the sperm. The mucus then becomes thick again, followed by dry days before the next period. The last day of the thin mucus is called *the peak symptom* and, to avoid conception, the couple should wait until the fourth day after the peak symptom has passed.

A combination of these two methods enables the couple to establish when ovulation has taken place, and thus to plan a pregnancy if they wish to conceive, or to abstain from intercourse if a pregnancy is not wanted.

• **Cervix**
The neck of the womb

The diaphragm or cap   This is a soft rubber cap with a flat or coiled spring in the rim. It is inserted into the vagina to cover the cervix.

It can be inserted for up to three hours before intercourse, but must be left in position for six hours afterwards.

The woman is taught how to insert the cap, check its position, remove and care for it. She must return to the clinic six-monthly, after childbirth or after a loss or gain in weight of 3 kg, to ensure the fit is still correct.

Spermicides These come in the form of jellies, creams, pastes, pessaries and aerosol foams. Their purpose is to inactivate sperm. They should *always* be used in conjunction with the cap or sheath, as they are not an effective method of contraception on their own.

Intrauterine contraceptive devices (or coils) These are small plastic devices which are inserted into the womb by a doctor. Some have copper added to increase their efficiency. IUCDs work partly by preventing the egg from implanting in the womb by causing changes in the uterine wall. They also produce extra hormones causing uterine activity and so expelling the fertilised egg.

The coil should be inserted during or just after a period, not only for ease of insertion but also to exclude the possibility of pregnancy. You will be taught to feel for the threads of the coil in the vagina, to check that it is still present. It is not recommended for nulliparous women. Heavy prolonged periods may be experienced for some months after insertion, but later subside. Pelvic infection can be a complication.

- **Uterine wall**
  The wall of the womb

- **Nulliparous women**
  Women who have never been pregnant

Oral contraception (the Pill) Oral contraception includes both the combined pill (oestrogen and progesterone pill) and the progesterone only pill (the mini pill). Oestrogen acts by inhibiting ovulation. Progesterone alters the consistency of the cervical mucus making it impenetrable to sperm, reduces the motility of the ovarian tubes so that the sperm have difficulty passing along them, and causes a change in the lining of the womb making it hostile to implantation.

The combined pill must be taken daily for 21 days with a break of seven days when a withdrawal bleed occurs. If, however, more than twelve hours has lapsed before taking a pill, another form of contraception must be used. It is not recommended for women over the age of 35, those who smoke and those who are overweight. Minor side effects include weight gain, breast enlargement, nausea and headaches. Serious complications are rare.

The mini pill is recommended for women over the age of 35 and for breast feeding mothers who should not take oestrogen. Periods may become irregular and breakthrough bleeding may occur.

Injectable contraceptives Progesterone can be given as an injection and its effectiveness will last for three months. Depo-provera is commonly used. It is suitable for poorly motivated women or women for whom other methods are unsuitable.

Female sterilisation   This is a permanent method of contraception in which the ovarian tubes are either cut or tied, so that the ovum is prevented from meeting the sperm. A general anaesthetic is necessary at most centres, but the procedure is often carried out as day surgery.

Sterilisation is ideal for couples who are absolutely certain that they have completed their families, and screening of these couples by careful counselling is important. Occasionally a pregnancy can occur if the tubes rejoin.

Male contraception

The condom (sheath)   This is the most common form of contraception as condoms are cheap and easily available. They are made of thin rubber and are worn over the erect penis to trap the sperm.

Condoms are recommended for protection against sexually transmitted diseases, AIDS, and cervical cancer. Occasionally they may slip off or become damaged allowing sperm to leak out. Some people object to using the condom as they find it aesthetically undesirable, and some men report a loss of sexual sensitivity.

Withdrawal or coitus interruptus   This involves withdrawing the penis from the vagina before ejaculation takes place. It is not recommended, being an unreliable form of contraception as a small amount of seminal fluid is released before ejaculation. It often leads to sexual frustration in both partners.

Male sterilisation (vasectomy)   This is a permanent method of contraception where the *vas deferens* are cut and tied, preventing the passage of sperm into the seminal fluid. As with female sterilisation the couple must be thoroughly counselled before a decision is made about surgery. Vasectomy is now carried out under local anaesthetic as a day patient. The couple are advised to use another form of contraception after the operation until two semen specimens are without sperm.

• **Vas deferens**
Tubes from the testes to the penis, carrying seminal fluid

4.1(b)   PRECONCEPTION CARE

Preconception care bridges the gap between family planning and the antenatal service. It is an attempt to reduce, and if possible to eliminate the known potentially harmful influences that can compromise the quality of a baby during its earliest days of life. Ideally, preconception care should start 3–6 months before thinking about a pregnancy. The diagram below summarises the aspects about which some couples may be worried.

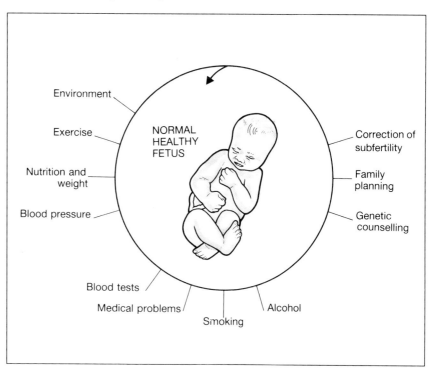

Optimising the environment for the unborn baby

See also Chapter 7, section 10(d) on Occupational disorders

See also Chapter 1, section 2 on Exercise

See also Chapter 1, section 1 on Diet

Environment

It is a good idea to check with the work place that any health hazards (e.g. poisonous gases and toxic fumes) are identified and can therefore be avoided. Sperm can be affected by the environment so this check should also include the male partner.

Exercise

Daily exercise in moderation is advised so that you are fit and healthy for your pregnancy. In contrast, time should also be allowed for adequate rest and relaxation.

Nutrition and weight

Eat a good, well balanced diet to include bread and cereals, meat and alternatives, milk and dairy products, vegetables and fruit. Any dietary problems should be assessed and treated as necessary. Do not go on a crash diet. Weight should be corrected by good food and exercise.

Blood pressure

Blood pressure should be checked by your doctor and an attempt should be made to lower high blood pressure by medication, loss of weight and exercise.

4

- **Haemoglobin count**
  Measurement of the iron content of blood

- **Rubella**
  Commonly known as German measles – can have serious consequences for the unborn baby

- **Fetal alcohol syndrome**
  Affected babies may be smaller than they should be, mentally retarded and suffer from a variety of physical defects

See section 4.1(c) below

See section 4.1(a) above

See section 4.2 below

Blood tests

Haemoglobin count should be checked and, if it is found to be low, diet can be modified or iron supplements given.

Rubella immunity should be checked. If no immunity (or low immunity only) exists an injection can be given, after which pregnancy must be avoided for three months to ensure that the developing baby is not affected as mental retardation, blindness and deafness can result.

Medical problems and medication

Anyone suffering from a medical problem such as mental illness, epilepsy or diabetes should visit their doctor before becoming pregnant to ensure that any medication is safe to take during pregnancy.

Tobacco and alcohol

Cut down smoking and aim to stop altogether before trying for a baby. Smoking in pregnancy can cause growth retarded babies. Cut out alcohol entirely or at least to no more than one drink a day. Excessive alcohol intake during pregnancy can cause fetal alcohol syndrome. Both alcohol and tobacco use may increase the risk of miscarriage or premature birth.

Genetic counselling

Anyone concerned that a medical problem in the family may be hereditary should seek a referral to the genetic counselling service through their doctor.

Family planning

Allow between three to six months to prepare yourselves for a pregnancy. Contraception should be used during this period. Wait at least one year after the birth of one baby before trying for another.

Subfertility

If you have been trying to become pregnant for more than six months, seek an appointment with your doctor. A consultation with a gynaecologist may be necessary.

4.1(c)   GENETIC COUNSELLING

Anyone concerned about a medical condition in their family that may be hereditary should be referred to a genetic counselling clinic. They will be advised of the consequences of the disorder, the probability of developing or transmitting it, and of the ways in which it may be prevented or reduced.

At the clinic detailed family information will be obtained. In some circumstances a genetic counselling nurse may visit the family to gain as much information as possible before the consultation. Blood samples may be required.

Before the counselling may begin appropriate hospital notes, post-mortem reports, chromosome and DNA results are necessary to confirm the diagnosis.

At the consultation a medical examination of the affected member of the family may be required. The genetics of the condition and the risks of the disorder occurring in other members of the family, born or unborn, are explained. Options available to the family are discussed. These may include:

- Prenatal diagnosis (e.g. scanning, amniocentesis, chorionic villus sampling) with possible termination of an affected fetus;

- Artificial insemination by donor (D.I.);

- Adoption;

- Sterilisation;

- Future approaches for further generations, for example new tests.

See section 4.3(a) on Termination of pregnancy, section 4.4(b) for information about tests during pregnancy and Appendix VII for Addresses of useful organisations

Follow-up support

Genetic counselling should always include follow-up support. It must be established that the individuals counselled have clearly understood all that has been discussed with them. This includes the risk estimate, the nature of the disorder and the options available. Often information given in the clinic is very detailed and further explanation is important and necessary.

An effort to contact other family members who are at risk of the condition is made, and appointments for them can be arranged. Support group addresses are offered.

- **Nucleated somatic cells**
  These are non-sex cells, i.e. all body cells except ova or sperm (see below)

Chromosomes

In every nucleated somatic cell there are 46 chromosomes, in 23 matching pairs. The chromosomes are numbered in order of decreasing size. Numbers 1 to 22, *autosomes* or non-sex chromosomes, are similar in males and females. The remaining pair are the *sex chromosomes*. Females have two X chromosomes, and males have an X and a Y chromosome. Each individual receives a set of 22 autosomes and a sex chromosome from each parent.

Gametes have only 23 single chromosomes.

- **Gamete**
  An ovum or a sperm cell

Genes

The chromosomes carry genes which are are responsible for all inborn and inherited characteristics. Most single gene disorders follow a recognised mode of inheritance and most commonly they are autosomal dominant, autosomal recessive or X-linked.

Autosomal dominant inheritance   With all autosomal dominant conditions there is a 1 in 2, or 50 per cent, chance that an affected parent will pass on the gene for the condition to his or her offspring who will also be affected.

Autosomal recessive inheritance   With autosomal recessive conditions there is a 1 in 4, or 25 per cent, chance that parents who are both carriers will pass on the gene for the condition to any offspring who then will be affected.

X-linked inheritance   With X-linked conditions there is a 1 in 2, or a 50 per cent, chance that a carrier mother will pass on the gene for the condition to her sons, and the same chance that her daughters will be carriers. All the daughters of affected men will be carriers, but their sons will be unaffected.

Multifactorial inheritance   This refers to a large group of disorders in which there appears to be no clear pattern of inheritance and no identifiable chromosomal abnormality. They can result from a number of influences, some genetic, environmental, or unknown. The recurrence risk in this group is usually greatest amongst close relatives and decreases rapidly with more distant relatives.

See section 4.4(b) for more information about tests during pregnancy

Chromosomal abnormalities   There is a well recognised relationship between increasing maternal age and chromosomal abnormalities. Any women who is over the age of 35 and considering a pregnancy may be concerned about her chance of having a baby with a chromosomal abnormality such as Down's syndrome. She should be referred for genetic counselling so that the risks and appropriate action can be discussed.

Some examples of genetic disorders

Autosomal dominant	Autosomal recessive	X-linked	Multifactorial
Huntington's chorea	Cystic fibrosis	Duchenne muscular dystrophy	Spina bifida
Adult polycystic kidney	Phenylketonuria	Becker muscular dystrophy	Heart defects
Neurofibromatosis	Tay Sach's disease	Fragile X mental retardation	Diabetes mellitus
Achondroplasia	Sickle cell disease	Haemophilia	Pyloric stenosis
Myotonic dystrophy	The thalassaemias	Colour blindness	Cleft lip/palate
Marfan's syndrome	Galactosaemia	Ocular albinism	Epilepsy

SUBFERTILITY

Subfertility is acknowledged when a couple have failed to conceive following 12 months or more of unprotected sexual intercourse. Although they may consider their problem unusual, subfertility is more common than most people imagine. Survey results confirm that approximately one couple in every six will have difficulty starting a wanted pregnancy at some point although, given time and treatment, a proportion of these will eventually achieve pregnancy.

Accepting that a problem exists can be painful for both partners. Most people expect to become parents and failure to conceive may cause them to feel as though they have lost control over an important aspect of their lives, especially if the dawning realisation of subfertility follows years of careful contraception. In some cultures and religions childlessness is a disaster. Even in societies where views are less extreme, inability to have a baby is likely to generate keen disappointment.

See Appendix VII for Addresses of useful organisations and support groups

Everybody has a right to treatment but availability and quality of the service offered vary considerably. In the United Kingdom, some family doctors are willing to undertake more tests than others. In many cases couples are referred to a clinic specialising in fertility problems soon after consulting their general practitioner. Although more travel may result, inconvenience is compensated by the expertise of doctors and nurses who meet this type of patient every day. Also, the sight of others in the same position emphasises to the couple that they are by no means alone in their predicament.

When a couple first seek medical advice, both partners can expect to be given a full physical examination and to be asked about their general health. For men, a history of mumps after adolescence may indicate damage to the testes. Operations for undescended testicles or repair of hernia will also be regarded as relevant. The doctor will enquire about occupation and working conditions as, for example, the intense heat necessary in a boiler house or blast furnace may be sufficient to reduce sperm production, damage that is reversible. The woman will be asked about any infections she has had in the past, especially those involving the pelvic organs. Surgical intervention such as appendicectomy may cause adhesions of the pelvic structures, reducing the normal, healthy motility of the fallopian tubes, and this can make pregnancy harder to achieve. Mumps in women occurring after adolescence can damage the ovaries.

- **Adhesions of the pelvic structures**
  Attachment of the various structures to each other

- **Ovulation**
  The production of eggs

Information about the menstrual cycle is of obvious importance. The woman will be asked the age at which her periods started, their frequency and the character of menstruation, as irregular scanty periods may be an indication of failure to ovulate, especially if periods are pain free and not accompanied by breast tenderness.

miscarriage and terminations. Even when couples have a very close relationship which has endured several years they may not wish to share *all* their secrets, so opportunity should be provided for each to spend some time alone with the doctor, although in other respects they will be considered as two people who share a problem. Finally it is important to establish that sexual intercourse is taking place correctly, that the man is achieving orgasm to ensure the release of sperm and that the couple understand that in order to conceive, intercourse should occur in the middle of the woman's cycle, when ovulation is most likely to take place. For a 28 day cycle this would be around days 13–18, counting the first day of menstruation as day one of the cycle.

In approximately one third of cases a fertility problem affects the man and in another third the woman. In the remaining cases both man and woman contribute to subfertility.

Sometimes difficulties can be resolved with relatively little intervention. It is possible that when a couple do not have intercourse frequently and the woman's periods are very far apart the sperm and egg simply lack opportunity to meet. A woman can be taught the signs and symptoms of impending ovulation and intercourse planned to coincide. In most cases, however, further investigations will be necessary to establish a cause.

Following physical examination to rule out structural abnormality of the the reproductive organs the man will be requested to provide a specimen of semen, in order for sperm count and motility to be estimated. Any ejaculation will contain a proportion of inactive and damaged sperm, but their total number should not exceed a certain minimal level if conception is to occur. Although providing these specimens is often very stressful it is vital for the couple to appreciate their importance and to accept that one or two poor results are not definitive. Sperm count and size of ejaculate vary considerably, so it is often necessary for several specimens to be analysed. Where a count is genuinely low little can be done to improve it, but careful timing of intercourse and sometimes artificial insemination may be employed to achieve pregnancy.

Most women experience the odd anovulatory cycle occasionally, but continued failure to ovulate requires treatment with hormones. This is usually successful, although some women worry about the risk of multiple pregnancies which, in the past, have resulted through the administration of large doses. Today this risk has been reduced considerably.

The time of ovulation as well as ovulatory failure is detectable by the woman keeping temperature charts as there is a slight, but perceptible increase when the egg is released. However, more modern and sensitive methods involve monitoring blood or urinary levels of the hormones responsible for ovulation.

- **Anovulatory cycle**
  A menstrual cycle in which no egg is produced

- **Appendicectomy**
Surgical removal of the appendix

Sadly, one of the most common causes of subfertility in women is damage to the fallopian tubes, usually scarring which has followed infection, inflammation or pelvic surgery. The delicate tubes are easily damaged and in cases where infection was mild, or an appendicectomy was performed long ago, the incident may be forgotten or dismissed as unimportant and not mentioned. A variety of surgical techniques exist to break down adhesions to restore tubal potency and motility. Until recent years this met with limited success, but today, with refinements in microsurgery and the growing experience of gynaecologists, the chances of achieving pregnancy are increasing all the time, although it can never be guaranteed. In general, the greater the tubal damage, the more difficult it will be to restore normal function.

The media has given much attention to the technique IVF (*in vitro* fertilisation) which involves fertilising eggs outside the woman's body, then returning them to the womb bypassing damaged tubes. IVF is not suitable for every couple and may have to be repeated several times, sometimes still without achieving pregnancy. A new technique, GIFT (gamete intra-fallopian transfer) which involves mixing eggs and sperm then returning them to the fallopian tube, the usual site of conception, is now used increasingly as it is easier to perform and has been reported to have a fairly high rate of success, although again, pregnancy is not inevitable.

There is no 'magic' cure for subfertility, but newer treatments are becoming available and as gynaecologists gain more experience with each, more couples are able to have a baby than was possible a few years ago.

4.3 WHEN PREGNANCY FAILS

Pregnancy ending before the 28th week of gestation is technically known as abortion. This may occur spontaneously (accidental abortion or miscarriage) but may also be induced as the law presently operates in the United Kingdom. A third situation in which pregnancy is lost occurs when the developing embryo embeds itself in the wall of the fallopian tube, or, more rarely, at some other site outside the uterus (ectopic pregnancy). Loss of a baby after the 28th week of pregnancy is known as intrauterine death or stillbirth.

4.3(a) TERMINATION OF PREGNANCY

Unplanned pregnancy is frequently regarded as unwanted pregnancy, but this is not always the case. Women whose lives seem already to be full, with career, other children or even both, may initially react with dismay, but adjust as the pregnancy progresses. For other couples the financial or social situation may be such that unplanned pregnancy constitutes disaster, providing little alternative to termination.

In 1970 when the British law legalising termination of pregnancy was passed, it was believed that demand would always be low and that in most cases abortion would be performed on medical grounds. However, government records reflect a gradual increase in abortions undertaken mainly on social grounds, not restricted to the young or unmarried. Most abortions take place early in pregnancy (before 12–14 weeks gestation). Later terminations are more likely to be performed because of fetal abnormality, in most cases through failure to detect a problem at an earlier stage. After the first three months, pregnancy is technically more difficult to terminate and the situation will be harder for the woman to accept, as she will be visibly pregnant and will probably have felt the baby move.

Fetal abnormalities such as Down's syndrome are statistically more a risk among women after the age of 35. Currently the main method of detection is by a procedure called amniocentesis, in which a sample of fluid surrounding the fetus is obtained after the woman has received a local anaesthetic. The fluid contains cells shed from the surface of the fetus, which can be grown in the laboratory and subjected to genetic and biochemical tests. Amniocentesis is difficult to attempt until around the 16th week of gestation and the results are not available immediately because the cells must have time to grow. Occasionally the cell culture fails and amniocentesis may have to be repeated. Under these circumstances a termination necessary through fetal abnormality will inevitably be performed late. In some centres, a newer technique called chorionic villus sampling (CVS) is offered. This test can be performed as early as seven weeks gestation to produce results without the need for cell culture, but is not yet available everywhere.

No couple will be subjected to either of these tests unless they consent, although the service may be offered on grounds of maternal age or because the family has a known history of genetic or congenital disorder. Both partners should have been encouraged by their doctor or midwife to consider how they might react to a positive result and to have discussed their options, as a decision may have to be taken quickly.

The first step if pregnancy is suspected, is confirmation either by arranging for a test to be performed by your family doctor, a chemist, a family planning clinic or by using a kit to perform the test yourself. Modern tests detect the presence of human chorionic gonadotrophin (HCG) the pregnancy hormone, within the urine and most are now sufficiently sensitive for use on the same day that

See also section 4.1(c) on Genetic counselling, and section 4.4(b) for information about tests during pregnancy

your period was due, giving a result in as little as five minutes. Kits are expensive but usually provide sufficient materials for two tests to be performed. If you are in any doubt repeat the test: remember that its result will only be as good as your technique, which could be poor owing to shaking hands. Before you purchase the kit look to see exactly how many tests can be attempted, and if the result does not seem definitive repeat it with a specimen of early morning urine. Urine that has been in your bladder all night will be concentrated (less is produced at night), so its HCG content if present should be correspondingly higher.

A woman who is unhappy about being pregnant can seek help from her doctor or family planning clinic, which can arrange a hospital referral. Alternatively she can contact a private agency by obtaining the number from the yellow pages of the telephone book and making an appointment for herself. Whatever action she takes, she should expect a doctor to acknowledge the pregnancy by looking at the evidence provided by the test (she can take this with her) and by performing a gentle vaginal examination. Her breasts will be examined and she will, of course, be asked the date of her last menstrual period and its character: sometimes a slight bleed can occur at the expected time of menstruation although pregnancy has already been established during the previous cycle. A woman who is contemplating termination will need to talk this over with someone in addition to her partner. In hospital this will probably be a social worker. Privately run establishments usually employ their own counsellors. Post-abortion counselling is sometimes offered and a telephone service may be available.

See Appendix VII for Addresses of useful organisations and support groups

If a decision to terminate pregnancy has been taken the woman may be admitted to hospital or a clinic overnight. Alternatively, if she can be collected and has someone at home to look after her, she may undergo the procedure as a day patient, having been asked to arrive fasting (no food or fluids) for at least six hours. She will probably be advised to bring overnight requirements just in case she is not well enough to go home.

In the United Kingdom, pregnancy is usually terminated after the woman has been given a light general anaesthetic, although some clinics offering day care facilities will offer local anaesthesia and a sedative instead. Afterwards the woman will rest in bed for a few hours and her pulse and blood pressure will be checked several times to ensure that excessive bleeding is not occurring. Pains similar to period pains may be experienced and can be controlled by a mild analgesic. Nausea and sickness are exceptional because anaesthesia is so light. She can get out of bed a few hours later, taking care as she may feel dizzy at first. As she stands up, any blood left in the vagina will drain away through gravity so, unless forewarned, she may believe that she has had a sudden loss of blood.

When she goes home the woman should rest for a few days before returning to work. Heavy or strenuous work should not be resumed for a week. Bleeding should never be more than slight, soon becoming a yellow coloured discharge and clearing up altogether in a few days. Tampons should not be worn for this bleeding, nor for the next period, because the neck of the womb has been opened and there is a chance of introducing infection. In the event of blood loss that becomes heavy, bright red or smells offensive, she should contact her family doctor or the ward or clinic where the operation was performed. A course of antibiotics may be necessary. The signs and symptoms of pregnancy should gradually regress as HCG remaining in the body is lost via the urine. If symptoms persist, medical help should again be sought promptly as it is very occasionally possible to 'miss' an early pregnancy at a stage when it is still tiny.

Today, termination of pregnancy is usually effective and very safe. The complications described above are rare and there are seldom any physical effects later: it is not necessary to stretch the neck of the womb very much to remove the products of conception, ensuring that future pregnancies are unlikely to fail. However, a new menstrual cycle will commence within a few days, and unless adequate contraceptive precautions are taken, another pregnancy could occur straight away.

4.3(b) MISCARRIAGE

'Miscarriage' is the layperson's term for interrupted pregnancy. It does not have the same unpleasant connotations as the word abortion but, technically, expulsion of the fetus before the 28th week of pregnancy constitutes an abortion even if it is accidental. Couples who are unaware of this may be distressed if they hear medical staff refer to their lost but much wanted pregnancy in this way.

The first sign that something is amiss usually occurs when the woman notices vaginal loss. Bleeding comes from the placental site and may be accompanied by pelvic pain or backache of variable intensity. At this early stage it is not usually possible to predict whether the pregnancy will definitely be lost (inevitable miscarriage) or whether it will continue (threatened miscarriage). Recommended action is to rest while medical aid is summoned, or, if there is any doubt about the doctor's willingness to perform a home visit, to go to the Accident and Emergency Department of the nearest hospital. Any blood clots or other tissue passed should be saved for inspection.

The doctor will perform a gentle vaginal examination to determine whether the cervix is open or closed. If it is open, pain is moderate or severe and there is fairly heavy bleeding, it is likely that the

• Cervix
The neck of the womb

pregnancy has ended. Mild pain, spotting and a closed cervix indicate that all may be well. Further information is provided by an ultrasound examination, as it is possible to detect the developing baby and to determine whether or not it remains viable from the fifth week of pregnancy. The woman may also be asked to provide a specimen of urine so that a pregnancy test can be performed, but the results are not likely to be very helpful at this stage. Human chorionic gonadotrophin, the hormone detected, takes a few days to leave the body when pregnancy fails, so a positive result may occur for a short time after a miscarriage has become inevitable.

Types of miscarriage

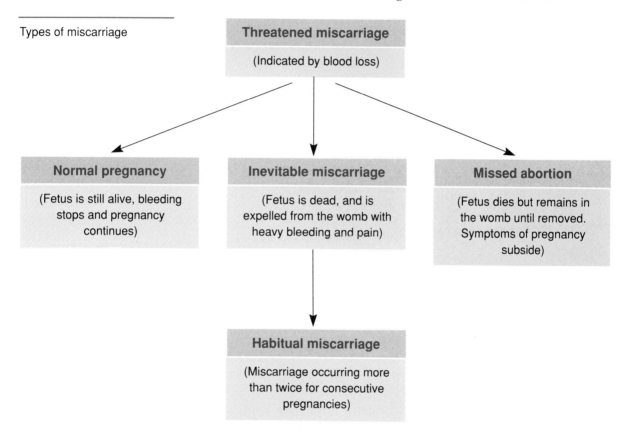

Threatened miscarriage

(Indicated by blood loss)

Normal pregnancy

(Fetus is still alive, bleeding stops and pregnancy continues)

Inevitable miscarriage

(Fetus is dead, and is expelled from the womb with heavy bleeding and pain)

Missed abortion

(Fetus dies but remains in the womb until removed. Symptoms of pregnancy subside)

Habitual miscarriage

(Miscarriage occurring more than twice for consecutive pregnancies)

If the pregnancy has been lost it may be necessary for the woman to be admitted to hospital to undergo a minor surgical procedure under general anaesthesia to remove remaining tissue and blood clots from the womb. If this is omitted, she may be at risk of infection and possible haemorrhage, but the doctor will assess the risks and needs for the individual woman.

See Chapter 7, Section 10(a) for more information about 'D and C' (dilatation and curettage)

After this operation, which is really no different from a 'D and C', the woman will probably feel tired and a little shaky as well as emotionally upset. She will be allowed to get out of bed a few hours later, but must take care as she may feel dizzy. When she stands up blood pooling in the vagina will trickle out and this may be distressing as she may believe that she is still bleeding. Pain is usually mild to moderate and pain relief will be provided by the nurses, who will also check that she has been able to pass urine. The next day she will be allowed to go home provided she has not got a temperature and vaginal discharge is slight.

After a miscarriage the symptoms of pregnancy will regress over a few days and the menstrual cycle will often resume very swiftly, so contraceptive precautions are advisable unless the couple wish to establish another pregnancy straight away. Until vaginal discharge has ceased, sanitary pads rather than tampons should be worn and also for the next menstrual period, as the cervix has been dilated and there is some risk of infection. Continued bleeding, especially a heavy or offensive discharge accompanied by pelvic pain or backache suggest that infection has occurred and the woman should seek medical help.

If ultrasound results suggest that the pregnancy is viable the woman will be admitted to hospital where she will be prescribed a regime of bedrest until bleeding and pain has ceased. No specific drugs exist to treat threatened miscarriage and no other special treatment has ever proven helpful. Treatment by bedrest itself is controversial: when the woman leaves hospital it is highly likely that she will be told to resume her previous active lifestyle and not make herself into an invalid, for there is no evidence that physical exertion is in any way responsible for threatened or inevitable miscarriage. However, treatment of threatened miscarriage by bedrest is almost universally advised at the present time.

Couples react to the loss of a baby with disbelief and grief, no matter how early their pregnancy: even if miscarriage is only threatened and pregnancy then progresses safely they may spend the remaining months worried and possibly bewildered that apparently so little positive action could be taken on their behalf. Many couples feel alone, not realising that miscarriage is extremely common, especially during the early months. Estimates vary, especially as an extremely early pregnancy lost around the time that menstruation was due may be mistaken for a late, heavy period, but some doctors believe that one in every six or eight conceptions (and perhaps even more than this) is lost.

See section 4.3(e) below on Loss and grief

Despite the very large number of women who have miscarriages, the topic has attracted remarkably little medical research. Usually it is not investigated unless recurrent. One problem that is open to treatment, however, is incompetent cervix: the neck of the womb is not sufficiently strong to 'support' the developing pregnancy. A non-dissolving stitch (MacDonald or Shirodkar suture) may be inserted, drawing together the lips of the cervix to provide extra support. The stitch is removed towards the end of pregnancy near the time the woman is expected to go into labour.

The reason for most miscarriages is never known. Loss is most likely at 10–12 weeks, a time when the maturing placenta is known to take over secretion of the hormones needed to maintain pregnancy from the cells (corpus luteum) left in the ovary which originally surrounded the egg. It has been suggested that miscarriage is threatened or occurs when the placenta is not quite ready to take over this function, allowing hormone levels to dip too low to continue pregnancy. However, hormone therapy does not improve the chances of a threatened miscarriage being saved. Infection has been known to result in miscarriage with pregnancy successful once it has been resolved. Genetic abnormalities have been detected in fetal tissue after miscarriage on many occasions, leading doctors to suppose that in such cases the baby was probably too imperfect to survive and that the maternal immune system is somehow able to detect this, causing rejection of the fetus. Emphasising that the pregnancy was unlikely to succeed is not helpful to couples mourning their loss, however, as discussed in section 4.3(e) below.

4.3(c) ECTOPIC PREGNANCY

Ectopic pregnancy occurs when the fertilised egg embeds itself outside the womb. Extrauterine implantation is most common in the fallopian tube, but has occasionally been reported on the ovary, cervix or within the pelvic cavity, although this is very rare.

See section 4.1(a) for more information about the IUCD and the progesterone only pill

The incidence of ectopic pregnancy within the fallopian tube is known to be becoming increasingly common, especially among women in their late 20s and 30s. Associated risk factors include use of an intrauterine contraceptive device (IUCD) or the progesterone only pill; both forms of birth control are believed to alter normal function of the fallopian tubes. The figure overleaf shows that the delicate fallopian tubes are not of uniform diameter along their length as they lead towards the uterus. They end in tiny tubes of very fine bore capable of free movement. Mobility tends to increase at certain stages of the menstrual cycle. When an egg is released, the tubes apply themselves closely to the surface of the ovary. Since they are open-ended, the egg travels into them soon after it is released, then moves down the fallopian tube towards the uterus. If fertilisation occurs, it will usually take place in a slightly expanded part of the tube (the ampulla). Passage is facilitated by muscular contractions of the walls of the tube and by wafting movements of very fine hairs called cilia which line it.

If for any reason the fertilised egg is delayed in its journey it will burrow into the wall of the fallopian tube instead. After fertilisation the egg begins to divide quite rapidly and within five or six days is already a mass of cells gradually increasing in size and requiring

4

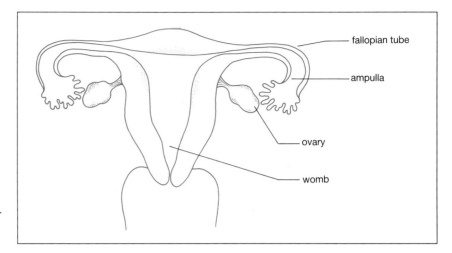

The womb, ovaries and fallopian tubes

- **Endometrium**
  The thickened vascular lining of the uterus

nourishment for further development. This is usually provided by the endometrium which develops to receive a possible pregnancy during the second half of the menstrual cycle. When the egg fails to reach the uterus it embeds itself into the wall of the fallopian tube instead.

The fallopian tube has a particularly generous blood supply as it carries along its length the main blood vessel supplying the rest of the reproductive organs. Erosion of the tubal wall by the developing egg rapidly causes bleeding. The amount and consequent symptoms experienced by the woman vary according to the degree of damage caused to the fallopian tube.

If the embryo implants itself at a site away from a major blood vessel it will soon die through lack of nourishment. A blood clot forms locally. The woman will experience some pain and tenderness, but the very early signs and symptoms of pregnancy which she might just have begun to notice will regress. Pregnancy hormone ceases to be produced and a test performed at this time would be negative. Up until now the uterus has continued preparations as though housing a normal pregnancy, but the thickened lining is now shed.

If the egg embeds itself in the region of a large blood vessel development will proceed until a slightly later stage and the vessel, when eventually eroded, will bleed more profusely. Haemorrhage may be sufficient to result in shock (see below) and blood escaping through the damaged wall of the tube will carry the products of conception into the pelvic cavity. Gravity causes the fluid to drain downwards into the pouch formed by the juxtaposition of the rectum and vagina. Treatment in hospital for haemorrhage and surgical removal of the blood clot are necessary.

A third, more dramatic outcome occurs when the egg erodes a major blood vessel, causing a rupture with major haemorrhage. Profuse internal bleeding occurs suddenly, causing the woman to collapse in pain with a low blood pressure and weak, rapid pulse. She will be pale, her skin will be cold and clammy to touch and her respirations may become deep and sighing as less blood remains in the circulation to carry vital oxygen supplies to the rest of the body. These are the classic signs of shock which every doctor and nurse is taught to recognise, though of course, at this stage it would not be possible for medical staff to diagnose the exact cause of bleeding. This is an emergency situation demanding the most urgent medical attention. The woman must be sent to hospital by ambulance *at once*, so that bleeding can be controlled and its cause established. While you are waiting for the ambulance it is a good idea to cover her with a coat or blanket to preserve warmth and try to establish how the hospital can contact her family. You will not see any bleeding: haemorrhage is internal and surgical intervention will be required, so no attempt must be made to give her anything to eat or drink.

Official statistics in both the United Kingdom and North America show that ruptured ectopic pregnancy remains the most common cause of maternal mortality, although it occurs so early in pregnancy that the woman has probably not yet suspected that conception has occurred. However, this dramatic picture is not the most frequently seen. The results of a recent survey indicate that over half the women affected present with pain but less severe haemorrhage. Hospital admission is always necessary, for even if the fallopian tube has not already ruptured, it may still do so and surgery will still be necessary.

Thus, if there is any possibility of ectopic pregnancy the woman will be prepared for theatre swiftly. All or part of the affected tube will be removed, depending on the degree of damage. If any of the tube can be preserved it will be surgically reconstructed.

The woman can expect to wake up to find that she has an intravenous drip in progress, which will be removed sometime the following day when she is able to drink clear fluids without experiencing nausea. Initially pain will be controlled with injections, then with paracetamol or aspirin. She will be encouraged to perform deep breathing exercises to reduce the chances of developing a chest infection after the anaesthetic, especially if she smokes, and will be reminded by the nurses and physiotherapist to move her legs to avoid circulatory complications. She will be helped out of bed to sit in a chair the day after her operation and can expect to eat and drink normally within 2–3 days. Stitches are removed around the fifth or sixth day post-operatively in most hospitals. The woman can expect to go home a day or so afterwards, although 2–3 weeks convalescence will be needed before resuming work with perhaps an extra week if she has a strenuous job. Other activities such as sport are safe at around the same time, providing she feels fit, but heavy lifting should be avoided for several months, because the scar, although superficially well healed, will still be undergoing a degree of tissue strengthening and repair.

Women who have had an ectopic pregnancy are bound to worry about this happening again and may have fears about future fertility. These should be discussed with an appropriate member of staff before leaving hospital, as it is likely that some alternative form of contraception to the IUCD or progesterone only pill may have to be found. It is possible to conceive and have a normal pregnancy when left with only one fallopian tube, but expert advice is needed, as chances vary with the extent of surgery performed.

4.3(d) INTRAUTERINE DEATH

This tragic event is the death of a baby within the uterus occurring during or after the 28th week of pregnancy (it is very likely that this will soon be changed to the 24th week of gestation). When the baby is delivered it is said to be stillborn. In England in 1988 there were five stillbirths amongst every 1,000 babies born but the comparative rarity of the situation will be of no comfort to the families involved.

Prevention

It is rare that any blame can be apportioned in relation to intrauterine death but an awareness of certain factors can be helpful.

- Pregnant women of this gestation should feel their baby move at least ten times daily.

See section 4.5(c) below for a description of the 'show'

- Vaginal bleeding in pregnancy is not normal (apart from the bloodstaining which may accompany the 'show').

- Acute or persistent abdominal pain is not normal.

Any deviation from normal should quickly be reported to the maternity hospital, community midwife or family doctor. Regular attendance for antenatal care will also enable a check to be kept on the baby's well-being. Smoking and excessive alcohol consumption are not advised during pregnancy.

Investigation if there is concern

Should there be concern about a baby's condition a cardio-tocograph (CTG) recording will be attempted; this is a simultaneous recording of the baby's heart rate and any contractions of the uterus which may be taking place. The reaction of the baby's heart rate to any movements he may make or to contractions can give some indication as to whether he is short of oxygen. If the heart rate cannot be heard, the baby's death will probably be confirmed by an ultrasound scan. It is best if the woman has a companion of her choice at this time. This may well be her partner and for simplicity's sake will be considered to be so for the remainder of this section.

Care following intrauterine death

If intrauterine death has occurred it is usually suggested that labour should be induced fairly soon but for psychological reasons some women prefer to go home first before being admitted to the maternity hospital for induction. A substance called prostaglandin which is normally produced by the uterus during labour is most likely to be used, and is inserted into the vagina as a jelly or pessary. Sometimes an intravenous infusion (drip) containing syntocinon is also needed to cause contractions of sufficient strength to dilate the cervix. Occasionally an intrauterine death may occur after labour has already begun.

See section 4.5(b) for information about care during labour

The care given during labour will differ very little from that given to a woman with a live baby, but of course the baby's heart will not be recorded. The choice of methods to relieve the pain of labour is the same but injections of diamorphine may be offered instead of pethidine as it is perhaps a better analgesic and produces more of a sense of well-being and detachment. It is however important that the mother perceives the birth of her baby as having been a reality so that her grieving is not inhibited. Every effort will be made to limit the number of people providing care during labour and the baby will be handled as carefully at delivery as if he was alive. A forceps delivery is unlikely to be necessary.

See section 4.3(e) below, discussing the importance of grieving

It is very difficult to grieve for a person of whom one has no memory and evidence suggests that parents often find it very helpful to see and hold their baby. The midwife will discuss this with them and, if they wish to do so, will describe the baby's appearance. It is usual to suggest that any abnormalities should be covered initially and the coverings removed when and if the parents choose. Most parents find their baby very beautiful and may want to have time alone with him both now and during the next few days.

Many hospitals take a photograph of the baby which they keep in the mother's notes if she does not wish to be given it at the time. A lock of hair is another momento which may be treasured. Naming the baby can also help parents to acknowledge the reality of what has happened.

The mother may be offered the choice of being transferred to either an antenatal or a postnatal ward and some women prefer to face the trauma of seeing and hearing other people's live babies for the first time while they are still in hospital. It is usual to give the mother a single room and it may be possible for a double bed to be made available; some couples welcome physical closeness at this time, for others it may not feel appropriate.

The mother will decide how long she wishes to stay in hospital after delivery. Once she has gone home, the midwife will continue to visit her at least until the 10th day after the baby was born. Despite the fact that she has no baby to feed, the mother will still find that her breasts fill with milk about three or four days after delivery; tablets can be prescribed to prevent this from happening but if this is not considered desirable the situation will resolve itself quite naturally within a few days provided that a firm brassière is worn and no milk is removed.

The mother or father will have to register the stillbirth of the baby and it is fairly common for the Registrar to have an office within the maternity hospital. The Registrar will provide both a Certificate of Registration of Stillbirth which the parents can keep as official acknowledgement that their baby existed and a Certificate for Burial or Cremation which must be given to the undertaker. Parents can either choose to make their own arrangements for burial or cremation or ask the hospital to do this for them. Even if they do the latter, it is usually possible for a Minister of Religion to officiate if this is what they wish. Parents may find that attending the ceremony helps them to focus their grief and erecting a memorial plaque may provide comfort later. No other baby will ever take the place of the one which has died and time should be allowed for some some emotional healing to take place before any further pregnancy is embarked upon.

Several weeks after the delivery the parents will be offered an appointment with a doctor (usually the Consultant Obstetrician) to discuss any information available as to why their baby died (permission for a post-mortem examination will have been sought soon after delivery). It is helpful if this information is also provided in writing, as people under stress often have difficulty in remembering what has been said to them.

4.3(e) LOSS AND GRIEF

Infertility, miscarriage, termination of pregnancy, pre-term delivery, the birth of a handicapped baby or one of the 'wrong' sex, giving a baby up for adoption, stillbirth or the death of a young child are some of the possible causes of grief which may be related to childbearing. Grief may be no less if pregnancy has only lasted a short time, for dreams and self-esteem have often been lost and replaced by feelings of inadequacy and a lack of control over destiny.

Grieving is often described as having several stages but not all individuals will experience the same reactions and it is impossible to give any guidance as to how long each stage is likely to last. Sometimes more than one stage is experienced at the same time.

What grieving people have in common however is that they need to work through their grief so that they may regain a degree of self-acceptance and have enough emotional energy to invest in other relationships.

The grieving process

The first stage of the grieving process is disbelief. After the initial shock there is numbness, as if the person is being being protected from emotions which would otherwise be overwhelming. The person denies that the event has occurred and this is probably a psychological defence mechanism which occurs whilst the subconscious is adjusting to the news and preparing to defend itself in other ways.

The second stage is one of developing awareness. Anger is expressed, often against those who have done nothing to deserve it. God, medical and midwifery staff, the partner and the baby are often the targets of the rage and valuable friends may be alienated, becoming angry in return. There is likely to be envy of those who have borne children successfully and a deep sense of guilt may be felt even though this is usually quite unjustified. Bargaining may take place, in which the grieving person promises (often to herself or to God) that she will do certain things if only the tragedy can be reversed. A great sense of loss is felt along with depression, emptiness and pining and there may be physical manifestations such as arms which ache to hold the baby.

The third stage is acceptance and readjustment. It may take two or three years to achieve this, but even then it is still quite usual for deep feelings of sadness to return on significant anniversaries or at certain family events.

It is worth mentioning that the health care professionals may also feel that they have failed and undergo a form of grieving process.

Care of those who are grieving

Probably more than anything else, those who are grieving need someone who is prepared to spend time with them, listening to what they have to say, or maybe just in silence. If parents are very deeply distressed it may be necessary to maintain some sort of physical contact, such as an arm around their shoulders, if they are to remain aware of their companion's presence. It is important to be non-judgmental even if sentiments are expressed with which one does not agree.

Support societies may be able to provide help through counselling as this may be a role which relatives and friends find especially difficult as they too have feelings of grief which they need to work through. Some friends have no idea what to say and handle the situation by pretending that the baby never existed; parents can find this especially hurtful.

See also Chapter 3, section 10, Bereavement and loss

See Appendix VII for Addresses of useful organisations and support groups

In the case of both miscarriage and adoption the same difficulty exists as for parents of stillborn babies – it is very difficult to grieve for someone of whom one has no memory. Mothers who are giving their babies up for adoption are now encouraged to see and hold them, if not to care for them for a few days, and many women who have miscarried wish to see their babies. It is important that the sex of a miscarried baby is known so that the parents can name it. It is becoming more common for parents who have undergone a miscarriage, or in some circumstances a termination of pregnancy, to request the burial of their baby.

Care of brothers and sisters

Children's questions should be answered honestly as they will usually sense that something is wrong and will become distrustful of adults who seek to protect them from the truth. It is not unusual for children to have had very mixed feelings about the impending birth of another baby, and they may now experience considerable guilt for having felt angry or jealous; they may in fact feel responsible for the tragedy. Children are thought not to accept the finality of death until they are about four or five years of age, and an adult understanding of death is probably not reached until the age of puberty.

4.4   ANTENATAL CARE

Having a baby is usually one of the most important events of a woman's life and one that will be remembered and talked about a great deal. Most of pregnancy is taken up with thoughts of the labour and, once this has passed, the future of the rest of parenthood begins. The whole process is awesome – and rightly so – the responsibility of the parents for their child starts before conception and lasts until the child is at least 18 years old.

Antenatal care, which has developed into a speciality since the beginning of this century, has as its aim a healthy, happy mother who will give birth to a thriving baby. 'Parentcraft' (education for parenthood, as well as preparation for the birth itself) is also an important feature of the antenatal period.

4.4(a)   THE PEOPLE YOU WILL MEET

There are three groups of health professionals who specialise in the care of pregnant women and their babies – midwives, doctors and health visitors. In order to give effective care, they liaise with each other and work as a team. Of course not all doctors are male – and, indeed, not all midwives or health visitors are female.

Midwives   A midwife (literally 'with woman') is a specially trained professional, skilled in the conduct of normal pregnancy and childbirth, who is capable of looking after you without reference to the doctor unless complications arise. Her role is also that of educator, so she will be involved in parentcraft classes and teaching individual mothers about baby care.

In the United Kingdom, a midwife will continue to visit you at home for some days following the birth. This will enable her to ensure that both you and your baby are coping well.

Doctors   The doctors whom you meet will have different specialities. Your general practitioner (family doctor) whom you already know may or may not give you maternity care. If he does not, then he will refer you to one who does, probably in the same practice. Maternity care is only part of the work of the family doctor but the hospital doctor will specialise in maternity work or obstetrics. You will probably meet doctors at different stages of their careers, from juniors to consultants. Other specialists whose work brings them into contact with childbearing women or their babies are paediatricians, who work with babies and children, and anaesthetists, who are involved with pain relief and operations.

As well as referring you to the hospital, and perhaps giving some of your antenatal care himself, your family doctor will always be available if you need a visit because you or your baby are unwell.

Health visitors   The health visitor is a nurse with an extra qualification in her specialist field. She may or may not be a midwife too. Her role is to help you to adapt to parenthood and to monitor your own and the baby's physical and emotional well-being. You may meet her at the antenatal clinic, parentcraft class or when she comes to see you at home after the birth. She will be able to visit as often as necessary and will introduce you to the baby clinic and tell you about immunisations to protect your baby from certain infections. She will also perform regular developmental checks on your child up to the age of five.

See Appendix IV for more details about Immunisations

4.4(b)   PREPARING FOR PARENTHOOD

The antenatal clinic

The exact pattern of antenatal care varies slightly in different areas but the principles are the same. At the first visit to the hospital, at what is called the booking clinic, a detailed medical history is taken to see if there are any conditions which need special attention. You will be asked about the health of close members of your family as some conditions can be carried down to an unborn child. If you have children already, you will be asked about those pregnancies and deliveries so that a full picture can be built up of you as an individual and you can receive the best possible care. Sometimes these details are taken by a midwife visiting your home. You will be asked to have a blood test for routine purposes. At this and every visit you will be weighed, asked to produce a specimen of your urine and have your blood pressure checked.

Records are kept on paper or cards and you will probably have a copy to take away with you. Some of the terms that may be found in your notes are explained in the box below.

Antenatal care can be given by a midwife, family doctor or hospital doctor (obstetrician). It can be given in your own home, at the local surgery or health centre or at the hospital. Visits usually take place monthly at first until 28 weeks, then fortnightly until 36 weeks and then weekly until you have your baby.

See the section below on Tests during pregnancy

Understanding your notes

The chart gives some of the terms and abbreviations you may find in your notes, together with explanations

---

DATE: of your antenatal visit

WEEKS: the duration of your pregnancy

WEIGHT: given in kg. The average weight gain for the total pregnancy is 9–14 kg

URINE: tested at each appointment for protein and glucose.'NAD' means 'nothing abnormal detected'

B.P.: blood pressure. Monitored at every visit

HEIGHT FUNDUS: the height in cms of the top of your growing womb

PRESENTATION OR POSITION: 'Ceph' is short for 'cephalic', i.e. head down. 'Breech' means that the baby's bottom is downwards

RELATION OF P.P. TO BRIM: the position of the presenting part (i.e. the head in a baby whose presentation is cephalic, the bottom in a baby whose presentation is breech) in relation to the brim of your bony pelvis. 'Not eng' or 'Free' means that the presenting part has not yet 'engaged' or dropped down into your pelvis. Engagement is measured in fifths

F.H.: 'fetal heart'.FHH means 'fetal heartbeat heard'

OEDEMA: swelling – usually of the fingers, feet, ankles, or face

Hb: Haemoglobin level; if this is low (below about 11) your doctor may prescribe iron supplements

Your blood group will be noted, along with whether you are rhesus positive (Rh+) or rhesus negative (Rh–) and the results of specific blood tests

---

Progress through pregnancy

Pregnancy is defined as the period of time from conception to the birth of the baby. However, because the exact date of conception is not often known, it is more convenient to calculate it from the first day of the last period (see the box opposite). Using this measurement, it is 40 weeks long, give or take a couple of weeks.

Formula for calculating the estimated date of delivery (EDD)

- Take the date of your last menstrual period (e.g. 22 August 1992)
- Add 7 days (29 August 1992)
- Now add 9 calendar months
- EDD is 29 May 1993

NB.   Do remember that the EDD is not a certain prediction of when your baby will arrive – an estimated 3% only will actually be born on this date. Babies can arrive quite happily and safely for two weeks either side of the EDD, and are more likely to be late than early.

At the first visit to your doctor, he will work out an estimated date of delivery for you. Doctors and midwives break pregnancy up into three equal parts called trimesters for convenience. Each trimester therefore represents just over three months.

You will be well into the first trimester by the time your pregnancy is confirmed. You may be experiencing morning sickness and changes in your breasts. It is also usual to need to go to the toilet to pass urine more frequently. Although you do not look pregnant, your body is changing quite rapidly and you need plenty of rest. You will meet the professionals who will look after you through your pregnancy, delivery and afterwards and be asked to attend an antenatal clinic so that your well-being and that of your unborn child can be monitored carefully. You should also be given the chance to come to classes which offer you education for your new role as a parent. Mothers-to-be are entitled to time off work without loss of pay for visits to antenatal clinics and parentcraft classes.

The second trimester is usually a period of growth and adjustment to your new situation. During this time you will change into maternity clothes as the baby in your womb grows and develops. Many women describe feeling very well with hair and skin condition improving.

Into the third trimester the unborn child is fully developed with a good chance of survival outside the womb if it is born early. All that remains is for it to reach maturity and lay down some useful fat stores which will keep it warm after birth. The mother's weight increases at about 0.5 kg or 1 lb a week at this time. Overall, the average weight gain is 9–14 kg. The mother's body is also preparing for the pleasant task of feeding the baby and drops of a creamy fluid, colostrum, may be seen on the surface of the nipple.

See Chapter 5, section 1(a) for more information about colostrum and early feeding

The womb makes some practice (Braxton-Hicks) contractions which are felt as tightening up and hardening of the abdomen, without being painful. As the bladder has less room to expand, there is a need to go the toilet more frequently, including at night.

At the end of pregnancy your body is ready for the processes of birth and feeding, and your baby is ready to be born.

Tests during pregnancy

When first attending the doctor or hospital antenatal clinic, you will be offered a number of tests which have been developed in order to try to make sure that you and your unborn baby are in the best possible health. Some tests are performed only once, others may need to be repeated as the pregnancy progresses.

Tests on the mother   The very first test is usually the pregnancy test itself which is a straightforward urine test. At the booking clinic, the midwife or doctor will ask for another specimen of urine which will be tested for the presence of sugar, protein and micro-organisms or germs which may cause an infection in the bladder. This urine test will be repeated at every visit.

It is usual to have a specimen of blood taken at the first clinic visit from a vein in the arm. The midwife or doctor may do this or you could be asked to go to the laboratory to have it done. The blood specimen is examined for several reasons. Firstly, the blood group and rhesus factor will be noted; 15 per cent of women are rhesus negative and if the baby they are carrying is rhesus positive, special treatment may be needed. If this applies to you the staff will explain it all fully to you. The blood is also checked to see that you are not anaemic. All pregnant women need to increase their iron intake by eating foods such as red meat and dark green leafy vetables. Some will also need iron tablets. This test for anaemia will be repeated later on in the pregnancy.

It is also routine to test the blood for rubella (german measles) which can affect an unborn baby. If you are not resistant to rubella because you have never had it nor been vaccinated, you will be offered the vaccination *after* you have had your baby. Another routine test is for syphilis which can be treated successfully in pregnancy so, although only a tiny number of women are affected, it is worthwhile. It is not routine to test for the AIDS virus, although blood samples may be taken anonymously as part of a national screening programme to see how the disease is spreading. You are not obliged to have any of these tests and if you are at all concerned you should discuss your anxieties with your doctor or midwife.

As well as the tests mentioned above, your breasts may be checked for normal growth and the baby, or fetus as it is called, will be felt through your abdomen as the weeks progress. The size of the fetus can be assessed by ultrasound scan which is offered routinely in many hospitals. You will have an opportunity to ask any questions and obtain advice about health matters, financial problems or any worry you may have. If you need to have a female doctor, that

- **Anaemia**
  Reduced oxygen carrying capacity of the blood due to a low level of haemoglobin (the oxygen carrying pigment in the red blood cells). Haemoglobin levels can be raised by increasing your iron intake

can be arranged for you too. Parencraft classes will be offered and, if you are able to attend these, they should be helpful. Many hospitals will offer the opportunity to see the delivery ward before you go into labour and this can be reassuring.

Monitoring the well-being of the baby   When the baby has grown to about 12 weeks size, the top of the womb can just be felt above the pubic bone in the front of the abdomen. At each visit, the doctor or midwife will feel the top of this bump as it grows and record their

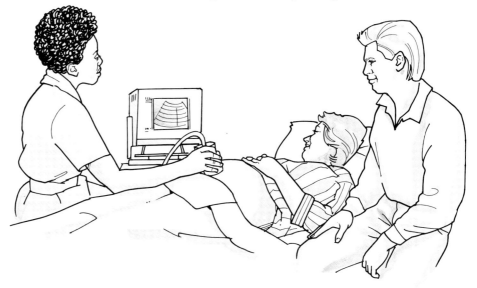

findings. As the baby gets bigger, movements can be felt and limbs or bottom can be identified. The heartbeat can be heard in several ways, through a trumpet style stethoscope, with the help of a little microphone which you can hear too, or you can see the heartbeat when you have a scan.

An ultrasound scan is often performed at or around the time of booking. A very accurate assessment of the fetus's age can be made from the scan. The operator will also be able to see whether certain key organs are developing properly. Some hospitals perform a second ultrasound scan later on in the pregnancy to check the baby's size.

One of the blood tests performed at about 16 weeks is to check the level of a certain protein (alphafetoprotein) in the baby. Very high or low levels may indicate a rare but serious abnormality which would require further investigation.

Finally, some women – such as those over 35 or women who have a family history of certain abnormalities – will be offered specific extra tests. Perhaps the most common of these is amniocentesis which involves taking a sample of the fluid from around the baby through a needle which goes into the womb as shown in the figure.

Amniocentesis

This test involves the taking of a sample of the amniotic fluid which surrounds the baby in the womb

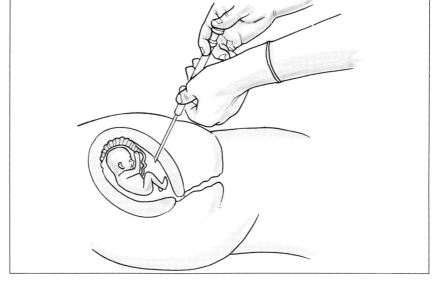

The cells in this sample can be cultured and analysed. A newer test, chorionic villus sampling (CVS), can be performed much earlier as the placenta or afterbirth develops but this is not available everywhere. A further, noninvasive test (involving the checking of levels of several different hormones in a sample of blood) has been developed recently and is gradually coming into use.

Tests to screen for fetal abnormalities should be accompanied by counselling in case they should be positive and the question of terminating the pregnancy arises. Never be afraid to ask for more information from the midwife or doctor if you do not understand fully what is being offered to you.

See section 4.3(a) for more information about Termination of pregnancy

See Appendix VII for Addresses of useful organisations and support groups

Parentcraft

Parentcraft classes are offered by health authorities to some, if not all, pregnant women who book for delivery in the area. In addition, private classes are usually available through organisations such as the National Childbirth Trust. Classes are designed to increase your knowledge about the processes of childbirth and child rearing, to enable you to ask questions and offload anxieties and to maintain or improve your physical well-being. The health service classes are usually organised by a midwife or health visitor although other members of the health care team may be brought in from time to time. Private classes are run by specially trained women who are parents themselves.

One important feature of the classes, wherever they are held, is that you have the chance to meet and share your experiences with others from your neighbourhood who are going through them too. Friendships can be forged which will last right through your children's school life, providing a great deal of support.

Some teachers offer an early class at about 12 weeks of pregnancy in order to discuss the points which are relevant at the time and the problems which have disappeared by the time the later classes come along. Otherwise they usually begin at about 30 weeks and will take place weekly for 6–8 weeks. Daytime classes are usually for mothers only and evening ones for couples.

In class, you will learn about how your body is changing with pregnancy and how a fetus grows. Labour will be explained – how it starts and what you should do about coming in to hospital. Pain relief will be discussed fully and most women find this an important and helpful session. Once your baby is born, he will need to be fed and this topic usually takes up another complete class. Sometimes it is possible to mix with women who have had babies before so that there is an exchange of experiences, or to get newly delivered mothers to attend and talk about what they have found helpful. It is by sharing and discussing that any fears can be brought out into the open. It is usual to find that your concerns are shared by many others and this can be very reassuring.

Some simple exercises to keep you supple are likely to be taught, as well as breathing and relaxation techniques for labour. These can be very helpful, especially if they are practised at home as well. You will also be taught exercises for the muscles of your pelvic floor.

Smoking, alcohol and drugs

The idea of this section is not to alarm you but to make you aware of the danger of smoking, alcohol or drugs both to you and your baby. Help, if you need it, will be available from your midwife, doctor or health visitor.

Smoking has been associated with chest and heart disease for many years now, yet people still smoke and find it difficult if not impossible to stop because nicotine is addictive. Unfortunately, the unborn baby has no choice but to take in nicotine when his mother smokes and this, together with gases which deprive him of oxygen, can lead to a situation where his growth is stunted and his mental development can be affected. It has never been possible to say what is a safe number of cigarettes to smoke because babies are individual and some are more susceptible than others. Obviously it is best not to smoke at all but if that is not possible, try to reduce to the lowest level you can manage. There are special groups in some areas which offer support and may be helpful. You could try putting the money you would spend on smoking in a jar to buy something for the baby or for yourself. Talk it over with someone who has had a similar problem and learn how they coped with it.

We now know that alcohol harms the developing baby's brain and like smoking, drinking should ideally be discontinued while you are pregnant. Again, we do not really have a safe level, but at the

See section 4.5 below for more information about labour and pain relief

See Chapter 5, section 1(a) for more information on feeding the newborn baby

See section 4.6(c) below for more information about pelvic floor exercises

See Chapter 7, section 10(k) for more information about the health problems associated with smoking, alcohol and drugs

See section 4.1(b) above on Preconception care

moment it is thought that the occasional social drink is probably not harmful. Regular, heavy drinking is dangerous but difficult to stop as the addiction is very powerful.

Addiction to drugs is a problem which requires urgent and professional help if the baby is not to suffer. Babies of addicts will need special care at birth as they themselves will have to be weaned off the harmful substance.

Prescribed drugs   It is important to take only drugs which have been prescribed for you personally, by a doctor who knows that you are pregnant. Certain drugs which are in common use are known to harm unborn babies and you should never take tablets belonging to someone else or old ones given to you before you were pregnant.

Sex during pregnancy

There is sometimes a reluctance to discuss the question of sexual intercourse during and after pregnancy with medical and midwifery staff, although a concern with this question is the most natural concern in the world for two people who love each other and have expressed that love in the conception of a baby.

There is no reason why most couples should not continue to make love as and when they want to. A small number of women who have had problems with miscarriage in the past will be advised to avoid lovemaking when their period would have occurred for the first 3–4 months of pregnancy.

The pregnancy will cause certain changes however. The sex drive can change during this time, either increasing or decreasing. Hormonal changes can give a pregnant woman mood swings which may be unpredictable and this can make communication difficult. It is important to try to keep talking about feelings so that both partners can understand the changes which are taking place.

Lovemaking may become uncomfortable in late pregnancy, especially if the usual position of man on top is used. Instead of discontinuing sex altogether, you could try different positions to get more comfortable – for example, lying on your side with your partner behind you. You may find that the normal vaginal lubrication is lacking (although this is more commonly the case after delivery than before). A safe and effective lubricant (e.g. K-Y jelly) can be bought from the chemist to help this problem.

Some men express the fear of hurting the baby during lovemaking, especially when the birth is close, but this is almost impossible within the normal range of activities.

Of course, you may both decide that you do not feel like vaginal intercourse at this time and if that is the case then you can still enjoy being close to each other and having a cuddle or caressing each other to a climax.

4.4(c) MINOR DISORDERS OF PREGNANCY

Being pregnant affects all the systems of the body. Some of the changes which occur are experienced as strange and uncomfortable just because they are unusual. Feeling the baby move and kick, for example, is a sensation which is unique and hard to describe. While this is not actually painful, it may cause some discomfort at times.

There are some well known minor disorders which would not send you to a doctor but respond well to a little explanation, reassurance or simple remedies. Some of these are described below. Remember, though, that if you are worried about any of your physical or psychological feelings during pregnancy, your doctor and midwife will be able to help and advise you.

Constipation

This is perhaps the most common minor disorder of pregnancy. It is caused by the slowing down of waste products passing through the digestive system which is affected by a hormone, progesterone. This hormone affects all the tubular structures of the body, making them dilate slightly and relax. Thus pregnant women may find themselves not only constipated but also suffering from haemorrhoids (piles).

Constipation can be prevented to an extent by altering the nature of the food you eat and drinking plenty of fluids. Fibre in the diet is an important feature. This can be obtained from breakfast cereals high in fibre such as ones containing a high proportion of bran. Fresh fruit and vegetables, especially with the skin on, are preferable not only for their fibre content but also for the conservation of vitamins.

Pregnant women often cut back on the amount of fluids that they drink because they are worried about putting on weight or getting swollen legs. Also, they do not want to be going to the toilet all the time. However, it is important to drink plenty of liquid. This does not have to be sugary or milky and thus high in calories. You could try mineral water, diluted fruit juice, drinks made from vegetable or meat stock cubes or low calorie fruit squashes.

It may be necessary to use a laxative occasionally but this should not be habitual. If you find that the problem persists in spite of the simple measures outlined above, do discuss it with the midwife who will advise you of the safest forms of laxative to take. You should avoid oily preparations, such as liquid paraffin, as they coat the gut and prevent the absorption of valuable food substances.

Morning sickness

This is one of the least pleasant aspects of being pregnant. It affects at least 45 per cent of women and can cause a lot of disruption to your daily routine and to that of your family.

Nausea is more common than actual vomiting. Both are characteristically present in the mornings because the hormone levels responsible for the condition are highest in the mornings. Some women find that sickness occurs at other times of day too.

Gradually, your body becomes accustomed to the new hormone levels and the symptoms subside. For a few unfortunate women sickness persists beyond 10–12 weeks and an even smaller number experience it throughout the pregnancy. Fortunately, once the baby is born, all symptoms disappear.

Feeling sick like this can certainly make you feel low and off your food, so weight loss may occur. Some suggestions for coping with nausea and vomiting are given below.

- If you are working, ask your employer if you could work in a more flexible way for a few weeks so that you could avoid rush hour travel as hot crowded trains or buses are the worst environment for you.

- If you are at home try to get help with the early morning routine of getting other children up and dressed and possibly off to school.

- When you wake get a cup of tea and a dry biscuit or piece of dry toast, or persuade someone else to do this for you.

- Get up slowly.

- Have plenty of drinks throughout the day and small frequent snack meals rather than one or two large ones.

- Always consider your food intake sensibly and avoid gimmicky foods or too much of the same thing. A balanced diet is always best for you and your unborn baby.

- Some women find eating dry crackers, or ginger biscuits, or drinking fizzy drinks such as carbonated mineral water, is helpful in staving off nausea.

Vomiting in pregnancy: when to call your doctor

- If you are more than 14 weeks pregnant and vomiting is still causing you to lose weight.
- If you are really not managing to keep anything down, or if vomiting is accompanied by diarrhoea – you may become dehydrated.
- Sudden onset vomiting accompanied by other signs of being unwell may be due to an infection which will need treatment.
- Persistent nausea and vomiting after 12–14 weeks may have an additional cause – for example, if you are taking iron supplements these could be disagreeing with you. Your doctor will prescribe an alternative preparation.

There are no easy cures for this condition. Tell your midwife or doctor when you see her; she may make further useful suggestions. In certain, particularly acute, circumstances you should contact your doctor without waiting for your next antenatal appointment. There are some treatments available which will reduce the sickness but they often make you feel very sleepy and dry mouthed. Such medication is only available on prescription and you should never take anything given by a friend but only if it has been prescribed specifically for you.

Heartburn

Heartburn is an unpleasant sensation which can be felt when the acid contents of the stomach pass into the gullet, or when bile passes upward from the small intestine. This can happen to anybody but it is common in pregnancy, especially in the second half. It is usually felt when you are lying down so it is common at night and may prevent you from sleeping.

It is due to the following changes which take place in your body in pregnancy. Firstly, the growing uterus pushes the stomach out of place and squashes it so that it cannot hold so much food. The contents of the stomach are therefore more likely to be in the upper part of the stomach. Secondly, the ring of muscle at the top of the stomach which normally holds the stomach contents in, relaxes a little under the influence of the hormones of pregnancy. This means that reflux of the stomach acid or bile can occur causing the heartburn.

The condition disappears completely when the pregnancy is over but that may be some time away. There are some things that you can do to decrease the chances of heartburn and to relieve it when it occurs.

- Eat small frequent meals rather than large ones once or twice a day and experiment with the type of food you eat. You may find that hot, spicy food is not good for you whereas bland foods and milky foods are better tolerated.

- A milky drink last thing at night helps in some cases.

- Give yourself an extra pillow or two so you are not so flat in bed (see the left hand figure overleaf).

- Do tell your midwife or doctor when you go to the clinic as they may have more useful advice. They may also wish to give you some antacid tablets or medicine to take but you should not use these without medical advice on a regular basis as they can impair your absorption of valuable foodstuffs.

- The occasional use of over the counter antacids is permitted but do tell your midwife when you see her.

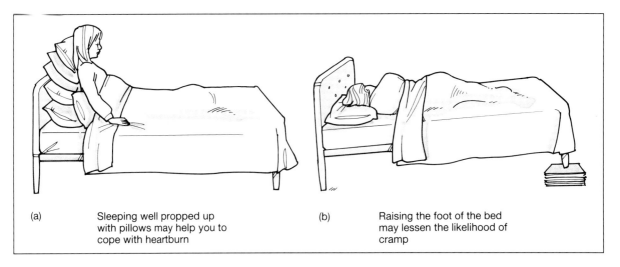

(a) Sleeping well propped up with pillows may help you to cope with heartburn

(b) Raising the foot of the bed may lessen the likelihood of cramp

Cramp

Cramp is an unpleasant and painful muscle spasm which can affect anybody but is especially common in pregnancy.

Characteristically, it occurs at night when you are lying down and straightening the legs. The muscle at the back of the calf goes into spasm causing a pain which wakes you up if you were asleep and for a moment you are taken by surprise and do not know what to do. Unfortunately the cause of this is not fully understood and therefore treatments can only be aimed at relieving the symptoms rather than curing the condition. Some authorities think that cramp may be due to changes in the rate of blood flow within the veins of the legs as the pregnancy progresses. Others have suggested that there may be a shortage of certain minerals in the blood in pregnancy but no dietary adjustment seems to bring relief.

It may be helpful to elevate the foot of the bed a few inches by putting large books such as telephone directories under the legs of the bed. This must be on both sides, obviously, to prevent damage to the bed (see the right hand figure above).

When an attack occurs, sit up and pull your foot up towards your shin slowly and deliberately. This should have the effect of stretching the muscle and removing the spasm. Getting your partner to massage the affected leg is also beneficial. Although cramp is unpleasant for you and disturbs your sleep it is not a harmful condition and will pass once the baby has been born.

Stretch marks

Stretch marks can appear in certain medical conditions or as a result of treatment but they are a common occurrence in pregnancy when they are known as *striae gravidarum* – stretch marks of pregnancy. They are thought to be due to the extra weight which you put on during pregnancy which stretches the underlying tissues of the skin. The hormones circulating in your bloodstream may assist in this process and there also seems to be a familial tendency as two women of the same weight will not necessarily have the same amount of stretch marking. Striae may be seen on the abdomen, usually low down at first and also on the breasts, buttocks and upper thighs. Some individuals are not affected at all, others have only a few, but some women are badly affected and feel their stretch marks are unsightly.

The good news is that they fade from a deep pink colour in pregnancy to a silvery shade that is almost invisible a few months after the birth.

As far as preventing stretch marks is concerned, there is little you can do except keep your skin moisturised by using a cream or oil every night on your abdomen and breasts. This will reduce itching which is produced by the stretching skin and can be very uncomfortable. There is no proof that any particular product is better than another so there is no point in spending a lot of money when an ordinary moisturiser will do just as well.

It is important get a brassière which will support the breasts well and this will help to prevent sagging as well as stretch marks. You may feel a support pantie girdle would be helpful if you are a large size or expecting more than one baby. You should always try these on before buying to see that they are comfortable and the right size.

Remember even if you have quite noticeable stretch marks now, they will fade later. A little flesh coloured make up can be used if necessary on the beach if you feel they are very obvious.

4.4(d) COMPLICATIONS OF PREGNANCY

Pregnancy is not an illness and most women experience little more than the occasional minor disorder. True complications of pregnancy are not nearly so common and attendance at the antenatal clinic should serve to monitor your well-being and alert the midwife or doctor to any health problem so that it can be sorted out quickly.

Sometimes, however, a woman becomes pregnant having a condition (diabetes mellitus, for example) which has already been recognised and treated. On the other hand, complications may arise as the pregnancy progresses, necessitating treatment in or out of hospital. In a book such as this, it is not possible to discuss all the complications which may occur and if you are unfortunate enough to encounter a major complication, the health professionals looking after you will be able to explain the condition and the treatment at the time. It may be helpful, however, to consider some of the complications which can occur while you are at home and therefore alert you to calling for further help.

Urinary problems

Anatomically, the urinary tract and the reproductive organs lie extremely close to each other in the pelvis. They actually share the same nerves and blood supplies so it is not surprising that, when the reproductive system is undergoing the major changes associated with childbirth, the urinary tract gives some unusual sensations. It is also more susceptible to infection at this time.

The first thing you may notice when you become pregnant is that you want to go to the toilet more frequently. This feeling will wear off after a few weeks as your body gets used to the hormones of pregnancy and the growing womb moves up and out of the pelvis, but it is likely to return in the last few weeks. When the baby's head, settled deep in the pelvis, presses on the bladder, it will give you the urge to urinate. This may occur frequently during the day and, unfortunately, during the night too. There is little you can do about it except get up and go, for if you lie in bed hoping it will pass off, it will not and you will not be able to get back to sleep.

That is simply a nuisance but there is another common problem which afflicts pregnant women which can be rather more embarrassing. Stress incontinence is the name given to the condition when coughing, sneezing, running or the like causes you to leak some urine. Obviously, getting wet can be uncomfortable and may cause embarrassment. It does not happen to everyone, but if you find that you are affected you should try extra hard to master pelvic floor exercises which will improve the tone of the muscles which control the bladder. The earlier in your pregnancy you can start these, the better. Keep doing them after the baby is born as well in order to maintain good muscle tone.

See section 4.6(c) for a full explanation of pelvic floor exercises

Urinary tract infections   Such infections are not only unpleasant, they can also be dangerous in pregnancy as kidneys will be more easily affected than at other times. The symptoms of such an infection are a frequent need to visit the toilet, a burning sensation when passing urine, and urine which is cloudy and smelly or even blood-stained. You may have pain in the lower abdomen or back and feel generally unwell with a temperature. You will need to see your doctor as soon as possible and, in the meantime, drink at least one glass of water each half hour in order to dilute the urine. A mild painkiller such as paracetamol may be taken and a hot water bottle is very soothing. If symptoms are very severe, ask the doctor to call and put yourself to bed. Save a specimen of your urine as he may want to send this for testing before prescribing antibiotics for you.

See section 4.3(b) for more information about miscarriage and threatened miscarriage

See section 4.5(b) for more information about the start of labour

Vaginal bleeding

Bleeding from the genital tract at any stage of pregnancy is abnormal and should be investigated. In early pregnancy, it may be the first sign of a miscarriage. At the very end of pregnancy, a mucousy, bloodstained loss called the 'show' can herald the start of labour but this is not usually heavy or prolonged. A call to the midwife will usually put your mind at rest. Bleeding in late pregnancy may be due to an infection which is easily cleared up with antibiotics or it could be something more serious.

Sometimes, the placenta or afterbirth forms in the lower part of the uterus or womb instead of in the upper part. The condition is called *placenta praevia* which means 'placenta in front'. As the baby grows and moves, the placenta can become partly separated and blood is lost. This takes place at or after six months of pregnancy and, characteristically, is a sudden and painless blood loss. It is a potentially serious situation for the baby and the mother must call for medical help at once. The bleeding may settle down and the pregnancy be allowed to continue once it has been established that the baby is well. Sometimes, however, it is necessary to deliver the baby and usually this will have to be achieved by caesarean section. In most cases, delivery when the pregnancy is fully advanced will also have to be by caesarean section as part of the placenta may be lying over the cervix.

- **Cervix**
  The neck of the womb

Causes of vaginal bleeding in pregnancy

Time	Cause
Early/mid pregnancy	Threatened miscarriage
Mid/late pregnancy	Placenta praevia (placenta lying near or over the neck of the womb) Infection or placental damage
Term (if brown or mucousy rather than bright, fresh blood)	The 'show' – indicating that labour is about to begin. The 'show' consists largely of mucus and should not contain more than a teaspoon of blood

In other cases, the placenta is correctly situated but separates from the wall of the womb, possibly due to high blood pressure. Again, the doctor must be called and he will want to transfer the mother to hospital where the condition of the baby can be ascertained and the correct investigations and treatment carried out.

Significant bleeding from the genital tract occurs in only 3 per cent of pregnancies but it must always be taken seriously and medical help sought.

High blood pressure

Your blood pressure is measured at each visit to the antenatal clinic. Measurements in early pregnancy are used as a baseline for later on and usually there is a slight fall in the middle months with a resumption to the earlier level at the end. Sometimes the level rises and may be accompanied by swelling of the feet, hands and even face. Some slight swelling of the extremities is common in pregnancy, especially in hot weather. However high blood pressure is always taken seriously and even more so if protein is found in the urine. The condition described by these findings is now called *pre-eclampsia* or *pregnancy-induced hypertension*. ('Toxaemia' was an earlier term, but this implies a poisoning of the blood which is misleading.) The cause is not fully understood but it is thought to be a condition of the placenta or afterbirth. It is certainly found more often where there is a large placental site, such as in a multiple pregnancy or when a large baby is expected, and it is also found more commonly in younger women expecting their first baby. About 5 per cent of all pregnancies are affected in this way.

There is a risk that the baby will not grow adequately as the nutrient supply from the mother to the baby is insufficient. The mother's health can also be jeopardised by her very high blood pressure; in extreme cases, fits of an epileptic type may occur.

If the blood pressure is taken regularly and a moderate rise is discovered, then resting at home may well have a beneficial effect. Sometimes this is not possible because of the home circumstances, or it does not work, and admission into hospital is recommended. If the situation continues to worsen, drugs will be used to bring the blood pressure down.

The condition of the baby is monitored carefully by CTGs (cardio-tocographs – graph-like recordings of the fetal heartbeat) and by ultrasound scanning to see that it is continuing to grow satisfactorily. If there is any doubt about the well-being of the baby, then delivery will be brought about, either by inducing labour or by performing a caesarean section.

It is usual for a woman to feel perfectly well if she has high blood pressure and it is not until it reaches a potentially dangerous level that she would have symptoms such as severe headache, vomiting and visual disturbances. This means that she finds it difficult to believe that the condition is serious and is inclined to 'carry on as usual' when she should rest.

If any of the above symptoms occur, especially in the last three months of pregnancy, then you should go to bed and call the doctor or midwife who will take the appropriate action. It may be just a false alarm but, because the risks – to you and your baby – are significant, they will not think that you are wasting their time and it will put your mind at rest.

HAVING THE BABY

The birth of a wanted baby is a joyous occasion, and a happy end to the many months of waiting. It is also, of course, a beginning: the first day of a lifetime of parenthood.

The birth of the baby invariably lasts less than one day, so it is important to prepare in whatever way you wish to make that day special. There are a number of choices which can be made about the 'birth experience' and it is important that the pregnant woman and her partner exercise their right to choose where and what is to happen at this experience. The pregnant woman ought to feel she has control and that giving birth is not just a series of 'things being done' to her. She must also feel that she has every right to change her mind if any of her decisions cease to feel appropriate.

4.5(a) WHERE TO HAVE YOUR BABY

There are a number of options as to where to have your baby and the decision will depend on the availability of choice and services in your particular area. Most babies in the United Kingdom are born in hospital (about 99 per cent, in fact and 1 per cent at home). In some other countries, for example Holland, many more babies are born at home. The decision of where to have your baby is discussed at the initial visit to your family doctor unless you have decided to commission an independent midwife, who would then be your first contact.

To find a local independent midwife you should contact one of the midwives' organisations listed in Appendix VII

There are a number of different schemes or options available when having your baby in hospital. Most women in Britain have what is known as 'shared care' whereby, once pregnancy is confirmed, visits are 'shared' between a suitably qualified general practitioner and a hospital team, normally headed by a consultant obstetrician (known as Mr not Dr) supported by a tier of doctors and/or midwives. The general practitioner often has a midwife attached to the practice and she may perform the antenatal examination instead of him.

Women who have known diseases which complicate pregnancy, such as diabetes or epilepsy, or where pregnancy exacerbates the condition such as heart disease, are usually seen only by the hospital obstetric team. If the hospital is many miles away, or nearer but difficult to get to by public transport, other arrangements are sometimes made. Satellite clinics are held in some inner city areas where the hospital obstetric team go out to clinics located within the community.

When medical complications arise in pregnancy the option of where to have the baby is usually restricted to a hospital consultant unit, which is frequently located alongside a general hospital. This has the advantage that physicians and surgeons are available to help control or correct complications as they occur, and can more easily keep the pregnancy under closer surveillance. If however physicians and surgeons are at another site, then unfortunately much time can be spent at outpatient appointments in two places. This may not be so bad if this is the first pregnancy, but obviously for those with other children it can become a real problem.

If this is not the first pregnancy and complications arose in previous pregnancies (including at the birth necessitating, for example, a caesarean section or difficult forceps delivery) then the choice of place of birth may be restricted to the consultant obstetric unit.

For the first pregnancy most women and virtually all doctors prefer the place of birth to be in a consultant obstetric unit. The reason for this is said to be that birth of a baby cannot be considered normal or uneventful except in retrospect. To put this in proportion, however, 80 per cent of births in this country are normal and only 20 per cent, one in five, require intervention by an obstetrician.

In some areas there are isolated maternity units run by general practitioners and midwives. These are becoming less common in the United Kingdom since a government report in 1980 suggested they be phased out. Often these are small local units, ideal for the uncomplicated pregnancy and therefore expected birth. They may be closer to the woman's home than centralised obstetric units, making it easier for visits by other children, family and friends. These units do not contain the advanced technology which may be required for the complicated birth but if one does arise unexpectedly, transfer to a consultant unit can be arranged.

Some such units are not isolated but are attached to consultant units, often taking up a floor of the same building. Women stay under the care of their family doctor and do not usually see a member of the consultant team unless complications arise, in which case care is transferred to the consultant obstetric team which is close at hand physically. The family doctor and his attached midwife, or a midwife from a team known to the woman, are present at the birth. Again in this type of unit equipment tends not to be very highly technological, but obviously if such equipment becomes necessary then the consultant unit is much nearer and transfer is easy.

Domino schemes are other options and can mean different things depending on the local system. The Domino usually refers to a birth which takes place in an obstetric unit, but which is attended by the woman's own family doctor and community midwife, usually with a short stay of six hours after the birth before returning home. Variations on this scheme include arrangements where only the community midwife is at the birth, with possible obstetric cover, or a longer hospital stay of up to 48 hours.

• 'Domino'
Stands for 'Domiciliary Midwife in/out' and affords a 'halfway house' between a home birth and full hospital care

Many progressive hospitals have a 'birthing room' or 'alternative' suite where the birth of the baby can be in non-medicalised surroundings, without the 'high tech' equipment found in the standard delivery rooms of a labour ward or central delivery suite.

The other place where you may choose to have your baby is at home. There has been much debate since the 1950s as to the safety of home births. If we remember that 80 per cent of births are normal and uncomplicated, then many more than the 1 per cent of babies who are now delivered at home could be. Providing again there are no complications of pregnancy, and no obvious foreseen complications of labour, there is no reason why birth should not be carried out at home. Obviously not all women or their partners may feel comfortable with this option, but it is an option. Unfortunately some family doctors may have had little experience of home births these days and are therefore reluctant to take on the responsibility. In the United Kingdom, however, providing a midwife is in attendance to a woman, there is no legal requirement to have a general practitioner present if one will not take on the case. It is often the policy of the district that two midwives are present at the home birth, or indeed any birth. Home births are usually provided with a back up service in case of an emergency, in the form of a Flying Squad/Emergency Obstetric Unit – an ambulance containing a senior obstetrician, an anaesthetist, senior midwife and possibly a paediatrician, with all the equipment necessary for most eventualities. However this service is being curtailed in many areas, for economic reasons, and with the move to encourage all births to be in hospital.

There are a growing number of independent midwives who offer to provide a complete 'package' of service from booking of pregnancy, home birth (usually) and postnatal care. These midwives are private and therefore charge a fee, which varies in amount. This arrangement of care ensures continuity and the one to one care throughout the birth experience, with someone whom you get to know quite well over a period of time, is ideal. If complications arise, transfer to hospital is obviously available and some independent midwives have an honorary contract with the local hospital to enable them to continue with your care once you have been admitted to hospital, if this is appropriate.

The choice of where to have your baby should be yours, providing there are facilities available to meet your needs. Throughout pregnancy or even in labour there should always be an option to change the intended place of birth in case of complications occurring in either mother or baby.

In some instances where labour progresses quickly the baby may be born at home, or elsewhere (in a shop etc.), when the intended place was not at home. In that case it is usual for an ambulance to be called, and this process will also alert a midwife. Once the midwife arrives, she will be 'in charge' and take over from whatever the ambulance personnel may have done. In most circumstances even if the baby is delivered before or with the ambulancemen, the midwife will deliver the placenta (afterbirth). In this instance, if the mother and baby are well, the choice of whether to stay at home or transfer to hospital should be the woman's.

4.5(b) ## WHAT HAPPENS IN LABOUR

The cause of onset of labour is unknown for sure, but once it has started there are three stages.

The first stage of labour is said to be from the onset of regular contractions, which have an effect on the cervix, to full dilation of the cervix. This stage can vary in length enormously and even once it is established it is impossible to predict how long it will last. During this stage there may or may not be a 'show', which is a plug of

• Cervix
  The neck of the womb

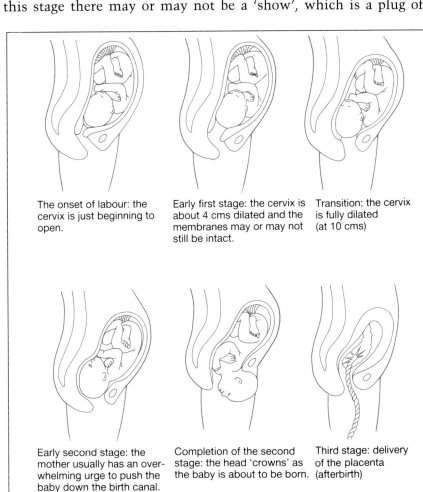

The onset of labour: the cervix is just beginning to open.

Early first stage: the cervix is about 4 cms dilated and the membranes may or may not still be intact.

Transition: the cervix is fully dilated (at 10 cms)

Early second stage: the mother usually has an overwhelming urge to push the baby down the birth canal.

Completion of the second stage: the head 'crowns' as the baby is about to be born.

Third stage: delivery of the placenta (afterbirth)

Labour: stage by stage

mucus which is in the cervical canal during most of pregnancy and comes away sometime near the end of pregnancy. There may or may not be draining of fluid (liquor amnii), the 'waters' which have surrounded the baby and given it protection during pregnancy.

The second stage of labour is from full dilation of the cervix to the birth of the complete baby. The baby descends the birth canal, the 'powers' of the contracting womb moving the 'passenger' (the baby) along the 'passage', the birth canal. The baby is born, usually head first and usually head tucked in so that the back of the head presents at the vagina first. Then the head is said to 'crown', which is when it stops receding with contractions, and at this point, if at all possible, it is best to listen to what the midwife is saying and stop pushing, by either panting or blowing while the head is born. The shoulders then rotate into the correct line for birth. Once the shoulders are born the body slips out easily as the biggest parts (usually the head, but sometimes the shoulders) are already clear. Left to nature this can take a varying length of time, but if delivery is being managed in a hospital a limit may be set after which artificial means may be used.

See section 4.5(e) below on Emergency or assisted delivery

The third stage of labour begins with the birth of the baby and continues until complete expulsion of the placenta and membranes (afterbirth), and includes the body's natural initial control of bleeding. During this stage the uterus continues to contract and various mechanisms come into force naturally to help expel the afterbirth and help curb bleeding effectively. In many hospitals, an injection may be given to the woman, usually in the leg, with the aim of speeding up this stage. The third stage takes anything from a few minutes to up to half an hour.

If any tears to the birth canal have occurred during the birth, the midwife or doctor will stitch them if necessary. A local anaesthetic injection may be used to numb the area.

How any labour will be managed will very much depend upon the progress of that particular labour, as they are all very individual. Management of labour will vary according to where you have your baby and according to the practice of the midwife and/or doctors.

- **Episiotomy**
  A surgical cut of skin and muscle between the vagina and anus

During labour, wherever it occurs, you should be given the choice about certain procedures. This should be accompanied by relevant information. Such procedures include whether or not the membranes should be ruptured (the waters broken), whether you should be mobile in labour, whether you want a bath in labour, whether you would prefer to tear or to have an episiotomy, whether you want your baby to be delivered onto your stomach, what you want to happen in your third stage, and whether you want your baby to have a vitamin K injection or drops after he is born. There is not space here to discuss all these aspects fully, but if you feel you want more control or say in what is to happen in your labour it is worth finding

See Appendix VIII for Suggested further reading

out more about these particular issues. All choices should be unbiased, researched, and well informed. However it is important to remember that the professionals caring for you during the labour should have your best interests at heart and, where you do not have the knowledge or strong feelings about something, then it is best to conform to their advice.

Throughout labour your partner, if present, should be able to comfort and support you in whatever way you both wish.

4.5(c)   KNOWING YOU'RE IN LABOUR

This is not always as easy and straightforward as one may think. Beginnings of labour are different for different women and for each labour. Often you may consider that labour is starting when it is not, but if there is any doubt then telephone the relevant place or people. Even after all these thousands of years of women having babies, it is not really known why labour begins. There are many different theories but none of them is proven.

See also section 4.5(e) below on Emergency or assisted delivery

There are a number of signs which you may or may not notice in yourself. Labour usually starts naturally between the beginning of the 37th week and the end of the 42nd week of pregnancy. However as with all things there are exceptions to the rule and some babies are born before this time and some may need to be induced (started artificially) for medical reasons.

The baby may be noticeably more active or very still when or just before labour commences. If your baby is very still for longer than is normal in this pregnancy, and does not move if you gently prod your bump, then it wise to have a check by a midwife or doctor.

Nausea, vomiting or diarrhoea may indicate that labour is starting. There may be a 'dragging' feeling in the vagina which may be accompanied by pains down the inner thighs. Backache, which may be continuous or intermittent, might also indicate the start of labour.

More commonly the obvious start to labour is the presence of a 'show', a plug of mucus which has been in the cervix from early pregnancy. This may be red in colour from blood, or it may be brown which is old blood like the end of a period, or even clear. The 'show' should not contain more than a teaspoon of blood – if it does, phone your midwife or doctor. A 'show' on its own is usually not a sign of the start of labour, but if it is accompanied by another sign, it may well be the start.

Some labours start with the 'waters' (liquor amnii) 'going'; this is a leak from the bag of fluid which protects the baby in pregnancy and in labour. The 'waters' may 'pop' and flow in a gush, or there may be a trickle indistinguishable from urine leaking. If in doubt, telephone for advice. It is usual to be asked to go straight to hospital, if this is the intended place of delivery, once the waters have gone. If the waters are greenish in colour, it is even more important that you go to the hospital as this means that the baby has been or is in some distress and has opened its bowels. It may be easier to use a rolled up or folded hand towel instead of numerous sanitary towels, especially if there is a large amount of fluid.

It is usual for the womb to 'practise' contracting from 37 weeks onwards, which you may be aware of. If you place the flat of your hand on your abdomen it will feel harder than normal. These are called Braxton-Hicks contractions or tightenings and should be painless. Contractions, which may be your only sign of the start of labour, are usually more painful forms of tightenings. Some women are fortunate not to feel contractions as pain, others not so fortunate may feel contractions either at the top of the uterus or the bottom, the sides, the back or over the thigh region. For labour to have started these contractions need to be effective, by dilating (opening) the cervix. If contractions are not doing this then unfortunately, although you can feel them, labour itself has probably not started.

Because dilation of the cervix cannot be seen with the naked eye, it is difficult to determine whether labour has started or not, both for you and for the midwives or doctors. The only definite way to know whether you are in labour or not is for an internal examination to be performed to assess dilation of the cervix.

Some women just 'feel different' at the start of labour and cannot describe it any more than this. Knowing that you're in labour is not as easy as it may sound and because of this onset of labour is often missed, or it is assumed when in fact it has not started.

4.5(d) HOME DELIVERY

Preparation

If the intended place of delivery is at home and the pregnancy has progressed well, then there is usually some preparation of the home to be made prior to the onset of labour.

It is usual in most pregnancies for women to get what is known as a nesting instinct near the time of the birth, when more housework is done and the cot or crib is prepared for the baby.

In some areas 'home birth boxes' are left in the home from about the 36th week which contain different things according to where you are. Very absorbent sanitary towels, plastic sheets for the protection of the bed or floor area where you are to give birth, and large absorbent pads may be included in such a box. Other equipment is usually brought by the midwife when she comes to the home when you have called for her when you think you are in labour.

Usually, the midwife will be known to you, as midwives attached to general practices work in small teams, and ideally you should have had an opportunity to have met them all in your pregnancy. If there is no general practitioner covering your birth then you will be likely to know your midwife very well, as she will have provided your antenatal care, either individually or as part of a team. Before the onset of labour you will know how to contact your midwife.

Once you think you are in labour, contact the midwife and those you want to be with you, including someone who is able to look after your other children while you are in labour, or if you have to be transferred to hospital. It might be useful to have a small bag packed with nightshirts, sanitary towels, washbag, clothes and a couple of nappies for the baby, in case of the need to transfer to hospital. Your partner might also want to be prepared, if only with a sandwich and a book.

CHECKLIST

What you need for home birth	Plastic sheeting for mattress (from about 37 weeks if it is not too hot)
	Thick plastic for any surface you may deliver on, or for any soft furnishings you may like to sit on during labour
	Extra pillows or scatter cushions
	Old sheets and old towels (fresh old sheets and towels will be needed after the birth)
	Plenty of absorbent cotton sanitary towels and old knickers
	Something to wear for labour if desired
	Cot/crib and clothes for baby, plus hot water bottle to air them
	Nappies for baby
	Spot light which can be used for suturing if it is necessary
	Space under bed or on chest of drawers for midwife's equipment
	Extra heater if required for room

It is usual to have decided upon a room in the house where you want the baby to be born, either because it is special to you or because it is practical, for instance not expensively carpeted, not too far from the bathroom or not overlooked. Your criteria for choice of room will obviously be personal to you. Certainly after the birth that room will be incredibly special to you. If possible or if needed, protect any soft furnishings with plastic. Remember that plastic covered things are very hot to sit or recline on. You may also want to give thought to what you are going to wear – just remember that labour is hot work. You may choose what noises or sounds you want around you. Some women use a selection of music as a distraction as a form of pain relief. Lighting of the room may need some prior consideration. It is thought that a baby prefers to be born into a dimly lit area, after all this is what he has been used to over the last nine months and there are enough changes of stimuli to get used to without bright lights if possible. The baby will require a warm place to be, once born. If this is not in the bed with you, remember to put a hot water bottle in the crib or cot to warm the clothes and blankets whilst you are in labour – and to remove it before placing the baby into it. Clothes can also be warmed over a radiator.

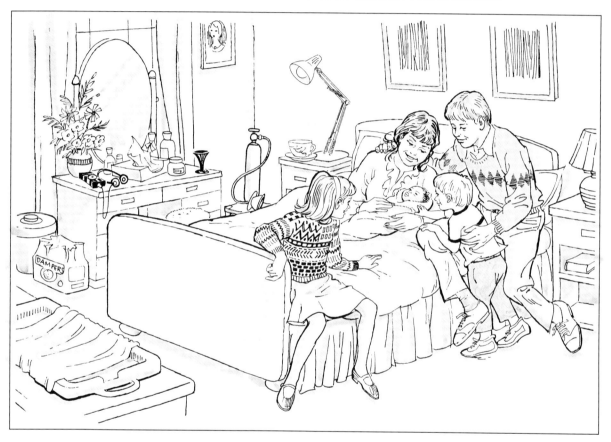

The room where you have your baby will become very special to you

The birth itself

Once the midwife has arrived and established that labour has begun she will not leave, unless a replacement is there. She may call the doctor who may or may not choose to visit. The midwife may call a second midwife at some point in the labour if this is the policy of the area. Labour will progress and you should be able to do as you please with the midwife taking care of you and your baby, by doing certain observations hopefully in an unobtrusive manner. Remember professionals are guests in your own home.

Once you are in second stage, the midwife will probably contact your general practitioner if he was involved with your care during pregnancy, who may be able to come to be with you, although not necessarily to do anything. If no problems have occurred, you will deliver your baby, with the midwife's help, in whatever position you wish. If you have decided to have your baby at home, you may have given thought to how you want your baby to be received by you and your partner and how you want your third stage (the delivery of the placenta) to be conducted. The midwife may well invite you or your partner to cut the cord and you may have other wishes about the timing of when this is done. It is easier to have discussed these things with your midwife beforehand if possible, or at least to have them written down for her to read at some point so that she can appreciate your wishes and help you to execute them where possible. If any stitches are needed, the midwife usually will be able to do them where you are, as long as there is an adequate light source. Torches and/or spot light lamps are more useful than main lights in the room for this purpose. The midwife will probably use a local anaesthetic to numb the area first.

See Chapter 5, section 1(a) for more information on infant feeding

You will have given thought to the method of feeding your baby and this may be done as early as you and your baby wish. It is a good idea for you to take a bath (possibly with the baby), or a shower if you feel able and this is an ideal time for the midwives to make up your bed afresh and clear away any equipment and any rubbish that has accumulated. For the first few days, it is advisable to use old sheets rather than your best ones. Some women like to sit on a large towel during this time in case of any soiling. It might also be wise to continue with the plastic sheeting for a few days.

The midwife will stay in your home for at least one hour after the birth to make sure that you and your baby are well. You will be left with a telephone number to enable you to contact a midwife at night or day during your postnatal period, which extends up to 28 days, although visits will not necessarily occur on all these days. If all is well the midwife usually stops calling after about 10 days.

If any intervention is needed during labour or birth, the midwife can make arrangements to transfer you to hospital. If this happens, you will usually switch from her care to the care of a hospital team of midwives and doctors. In some instances, however, the community midwife (or the independent midwife if you are using one) will have an arrangement whereby she can continue with your care, which is obviously much nicer for you and your partner. If it is deemed that a transfer is not suitable, then an Emergency Obstetric Unit/Flying Squad (if there is one in your area) may be summoned. The medical team on board can deal with most emergencies in the home until transfer to hospital is suitable or appropriate. It is usual in such a case for the partner to travel independently of the ambulance. The midwife will be trained to deal with emergencies and will have equipment to give oxygen to mother and baby as well as equipment to help the baby to breathe should it be necessary.

Dealing with pain

As far as pain relief is concerned, having a baby at home obviously reduces the options. Most community midwives and independent midwives will carry 'entonox' (a gas and air mixture) and will or can carry pethidine – a much used relaxant injection. But epidurals, spinal blocks (both regional anaesthetics, numbing pain from the waist down) and general anaesthetics are of course not available, due to the specialist equipment and skills required. Complementary therapies such as hypnotherapy, reflexology, massage, aromatherapy and homeopathy lend themselves very much to home settings. TENS (transcutaneous electronic nerve stimulation) is a self-administered method of pain relief consisting of small pads on the back connected to a small control box. This works by stimulating the release of natural pain-relieving substances (endorphins) within the body, and can be an option of pain relief for home. It may be argued that because the surroundings are familiar in every way there is a higher level of natural endorphins released, altering the pain felt, and so less other pain relief will be required.

WAYS OF RELIEVING PAIN IN LABOUR	
At home/in hospital	Relaxation and breathing techniques
	Meditation/yoga
	Warm baths
	Massage
	Music therapy/distraction
	Entonox (gas and air)
	Pethidine
In certain hospitals only or at home with specialised instruction/help	Hypnotherapy
	Aromatherapy
	Reflexology
	Acupuncture
	TENS
In hospital only	Epidural anaesthesia
	Nerve blocks
	General anaesthesia

After the birth

The room into which the baby will be born should ideally be at 21°C (70°F), or warmer if the baby is not going to be wrapped straight away. The baby has been in a much warmer temperature and, being wet, will lose a lot of heat by evaporation. Babies are not able to shiver to help maintain their temperature and can use up a great deal of much needed energy in trying to keep warm. Your body will be producing heat and is the perfect source of warmth for your baby, if you feel you want to cuddle him (not all mothers do straight away). Otherwise as mentioned earlier a preheated sleeping place with a hot water bottle (which should be removed before placing the baby into the cot) is ideal.

The placenta (afterbirth) will generally be disposed of by the midwife, unless you particularly want to keep it. If you are not squeamish, then it is fascinating to look at this sac of membranes and the placenta itself to see what has nourished your baby over the last nine months.

Birth in an unexpected place

If the baby is born at home, by accident as it were, or in any place other than the hospital, then fewer precautions are likely to have been taken in protecting the furniture and preparing a room etc. In such circumstances it is a priority to ensure that the room or place is heated, in some way or another, to as near 21°C (70°F) as possible – babies lose heat so quickly and this can lead to other problems. If the very unfortunate happens and the baby is born when you are out shopping or somewhere similar, obviously try to get to a private room of the shop floor. If the shop cannot provide towels or garments suitable to wrap the baby in then the warmest place for your baby will be snuggled in against your skin, until the ambulanceman or midwife gets to you.

If the birth has been very quick, it is quite likely that the baby will look bruised around the face. This will generally disappear within the first week.

Having the baby anywhere other than in the intended place is likely to be distressing for you. Fortunately, this very rarely happens but if it does just remember that if your baby comes quickly the chances are that you have had a good labour and that you have a healthy baby.

The box opposite gives guidelines on what to do if you are with someone who starts to give birth unexpectedly.

4.5(e) EMERGENCY OR ASSISTED DELIVERY

As mentioned above, only 20 per cent of births in this country need medical intervention. Of those 20 per cent, many end with a normal delivery but some need emergency deliveries, usually performed by an obstetrician. In such cases there is usually a paediatrician present in case of the baby needing medical attention.

- **Paediatrician**
  A doctor specialising in the care of babies and children

UNEXPECTED DELIVERY

What should you do?

Stay calm

If you are at home, encourage the woman to adopt whatever position is most comfortable for her and telephone for a midwife or ambulance

If you are elsewhere, co-opt bystanders to telephone the emergency services so that you can stay with the mother

Try to provide warm, clean wraps for the mother and baby (coats, towels etc.) – get bystanders to help you

Try to ensure as much privacy as possible

Wash your hands

DO NOT INTERFERE WITH THE COURSE OF NATURE. IT IS DANGEROUS TO GET THE MOTHER TO CROSS HER LEGS OR TO ATTEMPT TO PUSH THE BABY BACK IN!

As the head emerges, support it gently with your cupped hands. DO NOT PULL THE BABY'S HEAD

If the cord is round the baby's neck, slip it over his head

Deliver the baby onto the mother's body. Put clean warm wraps (e.g. towels) over him

DO NOT ATTEMPT TO CUT THE CORD – WAIT FOR THE EMERGENCY SERVICES

Wipe any mucus from the baby's mouth with a clean cloth

If the baby does not start to breathe immediately, stimulate breathing by holding him with his head lower than his body. DO NOT SLAP THE BABY ON THE BACK

The placenta (afterbirth) should come out by itself within about 15 minutes

DO NOT PULL ON THE CORD TO DELIVER THE PLACENTA. If it does not come out and the mother appears to be losing a lot of blood (about two cupfuls or more) put the baby to her breast

Once the placenta has emerged, put it in a clean plastic bag for inspection by the midwife

DO NOT GIVE THE WOMAN ANYTHING TO EAT OR DRINK BEFORE THE EMERGENCY TEAM ARRIVES

There are a number of reasons why a baby may need to be delivered in an emergency, but they fall into two main categories – either the mother's health warrants the baby to be delivered, or the baby's health would be adversely affected by undergoing the stress of more contractions of labour.

If an emergency arises, the speed and skill of the operators are of the essence and this is what the obstetrician is trained to do.

Assisted delivery

If the baby is very nearly born and needs a quick delivery, a change in the mother's position and an episiotomy may be the only require-

- **Episiotomy**
  A surgical cut of skin and muscle between the vagina and anus

- **Cervix**
  The neck of the womb

- **Epidural anaesthetic**
  A regional anaesthetic which numbs from the waist down by means of injecting a drug into a space outside the spinal column

- **Pudendal block**
  An injection of anaesthetic into the part of the vagina at which the nerve fibres for pain emerge

ments. If stronger, longer contractions are required, the addition of a synthetic drug, which is injected into an intravenous infusion (drip in the arm), may prove useful. A local anaesthetic injection may be used into the area to be cut if there is no other pain relief affecting the area at the time. The episiotomy or any tear sustained may be sutured (stitched) after the birth by the midwife or doctor.

In the case where the cervix is fully dilated and the baby therefore is somewhere along the birth canal, forceps may be applied to the baby's head, which act as a protection for the baby's head to aid a quicker delivery. There are different types of forceps, depending on where in the birth canal the baby's head is, and on which hospital you are in. They are commonly called low or 'lift-out' forceps, mid cavity or rotational forceps. It is usual to have an episiotomy with all forceps deliveries.

Ventouse extraction, which is a suction cap applied to the head of the baby, can be used to expedite delivery when the cervix is not quite fully dilated, or when it is fully dilated but the baby does not need to be rotated by much.

The pain relief used or required for forceps is usually an epidural, which is fine if one is already sited, but is rather slow to put up if speed is important. Epidurals are put in by anaesthetists. If there is no epidural service, a spinal anaesthetic may be used, which is similar to an epidural and inserted by an anaesthetist, but the drug is inserted into a slightly different place. This is a quicker procedure and the same area is numbed more quickly. Another quick form of analgesia is a pudendal block. This is performed by the obstetrician and acts just on the vagina and surrounding tissue.

Caesarean section

If none of the above methods is appropriate and the baby needs to be delivered with speed, a caesarean section is the only answer. This is usually performed in a different room to where the labour has taken place. Pain relief for this operation may be either an epidural, a spinal block (see above) or a general anaesthetic. In very few units acupuncture and/or hypnotherapy may be used. For a general anaesthetic, the woman is put to sleep by an anaesthetist by means of drugs into a drip and use of gases via a mask. The operation entails a cut along the top of the pubic hair about 15 cm or 6 inches long. A cut down the abdomen is now much less usual. The baby is born within the first 5–7 minutes and the operation in total lasts about 30–40 minutes. There will be a paediatrician present who will take care of your baby along with a midwife or a nurse trained in the special care of babies. Depending on hospital policy, it is usual for partners to be offered the opportunity to go into the theatre if an epidural or spinal block is the method of pain relief. Obviously if the partner doesn't wish to then he must not feel obliged to. He will not see the operation in progress, but sit beside his partner's head with a screen in place so that he cannot see.

Adequate explanation should always be given to both parents of what is going to happen and why. In the rare case of an emergency occurring when no or little explanation is given at the time, it is important to ask after the event, if not in the first few days then at your six week check. Always remember that it is your body and your baby that are having things done to them, with little control from you at the time over what happens. It is important to understand what was done and why, if only for your own peace of mind.

It is perhaps important to mention also that caesarean section may need to be performed without labour having started at all. Either the mother's condition warrants the baby to be delivered or the baby is showing signs of stress without any contractions and therefore should not be allowed to undergo labour which would cause more stress for the baby. Caesarean sections are sometimes performed too when the baby is not coming head first. Also in some instances the placenta grows over the opening of the womb (placenta praevia) and in such cases the only method of delivery is by caesarean section.

See section 4.4(d) for more information about placenta praevia

4.6 AFTER THE DELIVERY

During the first six to eight weeks after delivery your body returns as near as possible to the way it was before pregnancy. Throughout the first 10 days a midwife will check you and your baby thoroughly. Depending upon local health policy and individual needs, the midwife may continue her visits up to the end of the first month. Midwives are experts in normal childbirth and the care of the newborn baby, and will advise and help you in your role as a mother of a new baby. Midwives work closely with general practitioners, to whom they will refer if they spot any problems – actual or potential.

Midwives also work closely with health visitors, nurses specialising in the care of babies and mothers outside of the immediate postnatal period. It is likely that your health visitor will come to see you at home when the baby is about two weeks old, and she will continue to see both of you at clinics (or at your own home if necessary).

4.6(a) HOW YOU WILL FEEL

Women's reactions and feelings after childbirth will vary enormously. There are, however, emotions that are common to most women. It is usual, for example, for women to have swings of emotion in the first few days and most will find that, for no accountable reason, they become tearful on the third or fourth day. This is a reaction to hormonal changes and also to a major event in their lives. They should be reassured that it is normal to feel like this and that the feeling will pass soon.

Many women experience profound relief when the labour has ended, and they know that they have a healthy baby. It is also common to feel excited, in some cases to the point of euphoria, and this feeling can last for several months. On the other hand, there are some individuals who feel trapped, anxious, depressed and worried about their ability to cope (sometimes these emotions affect a mother some weeks or months after the birth of her baby). In most cases, these are realistic anxieties about a major change in lifestyle. If, however, the feelings become extreme or persist, professional help should be sought as they may be indicative of postnatal depression. It may be easier for another person (e.g. a close relative or partner) to be aware that there is a problem.

See section 4.6(f) below for more information on postnatal depression

Factors affecting a woman's emotions

If a woman has prepared and hoped for a normal delivery, it is understandable that she could feel disappointed and, in some cases, guilty (due to societal expectations) or resentful if there are any complications. In addition, problems during pregnancy or birth can leave a woman feeling tired, unwell or so worried about potential problems with the baby that she is unable to 'bond' for a while. It is essential that these women are given support and reassurance while they are going through this period.

A long and difficult labour, instrumental delivery, premature labour, caesarean section or postpartum haemorrhage are a few of the problems experienced by some women. Any of these events could, and often do, leave a woman feeling shocked and exhausted. One of the major regrets expressed by those who have experienced such problems is that they were too tired (often as a result of drugs given to them) to remember the first few precious moments with their new baby – and partner if he is present. Perhaps midwifery staff should emphasise the importance of taking photographs so that there is, at least, some memory later of the immediate moments after birth.

Other factors affecting a woman's feelings after delivery include the amount of support she will receive, whether the pregnancy was wanted or not, environmental and social factors, and financial problems. Inevitably, a mother who has any of these difficulties could find that she resents the new baby and that she feels anxious and depressed. It is important, therefore, that these women are given advice about the help and benefits they could receive.

See Appendix VI for information about Benefits

First pregnancy and birth

Parenthood represents a significant change of lifestyle, and many women will comment on the adjustments they have to make. Their initial feelings can include those of disbelief, wonderment, anxiety about their ability to cope and worries about the baby's health. Many women will say that they experienced a 'foggy' period when they seemed unable to concentrate on events and conversation for sustained periods of time. All of these feelings are normal. Adjustments to parenthood can last for as long as 12–24 months.

However, it is only when the adjustment takes longer or when women experience extremes of emotion that further help need be sought. Regular contact with the health visitor, such as monthly visits to the child health clinic, will help to overcome the many minor difficulties experienced by most mothers.

See the section on Postnatal depression in 4.6(f) below

Second and subsequent births

It is common for women to feel different after each birth. Some women, for example, 'fall in love' with their first child, but have stronger nurturing feelings towards the second. Some find it easier to 'bond' with the second child, while others do not as they have subconscious worries about the first child's emotions. On the whole, though, women are generally more confident about having their second and subsequent children.

Professional and/or older women

Although generalisations cannot be made, it is important to realise that women who have had careers or who are older may experience specific problems more acutely. Of course, this does not imply that other women never have these problems. However, a woman who has had a responsible job or who has been used to being competent in a well established lifestyle may find motherhood especially difficult at times. There may be a tendency to attempt to be 'wonderwomen', in an artificial attempt to recreate professional status. Also, some slightly older women may feel more tired than their younger counterparts. In addition, there are aspects of motherhood that could be found boring (this, of course, could affect anyone), and a mother could feel guilty for feeling this.

Partnership problems

Some women become less interested, or completely uninterested, in sex for about 12 months after having their first child. After a second or subsequent child, this period of time can last for considerably longer. This, in addition to the fact that women are often preoccupied with their baby for at least the first six months, can create jealousy and discord in the relationship. It is important to discuss these feelings openly, and to seek further help if necessary.

See Appendix VII for Addresses of useful organisations

Although some people can have difficulties with parenthood, most will find it a rewarding (albeit somewhat tiring) experience. It is no surprise that most mothers think that they've got 'the best baby in the world'.

4.6(b) SLEEP AND REST

Sleep and rest are not necessarily synonymous with parenthood!

It is very difficult for a woman to get sufficient sleep and rest once she becomes a mother. This is especially true if she has more than one child, or if she has a hyperactive child or one who does not sleep. Women who must continue working, for whatever reason, will find it difficult to get enough sleep and rest. This is also true for single women and those who do not have support. However, an individual's energy requirements will be increased dramatically once she becomes a mother, especially if she is breast feeding. It is important, therefore, to give practical consideration to ways in which sleep and rest can be achieved.

The early weeks may be very exhausting and it is not unusual for the new mother to feel she is unable to cope, especially if the baby is unsettled and cries a lot. Most new mothers experience some tiredness and many much more than this. If you become overtired you are more likely to be irritable, anxious and depressed, and this may transmit itself to the baby who in turn may become restless and demanding, tiring you even more. Thus a vicious circle may develop. There are various organisations that may offer advice and support and of course your midwife and health visitor are also there to help.

See Appendix VII for Addresses of useful organisations

The immediate postnatal period

During the few weeks immediately after delivery it is particularly important for the new mother to have enough rest. It may not be easy for this to be achieved, especially if the baby is wakeful at nights. Nature partially compensates for this alteration in sleep pattern in that although the actual amount of sleep may be reduced it tends to be more efficient, thereby enabling you to make better use of a smaller amount of sleep.

Pregnancy and delivery tend to deplete the body's iron stores and any anaemia resulting may make you feel tired. It is therefore important that you replenish these stores by eating a diet containing plenty of iron (for example, dark green leafy vegetables, lean red meat, dried apricots). If anaemia is a problem, some doctors may prescribe iron supplements too.

Neighbours and relatives will probably want to see the new baby as soon as possible and having lots of visitors may make it difficult for you to obtain uninterrupted rest. It may help to attach a note to your front door to the effect that 'Mother and baby are resting – please do not disturb'.

Partners may act as 'gatekeepers' to ensure that the new mother is not overtired by too many visitors. This also applies to visitors when the mother is in hospital. Many mothers become overtired with the strain of talking to too many people. Visitors to new mothers should not feel they have to stay for long periods of time, ten minutes is often quite long enough.

Most mothers have someone to help them for the first week or so after returning home, often their partner or a close relative. The duties of the helper should be to carry out the routine household tasks, freeing the mother to care for the baby and give attention to the baby's brothers and sisters. Particularly if a relative is the helper, this help should be as unobtrusive as possible and should allow for the mother, father, baby and other children to have time together. It may be difficult for the helper to achieve a fine balance between helping and 'taking over'; the helper's task is not an easy one but it can, nevertheless, contribute enormously to the well-being of the new mother.

Planning ahead

One of the major advantages of the extended family was that a woman could rely on family members to give support. It was usual for a sister or grandmother, for example, to look after the baby while the mother had some rest. Now, however, this is not generally the case and, after the first couple of weeks she may well find herself on her own with the new baby for most of the time. As this is likely to happen before the baby establishes a routine for sleeping through the night and, in many cases, before the mother feels fully recovered from the birth, it is important that she feels able to ask for help. Although she may find this embarrassing, many people will be delighted to give support. For example, a friend might take the baby for a ride in the pram or pushchair while the mother rests. Often, neighbours who are going shopping anyway will not mind doing a little extra and, if it is handled tactfully, an older child may benefit from the individual attention given on a special outing with doting grandparents.

Other possible means of getting more sleep or rest include the following:

- Prioritise workload – do only essential tasks;

- Share domestic chores etc. with your partner;

- Try to spend a portion of each day on your own;

- Wake your baby for a feed just before you go to bed;

- If your baby is a poor sleeper, try to get him used to background noise, and reduce daytime sleeping;

- Try to differentiate (for your baby) between night and day routines;

- Try to go to bed early;

- Try to get some rest when your baby sleeps;

- If possible, share getting up for the baby with your partner;

- Try to make reciprocal arrangements with a friend you trust who has a child of the same age (i.e. one day arrange to look after her child and on the next occasion she can care for yours).

There are many other suggestions for ways in which a woman could try to get sufficient sleep and rest. However, the fact remains that it is difficult to achieve this. Fathers, too, can become sleep deprived. Eventually, however, it is in the child's interest to get as much sleep and rest as possible as tired parents will become stressed, irritable and unable to care adequately for their child.

4.6(c) PHYSICAL RECOVERY AND EXERCISE

Your midwife will advise upon exercises designed to tone up the abdominal and leg muscles after childbirth. A basic early exercise plan is outlined in the box but your own regime should take into account the type of delivery you have had and your general level of fitness. Many mothers find that doing these exercises just before starting their rest period is quite relaxing and conducive to rest.

More energetic exercises should be resumed gradually; again the midwife will advise on this. Most mothers are able to go out for a short walk towards the end of the first week. After a few weeks other forms of exercise may be started, such as swimming. This exercise should however be gentle and more vigorous exercise (such as cycling, weight training or digging the garden) should not be indulged in until after the final postnatal check, and then only gradually. As normal household tasks are resumed, such as bedmaking and cleaning, the bending and stretching these involve can also be good exercise.

It is advisable for you to continue to take care of your back at this time, avoiding stooping and heavy lifting. Attention should be paid to good posture so that backstrain is avoided. For instance, backache may be reduced by tucking a small cushion in the small of your back whilst sitting to feed the baby. Remember to bend at the knees instead of bending your back when lifting, keeping the burden as near to you as possible.

EARLY POSTNATAL EXERCISES

	On the first day after you have had your baby, or as soon as you feel ready, you can start the following: **Pelvic floor exercises** (see Exercise one on the following page)
Deep breathing	– Lying on your back with your legs relaxed and your feet apart, breathe in deeply to the count of five, hold for a second and breathe out slowly.
Foot pedalling	– This helps improve circulation and is especially beneficial if you have swollen ankles. Lying on your back with your legs outstretched, move your right foot from the ankle so that your toes point up to the ceiling. Then move it in the other direction so that your toes point away from you. Repeat five times and then do the same with the left foot. You can also do this exercise sitting in a chair.
Tummy toning exercise	– Lie on your back with your knees bent and your legs slightly apart. Take a deep breath in. As you breathe out, pull your tummy muscles in towards your spine. Hold for a few seconds and then relax. (WARNING: You should not do this exercise yet if you have had a caesarean; indeed in this case you should discuss all exercises with your midwife). As you start to feel stronger, you can add a variety of other exercises. The ward staff, the hospital's obstetric physiotherapist or your community midwife will advise you, taking into account your individual needs and requirements.

Certain exercises such as 'cycling in the air', sit-ups or lifting both legs together while lying on your back should not be done until at least three months after delivery (or longer if you have had a caesarean) as these may strain abdominal and other muscles and do far more harm than good.

Pelvic floor exercises

These exercises are important to restore the tone of your pelvic floor muscles and to prevent the development of stress incontinence.

The box overleaf gives three versions of the standard pelvic floor exercise. The first of these may be performed as soon as you feel ready after the delivery. It is an easy exercise to do and can be performed while you are standing, sitting, lying in bed or even waiting in a queue. No one will know you are doing it and it is a good exercise to continue throughout your life to keep your pelvic floor strong.

As you feel your pelvic floor muscles regaining some strength following delivery, try the second exercise and repeat it a few times every week. This second exercise is quite a difficult exercise to do but, when you are successful, you will know that your pelvic floor muscles are strengthening.

PELVIC FLOOR EXERCISES

Exercise one	Clench your pelvic floor muscles around your back and front passages as though you are stopping yourself from passing urine and draw them up inside you. Hold this for five seconds and relax. Repeat this a few times.
Exercise two	As you are passing urine, try to stop in mid-stream by clenching the muscles around your vagina. Hold for a second or two before resuming passing urine.
Exercise three	With a full bladder, stand with your feet apart and jump up and down a few times, coughing as you do so. If urine leaks, continue your pelvic floor exercises and try this again in a few weeks.

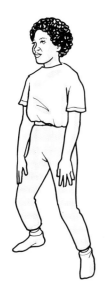

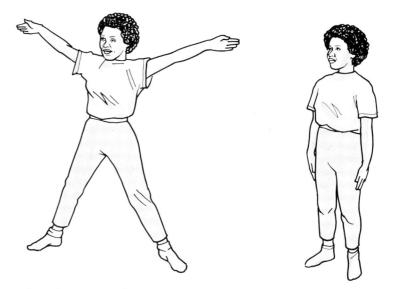

Testing your pelvic floor muscles

Besides these specific exercises, other forms of exercise are at least (and possibly even more) beneficial. These may include swimming, dancing and keep fit programmes, all of which may be resumed gradually as soon as you feel fit enough. But it is important not to overtire yourself. Go slowly at first as straining weakened muscles will not help them to regain their strength. After a few months, try exercise three as a final test of the strength of your pelvic floor.

If after a few more months urine is still leaking, consult your doctor as you may require more treatment to stop stress incontinence. This is most important as some women find stress incontinence persists for years if not treated adequately, considerably reducing the quality of their lives. It is, however, never too late to receive treatment for this most unpleasant condition.

Final postnatal examination

This is carried out from the sixth postnatal week onwards, usually by your general practitioner. He will check that your body has returned as far as possible to the way it was before pregnancy, and that you are feeling well in yourself. This is a worthwhile examination because problems identified and dealt with at this point (for instance, depression or stress incontinence) may save a great deal of trouble later. For this reason, if you have any problems at all don't hesitate to mention them to your doctor.

4.6(d) SIBLING RIVALRY

It would be rare to find a child who showed no jealousy at the arrival of a new baby to the family. Sibling rivalry could, therefore, be regarded as an inevitable consequence of having more than one child. Indeed, it could even be argued that it would be unnatural for there to be an absence of it. However, the degree of jealousy shown, its duration and the way in which it manifests itself, will vary enormously from one situation to another.

If there is more than one child in the existing family, it is usual for the youngest child to show the most jealousy, although this is not always the case. In general, it is impossible for parents to predict accurately the nature of their child's jealousy. However, one thing is certain, it will emerge at some stage and it must be treated firmly, but with sympathy and understanding.

Causes of sibling rivalry

It is important to realise that small children do not have the maturity to cope with powerful emotions. Therefore, in certain situations they will react in uncontrolled and, sometimes, extreme ways. The arrival of a new sibling to the family is one such time when a child can view the event as a personal threat. If, as in the case of an only child, she has received the individual attention and love of her parents, she can feel rejected, insecure and jealous when a sibling is born.

In a larger family, the 'baby' of the family, or a child who has been shown favouritism, can experience the same emotions and feel that his status has been changed and that he will not, therefore receive as much attention. Also, it should be remembered that the older children in a larger family can experience jealousy as well, although this is often to a lesser degree.

Emergence and manifestations of jealousy

Sibling rivalry can begin immediately the new baby is born. However, it is more common for it to emerge some months later when there is the realisation that the baby is a person in her own right and not just a visitor. (It has been known for a child to ask her mother when the baby is going to be taken back to the hospital!)

Some jealousy passes in a few weeks or months, some persists for life. Usually, the frequency and intensity of the jealous attacks becomes less as time goes by.

There is an endless list of the manifestations of sibling rivalry as children can be very innovative. However, certain generalisations can be made. Children will often show their jealousy by angry, aggressive, regressive or subdued behaviour. This is not always appropriate to a child's personality, and parents can be shocked by the Jekyll and Hyde changes of behaviour. For example, an otherwise passive child might become quite violent, whereas the more aggressive child might become withdrawn.

Although it can be upsetting for a parent to witness this, it is best to try not to become too anxious about the problem. If possible, parents should be as pragmatic as possible and try to remain consistent, loving and reassuring. Advice and help can be sought from the health visitor and, in extreme cases, further help may be necessary.

Jealousy can be directed at the new baby, a parent (especially the mother) or, in some cases, a close friend or relative. If it is directed at the baby it is usual for it to take one of two main forms. In the child's eyes, she has lost some of her mother's love and attention. In order to regain this, therefore, she will attempt to make the baby

Meeting the new baby

Even if this is handled tactfully by the parents it can still make the child feel a little insecure

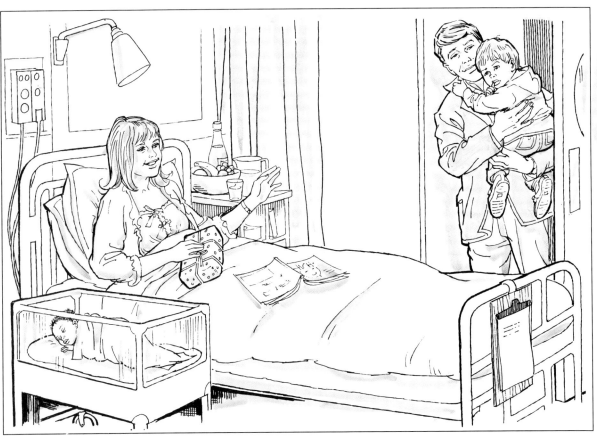

seem irritating or bad. This can be achieved by pinching a baby to make it cry or by other similar activities. Another, more worrying, form of jealousy directed at the baby is the subconscious desire to get rid of it. Of course, it is only in extreme cases that a child would be aware of the implications of her behaviour. However, it is necessary to be vigilant if a child manifests this kind of behaviour. In such situations, the older child could, for example, attempt to stab the baby or to suffocate him with a pillow.

Some children direct their anger at the parents, especially the mother. There are many different ways that they can show their feelings. These include: hitting, shouting, insolence, playing one parent off against the other and frequent tantrums or crying attacks. These behavioural changes are all perfectly understandable and are a cry for attention. Eventually, with reassurance, they will diminish and finally stop.

Regressive behaviour is another way that some children show their jealousy. This can take the form of recommencing bed-wetting or drinking from a bottle when both activities had previously stopped. Difficulties at nursery or school are also commonplace, and some children will not want their mothers to leave them. In general, all of these manifestations are intended to make the child seem more 'babylike' and, therefore, are a demand for attention. In these situations, no child should be made to feel foolish as this may be their only way of expressing their emotions.

Coping with sibling rivalry

It is important to remember that no one is perfect and, therefore, all parents make mistakes. They will find it difficult to remain calm and to retain their ideals all the time when coping with sibling rivalry. A busy and tired mother who is, for example, attempting to do a week's shopping in a crowded supermarket, holding a baby and coping with one or more children may show more than a touch of irritation if a jealous tantrum takes place at the checkout till. However, the important point is to give the child explanation and reassurance after the event, rather than ignoring the episode.

Ideally, the preparation for sibling rivalry begins before the birth of the new baby. It is useful to discuss all the facets of jealousy and to explain to the child that she will feel jealous, but that there is nothing wrong in having these feelings.

It is also important to discuss the needs of the baby and to say that she will demand a great deal of attention. At the same time, it is essential to make it clear to the child that he will be loved as much as before even though the baby will receive much attention. These discussions and reassurance should continue for a long time after the birth of the baby. It can be useful to enlist the help of the child's father who could discuss his own jealousy when she was born.

Each parent will find their own way of coping with sibling rivalry. However, there are a few practical tips which could be helpful.

- When the child first comes to see the new baby, it is tactful to avoid breast feeding at that moment.

- Give a present, such as a doll, to the child, and say that it is a gift from the baby.

- Encourage friends and family who are visiting the baby to acknowledge the presence of the older child or children first.

- Some of the individuals who wish to bring presents should be encouraged to give the present to the older child, or to both if they can afford it. Alternatively, the older child could be allowed to open the presents for the baby.

- Encourage activities with the older child at intimate times, such as breast feeding. Reading books can be fraught with difficulties as it is almost impossible to feed a baby, cuddle a child and turn the pages of a book at the same time. Additionally, a jealous child may try to sit on the baby. However, other activities, such as drawing can be successful. Provided the area is prepared beforehand, it is possible to give the baby full attention while, at the same time, admiring the older child's work.

- Allow the child to participate in certain areas of baby care, such as bathing the baby while the mother holds him. Alternatively, she could be encouraged to mimic certain activities, such as changing a doll's nappy while the mother is changing the baby's.

- Develop 'special' activities with each parent. This will enable the child to have time on her own with the parent, developing the relationship between them and helping the child to feel important and loved.

- If the child is old enough, encourage him to discuss his feeling. Although it is tempting for a busy parent to brush off a comment with 'don't be silly . . .', this will not help the child and could further emphasise his feelings of insecurity.

- A child should not be shouted at or smacked when she has an episode of jealousy. This will only reinforce her feelings of rejection. Instead, there should be firm handling of the situation, and discussions about why she should or should not do certain things.

- Sometimes, a well-managed discussion about difficulties with the baby can help. For example, enlisting advice from the sibling about crying or sleeping problems can make her feel important. However, this type of discussion must be carefully handled so that the child does not feel inclined to punish the baby.

There are many other methods that could be used to cope with sibling rivalry, but by far the most important will always be reassurance and love.

Adopted and fostered children

These children will need as much, if not more, reassurance and love than 'natural' children, especially if they were adopted or fostered at an older age from a family in which abuse took place. Additionally, they have not had the nine month adjustment phase before the arrival of a new baby or child to the family, if the new sibling is also adopted or fostered.

4.6(e)   PHYSICAL PROBLEMS IN THE POSTNATAL PERIOD

Given the very close eye kept upon the mother's progress by the midwife it is likely that any problem will be identified quickly and the appropriate action taken. Sometimes problems arise quickly however and action may need to be taken whilst awaiting the arrival of the midwife or doctor. In the rare event that a doctor or midwife cannot be contacted immediately, and advice is needed urgently, the nearest hospital maternity unit could be contacted. There will always be a midwife on duty who will provide advice in an emergency.

The uterus (womb) during the postnatal period

In the first few days after delivery the hard bulk of the uterus may be felt just below the navel. The uterus will gradually shrink until by approximately the tenth day it may no longer be felt.

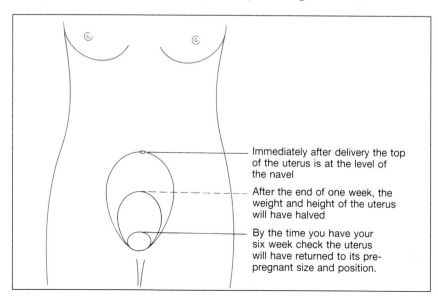

Immediately after delivery the top of the uterus is at the level of the navel

After the end of one week, the weight and height of the uterus will have halved

By the time you have your six week check the uterus will have returned to its pre-pregnant size and position.

Changes in the size of the womb after delivery

Normal vaginal loss and haemorrhage   During the early postnatal weeks the raw area to which the placenta (or afterbirth) was attached heals. A little blood will seep from this placental site, but the uterus itself stops any heavy bleeding by wrapping and clenching its muscle fibres around the severed ends of the blood vessels leading to the placental site. Together with some of the now unwanted lining of the uterus and the general debris of childbirth, this blood escapes via the vagina and is known as lochia. The colour of normal lochia is red for the first few days, gradually turning to pink as bleeding lessens, and then brown as the blood becomes stale. Over the next week the lochia will become a whitish yellow and indistinguishable from normal vaginal discharge. Particularly in the first few days the lochia may contain small shreds of tissue but these should be no bigger than a small fingernail. At no time should the lochia contain blood clots. Normal lochia often possesses a rather pungent odour, but it should not smell offensive. During the first few days after delivery the amount of lochia should be about the same as a rather heavy menstrual period but should quickly reduce thereafter.

Red lochia after the sixth postnatal day is abnormal as this indicates that bleeding is still occurring and the advice of a midwife or doctor should be sought at once.

Vaginal bleeding in the days after childbirth is excessive if sanitary pads quickly (i.e. within an hour or so) become soaked with fresh blood, particularly if blood clots larger than a thumbnail are also passed. In this event, all the pads and clots should be saved for inspection by the midwife or doctor (who should be contacted urgently), as it is possible that they may contain fragments of placenta which may need to be removed.

Very rarely the bleeding may be so heavy that the mother feels faint and eventually she may collapse if it continues. In order to stop the bleeding (having sent for the midwife or doctor), firstly try to enable her to pass urine as a full bladder may be adversely affecting the power of the uterus to control bleeding. If the bleeding continues lay her flat (preferably protecting the surface underneath with old towels) and gently massage the area of her abdomen just below the navel until you feel her uterus harden under your hand. If the uterus hardens then it should be capable of controlling the bleeding which should then diminish. If it does not, and the woman is in danger of collapsing, keep massaging and send someone to call for an ambulance as she needs immediate hospital attention.

Infection of the uterus   Usually the raw placental site heals without problems but occasionally infections may occur, particularly if fragments of placenta remain in the uterus. If the placental site becomes infected then healing will be delayed, bleeding will continue, the uterus will feel tender and the lochia will remain red. Blood clots may be passed; these may contain pieces of placental tissue. The lochia may become heavy (see above) and may smell offensive. The temperature may be raised (often only slightly to about 38°C/99.5°F although it could be higher) and the pulse rate increased from its normal rate of about 70 to 80 beats per minute.

It is important that the infection is treated as soon as possible before it spreads.

It will be necessary to get rid of any placental fragments from the uterus causing the infection. The doctor may prescribe drugs to make the uterus contract and expel the placental tissue. Alternatively the new mother may be admitted to a gynaecological ward, an anaesthetic given and the fragments removed via the vagina. This procedure is termed 'evacuation of retained products of conception' and is likely to necessitate at least an overnight stay in hospital. Many hospitals have facilities for the baby to stay with the mother; this is particularly valuable if she is breast feeding.

Infections may arise when no placental tissue has been retained, although this is very rare. The healing placental site is ideally suited for various bacteria to flourish. It is therefore important for hygiene to be adequate to prevent bacteria spreading up the vagina to the inside of the uterus. For example, pads should be changed frequently and the general area of the vulva and perineum kept clean and dry (a moist environment encourages infection). However, such infections are unlikely to arise after the midwife has stopped her daily visits and she will identify any potential problems and stop them from developing.

The perineum, vagina and vulva

The perineum is the area between the vagina (front passage) and the anus (back passage). During childbirth the perineum becomes temporarily stretched to several times its normal length and may become bruised, swollen and torn. An episiotomy may have been performed. It may have been necessary for the midwife or doctor to stitch the perineum following delivery and these sutures are likely to add to the discomfort and distress experienced by many women at this time. Not every woman will suffer in this way, but even an apparently undamaged perineum may feel sore for several days. There may be minute abrasions which can sting, particularly when urine is passed. These abrasions may be situated in the front part of the vulva rather than the perineum but, wherever they are, they tend to heal quickly and should not be sore for more than a few days. Warm water bathing immediately after passing urine may help in this case.

If the perineum has been stitched, care needs to be taken to keep the area clean and dry so that healing is encouraged and infection

- **Episiotomy**
A surgical cut of skin and muscle between the vagina and anus

prevented. Warm baths or showers are often soothing (there is no need to add salt or any antiseptic to the water) and the perineum may be patted dry with tissue paper or a soft towel, or dried with the gentlest heat of a hair dryer. Care needs to be taken that the dryer is not too hot, and that it is not blowing too hard as this may delay healing instead of encouraging it. Talcum powder should not be used as it tends to clog. Cotton pants allow better air circulation than nylon (thus helping to keep the perineum dry). Exposing the perineum to the air may also help healing.

Some suture materials are dissolvable and do not require removal. These stitches tend to drop out after a week or so, and look like small brown worms when they do so. Other stitches need to be removed towards the end of the first week; often this procedure affords instant relief.

Painful perineum   Paracetamol is recommended for perineal pain. If this is ineffective then other painkilling tablets may be suggested by your midwife or doctor. There are many products available for application onto sore perineums, but few have been properly evaluated. It is possible that some (including herbal remedies) may do more harm than good; your midwife is the best person to recommend which preparations you should use.

Ice packs are frequently applied to painful perineums. Care should be taken that they are applied properly otherwise ice burns could result. Ice packs are probably best prepared as crushed ice between gauze pads, applied when you are resting so they do not slip as you walk about. They should be used for only a few minutes at a time to prevent excess cooling and over-constriction of blood to the perineum, which would be likely to delay healing. Application of a pad soaked in tap water and witch hazel may prove as effective as an ice pack. Local anaesthetic sprays or gels may also be useful; again, your midwife will advise you on these and any other treatments that may be available such as ultrasound or pulsed electromagnetic therapy.

Sexual intercourse can be resumed as soon as you want to; sometimes vaginal dryness is a problem which a lubricant cream (e.g. KY Jelly) will help. Different positions for intercourse may need to be tried to avoid pressure if your breasts or perineum are still tender. Many midwives and doctors would advise that you try intercourse before your final postnatal check-up so that any problems such as pain can be mentioned to your doctor.

Constipation and haemorrhoids

Many women find that they do not have a bowel movement for a few days after delivery. This is probably because they have not eaten very much during labour (and often the bowels will have been opened during labour).

Passing a motion may be uncomfortable during the early post-natal period, particularly if the perineum is sore. It is important to realise, though, that perineal stitches will not be damaged. Keeping the stool soft will help to reduce any discomfort. This may be encouraged by increasing your intake of fibre and drinking plenty of water. A mild laxative may also be effective – but do ask your midwife for advice.

Haemorrhoids (piles) will add to the discomfort of a sore perineum, leading to reluctance to pass a stool, and to constipation. Most newly delivered mothers find that haemorrhoids (which may have appeared in pregnancy) are at their worst straight after delivery but get better quite quickly. In the meantime various ointments are available such as Anusol – again, your midwife will advise you. The treatments described above for sore perineums (for example, cold compresses and warm baths) will also soothe the pain of haemorrhoids.

Urinary problems and thrush

Cystitis and thrush are not uncommon postnatally and both are painful and distressing conditions that need to be dealt with by your doctor. Frequently, they occur together.

Cystitis is an infection of the bladder, and is manifested by passing urine very frequently in small amounts, pain over the lower abdomen, and perhaps a slight rise in temperature. The urine often has a fish-like smell, and may be bloodstained. It may be helpful for you to increase your fluid intake to at least the equivalent of one glass of water every hour, and a hot water bottle over the lower abdomen may provide some relief.

Thrush is a fungal infection of the vagina. It causes intense itching, especially at night, making sleeping difficult. Vaginal discharge may sometimes (but not always) be increased, and the vulva and perineum may be red, swollen and sore. Sometimes the source of the thrush infection lies in the intestines. It may be difficult to eradicate and may keep re-infecting the vagina.

If you do suffer from thrush, it is important that you see your doctor so that appropriate medication can be prescribed.

Stress incontinence   Following childbirth as many as one woman in five experiences involuntary loss of urine when, for example, coughing, sneezing, laughing or exercising. This urinary stress incontinence is probably caused by over-stretching of the pelvic floor muscles (shown overleaf), or damage to their nerve supply during delivery.

See section 4.6(c) for Pelvic floor exercises

The pelvic floor muscles provide support to the uterus and bladder, and are used when trying to stop passing urine. If their effectiveness is reduced then they will be too weak to prevent involuntary loss of urine.

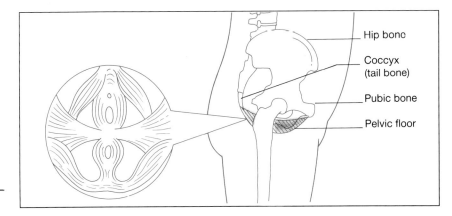

Hip bone

Coccyx
(tail bone)

Pubic bone

Pelvic floor

The pelvic floor muscles

Prevention and treatment of stress incontinence is aimed at strengthening these muscles and restoring to them an efficient nerve supply. Pelvic floor exercises are popular, but they need to be done well and frequently to be effective.

Breast problems

See also Chapter 5, section 1(a) on Feeding

Sore nipples and engorgement are common early problems for breast feeding women and, if you do not expect them, they can tempt you to give up this method of feeding. Both problems are certainly exacerbated by incorrect positioning of the baby at the breast so it is important to enlist the help of the ward staff or your community midwife to get this right. Once the baby's position has been sorted out, these problems will resolve.

There are, however, some simple self-help measures you can employ to get you through the period when sore nipples and engorgement may be a problem.

- Make sure that your nipples are dried properly between feeds – you can use a soft towel or a hair dryer on the gentlest setting to help achieve this.

- Expose your nipples to the air whenever possible – for example during your rest period.

- There are a variety of creams, lotions and sprays available for sore nipples, but do ask your midwife's advice first as some of them may do more harm than good.

- Some women find that expressing a small amount of milk and rubbing it into the nipple affords some relief.

- If the nipple is really cracked, it may be advisable to express milk from it for a day or two to allow it to heal, and to feed only from the other breast.

- If a breast is too engorged with milk for the baby to latch on properly, you may need to take a little milk off first, either by expressing it or by applying gentle downward pressure with a hot wet flannel (which will encourage the expression of some milk) followed by the application of a cold wet flannel as a compress.

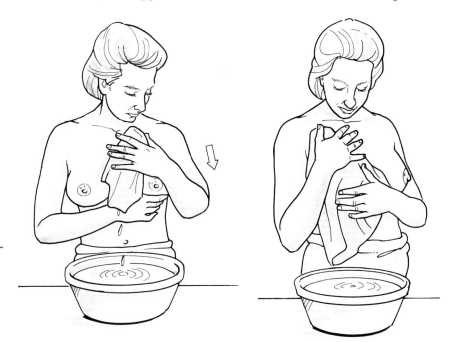

Relieving engorgement

Applying wet flannels to the breast, apply a hot flannel in a downwards motion (left) followed by a cold flannel as a compress

Women should feel reassured that these problems are temporary and easy to sort out, even though they may cause misery at the time. Certain more worrying problems can arise, however, as discussed below.

Mastitis   Mastitis is inflammation of the breast caused by infection tracking up from a cracked nipple, from rough handling of the breast (perhaps from over-enthusiastic expressing of milk from an engorged breast in the first few days of breast feeding), or from stagnation of milk. Mastitis rarely occurs earlier than the third postnatal week and is sometimes associated with weaning. A triangular wedge-shaped (or more diffuse) area of inflammation will be seen on a breast, and it will be painful and hard. The temperature may be raised and the mother will probably feel generally unwell, as though influenza is starting. She should rest as much as possible and drink extra fluids. Hot and cold compresses applied to the breast may be helpful.

See also Chapter 5, section 1(a) on Feeding

Medical advice should be sought in order to avert the possible formation of a breast abscess. Your doctor may send a sample of breast milk for culture to see if any bacteria are causing the inflammation and if so may prescribe antibiotics. However, in approximately 50 per cent of cases of mastitis no infection is present. Often, breast feeding can continue, but it is important to make sure the breasts are emptied at each feed, gently expressing excess milk if necessary. Keeping the breasts empty reduces the risk of abscess formation complicating the mastitis. Feeding technique should be good, so that the nipples do not become cracked and the breasts are emptied efficiently. The breasts should be well supported with an appropriate brassière and pain killers (as advised by the doctor) taken as needed until the inflammation subsides.

Breast abscess   Despite all treatment and precautions an abscess may develop in the inflamed area. The abscess probably will need to be treated under general anaesthetic, necessitating a short stay in hospital (the baby being admitted as well so that feeding can continue from the unaffected breast). Feeding can be resumed from both breasts after a few days.

4.6(f)   EMOTIONAL AND PSYCHOLOGICAL PROBLEMS

'The maternity blues'

On or about the third or fourth day after delivery (sometimes earlier) over a half of all new mothers experience the 'maternity blues', becoming very tearful. Crying may be brought on by problems occurring at that time: such as sore breasts, or a painful perineum, or perhaps problems with the baby such as neonatal jaundice. The tears may come on for no particular reason or may be precipitated by reading a sad story in a newspaper or seeing another woman crying. Frequently the woman may start crying upon the arrival of her partner or mother.

The actual cause of the 'blues' is not known; some believe it is due to the hormonal changes taking place at that time. Many patients undergoing surgery also seem to experience a similar condition a few days after the operation. Whatever its cause, the 'blues' is upsetting for the mother and for those caring for her.

There is no actual treatment except rest and sleep, and as far as possible alleviating any specific problem that appears to have precipitated the 'blues'. Some women experience nightmares the night before or after the episode which add to the distress. The 'blues' rarely last for more than 24 or 48 hours at the most and so, although a most unpleasant event, it is fairly short-lasting.

Postnatal depression

Approximately one in ten women experiences postnatal depression after childbirth. It may occur at any point from the second postnatal week to the end of the first year and lasts at least two weeks and possibly many months if unrecognised and untreated.

In most cases the depression is associated with problems such as tiredness, lack of help and support, or financial and marital problems when having a baby adds to an already stressed situation.

Many women in this situation realise only too well that they are depressed but may feel reluctant to tell the health visitor how they are feeling. It is most important that they do so, however. Health visitors are there not only for the baby, they also provide support and advice to mothers in all aspects of motherhood. It may be that the health visitor can offer specific advice about problems, or she may be able to refer to other specialists or organisations who can assist, or just talking about things with a sympathetic listener may help.

See Appendix VII for Addresses of useful organisations and support groups

There are also a number of support groups and organisations which help women suffering from postnatal depression.

Occasionally the woman may become depressed for no apparent reason. She may have enough money, a nice house, supportive partner, a beautiful baby but yet she is depressed. Sometimes the mother does not realise she is depressed and may be puzzled and guilty at the way she is feeling which is not at all how she had expected to feel. She may want to stay in bed all day, everything seeming too much trouble. Activities she used to enjoy hold no interest for her and she may feel continually lethargic and joyless. Again, it is most important firstly that the depression is recognised so that the mother understands why she is feeling as she does. This self-acknowledgement of the depression in itself is useful. Secondly, the depression should be mentioned to the health visitor or general practitioner so that treatment can start.

Postnatal depression is usually an easy condition to cure but treatment should start as soon as possible. Support and counselling may be sufficient, or the doctor may prescribe anti-depressants until the depression goes. Very rarely the depression is so intense that admission to hospital (along with the baby) is required.

The role of the woman's partner is crucial in recognising depression and supporting her through it. He (or another close relative) may be the first person to see that something is wrong and should not hesitate to contact the health visitor or general practitioner. Understanding and patience in the following weeks will contribute enormously to helping the new mother through her depression.

With the birth of subsequent babies the depression may recur. However this is by no means inevitable and steps can be taken to reduce significantly the risk of its happening again. Even if it does recur, it is likely to be recognised and dealt with more promptly than the first time.

Postnatal psychosis

This affects approximately 1 in 400 women after childbirth. Its most usual time of appearance is within the first two weeks after delivery.

The woman begins to behave strangely and may seem to be very suspicious of (and even aggressive towards) those attending her. She may also express bizarre ideas and seem to be not quite in touch with reality.

Postnatal psychosis is a dangerous condition because the woman may harm herself, her baby, or others. For this reason she should on no account be left alone for however short a period of time. She needs immediate medical and psychiatric attention and will probably be admitted to hospital for at least a few weeks. Often the baby will be kept with the mother, depending upon her condition. The illness is quite curable but the treatment may well extend over a period of several months. With subsequent babies, psychosis is more likely but by no means certain. Measures will be taken to prevent recurrence, or at least to diagnose it quickly so that treatment can be started as soon as possible.

4.7 BECOMING A PARENT

4.7(a) GETTING TO KNOW THE BABY

- **Trimester**
  A period of approximately three months, being one third of a normal pregnancy

During the months that the baby is growing and maturing in the womb, the mother will be conscious of its presence. The changes in her body will herald an awareness of this new individual making his own movements and becoming a separate person. An ultrasound scan, usually performed early in the second trimester, will give both parents a glimpse of their developing baby and for many (fathers in particular) this is the first time that the reality of the impending arrival registers fully. With the development of more sensitive pregnancy tests, particularly those that can be performed at home, some women will find themselves becoming intensely involved with the fetus from as early as one or two weeks after missing a period. With so many months to wait and plan for the baby's birth, it is perhaps inevitable that parents will fantasise about what their baby will be like. When he is finally born, the reality will certainly differ from this fantasy picture, to some degree at least. After the momentous experience of birth, the mother's first great task is over and, together with her partner, she must get to know her baby as he really is. It is crucial too, for the baby's survival, that he establishes a rapport with those who are to feed, protect and nurture him.

Ideally, the process of bonding and building a relationship between mother and baby should start in the delivery room. After the hard work of the birth itself, both the infant and his parents are often in a state of heightened awareness. If all is well, the midwife can deliver the baby onto his mother's body, she can touch him straight away and even put him to the breast if she wishes. Once the necessary observations and tidying up are out of the way, staff will usually leave the new parents alone with the baby – for perhaps an hour – so that they can all begin to get to know each other. This is of course dependent on both the baby and his mother being well enough. Women who have not had this opportunity (for example, those who have had a caesarean section under general anaesthetic, or whose babies needed immediate special care) may feel that they have missed out. They may worry too that 'proper' attachment will not take place. Other women, who expect to be overwhelmed by feelings of love on first sight of their baby, may feel guilty and unhappy if this does not happen. Fathers too may find that concern for their partner prevents them from responding immediately to the baby. Such parents should be reassured that, although they might be disappointed, their long term relationship with the baby is unlikely to be affected. Getting to know the baby, building and developing a rapport with him, will be a lengthy process.

The process of bonding is not initiated solely, nor even primarily, by the parent. The baby is born with the instincts and reflexes which equip her for survival. She must gain the attention of, or better still she must captivate, her carers.

A normal, healthy baby is born with the five senses operational, if not yet fully developed. Newborn infants and their parents often gaze intently at each other and eye contact is perceived to be important from the earliest minutes. A new baby's focal range is about 20–25 cms (8–10 inches) and this is the usual distance between her face and her mother's while she is being breast fed. Bottle feeding parents should try to maintain eye contact with their babies while feeding them too.

See also Chapter 5, section 1(a) on Feeding

From the age of about four days, babies appear to respond to human faces and will study them as if 'learning' them. Very early smiles (traditionally and somewhat inaccurately referred to as 'wind smiles') are physiological in origin, probably occurring in response to feelings of warmth, snugness and a full tummy. Real 'social' smiles usually start sometime between four and eight weeks and the parent may be bowled over by the first one. The parent's delight will 'reward' the baby who will soon realise that this is a good way to gain loving attention. A positive feedback circle is started: the more the baby smiles the more her mother responds, and the more response the baby can see, the more she will smile. This is the beginning of a real, interactive relationship.

See also Chapter 5, section 2(a) on Normal development

The sense of touch is important from birth. The newborn baby is bombarded with strange physical sensations and, after being held for so long inside the mother's body, may be able to recapture some of that security by being held closely in her arms. This will be particularly soothing if she can hear her mother's heartbeat as she could before birth. Both parents and babies enjoy the feel of each other's skin. The mother can stroke her baby or massage her using baby oil. The baby will probably want to caress her mother's breast or hold a finger while feeding.

The infant learns quickly to recognise his mother's voice and may turn his head towards her when she speaks. Babies enjoy being spoken to and, from the age of about two months, will smile, coo or gurgle in response. Parents will become attuned to different cries and will soon find themselves able to distinguish between screams of fear or pain, the whingeing of a tired baby and the hunger cry (which may be enough to stimulate the let down of milk in a breast feeding mother).

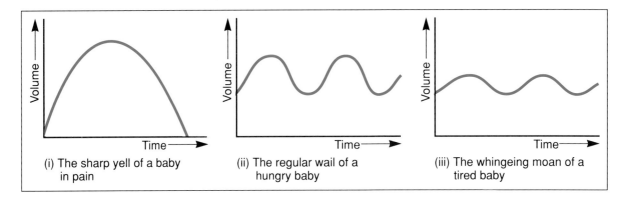

(i) The sharp yell of a baby in pain

(ii) The regular wail of a hungry baby

(iii) The whingeing moan of a tired baby

Different types of cry

The sense of smell should not be disregarded either. Babies become visibly excited by the smell of milk and at a very early stage can recognise their mother by her smell. Researchers in the 1970s discovered that four-day-old babies could distinguish the smell of their mother's breastpad from those of other women.

At the age of about eight months, babies enter what is generally referred to as the 'clingy phase'. They become passionately attached to their main caregiver (usually the mother) and will cry when she moves out of sight. Although flattering, this can be restrictive and annoying for the mother, but she can take comfort from knowing that this is a normal phase of healthy emotional development and will pass. Increasing the number of people who are important to the child (e.g. father, grandmother, childminder) will not mean that this phase will not occur, although it may be prudent either to ensure that she is settled with a childminder or other carer before this phase starts or to wait until the worst has passed before trying to do so (though this could involve a long wait).

Mothers who intend to return to work should be aware that if they leave their child with a conscientious and loving carer, as every working mother would no doubt wish to, the child will develop a close and affectionate relationship with this person too. Women who are unprepared for this can find themselves being quite taken aback by their feelings when they see their child apparently 'needing' them less at a very early stage. If this applies to you, you should take comfort from the knowledge that your child is likely to benefit from an extra important relationship. Babies' capacity for affection is not finite; you may feel as though you are losing out on your child's love but, as long as you have some time and attention for him, you will not.

See section 4.7(c) below on Parenthood and work

4.7(b) PRACTICALITIES

Registering the baby

It seems we never escape bureaucracy, even at birth. In the United Kingdom, one of the duties of the midwife attending the birth of a baby is to notify the authorities of this birth. In hospitals there will be a standard procedure for this but midwives, whether they are employed by your local health authority or independent, will have the same responsibility if your baby is born at home. The parents are responsible, however, for informing the Registrar of Births, Marriages and Deaths. This must be done, by law, within 42 days of the birth.

In some hospitals it is possible to register the birth with a visiting Registrar in the hospital itself on perhaps one or two specific days a week. Otherwise one or both parents must go to the nearest Registrar's office. If the parents are married, then only one parent need go even if the baby is to be registered in a different name (for example, a married women who has kept her maiden name may register her baby with his father's surname). If the parents are unmarried, registration of the birth can be a little more complicated. If they want the father's name to be on the birth certificate, then both parents must attend. It is not necessary to take the baby though; he can be left with a babysitter if you prefer.

Parental leave

The amount of time off work allowed to parents at or around the time of the birth varies considerably from country to country.

Current provision in the United Kingdom is low compared to that of some European countries – the Scandinavian countries are often held up as an example of excellence. The European Parliament is currently considering proposals for revised minimum provision, applicable to all Member States, which would become law in the early 1990s. If these proposals are accepted unchanged, they will greatly increase the financial benefits available to women taking maternity leave. The table overleaf gives details of current UK provision and the new proposals.

Maternity leave provision

	Current UK provision	EC recommendations
Available for	Women who have worked for the same employer for a minimum of two years before starting the leave	All women provided they have been working for the same employer since the beginning of their pregnancy
Paid and unpaid leave	6 weeks at 90% of salary 6 weeks at a fixed rate (in 1991 this was £39.25 per week) 12 weeks without pay	16 weeks at 100% of salary (the 2 weeks before the expected delivery date are obligatory)
Other benefits	Job security for 30 full weeks	Job security after the end of week 16 to be decided by individual Member States
	Time off with pay for all antenatal appointments and some classes	Should remain unchanged

At present, there is no statutory provision for paternity leave in the United Kingdom and some employers will insist that even the day a man takes off to be with his partner while she is in labour must come out of his annual holiday entitlement. Others are more flexible however, allowing between two days and two weeks paternity leave. If you are planning to start a family, it may well be worth talking to someone in the personnel department to find out exactly what your company's policy is.

Adoptive parents too need time to get to know their new child as well as to adjust to the momentous changes in lifestyle that parenthood brings. This is no less true if the child is a little older – indeed, although there may be fewer sleepless nights, there will be other demands and perhaps special problems. Most countries, unfortunately, have no provision at all for parental leave for adoptive parents. In such cases, it is particularly important to establish in advance how sympathetic and flexible your employer is likely to be and to plan carefully how you will organise your time off around the time of the child's arrival.

4.7(c) PARENTHOOD AND WORK

There are now over one million working mothers in Britain, and many millions more worldwide. If you are one of them, you will have special difficulties not experienced by your friends at home or by your childless colleagues. Even if your break for childbearing has been short, your life will have been changed completely. You may feel out of touch and you will certainly have lost confidence. Don't worry though. This is normal. All mothers returning to work have felt this way. You will be back in the swing of things within a few weeks or months.

Many women who have returned to work successfully say they would not have done so without knowing and having the support of other women who had done the same. You probably know other mothers who work already and now is a good time to get to know them better. They will all have experienced at least some of the problems you are facing now so you may find talking to some of them invaluable. Their solutions may not necessarily be your solutions, but it is good to know that problems can be overcome.

Childcare

Arranging a suitable person to look after her child (or, alternatively, finding a place in a nursery) will probably be the first concern of a new mother preparing her return to work. Most mothers feel very guilty and uncertain about leaving their babies in someone else's care. These feelings can be alleviated to some extent by allowing plenty of time to make childcare arrangements that you feel happy about. If your workplace has a nursery, go and look around it before your baby arrives. If you will be employing a nanny or taking your baby to a childminder, don't feel bad about interviewing as many people as you can. Talk to friends, take the advice of your health visitor, involve your partner in the decisions if at all possible and, above all, listen to your instincts.

There is no need to feel guilty provided that you have arranged good quality care for your child, and all mothers want to do that. In fact your child is likely to benefit in many ways by meeting and forming relationships with other adults and children.

Some studies indicate that the most unhappy women are those mothers of young children who want to go back to work but do not, while other studies have shown (and common sense would suggest) that unhappy mothers do not encourage happy, well balanced children.

Mothers' needs

The first days back at work are likely to be terrible for any new mother. You will worry and find yourself thinking of little other than your baby. This is only natural but when you rush home after work you will probably find her fast asleep or playing happily. Each day will become a little easier as your confidence in the person caring for your child increases and your belief in your professional abilities gradually returns. You may decide to ask your employer whether you can 'phase in' your return over a few weeks (or even months) to give you a chance to settle in again. This may be especially welcome if you go back to work early while wishing to continue breast feeding for a while longer. If you feel that you would prefer to work part time, it is worth exploring the possibility of a 'job share'. These are becoming more popular though, in many cases, it is still up to the employers themselves to 'sell' the idea. Do remember that recruitment and training of staff is an expensive business so any employer that has invested heavily in you in the past is likely to be open to ideas and discussion.

When you return to work, it is important not to do too much. You have nothing to prove. Your life has changed and, even if you have a minimal commute to work, have a baby who really understands that night time is for sleeping and have had an uncomplicated pregnancy and labour to recover from, you will still get more tired than before. Some women do everything superbly for a while then end up exhausted and at the end of their tether. This is definitely not to be recommended. You must be gentle with yourself, cook simply, cut corners with the housework for a while at least, and try to get enough rest. If your partner is helpful, let him do as much as he will. Similarly, if you have family members living nearby who can help out with some of the practicalities, don't be afraid to ask for help.

If something goes wrong – for example, if your childminding arrangements break down – don't immediately think of giving up work. A mother can usually buy herself a little time, perhaps by taking some of her annual holiday, and then work out solutions to her problems. Many employers will be sympathetic to such requests for time off as they are loath to lose valued staff members.

Some mothers may feel that they are criticised by friends and family members who have themselves remained at home to care for their young children. These same people may, however, secretly be rather proud of you for having the courage and the commitment to return to work after the birth of your baby. Don't feel that you cannot turn to them when you want advice or help. Remember that, in a few years time, some of them may well be asking for your help and advice when they plan to return to work themselves.

4.8 SPECIAL SITUATIONS

4.8(a) TWINS OR MORE

'I have some wonderful news for you – you are expecting twins (or triplets or more).' Modern antenatal care means that multiple pregnancy is usually diagnosed early, often at ultrasound scan in the early months of pregnancy. Reaction to the news will vary from elation to despair and it is a rare mother who does not wonder at some point how she will cope.

See Appendix VII for Addresses of useful organisations and support groups

Pregnancy

The pregnancy is a useful time for adjusting to the news and for preparing yourself, your family and your home for the arrival of your babies. It is worth while contacting your local Twins Club and the national Twins and Multiple Births Association (TAMBA) at this stage. This will enable you to make contact with other mothers of twins in your area and to avail yourself of other services offered (these usually include books and leaflets about twins and sales of second hand clothes and equipment).

Multiple pregnancy may be more troublesome than a single pregnancy with common complications more likely to arise. A weight gain of three or more stones (20 kg) is not uncommon and the final few weeks of the pregnancy may be extremely uncomfortable with two or more babies vying for space inside your body. Frequent visits to the antenatal clinic may be suggested so that your health, and that of your babies, can be carefully monitored. The need for adequate rest and a healthy diet will be stressed and you may be admitted to the antenatal ward for a short period for rest. The midwives and obstetricians will discuss the impending birth with you and outline the options available to you and the alternatives that may need to be chosen.

- **Obstetrician**
  A doctor specialising in the care of pregnant women

The birth

Twins are more likely than singletons to be born early and to have low birth weights. With higher multiples (triplets or more) this is even more probable. For these reasons, amongst others, twins may need to spend some time in the Special Care Baby Unit (SCBU) of the hospital. Other mothers will carry their babies to term and they will be of normal weight and transferred to the postnatal ward following delivery.

It is common to have a midwife and a paediatrician for each baby present at the delivery to ensure their safety and, in most cases, an obstetrician will be present as well in the delivery room. Twins will be delivered normally if this is possible though caesarean section is usually performed to ensure the safety of more than two babies.

- **Paediatrician**
  A doctor specialising in the care of babies and children

Attachment or bonding

Many mothers wonder whether it is possible to love two babies at the same time and with equal intensity, or even whether they will be able to tell which is which. Identical twins (those formed from one fertilised egg) may indeed be virtually indistinguishable in the early weeks but mothers seem to have no difficulty in loving them both. A 'favourite' may emerge but often this will change from time to time as the twins develop their own distinct personalities. If possible, try to spend a short time each day alone with each baby so that you can appreciate their individual characteristics.

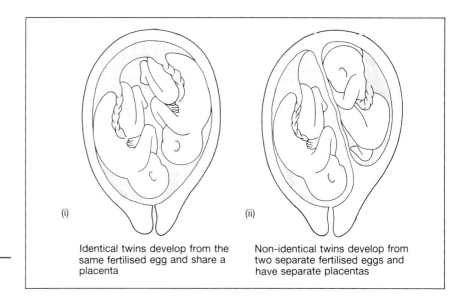

(i) Identical twins develop from the same fertilised egg and share a placenta

(ii) Non-identical twins develop from two separate fertilised eggs and have separate placentas

Identical and non-identical twins

Feeding

It is perfectly possible to breast feed two babies whilst reading a story to a toddler, but breast feeding twins is not always easy. The mother will produce sufficient milk for two babies but may become very tired – a nutritious, balanced diet and plenty of fluids are essential during this period. Twins may be fed together or separately. Individual feeding provides an opportunity to spend time alone with each child but can be very time consuming. Feeding together saves time but requires more organisation as the mother tends to be 'stuck' until the feed is over and both babies must be ready to feed at the same time. Babies may be held under the arms or across the lap and plenty of pillows or cushions will be required to support both mother and babies.

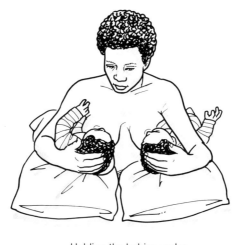

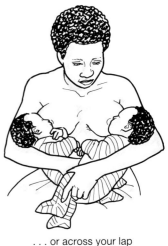

Breast feeding twins together

Holding the babies under your arms . . .

. . . or across your lap

Bottle feeding has an advantage in that partners and visitors can be called on to help but means that large quantities of equipment must be sterilised each day and milk prepared. Again babies may be fed separately or together. Many mothers of twins reach their own compromise and mix breast and bottle feeding, either by 'topping up' with formula milk after some feeds or by breast feeding one child each day and bottle feeding the other. Your health visitor will be able to advise you, and other mothers of twins will be happy to tell you how they managed.

Transport

Transport, both in the car and on foot, is another area for consideration. An up to date TAMBA leaflet is available outlining the advantages and disadvantages of the increasing selection of multiple transporters available. Many local groups and hospitals now organise loan schemes for baby car seats and you may wish to take advantage of these. Even the simplest outing seems to take a long time with twins; not only are there two babies and all their equipment to organise but once you are out it seems that everyone wants to stop to look at the babies and chat. This can engender feelings of great pride or of immense frustration in the mother.

Alike or different

Some mothers like to emphasise their babies' twinness by dressing them alike and encouraging them to do things together. Others prefer to emphasise their individuality by dressing them differently and encouraging their separation as much as possible. There is, of course, no right or wrong method and each family must adapt to suit their own needs. It may help others to identify each child if they are dressed differently or have different hairstyles. Separating twins, for example by sending them to different play groups, may work well for some families but will be totally impractical for others.

Twins as part of the family

See section 4.6(d) above on Sibling rivalry

The arrival of twins certainly causes an upheaval in family life and the mother may feel she has little time to spend with other family members. There is no evidence to show that sibling rivalry is any worse when twins arrive. Twins almost always prefer to be together rather than with anyone else in their early years and parents, siblings and friends can sometimes feel left out. This can be advantageous in that twins make their own amusement (or mischief) and will often play together for long periods allowing their mother a little more 'freedom'.

Twins and higher multiples involve a lot of hard work, particularly in their early years. You should be prepared to seek advice if you feel you need it and to accept help whenever it is offered. Your health visitor will be aware of your special needs and will help in any way she can. Contact your local Twins Club if possible and avail yourself of their services – it can be an enormous help just to chat to someone who has twins of her own. While no one would deny that twins are double trouble, there is no doubt that they are also double joy and fun.

4.8(b)   THE BABY WHO IS HIV ANTIBODY POSITIVE

See also Chapter 5, section 1

All babies have certain needs for warmth, love, nourishment and basic cleanliness. These apply equally to the baby who is HIV antibody seropositive.

But it is also important in the day to day care of your new baby that you look after yourself. Establishing a daily routine can help you both, as HIV is really a family health care challenge. Plan a schedule that allows for flexibility to suit the family, and also allows for you to have adequate rest and sleep.

How has the baby been infected?

HIV is a blood-borne infection and the virus can be transferred to the baby in the following ways:

See also Chapter 7, section 10(m) on HIV infection

- From the mother who is HIV infected herself;
- From receiving a transfusion of infected blood or blood products;
- Very rarely through infected breast milk.

The most common means of transfer of HIV to the baby is from the mother during pregnancy or during delivery. But not all babies who are HIV antibody positive at birth develop acquired immunodeficiency syndrome (AIDS), neither do the blood tests of all such babies remain antibody positive. The mother's antibody present in the baby's blood at birth may take 15–18 months to disappear.

Breast feeding

See Chapter 5, section 1(a) for more information on feeding and Chapter 5, section 2(b) for advice about weaning

If you wish to breast feed your baby this should be discussed with the midwife – before delivery of your baby if possible. This is in order to give you the opportunity to discuss fully all the implications, both for your own health and that of the baby.

Ongoing care

The paediatrician will usually suggest that the baby who has tested HIV antibody positive at birth should be seen more frequently on an outpatient basis. This is to monitor the baby's health and to detect early any problems should they arise. If you notice any change – perhaps an alteration of the baby's feeding pattern – or feel that progress is a bit slow, tell your health visitor or doctor. It may be a perfectly normal situation but should be mentioned just in case some early treatment is needed.

Immunisations

The recommended schedule for immunisation against the common infectious diseases of childhood will be advised by your health visitor or practice nurse.

See Appendix IV for more information about Immunisations

Consideration should also be given to reviewing the immunisation status of adult family members, as well as any brothers and sisters, in order to provide the best means of prevention of infection.

Family life

HIV is not transferred through hugs, kisses and cuddles nor through social contact. Play with, hold and hug your baby in the usual way. Physical contact between parents and their babies has been found to be a very important factor in development of all children.

Domestic cleaning

No special disinfectants are necessary. Household chores can be carried out in the normal way. The baby's linen and clothing can be washed in the domestic washing machine. If any is blood stained this should be washed separately at a high water temperature in the machine for not less than ten minutes.

It may be advisable to avoid disposable nappies because of difficulties in getting rid of waste. Disposable nappy liners can be flushed down the toilet.

4.8(c) THE HANDICAPPED BABY

See also Chapter 6, section 4 on The child with a physical handicap and section 6 on The child with a learning disability

Some babies have problems and handicaps that are noticeable before or soon after birth. Many handicaps are however only noticeable as the baby grows. Handicap means that a person is restricted or disadvantaged by his disability. Disability means restriction or reduction in what a person can do. There are huge variations in the types of handicap and disabilities that individual children have. It is impossible therefore to describe specific ones here. Rather this section is written in general terms and is intended to offer guidance to families on how to cope with the situation of having a handicapped baby.

Whenever parents are told of their baby's handicap it comes as a shock and many report that they remember vividly the moment the news of the handicap was broken but little of the information itself. It is quite common for shock and disbelief to block hearing the information. As the shock wears off you may find that you have lots of questions and a desire for information.

Finding out more

Your hospital specialist (if you have one) will be able to answer some of your questions and give you further information. If you don't have another appointment you should seriously consider arranging one. You may find you need to talk to the specialist more than once before you can take in all the information.

Your family doctor and health visitor may also be able to provide you with information. Remember though that nobody can answer all your questions, particularly about the baby's future.

There are many voluntary organisations for specific illnesses and handicaps. They provide useful leaflets and books about handicaps and illnesses and the help available. Some of these organisations have local branches, often consisting of parents in similar situations. You might also find your local library has books on specific handicaps – but be careful that they are up to date, otherwise you may get outdated and inaccurate information.

See Appendix VII for Addresses of useful organisations and Appendix VIII for Suggested further reading

Coping with feelings

Following diagnosis of the handicap, many parents are plunged into a period of emotional turmoil as they attempt to adjust to the new situation. Suddenly the hopes and dreams they had for their baby are replaced by an uncertain future, full of unknown problems. During this period, many parents find that they are helped to cope by knowing that others in similar situations have gone through similar emotional reactions and survived.

Common reactions experienced by parents are shock, disbelief, anger, guilt, feelings of failure and depression. If you are experiencing any of these and are upset by the strengths of your reactions, don't be, they are perfectly natural and justifiable. Whatever your feelings are it is vital for your complete well-being that you don't bottle them up but talk to someone – your partner, health visitor, doctor, social worker, a close friend, a minister, another parent of a handicapped child. Whoever it is, choose someone who is a good listener and remember that talking will help you understand your feelings and adjust to the new situation.

Some of the more common reactions experienced by parents are described here in detail.

Some experience intense *anger* which may be directed towards anything and anyone including other parents, children, the baby, doctors and God. Anger is a means of releasing emotional tension. Thus if you are finding that you lose your temper easily it is better to direct your anger away from people in case you say or do anything that you may regret later. Some people find writing down their feelings on paper and tearing it up afterwards helps, while others find help in channelling their anger into some strenuous physical activity.

Guilt is another very common reaction. This can have a number of causes:

- Worrying, on the parents' part, that the baby's problem might be their fault;
- A feeling of letting their partner and family down;
- Wishing the baby dead, and feeling that they can't love him;
- Feelings of rejection;
- Feelings of relief on having a diagnosis.

Whatever the cause of your guilt feelings it is important to talk them through. It is worth remembering that some parents of ordinary babies find it takes a while for their love to grow. Cuddling, looking at, talking and seeing your baby as an individual may help. Some parents experience very strong feelings of wishing that the baby would die now. This is particularly so if the baby has serious problems and is frail. These feelings may come and go but if they are very strong and you are worried that you may harm your baby it is vital that you talk to someone (e.g. your doctor, a social worker, health visitor, religious leader or someone from an organisation such as the Samaritans).

See Appendix VII for Addresses of useful organisations and support groups

Parents often have *regrets* ('What if I had not taken that drug in pregnancy'; 'What if I had called the doctor earlier' etc.). It is best to face up to these thoughts, talk them through and don't keep punishing yourself. A feeling of failure and jealousy of others who have 'normal' babies is common and often intense. Your health visitor will be sympathetic if you find attending the clinic difficult, and may offer to weigh the baby at home.

Some parents experience a feeling of *relief* on receiving a diagnosis after periods of uncertainty. This is quite natural and many parents find they are better able to cope with the future if they have a label for the baby's problem. Depression and frequent bouts of crying are also common, and are a normal part of the grieving process. Parents need to grieve for the expectations that they had for their baby before picking up the pieces and going on. So don't feel afraid to cry, it's a way of working through your grief. If the future looks bleak try and concentrate on today and don't be afraid to accept help in caring for your family and the baby when you are feeling low. However, some parents feel unable to cope or care for their baby. These babies are usually fostered or adopted – a decision taken only after careful discussion with the social services.

See also section 4.3(e) above on Loss and grief

It is worth noting that the feelings described here won't last for ever. Gradually you will begin to feel better, though you may find your feelings fluctuate. It is vital, however, that you do talk about how you feel.

Coping with feeding

The main aim in the self-help skill of feeding is to help babies to progress towards independence in eating and drinking as soon as possible. By the end of the first year, most babies are making some attempt to feed themselves, albeit somewhat messily. Feeding for some handicapped babies, may be problematic however. Problems encountered may be a very weak or absent sucking and rooting reflex, slow feeding, difficulties in weaning, difficulties in co-ordination leading to problems with independent feeding, slow weight gain etc.

See also Chapter 5, section 1(a) on Feeding the newborn and Chapter 5, section 2(b) on Weaning

Before considering some practical tips that may help you in feeding your baby certain general points are important. Firstly, all babies should have a healthy, nutritious and well balanced diet in order to grow. It is also important that babies learn to suck, chew, swallow and blow as these are very important functions for the development of speech. Making mealtimes relaxed, fun and a family occasion will also help.

See also Chapter 5, section 3(d) on Social development and nutrition

Practical tips for helping your baby to feed depend on the age of your baby, the stage he is at and his particular problem. Some handicapped babies are very contented and rarely cry for their feeds. Nevertheless, it is very important that they are woken up and given regular feeds. If your baby has a poor or absent sucking reflex it may help to use a larger-holed teat and give similar amounts of feed more often. However, do be careful that the hole is not too big or the baby may choke or swallow a lot of air and vomit. If your baby has persistent feeding problems you should contact your health visitor or doctor.

See Chapter 5, section 2(b) for detailed advice on Weaning

It is recommended that babies begin weaning at 4–6 months. It is particularly important to encourage chewing and for their speech development. Thus they should progress from milk to puréed food and lumpy foods as soon as possible and when they are ready.

Babies are ready to feed themselves with a spoon and drink from a cup when they have head control in a sitting position and can keep their balance when sitting in a chair, when they can reach out and grasp objects and take them to their mouth and when they want to feed themselves.

The position the baby is in when being fed is also important. If a baby's head is tilted backwards he will have difficulty in swallowing, therefore his head should be slightly forward, chin tilted down and hips bent. When your baby sits in his chair his bottom should be well back in the chair and his hips well bent as shown in the figure opposite. Some babies may need special chairs to help achieve this position.

See also Chapter 6, section 4 on The child with a physical handicap

If he has a problem with grasping a spoon or getting the food up to his mouth he may need a special spoon. Non-stick mats to prevent the dish moving around the table and special dishes may

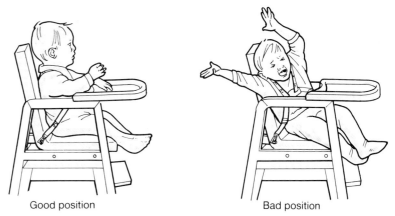

Good position

As soon as possible the child should sit on a chair. Her head should never be tilted back or to one side; always a little forward, with the chin tucked in.

Bad position

To correct – Bring head and arms forward and push bottom well to back of chair.

Positioning the older baby for feeding

Correct position is very important, especially for the baby with a handicap

also help. Make sure that the first food he starts with is easy to load on to a spoon.

If you are very anxious about feeding, and/or feel your baby needs special help speak to your health visitor. She may refer you to a speech therapist or occupational therapist for specialised help.

Stimulating your baby

Babies during the first year of life progress though various stages of development in order to acquire communication skills, self-help skills (e.g. independent feeding), gross motor skills (e.g. crawling, walking, sitting) and fine motor skills (e.g. reaching out and grasping toys). A handicapped baby, however, may take longer to pass through some stages and therefore may require extra help and stimulation to acquire these necessary skills. A baby's later development is based on his early learning, so stimulating and helping your baby in his early years will help his later development.

Helping your baby in this way does not necessarily take up a lot of time. It is often the quality of the help that is important. It is also valuable if the support of your family and friends is enlisted.

A valuable asset to helping your baby is a knowledge of the normal sequences of a baby's development. This information can be found in the early sections of Chapter 5 in this manual, or from any book on child development.

To help your baby learn you will find it more positive and beneficial to observe carefully what she can do rather than what she cannot do. This will help you to be aware of her progress and recognise what will be the next stage you should help her to reach. Breaking down each individual stage into small steps will help your baby to achieve the next step rather than expecting her to do something

See also Chapter 5, section 3

See Appendix VIII for Suggested further reading

which she may not be sufficiently physically or psychologically mature to achieve.

Health visitors, physiotherapists and occupational therapists have a wealth of knowledge about normal child development so do seek help if necessary.

Progress to speech

Speech includes:

- Words said, and an understanding of their meaning;

- Non-verbal communication such as gesture, facial expression;

- Intellectual use of language.

Babies in their first year usually progress towards the use of single words and understanding of simple commands such as 'wave bye-bye'. Before babies can speak words though they must be able to make a variety of sounds, make their voices rise and fall rhythmically, hear and locate sounds (attending to the important ones and ignoring the others), copy actions and sounds, use imagination in make believe, and recognise familiar objects in strange surroundings. Once they have mastered these skills they can progress to the use of words.

Some handicapped babies will be slow to develop their speech. This may lead to frustration later if they are unable to communicate their needs. It is important, therefore, to stimulate the babies' speech. You can do this by talking to your baby as you carry out ordinary everyday activities, such as feeding, washing, dressing. Tell her what you are doing so that she gets used to listening to the sound of your voice.

Listening is an important part of speech development. Musical mobiles, squeaky toys, rattles and bells will also help listening and locating of sounds. Right from the start, babies communicate by crying to get attention for food etc. Later they learn to smile. Copying actions or sounds back to her, particularly when she begins to make new sounds, e.g. cooing, gurgling, and then slightly changing the tone or sound will also encourage speech.

Holding your face close to your baby's face, so that she can watch your lips as you talk, is an important way of encouraging copying of lip movements and sounds. This can be enhanced, as her vision improves, by sitting her on your lap in front of a mirror. It is also important for meaningful use of words to match words with objects. It is important that babies understand the meaning of words before they can use words properly.

It is vitally important for all children, particularly those with specific speech and hearing difficulties, to encourage the use of gesture in order to help the process of communication. It also provides alternative methods of communication. Such gestures would be waving 'bye-bye', nodding the head for 'yes' and shaking the head for 'no'. Always use the words at the same time as the gesture and be consistent about using the same gesture with the same action each time.

Some babies may have to use sign language to aid communication. Speech therapists and specialist teachers will give advice and guidance on these and any other specific difficulties.

Progress to walking, use of eyes and hands

See also Chapter 5, sections 2(a) and 3

Gross motor development in babies generally consists of progress from lying, sitting, kneeling, standing to walking. During the latter stages they may also crawl or 'bottom shuffle'. Fine motor development consists of progress from seeing light and faces and moving arms haphazardly to looking at hands and feet, reaching out, grasping objects in a palmar grasp and later with fingers, taking objects to the mouth, transferring objects from one hand to another etc. Some handicapped babies may have difficulties in co-ordination, large movements and seeing.

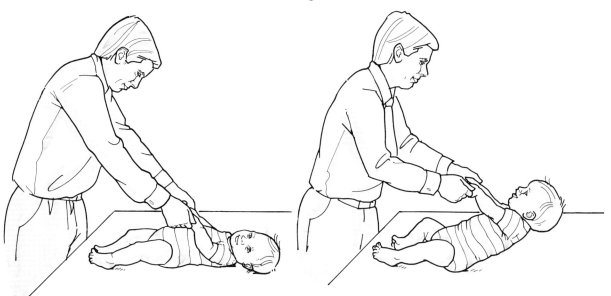

Active play and exercise 1

Helping the baby to develop head control and strengthen his neck muscles

To help babies progress in these areas of their development it is important that they pass through the normal sequences of development. It will also help if they are provided with opportunities to experience different positions. Thus for example, to help develop head control and strengthening neck muscles, lie the baby on his back with his feet towards your body and pull him up gently by his arms until you can just feel the weight of his head; eventually he will begin to hold his head himself. Don't be tempted to leave him in one position for too long. He needs the freedom of the floor to exercise. Thus, when he's awake put him on his back on the floor on a mat with his musical toys and rattles above him and later as he raises his head and leans on his forearms put the rattles in front of him on the floor. Sit the baby in an upright position in a chair as soon as possible, this will allow him to look around.

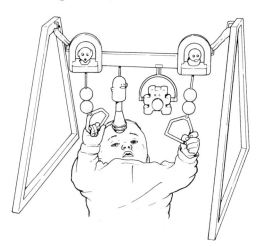

Active play and exercise 2

Your baby needs the freedom of the floor to exercise

See also Chapter 5, section 7 on Learning and exploring by play

See Appendix VII for Addresses of useful organisations.
See also Chapter 6, sections 4 and 5 for more advice on caring for the child with a handicap

If your baby has specific difficulties, such as problems with vision or hearing, specialist help may be sought from a paediatric physiotherapist and from the relevant support group or society. Your family doctor or specialist may also refer you to a physiotherapist.

Whatever the problem your baby has – whether it is physical, intellectual, emotional or connected with hearing or seeing – she will benefit from play for it is through play that a baby learns. Learning will be enhanced if you are relaxed and make play a time of active enjoyment for you and the baby.

This section has been written in very general terms, seeking to give you some hints on how to cope with your feelings, how to find out more about the condition and how to help your baby. Inevitably many parents will have a need for more specific help and information, which may be provided by the relevant specific organisation. Your health visitor will also be able to provide you with details of other services who can help. Other sections of this book which may help you have been listed as appropriate.

4.8(d) THE NEGLECTED OR ABUSED CHILD

Child abuse is as old as civilisation itself. Murder, maiming, wilful neglect, starvation, exploitation and abandonment of society's young have been reported throughout the ages. Children have been murdered for superstitious reasons – in Anglo Saxon times it was thought better to kill Friday's child than to allow her to grow up to a life of misfortune. There is plenty of evidence that extremely harsh discipline of children was sanctioned by society until fairly recently with many 19th century fathers referring to the verse in the bible which says 'He that spares the rod, spoils the child' to condone their actions. During Victorian times, however, British society was made aware of the plight of children by men like Dr Barnardo and Lord Shaftsbury. Improvements in child care generally continued during the 20th century and people really did think that child abuse was a feature of the past in Western civilisation. It was acknowledged that it still occurred in Third World countries through practices such as foot binding, female circumcision and the breaking of limbs to turn children into good beggars. So the description, in the 1950s, of the 'battered baby syndrome' shocked the world.

Battered baby syndrome referred to those children who had physical injuries deliberately inflicted. It very quickly became apparent, however, that this term was inappropriate as it became evident that:

- Not only babies were injured non-accidentally, but older children as well;

- Non-accidental injury was just one aspect of a whole spectrum of abuse.

This spectrum includes emotional abuse, sexual abuse, non-accidental poisoning, neglect (including nutritional deprivation) and a fairly rare form of abuse called Munchausen's syndrome by proxy. This refers to a situation in which a parent may fabricate illness in the child by describing to the doctor a false set of signs and symptoms. The child may then undergo painful, invasive procedures which are totally unnecessary.

It is common to find more than one form of abuse occurring simultaneously. For example a child who wets the bed may receive severe physical punishment e.g. having his buttocks placed in scalding water, together with being degraded by not being allowed to wear undergarments. Combinations of types of abuse may also be found in families. For example in one family a girl of eight was subjected to sexual fondling by the father, a boy of six was physically abused by him and a girl of two who had been neglected failed to thrive as she should do.

What follows is a brief discussion about some of the common forms of abuse.

Physical abuse

It is thought that several factors occurring together often lead to physical abuse of children. This mirrors the fire triangle in which oxygen, heat and combustible material cause fire only when they come together at the same time.

The factors involved in physical abuse involve particular problems for the parent, particular features about the child and a crisis which acts as a catalyst to the abusive incident.

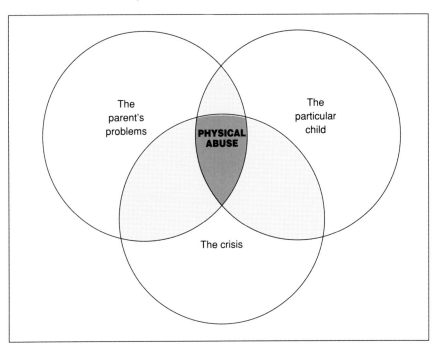

Various factors, coming together, are involved in physical abuse

Parents' problems may be many, including, for example:

- Parents being deprived or abused when they were children;

- Unemployment;

- Ill health;

- Youth and immaturity;

- Being a single parent;

- Marital problems e.g. violence in the home;

- Low intelligence;

- Drug or alcohol dependency;

- Frequent pregnancies perhaps leading to depression or exhaustion;

- Lack of family support;

- Aggressive tendencies;

- Unreal expectations of the child (for example that she be toilet trained by one year);

- Inadequate home and environmental conditions.

Any one of these on its own may not lead to physical abuse of children, but the chances of this increase if the following characteristics are also present:

- The child is the result of an unwanted pregnancy;

- There has been a difficult pregnancy and/or labour;

- The baby was pre-term resulting in prolonged separation from the mother and family, affecting the process of attachment;

- The child was ill during the neonatal period;

- Another child of the same sex had died earlier;

- The child is (in the parents' view) the 'wrong sex';

- The child is hyperactive, demanding much attention;

- A child who is just different from the rest of the family;

- A handicapped child or one who is slow to learn.

The crisis is the precipitating factor which results in the child being attacked by the parents. This varies from being something major like discovering another pregnancy or notice of redundancy to something minor like the milk boiling over.

Quite often the injuries which ensue are bruises and/or abrasions. It is important to remember that these also appear on a normal healthy child. They should not be viewed with suspicion unless:

- They are unusually severe;

- They occur in abnormal places (behind ears, on buttocks);

- Injuries are multiple and cannot be explained by a single accident;

- Bruises or grazes appear around the genital area;

- Injuries are inside the mouth particularly a torn frenulum caused by a feeding bottle being forced in or by a blow;

- Babies under one year old would not usually sustain bruises or abrasions;

- The cause of the injury can be identified by its appearance e.g. blows with belts and chains cause linear marks.

- **Frenulum**
  The skin flap between the inside of the upper lip and gum

Fractures Fractures are sometimes sustained following physical abuse. When a child has several fractures which are at different stages of healing, this would be seen as evidence of abuse. Children's bones are soft and supple and it is uncharacteristic for them to sustain a complete break unless by exceptional force – so the story as to how the fracture occurred is very important in determining whether the cause is abuse.

Intracranial injuries These can be caused by hitting the child about the head with a fist or instrument or by swinging the child by his feet and allowing the head to hit a wall. Shaking can be a very dangerous form of abuse which some parents think is an acceptable form of punishment. 'I never hit my child, only shake her', they say. In fact shaking can result in whiplash injury or in bleeding inside the skull which can lead to death.

When a child has been physically abused the parents may delay for hours or days before seeking medical attention. Hospital attendance might only be sought when the child begins to lose consciousness for example.

Emotional abuse

The child may be left alone for long periods without stimulus, and although he is adequately fed he will not thrive. We are reminded of this when we see pictures of underdeveloped children in Romanian orphanages, for example. In younger children who are left alone for prolonged periods, the tips of the hands and feet become cold and red. Older children may be made to perform degrading acts. Generally severe emotional deprivation results in a child who is unable to give love or show emotion, a child with frozen watchfulness who stares for prolonged periods with a blank expression. This child might even have been told that he is not loved.

Sexual abuse

This has only been recently recognised as a major problem. Most commonly sexual abuse is incestuous or the child will know the perpetrator personally – a neighbour or a friend's father. It is more common for girls to be abused sexually than boys, and the perpetrator is more likely to be male.

Sexual abuse is very difficult to detect. Sometimes this is because the child has trouble finding an adult who will believe the story and act on it on the child's behalf or because the child feels too guilty to divulge what is happening. The perpetrator may have said, for example, 'This is our secret and if you tell anyone Daddy will go to prison and Mummy will be upset and it will be your fault'. This guilt can be compounded if, when the sexual abuse is disclosed, the abused child is taken to a police station to be examined. This experience can reinforce any feelings of culpability which the child may have. It is preferable, therefore, for the child to be taken to a hospital for the necessary examinations.

CHILDLINE
Telephone no.
0800-1111

There is now a telephone helpline which any child can ring, free of charge and this service has done much to alleviate the suffering of sexually abused children.

There are behavioural and physical signs which are indicative of sexual abuse but any one of these should be viewed within the context of the total situation and never regarded in isolation.

Non-accidental poisoning

This is often another sign of stress in the house. The child may be given drugs not intended for him. Sometimes parents who cannot cope with a normal, lively child give him their sedatives or anti-depressants. Occasionally the reverse happens and a parent withholds drugs from the child who needs them e.g. for a heart complaint. The child subsequently develops symptoms of heart failure and is admitted to hospital.

Neglect

This often manifests itself as nutritional deprivation. The child may not be thriving developmentally as he should. Sometimes this is the result of an inadequate food intake caused when parents insist that their children follow particular dietary regimes like veganism or macrobiotics but without ensuring that all essential nutrients are included. The parents may not realise that such diets do not fulfil the needs of a growing child. Often a child who has been starved thrives when admitted to hospital where regular meals are taken.

Other ways in which neglect can occur include very severe nappy rash due to infrequent or non-changing of nappies. Skin infections and dirt can be signs of neglect but none of these on its own should be taken as evidence that neglect is occurring.

If you suspect abuse

The diagnosis of child abuse can be difficult. It may be hard to steer a course between falsely accusing innocent parents and failing to recognise and deal with a child who is genuinely at risk. When in doubt it is important that an experienced health professional is contacted. The names of appropriate health visitors can be obtained from the health centre or surgery or from the local telephone directory.

If health care professionals dealt with child abuse only by aiming to detect and treat it, then the incidence of such abuse would not fall. It is the aim of professionals to prevent child abuse occurring. Health visitors will be aware of families who are at risk and may be visiting quite intensively as a support to parents in that situation. It is sometimes the case that mothers have very aggressive feelings towards their child – this may be due to prolonged crying, coupled with sleep deprivation. The mother may be reluctant to tell a health professional or family member about it because she feels it would be an admission of failure. The risk is that she could end up having a violent outburst. Health visitors and general practitioners will listen very sympathetically and it is essential that mothers get this message from family and friends.

One important prevention strategy is to ensure that society's future parents are informed of the needs of growing children and that they do not have unrealistic expectations. As a consequence of advertising, for example, a mother might feel that 'the norm' is a continuously happy and contented baby whereas this picture often falls short of the reality.

Of course most children will sustain injury at some point in their lives. One in five children can expect to attend an Accident and Emergency department for this reason. To be grubby and dishevelled is a natural consequence of rough and tumble play, particularly if this occurs outside. While everyone should be aware of the possibility of malicious injury and neglect, overt suspicion should be avoided until there is definite proof; if you are in any doubt, then health professionals should be contacted.

The future for abused children

In the past many abused children were placed in care following incidents of proven child abuse and they languished in children's homes as a result without any real decisions being made for their future. This is no longer the case and options as safe places for abused children now include grandparents' home, foster parents, even the home of a close friend.

There is a rosier side to child abuse. We hear so much of tragedy that it is easy to forget that for many families who receive intervention from professionals the end is a happy one – with the children concerned blossoming with their foster parents, or indeed sometimes with their own parents.

FROM BIRTH TO FIVE YEARS

5.1 THE NEWBORN

5.1(a) FEEDING

Breast feeding is the ideal way to feed a baby and, if mother and baby are well, can be started in the delivery room itself. If it is successful, it is enjoyable, convenient, nutritious and economical. It also gives the baby a passive immunity to some diseases before her own immune system develops.

Some mothers are uncertain about breast feeding, but midwives and health visitors are there to advise and some women also gain excellent support from National Childbirth Trust or La Leche League breast feeding counsellors. The mother should be allowed to make her own choice but she should do so with the knowledge and understanding that a relaxed, private discussion with a trained person will provide. A reluctant breast feeder is unlikely to continue for long, and the tension generated by uncertainty or by fear of being considered a poor mother will be communicated to the child.

It must also be remembered that there are a number of mothers who, for one reason or another, cannot breast feed their babies. Such mothers should be reassured that a proper alternative, prepared with scrupulous attention to cleanliness and given with love, will ensure that their baby too has a good start in life (see the section on 'Artificial feeding' below).

See Appendix VII for Addresses of useful organisations and support groups

Breast feeding

For the first three days after the birth of the baby the breast produces colostrum to meet the baby's needs; milk follows when she is ready for the more substantial diet. The differing nutritional components of colostrum and human milk are shown in the table and compared with cows' milk.

The constituents of colostrum and milk

Constituent	Colostrum	Human milk	Cows' milk
Protein	8.0%	1.5%	3.5%
Sugar	3.5%	7.0%	4.5%
Fat	2.5%	3.5%	3.5%
Minerals	0.4%	0.2%	0.7%
Water	85.6%	87.8%	87.8%

Breast feeding should be an enjoyable experience for both mother and baby. There may be some difficulties in the beginning if the mother is inexperienced. The child may be incorrectly positioned at the breast or frustrated because the milk has not yet 'come in', and the mother needs the love and support of her family and friends, as well as help from the midwife, to help her build her confidence and remain relaxed. Colostrum is the ideal food for the baby during the first two or three days. In addition to the nutritional advantages of breast milk, the close physical relationship helps to establish the emotional bonding and the love that provides a foundation for a healthy family in the future.

It is important for the mother to be entirely comfortable for breast feeding. She may wish to go to the toilet and wash herself before arranging the items she may need for herself: a box of tissues or a glass of water for example. The baby too should be comfortable and, unless she is crying hungrily, the mother may change her nappy and spend a few minutes fondling and talking to her before starting to feed her. Most mothers choose to sit upright to feed their babies while others prefer to lie on their side, particularly if their bottom is tender.

Correct positioning of the baby at the breast is essential for successful breast feeding. The baby should be held close with her head and shoulders supported on the forearm, facing the breast, with her mouth at the level of the nipple. The mother may need to support a heavy breast with fingers held flat against the ribs, sometimes with her thumb at the top of the breast. If the baby grasps the

Positioning the baby at the breast

(a) Bad positioning – the baby sucks on the end of the nipple causing damage and failing to stimulate proper milk flow.
(b) Good positioning – the whole of the nipple and most of the areola is in the baby's mouth.

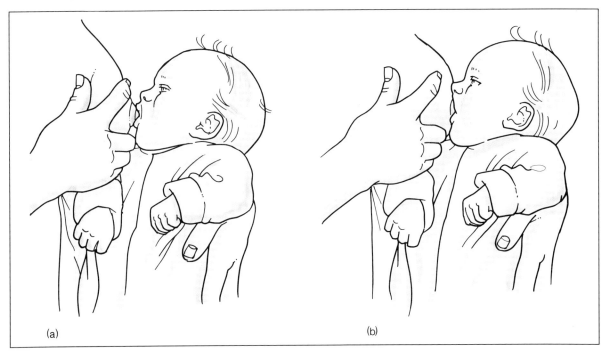

(a)   (b) nipple only, she should be removed gently from the breast and repositioned as illustrated. Allowing the baby to continue sucking when she is incorrectly positioned leads to sore nipples and a frustrated baby who has difficulty in getting enough milk.

There is much evidence now to support the opinion that babies should not be restricted in the time allowed for feeding at the breast, and that they should be fed when they wake up and seem hungry. When feeding starts, the baby receives the thirst-quenching fore-milk but the composition of the milk changes as the feed continues and the hind-milk has a higher nutritional value, with a higher content of fat and protein, and is more satisfying. Restricting the length of time the baby suckles may deprive her of the high calorie milk she needs.

Some babies obtain all the milk they need from one breast while others feed from both breasts. Alternating the breast first offered to the baby at each feed will ensure that each breast is emptied in turn.

BREAST FEEDING YOUR BABY

Positioning yourself	Either sit up in bed with pillows behind your back, lie on your side in bed, or sit in an upright chair or rocking chair with arms. You may find pillows useful for added support.
Positioning your baby	If you wish, undress your baby to promote comforting skin contact. A pillow on your lap can help support the arm holding your baby. Hold him gently and firmly with his head at the bend in your arm and his back along your forearm, your hand supporting his bottom. His head should be straight, neither bent forward nor arched back, and looking straight forward in relation to his body. He should be facing your breast so that an imaginary line from the middle of your breast passing through the nipple would go through the centre of his mouth.
Starting the feed	Cup your breast with your other hand, your fingers below the breast and your thumb on top but well away from the nipple. Stimulate your baby to open his mouth by touching your nipple to his lips. As soon as his mouth is wide open, draw him close so that all or most of the areola can be grasped. If he does not take enough into his mouth, and grasps the nipple only, break the contact by slipping your little finger into the corner of his mouth. Pull his chin down gently to allow more of the areola to enter his mouth. His tongue should be beneath your nipple. Be ready to take time and care to get the contact between his mouth and your breast right. Some babies need to be taught to do this, others take to the breast quite naturally.

Artificial feeding

A proportion of mothers choose not to breast feed or find breast feeding difficult to establish and decide to change to artificial feeding. Furthermore, there are some mothers for whom breast feeding is not an option, for example because they are taking medicines that would pass through their milk and affect the baby. Adoptive parents and certain others will need to use artificial milk too.

Infant formulae are artificial feeds which have been manufactured to take the place of human milk and to provide the sole source of nourishment. The formula is designed to be as close to, and as adequate as, human milk. There are many different brands to choose from. Most are based on cows' milk products but there are also infant soya based milks for babies who are allergic to cows' milk. The midwife and health visitor will advise you about which brand of formula is best for your baby.

Scrupulous cleanliness is essential when preparing formula feeds, and a steriliser is a vital piece of equipment. This can either be a large container in which the bottles and teats can be immersed in sterilising solution, or a steam steriliser. If the former is used, sterilisation solution granules or tablets are needed and (with most brands) the bottles should be rinsed with boiled water before they are filled. The sterilisation solution needs to be changed every 24 hours and care must be taken to see that no air bubbles are left in the bottles when they are immersed in the solution.

Mothers whose babies are bottle fed should have at least six wide-necked glass or polypropyline upright bottles with caps, teats and teat covers. Teats should be replaced regularly and the bottles and teats should be well scrubbed with a bottle brush and salt (which should then be rinsed off thoroughly) before they are put into the steriliser.

Some breast feeding mothers may wish to express some milk or collect it in breast shells. If this is the case, they too should have equipment for sterilising, collecting and storing milk, as well as a couple of bottles. Hand breast pumps and breast shells should be sterilised before use. Breast milk can be frozen and stored, but should be used or discarded within one month.

Formula milk should be made up by following exactly the instructions on the tin or packet. Cooled, previously boiled water should always be used and formula powder should be added in the proportions indicated. It can be dangerous to give your baby feeds which are either too dilute or do not contain enough water. Once prepared, bottles should be cooled by running under the cold tap and stored in the fridge for up to 24 hours. If they are not refrigerated, they should be used straight away. Unfinished feeds should always be discarded and never saved.

Just as for breast feeding, the mother (or father) and baby should both be comfortable and relaxed. The temperature of the feed should be tested by shaking a few drops on the wrist to make sure it is comfortable. The parent should hold the baby close when feeding him, should talk to him and maintain eye contact. In this way he will not miss out on the 'social' advantages enjoyed by breast fed babies.

5.1(b) KEEPING THE BABY CLEAN

In the early weeks, a baby's existence may seem to be one long series of physical demands. If she is not hungry or sleeping, the chances are that she will need her nappy changing and a wash or bath. It is important to keep babies clean and comfortable as far as possible. Nappies should be changed six to eight times a day and more often if soiled. It is not fair on the baby to leave her in a soiled nappy for longer than is absolutely necessary. Furthermore, soiled nappies may give rise to nappy rash and other infections.

There is much debate about the advantages and disadvantages of disposable versus terry nappies but no real evidence to suggest that one type is better or worse than the other. The choice should be the mother's and such considerations as cost and convenience are usually deciding factors. There is little point, for example, in investing in two dozen terry nappies if you have neither the space nor the facilities for drying them.

Topping and tailing

Newborn babies can be kept adequately clean by regular washing of the face and bottom. The baby's bottom should always be washed when her nappy is changed, regardless of whether or not she is soiled. The one exception to this may be when changing a merely wet nappy in the middle of the night when trying to encourage the baby to realise that night is different from day and a time for sleeping. Full topping and tailing should be performed at least once a day and more often if the baby gets very dirty or does not have a bath. Before you start, it is best to have everything you will need ready to hand. This will include the following.

- A 'topping and tailing' bowl with two halves, or two separate bowls, clearly marked. The same bowl or half bowl should always be used for the baby's face, the other for her bottom. They should contain water which is pleasantly warm (not too hot).

- Cotton wool balls or pieces.

- A clean nappy and, if appropriate, a change of clothing. It is wise to place the baby on her changing mat, in case of accidents. For comfort, put a clean, folded muslin square under her head. Wash your hands before you begin and at the end of each stage.

- Use the water in the 'top' bowl to clean her face, ears and neck. Change cotton wool balls often. Clean only the parts of the ears and nose that can be reached easily: never poke a cotton bud into your baby's ear or up her nose. Dry her face and neck with fresh cotton wool or a soft towel.

- Undo her nappy. If she is soiled wipe off the worst of the faeces with a corner of the terry nappy, cotton wool or prepared 'wet wipes'. If the nappy is a disposable one, put the wipes into it and fold it over. Now use the water in the 'tail' bowl to wet more pieces of cotton wool. Wash your baby's front, away from the genitals, and her lower tummy up as far as the navel.

- Now clean the genitals. A little girl should always be wiped from front to back to avoid spreading germs from the anus into the vagina. A baby boy's scrotum should be washed all over and care should be taken to clean the area under his penis thoroughly. The penis itself should be wiped away from the body. Never attempt to clean inside the lips of the little girl's vagina or to pull back the little boy's foreskin.

- Wash the baby's buttocks and anus, taking care that any remaining traces of faeces are removed. Dry carefully with fresh cotton wool, ensuring that no damp creases remain. If you use a barrier cream, be sure to rub it well in, then put on a clean nappy.

- Wash your hands again.

Bathing

Many babies enjoy bathtime and it can become a special time in their daily routine. Those who are not so keen, however, do not need to be bathed every day – they can be topped and tailed more often instead. It is probably as well to try reintroducing the idea of a full bath to the reluctant baby about every five or six days. You may find he loses his fears quite suddenly between attempts if he is allowed to become ready for real baths in his own time.

A baby bath is ideal but not essential for bathing your baby. A large, clean washing-up bowl or even the kitchen sink (providing the taps do not get in the way) can be used instead. A baby under four or five months old will feel lost in the big bath unless he goes in with a parent. If you do take the baby into the bath with you, do be careful to keep the water sufficiently cool.

Before you start bathing your baby, make sure that the room is warm enough. Ideally, it should be about 20°C (70°F). You will need a clean nappy and change of clothes, a bath or bowl with a non-slip mat in the bottom, baby soap – either as liquid or in a bar – and a soft flannel, one or two soft towels and equipment for topping and tailing as above.

Once the baby's face is clean, you may want to wash his hair. The most convenient way to do this is to squirt some liquid baby soap into the bath water checking first that, like most brands, it does not need to be rinsed off. Then keeping his nappy on, wrap him in a towel and hold him securely against you with one arm. Your hand should support his head, your forearm should be under his back and his legs should tuck under your elbow (see the figure). His head should be over the bath. Use your free hand to tip water over his hair, taking care to avoid his face (especially the eyes). Gently rub his scalp. Then cuddle him as you pat his head dry with the towel.

You can now finish undressing him and wash his bottom (see above) before putting him in the bath. It is important that he feels secure in the bath. Hold him firmly with one hand round his far shoulder while the wrist and forearm support the shoulder closest to you. Use your other hand to lift his bottom as you transfer him in and out of the bath. This hand can also be used to wash him.

Five minutes in the water is quite enough for a small baby. After taking him out, wrap him up in the towel and cuddle him to get most of the water off and ensure that he doesn't get cold. Then undo the towel and dry him carefully in all the skin folds and creases. Put a clean nappy on and dress him.

The young baby's bathtime

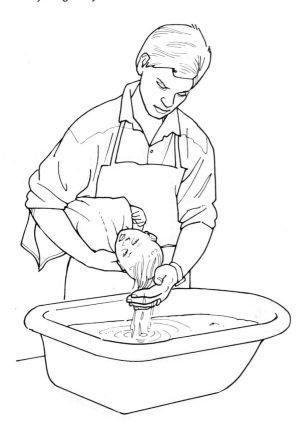

Washing the baby's hair . . .

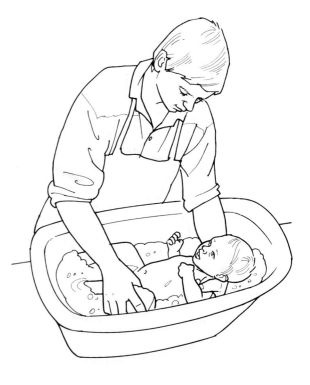

. . . and holding her securely in the bath.

5.1(c) MAINTAINING BODY TEMPERATURE

Adults can shiver and sweat. They can move about to warm themselves or can take off layers of clothing. A small baby is not so lucky. She cannot regulate her own body temperature so this must be done for her.

Newborns need to be kept at an even, warm temperature. The room the baby is in should be heated to 18–19°C (65–68°F) if the temperature in the house is below this. During a heatwave, you may need to use an electric fan to keep your baby sufficiently cool.

Warmth

A small baby needs to be kept warmer than an active older child or adult so, as a general rule of thumb, think about how many layers of clothing you are wearing and add one more for her. It should be stressed, however, that this is a rough guide only. If you are very tired or anaemic you may feel more than usually sensitive to cold, and if you are slightly feverish (for example if you have mastitis) you may think that the house is warmer than it really is. For the first few weeks after you bring the baby home, it may be helpful to have an ordinary wall thermometer in the same room as the baby.

It is particularly important to ensure that the baby does not get cold at night. Swaddle her in a blanket before lying her in her cot, and put further blankets over the top. Cotton or wool blankets are preferable to synthetic ones as they allow better temperature regulation. (You should not lose sight, however, of the dangers of overheating babies at night, which are discussed in the next section.) The best way to counter sudden night time drops in the environmental temperature is to have a thermostatted heater in the baby's room keeping it at around 18–19°C (65–68°F). If this is not feasible, it may be advisable to take her into your bed with you during a cold spell. Put her in between you and your partner (or if you are on your own, between you and a pillow) so that there is no danger of her falling out. It is extremely unlikely that you will roll over onto your baby unless you have been taking alcohol or drugs.

Do be sensible when taking a small baby out of doors. She should be wrapped up in an appropriate way for the weather. In particular, her head should be well covered to avoid losing body heat. Never leave her outside to sleep in her pram on a really cold day.

You can check that your baby is warm enough by feeling the back of her neck. Little hands become chilly quite quickly and should alert you, but if the back of the neck is cool, you should be concerned. Other signs that she is losing too much heat are listlessness, cool skin under her clothes and flushed cheeks. If you are in any doubt, take her temperature. If it is below 35°C, you should phone the doctor.

See Chapter 5, section 11 for advice on taking a young child's temperature

While waiting for the doctor to arrive, or if chilling is not quite this serious but still a problem, wrap the baby in an extra blanket and cuddle her close (alternatively, take her into your bed with you) and, most importantly, give her a feed.

Overheating

See Chapter 5, section 2(d) on Cot death

In the concern for keeping the baby warm, it is easy to forget that too much of a good thing can be equally dangerous. In 1990, a paper published in the British Medical Journal argued that overheating may interfere with the baby's ability to breathe, sometimes even leading to cot death.

On warm summer nights, babies should be dressed in a nappy and vest only and just a sheet or light cotton blanket put over them. Check the room temperature before you go to bed yourself to make sure it has not dropped unduly. On hot days, keep clothing to a minimum and try to make sure that cotton (not a synthetic fabric) is used. A very warm baby may feel better for being sponged down with tepid water and gently patted dry. An electric fan may help to keep the temperature down – so long as it is well guarded and not blowing directly at the baby. Alternatively, you may find a small paper hand fan useful. The baby will like the colour and movement as well as the gentle breeze. Take a hand fan with you when you go out as you may find it particularly difficult to keep him cool in an environment over which you have no control.

Babies can get very dehydrated during hot weather so offer plenty to drink. If your baby refuses to take anything other than breast milk, you may have to feed him more often, for shorter periods. Make sure that you drink extra fluids yourself if this happens.

Babies who produce six or eight wet nappies a day and seem cheerful are almost certainly getting enough fluids. If the number of wet nappies goes down, if your baby's fontanelle appears depressed and if he seems listless or floppy, you should phone your doctor immediately.

The 'soft spot' or gentle dip in the top of a baby's head, where the bones of the skull have not yet closed up. The fontanelle has usually disappeared completely by the time the baby is about 18 months old.

Babies' skin is very sensitive to the sun's rays so always keep him in the shade when out of doors on a warm day. Baby sunblock cream is an added precaution and, even with a pram shade or canopy, a sun-hat should always be worn. Never leave the baby to sleep out of doors unattended for long on a hot day as the sun can move faster than you expect, taking the pools of shade with it. Never leave your baby in an unventilated car, even for a few minutes. This could be fatal.

5.1(d) HOLDING AND HANDLING

Handling a newborn baby can be alarming – especially if you are not used to them. Many parents find holding and carrying their newborn particularly frightening once they get home. In hospital, the baby will be picked up and put down by hospital staff – all of whom know exactly what to do. Many mothers feel that they will seem foolish if they ask for advice on such basic procedures as picking their baby up, wrapping her up, winding her or changing her nappy. This is unfortunate – in fact staff are usually only too willing to help, advise and reassure.

Once you arrive home with your new baby though, the reality of her vulnerability and your responsibility hits you in a way that may feel quite overwhelming. Except for the visits in the early days from the community midwife and health visitor you are likely to be on your own. The baby is tiny. Her head rolls back if you don't support it and you may be terrified of hurting or dropping her.

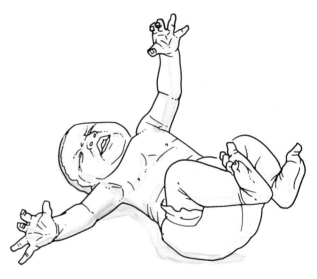

If handled too roughly, the newborn baby will throw up his arms and tremble – the 'Moro' response

If this is your first baby (and you are unused to handling other people's tiny babies) it may be some weeks before you feel really confident. You should be reassured at this stage, however, on two points. Firstly it is actually extremely unlikely that you will drop your baby (unless you fall yourself or have been taking drugs or alcohol), and secondly, small babies are usually a lot more robust and resilient than they look. In addition, your baby can be relied upon to let you know, either by yelling or by throwing her arms up and her head back in the 'Moro response' (illustrated above) if she does not like the way you are handling her. Remembering a few simple rules should make this unlikely however.

- It is important to be aware that your baby cannot support himself at all and is completely reliant on you. Use both your arms and your body to make him feel safe. Hold him against your shoulder, with one hand supporting his head and the other supporting his bottom, or cradle him snugly in your arms against your chest, with his head supported in the crook of one elbow and his back and legs supported by your other arm, as shown.

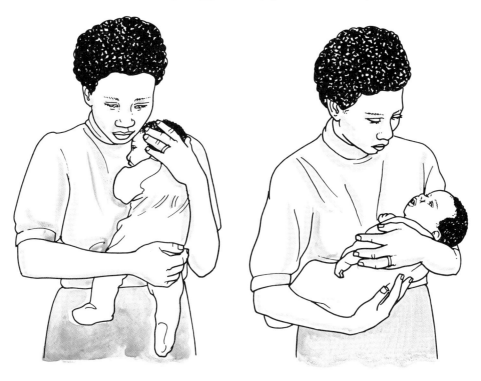

Hold your baby securely against your shoulder . . .   or cradle her in your arms

- Take your time over picking him up and putting him down. Try to make all movements as steady as possible. The transfer of his weight from mat to your arms and back to his cot should be entirely smooth. Don't let his head fall back or loll as you pick him up or put him down.

- Your baby should always be well supported in the bath (see section 5.1(b) above).

5.2 THE FIRST SIX MONTHS

5.2(a) NORMAL DEVELOPMENT

See also Chapter 4, section 7(a) for more information about bonding

The first six months of life is a period of very rapid growth for the infant, and often of as rapid an adjustment for the parents and family. Much has been written about the importance of early bonding of mother and child and the future adverse effects of early separation of mother and baby. It is important that parents do not become over anxious about early bonding to their child. Bear in mind the following points.

- Early studies on the effect of separation of mothers and newborn babies have been repeated using different methods and the original findings have not been confirmed.

- Premature and ill babies often need to be nursed in an incubator for a short period after birth and most of these babies develop normal loving relationships with their families.

- Perfectly normal parents often do not feel anything special for their new baby for several hours or days after the birth. The mother may be tired following delivery and the father over anxious about his new responsibility and perhaps even a little jealous now that he has to share his partner's attentions. It is important that these feelings are acknowledged and discussed.

The newborn infant

Behaviour Newborn babies sleep for about 20 out of 24 hours and when awake tend to cry or become restless, a situation which often frustrates anxious parents who feel that the child must either be hungry, require a nappy change or be in pain, often referred to as 'colic'. Usually a cuddle or a change of position will comfort a distressed baby if a feed is not imminent. When the baby is calm and wakeful, eye contact can be established between carer and child. It is thought that infants have rather immature vision at this age but research has shown that infants prefer to fix their gaze on patterns that resemble facial features, and prefer bright colours. Therefore, looking at your baby and also hanging brightly coloured mobiles within his field of vision are useful ways of stimulating his visual abilities. Hearing is also restricted to the immediate surroundings, but small infants do respond to the human voice and therefore it is important to talk to your baby from birth.

A social smile is observed in most infants at around six weeks. This important developmental milestone should be recorded.

Physical development At birth the average baby weighs 3.4 kgs and measures 50 cms in length. The newborn infant has a floppy head and neck and adopts a fetal position with arms bent and knees pulled up on the abdomen.

Following Department of Health Recommendations in 1991, parents are advised not to lie their tiny baby on his tummy. The position of choice for lying a newborn down to sleep is on his side swaddled in a blanket. A second rolled up blanket behind the baby's spine will stop him from rolling onto his back.

Older, stronger babies are likely to move themselves into the position they prefer, no matter how you lie them down.

See also section 5.1 above and section 5.12(a) below

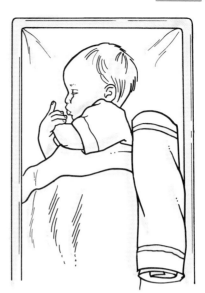

Position for sleeping

Your tiny baby will be safest swaddled and lying on his side with a rolled-up blanket behind him

Newborn babies have several primitive reflexes:

- *Grasp*   if an object is placed in the palm of the hand, the fingers will close tightly around it;

- *Startle (Moro)*   in response to a sudden noise or movement, the baby will fling his arms and legs wide and then curl up again (see section 5.1(d) above);

- *Walking*   if the baby's feet are placed against a firm surface, he will move his legs as if walking;

- *Supporting*   he will support his weight momentarily when held erect;

- *Sucking*   if his mouth is stroked, the baby will suck rhythmically;

- *Rooting*   stroking his cheek will cause him to turn his head to suckle.

These reflexes are strong in the early weeks of life but gradually disappear.

Three months

Behaviour   The baby is more wakeful and aware of her surroundings and vocalises using vowel sounds such as 'aa' and 'oo'. She begins to show excitement in anticipation of events such as feeding. She becomes interested in her hands and spends time watching and moving her fingers.

Physical development   She now has more control over the movements of her arms and legs. The following tells you what she can do in what position.

- *Prone*
  - Raises her head to an angle of about 60° and holds position for several minutes
  - Bears weight on her forearms
  - Legs stretched out and kicks one or both legs

- *Sitting*
  - Can balance her head in a sitting position but has little control over the upper part of her body
  - She has sufficient head control to allow turning and following of a moving object

- *Standing*
  - Can take some weight on her feet
  - Her head remains balanced in line with her body
  - Walking reflex has disappeared

- *Grasp*
  - Grasps an object placed in her hand, using a total fist grasp
  - She will loose her grasp after a few seconds but is not able to release grasp voluntarily
  - She is unable to reach and grasp, or to move her hand whilst grasping an object.

Six months

Behaviour   The baby will now turn readily when he hears his mother's voice across a room. He vocalises tunefully using double syllables such as 'da-da', 'ta-ta', etc. He will scream with annoyance and also react to differing emotional tones in the carer's voice. He is beginning to recognise familiar carers and to show suspicion of strangers.

Physical development   The range of activities the six month old baby is capable of is summarised below.

- *On his back*
  - He raises his head from the pillow to look at his feet
  - Lifts legs up straight and grasps one foot or (later) two feet
  - kicks strongly with alternate legs.

- *Prone*
  - Placed on his tummy, he lifts his head and chest well up, supporting himself on flattened palms and extended arms
  - Can roll over front to back and usually back to front
  - Moves his arms briskly and holds them up to be lifted.

- *Sitting*
  - Sits with support in cot or pram and turns his head from side to side to look around him

- When his hands are grasped, he braces his shoulders and pulls himself to sit
- When held sitting, his head is firmly erect and his back straight; he may sit alone momentarily.

- *Standing*
  - When held standing, with his feet touching a hard surface, he will bear his weight on his feet
  - Bounces up and down when held standing.

- *Grasp*
  - Immediately notices an interesting small object (such as a toy or sweet) within 15–30 cms (6–12 inches) and will stretch out both hands to grasp it
  - Puts most objects to his mouth
  - Uses his whole hand in palmar grasp and passes a toy from one hand to the other
  - When a toy falls from the hand, he will watch where it lands but, when a toy falls where it cannot be seen, it is soon forgotten.

5.2(b)   WEANING

For the first four to six months of life, milk, water and vitamins A, C and D provide babies with all their nutritional requirements, and the feeding of solid foods before this age is unnecessary. The general view is that the baby's digestive system is unable to cope with wheat proteins (particularly gluten, associated with coeliac disease) and the high salt content of many commercially produced foods. The previously held view that early introduction of solids pre-disposed to obesity in later life is unproven.

The objectives of weaning are as follows.

- To make the baby less nutritionally dependent on milk. By the age of one year, milk should still be an important food and ideally provide about 40 per cent of the calorie intake.

- To provide a variety of textures using puréed and finely diced food which will stimulate the baby's ability to chew.

- To establish the acceptance of a variety of foods and a wide range of flavours.

- Gradually to introduce regular family foods so that the baby may partake in social family meals.

- To introduce iron into the diet because human and unfortified cows' milk are poor sources of iron. During the first three to four months, a baby has sufficient iron reserves received from the mother during the final weeks of pregnancy. However, after four months, reserves are depleted and foods with good iron content need to be introduced.

- To train the baby to feed from a spoon and drink from a cup.

Introducing solid food

Weaning is often an anxious time for parents, particularly if this is a first baby. It is sometimes helpful to discuss introduction of solid foods with the local health visitor either during a home visit or on attendance at the child welfare clinic. Although commercially produced baby foods are convenient, they can prove expensive, particularly as the baby will take only small amounts initially, resulting in the remaining amount being wasted as it is unsafe to reheat food. Family foods can be adapted and, besides being cheaper, are often more nutritious.

Initially, half to one teaspoon of food should be offered before the normal breast or bottle feed. The morning or early afternoon feeds are usually considered to be the best time for introducing new foods, as in the early stages it is more time consuming. Parents should therefore choose a time when they are least pressured and thus make the experience enjoyable for themselves and their baby. If a baby shows a dislike for a particular food, another flavour should be tried and the rejected item tried again a few days later. Meal time battles should be avoided as they may result in protracted feeding problems and distortion of the carer/child relationships.

Most health visitors and dietitians recommend baby rice as a first food as it is easy to prepare and readily acceptable by most infants when mixed with milk, and is economical. It avoids introduction of wheat proteins too soon, as some younger babies do not tolerate this protein well. Unfortunately, cereal feeds are high in calories and can result in overweight if fed in excessive quantities. It is therefore recommended that no more than one cereal feed per day should be offered, the feed being prepared with milk with no added sugar and given from a spoon. The practice of adding cereal to the bottle should be strongly discouraged, as this upsets the milk formula and does not help the baby to learn to feed from a spoon.

Mashed vegetables, such as potatoes or carrots, mashed banana or finely-sieved chicken broth are all suitable first foods. A food blender or baby mincer can be used to purée family foods but from about six months onwards more lumpy food will be tolerated. About this time the first teeth begin to appear, but it is not necessary to wait for teeth before introducing lumpier foods.

Salt or spices should not be added to savoury foods fed to babies and sweet foods should be kept to a minimum to avoid the risk of dental caries when the teeth start to appear.

See section 5.12(b) for more information about Teething

	Stage 1 Not before 4 months	Stage 2	Stage 3 From 6 months
Foods to try:	Vegetable or fruit purées (e.g. potato, carrot, yam, plantain, spinach, apple, banana) Thin porridge (made from rice, cornmeal, sago, millet, tapioca) Puréed lentils (dhal) – mild spices may be used	Purées using lean meat (including liver), poultry, fish A wider variety of vegetables and fruit purées	Dairy foods, e.g. milk (whole milk not semi-skimmed or skimmed), yoghurt (bought or home made), cottage cheese Wheat-based foods, e.g. cereals, semolina Egg yolks, citrus fruits, smooth peanut butter
Still to avoid:	Milk other than breast or formula milk [1] Wheat-based foods [1] Eggs [1] Citrus fruits [1] Nuts [1,2] Sugar [3] and salt [4] Chillies [5]	Milk other than breast or formula milk [1] Wheat-based foods [1] Eggs [1] Citrus fruits [1] Nuts [1,2] Sugar [3] and salt [4] Chillies [5]	Sugar [3] and salt [4] Whole nuts [2] Chillies [5]

[1] May cause allergic reactions in susceptible infants

[2] Risk of choking

[3] May give a taste for sweet things, leading to problems with teeth and weight later

[4] A baby's kidneys, being immature, cannot readily excrete large amounts of salt

[5] Strong spices may irritate the gastrointestinal tract

Reproduced with kind permission of the National Dairy Council

Weaning schedule

As the quantity of solid foods consumed increases, the volume of milk intake should be gradually reduced. Breast milk or baby milk formula should be used until the child is at least six months old, and ideally throughout the first year. Although dietary guidelines recommend low fat milks, these are not suitable for babies and children under two who should be fed whole milk products.

A baby needs more fluid during hot weather and, to safeguard against dehydration, diluted unsweetened fruit juice or cooled boiled water should be offered.

From about seven months, pieces of hard foods such as crusts, peeled apple or a carrot should be given to help teething, but the baby should never be left alone with these foods because of the risk of choking. At this age, babies may want to take an active part in feeding themselves. Although this can be a messy business, it should be encouraged and suitable protection provided in the form of a 'pelican' or 'coverall' bib and plastic sheets on the carpet. By the time she is nine months, the baby will be sharing in most of the family meals.

5.2(c) HOW TO KNOW WHEN THE BABY IS ILL AND WHEN TO SEEK ADVICE

See also section 5.11 on Looking after a sick child at home

All parents worry about their children's health; it is a feature of being a parent. The family doctor, midwife and health visitor are available to give advice and should be accessible by personal contact or telephone. Common concerns about young babies usually relate to eating, sleeping, crying and bowel habits.

Eating

A baby's eating patterns may vary slightly from day to day, and as he grows he will tend to take larger feeds and sustain longer intervals between feeds. However, a normally healthy baby who refuses feeds for longer than 24 hours should be seen by a doctor. Loss of appetite can be an indication that the baby is suffering from an infection, particularly if this occurs with a change in bowel habits and/or vomiting. Although routine weighing is not considered necessary for otherwise healthy babies, parents often like the reassurance that their baby is thriving. Health centres and local clinics usually have open access clinics where the baby can be weighed and any concerns discussed with the health visitor.

Sleeping

Some babies sleep less than others, and there is a school of thought which suggests that potentially more intelligent children require less sleep. The problem is that young babies do not easily differentiate between day and night, and their sleep patterns may not accord with those of their parents. This causes the parents to become tired and more irritable, and this irritability may be communicated to the baby making her even more unsettled. An ill baby is more likely to be lethargic and sleep for prolonged periods, missing feeds, and as indicated this should constitute cause for concern. If the baby is unsettled during the night, it is wise to discuss with your health visitor how more regular sleep patterns can be established. This can often be achieved by varying feed times, giving the last feed at night as late as possible so that the parents can have six or seven hours of unbroken sleep.

Medication to promote sleep is not advisable except when all other methods have failed, and such treatment must be prescribed and supervised by the doctor.

Crying

A certain amount of crying is quite normal for all young babies. How much a baby cries will differ with individuals but the average is about two hours in 24. During the early days, a baby's cry is his only positive response to his environment and there may not be an easily found explanation.

See section 5.2(a) above for advice about positions for sleeping babies

The newborn baby has a strongly developed righting reflex, so that if he is placed on his back his arms and legs will fly out, invariably causing him to cry. He can usually be calmed by placing him on his tummy or wrapping him in a shawl or blanket. This is probably the reason why infants were swaddled in earlier times, and in some countries babies are still strapped to their mothers' backs.

Hunger is a strong stimulus for crying, but it should not be assumed that this is always the cause as overfeeding can lead to further crying owing to overdistension of the stomach with food. Babies do cry from boredom, and a change of position or a cuddle can often settle a distressed infant. Your baby will not be 'spoiled' if you pick him up – but the converse is also true and it does a healthy baby no harm to cry for a short period if you are not able to give him your immediate attention.

A wet or dirty nappy is frequently blamed for crying, but is seldom the cause. Although it is true that a baby will cry if he is cold, a wet nappy is more likely to have a warming effect (initially, at least). Babies should not be left too long in a dirty or wet nappy, however, as this can cause nappy rash.

Teething is not a cause of prolonged crying: if it were, we could expect individuals to be crying from six months to twenty years. It is often too easy to blame teething for the baby's distress at something more serious such as an ear infection.

A final point to remember is that it takes a considerable amount of energy for a baby to cry, and therefore a baby who is ill is less likely to cry.

Bowel habits

A baby's bowel movements will vary according to how he is fed. Breast fed babies often go for several days without having a bowel action, and this is quite normal. The stools of breast fed babies are soft and bright yellow, and if the baby is changed on to formula cows' milk the stools will become harder and more formed. This does not indicate constipation but just a change in the diet. Some formula milks cause the baby to have bright green stools, which is linked with bile metabolism in the gut, and is again quite normal. Babies have no control over their bowel movements and, although they may appear to be straining to fill their nappy, this is still a reflex action. If parents are still convinced that their baby has constipation, it should be treated by giving more diluted fruit juice or cooled boiled water and vegetables, and not by giving laxatives or extra sugar in the feeds.

See also section 5.12(h) below on Gastroenteritis

Diarrhoea in babies is much more serious, as this can indicate gastroenteritis. Where stools are very frequent – up to five or six dirty nappies per day – or they appear watery, slimy or excessively smelly, the doctor should be consulted immediately. Milk feeds will usually be suspended and the infant prescribed mineral supplements in water. Babies with diarrhoea rapidly become dehydrated, and therefore it is important to seek advice immediately, particularly where the diarrhoea is accompanied by vomiting.

Most babies regurgitate small amounts of food after a feed, and this is referred to as 'possetting'. Older babies may induce vomiting by cramming their fingers into their mouths, and, although this may be viewed by parents as a rather inconvenient habit, it is not serious provided the baby is otherwise well.

If vomiting is accompanied by diarrhoea or loss of appetite, or is extremely forceful, it should be treated more seriously and medical advice sought.

Health visitors are available for all families, and the golden rule is that if you are in any way worried about your baby, seek advice.

5.2(d) COT DEATH

This distressing occurrence may also be referred to as *unexpected death in infancy syndrome* or *sudden infant death syndrome* (SIDS).

A definition of cot death, adopted in the USA in 1969, refers to the condition as:

> 'The sudden death of any infant or young child which is unexpected by history and for which a thorough postmortem examination fails to demonstrate an adequate cause of death.

Cot death is therefore not a single condition and any baby's death may be the coincidental coming together of a number of trigger factors.

In the United Kingdom about 1 in 500 babies die unexpectedly each year. The most vulnerable age group is between two and four months with 75 per cent of cot deaths occurring in infants under six months of age. On average there is a higher incidence in January, February and March than in other months of the year.

Cot deaths have been recorded throughout history and the earliest mention is in the Old Testament. For many centuries such deaths were attributed to 'overlaying' and accidental suffocation; it was not until the 1950s and 1960s that researchers began to study the patterns of occurrence of cot deaths. In spite of a great deal of research over the last three decades no single cause for cot death has been discovered but several factors have been linked to the incidence of cot deaths. The evidence is in no way conclusive and a number of factors may contribute to the sudden death of an infant. Awareness of these may help parents to protect their infants.

Possible contributing factors

Undiagnosed disease   Retarded growth and failure to thrive may be a symptom of a long standing disease process.

Disorders of breathing   There have been reports of infants suffering from episodes of apnoea, most commonly during sleep. It must be stressed that episodes of apnoea are common among normal infants and extensive research has failed to show a significant connection between episodes of periodic or sleep apnoea and the incidence of cot death. These episodes are however distressing to parents and infants who display this tendency are usually kept under observation, sometimes by using an apnoea alarm.

- Apnoea
  Cessation of breathing

Disorders of the immune system   In the first two months of life infants are protected from infection by antibodies received from the mother whilst in the womb or transferred via the breast milk. It has been suggested that some infants fail to develop an efficient immune system and are therefore more vulnerable to infection.

A study in Oxford has shown that the mothers of infants who died were more likely to display allergic reactions than a control group. Various allergic responses have been suggested to substances such as house dust mite and cows' milk protein. It is known that cot death is less common in breast fed infants.

See also section 5.1(c) above

Disorders of temperature control   The body's natural temperature regulating system is inefficient in babies, particularly those of low birth weight. Cold and heat can therefore kill vulnerable babies. Low temperatures may contribute to underheating, and overheating – usually as a result of overclothing – has been shown to be a factor in some deaths.

Suffocation   Accidental suffocation, sometimes due to overlaying, is still a cause of some cot deaths. This has occurred in situations where infants have been put to sleep between two parents (one or both of whom has been taking drugs or alcohol) or other such inappropriate sleeping arrangements such as on a settee. It must be remembered that pillows in the cot or crib should not be used for infants under one year.

Infection   Many studies have shown a link between viral infections of the respiratory system and cot death. However, this may be linked with low birth weight and a depressed immune system which makes the infant more susceptible to infection. An infant with a feverish cold who is then overclothed by anxious parents has an increased risk of cot death.

Reducing the risk

Following the realisation that there are possible predisposing factors which make cot death more likely some health authorities have introduced a system of identification of infants thought to be more at risk of cot deaths. Such a system aims to score infants on such factors as age of mother, number of previous pregnancies, birth weight of baby, whether the mother smoked during pregnancy, feeding method, etc. High scoring infants are visited more frequently by the health visitor and are weighed on a one to two weekly basis for the first few months of life. Weights are carefully charted to detect any failure to thrive and parents are taught to monitor any symptoms of illness in their child. In areas where this system has been used the incidence of cot death has declined.

The parents' role in prevention

The Bristol Child Development Programme refers to the fact that there is a lower incidence of cot death in societies where babies are carried a great deal and seldom if ever left alone in the first few months of life. Although such evidence is useful it is important to remember that in such societies the level of reporting of deaths in infancy may be less accurate.

Based on this information the programme suggests that infants should be left alone as little as possible during the first few months of life. The infant should sleep in the parents' room preferably next to their bed. In the early months, when the baby is relatively light, she should be carried in a sling on the back or chest of one of the parents during the daytime and particularly when sleeping.

Premature infants will be monitored more closely by the doctor, midwife and the health visitor. Parents can work with professionals by assisting in monitoring of weight and consulting their doctor or health visitor early if their child shows any signs of illness or failure to thrive.

Parents who have experienced a cot death

Loss of any child is major tragedy but where the death is sudden and unexplained feelings of grief, anger and guilt may be overwhelming and may persist for many years. The support and understanding of family and friends can be most comforting but there are also specialist self-help groups with which your health visitor or doctor can put you in touch.

Decisions such as whether and when to have another baby are personal but counselling and support in such decisions is available from your doctor and health visitor or voluntary support groups. FSID (The Foundation for the Study of Infant Deaths) has a subgroup CONI which is particularly concerned with supporting parents who have lost a baby in their Care Of the Next Infant.

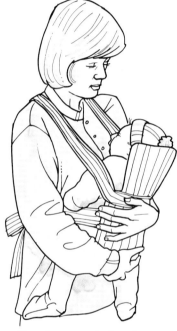

Keeping your baby close

A sling will enable you to carry the baby against your chest while he is sleeping

See also Chapter 4, section 3(e) on Loss and grief

See Appendix VII for Addresses of useful organisations and support groups

5.3 FROM SIX TO TWELVE MONTHS

5.3(a) GETTING ABOUT

During this stage, your child is likely to become very active. At the beginning, he will be able to sit without your help and roll over from his front to his back. A little later he will able to roll from back to front. When he is lying on his tummy, you will find he will pull his knees up and start to lean on his hands. This will very soon have movement added, and he will start to crawl – usually at about 9–10 months old. Some children will also learn to shuffle along on their bottoms, particularly if they want a toy that is out of reach. When he is crawling, you will find that he is always looking around for you, still needing the security of your presence.

Crawling

Most babies will learn how to get about on all fours somewhere around the age of 9–10 months

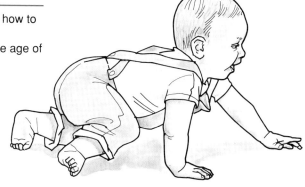

At around eight months old, your child may pull himself up to a standing position and he will get more used to taking his weight on his legs – almost in a bounding motion. Once he feels happy he will start to walk, while holding on to the furniture – probably around nine months old. This will be followed by him trying to go from one piece of furniture to another. How quickly he progresses to walking alone depends on how he reacts to falling. When walking, he will only take two or three steps before falling on his bottom and then getting up to have another try. However, some children are more cautious. Don't expect him to walk well on his own until about 12–15 months old or even later.

Most of the activity will happen because he wants to explore. Everything around him is of interest and acts as a stimulus to attract him to it. However, he cannot see any dangers, so it is important for you to think for him. Anything sharp, such as dressmaking pins or nails, should be picked up immediately. Glass ornaments which can be dropped and broken should be moved out of the way. But do remember that the thing that will help your child to walk or crawl is to have an object he wishes to explore slightly out of reach. By

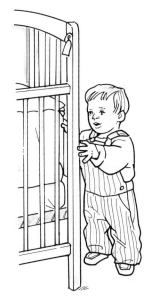

Standing and 'cruising'

Once he has learned to pull himself up into a standing position, he will enjoy 'cruising' round the furniture

removing *all* objects you are removing this stimulation. It might be useful to remove the valuable or breakable objects, but leave some colourful, less important ones to attract him.

It is also important to remember that everything will still go into his mouth, so do check that no very small items (parts of older children's games for example) are left within his reach.

During the later part of this time, he will also start to use his other senses, such as touch and smell. If the objects left to act as stimulation are of different textures, e.g. smooth wooden bricks, fluffy toys and ridged plastic blocks, this will encourage him to rely on more than what his mouth is telling him.

As he becomes more proficient at crawling and walking, you should consider other safety factors too, such as a gate at the top and bottom of the stairs so he can't crawl on the landing and fall, or attempt to crawl up a step. If you have a gas, electric or open fire, do buy a fireguard before he crawls and make sure it can be fixed to the fireplace or wall so that when he is able to pull himself up on the furniture, he will not pull it over on top of himself.

Many parents consider buying a baby walker or bouncer at this stage to help the child walk. These have proved to be a danger if your baby is not supervised carefully. The wheels of the baby walker can catch in the edge of a rug or against a hearth and tip over causing injury to your child. They also do not encourage him to walk unsupported, as he can get around without taking all his weight on his own feet.

See also section 5.8 below on Learning and exploring through play

See also section 5.10 below on Keeping your young child safe

5.3(b) MANUAL DEXTERITY AND CO-ORDINATION

During this second half-year your baby will develop quite a lot of skill with her hands and she will be able to understand a lot more of what is happening around her.

At around seven months, she begins to realise that she has two hands and will very quickly learn to hold a toy in each, bringing them together. Within a month, she will have learnt to pick up objects with thumb and forefinger, having much more control over her hands. She will also offer a toy to you, or will attempt to put a brick in a container but won't, as yet, be able to release it successfully. By the time she is a year old, a girl would be able to play a game of give and take. Boys take a little longer, but they are better at rolling a ball to you. To encourage all this activity, you will need some objects that are small enough to hold without any danger of being swallowed, as everything goes to the mouth still – although this gets less by the first birthday. Bricks, softly stuffed toys and pieces of cloth are ideal, as are very soft balls.

See also section 5.8 below on Learning and exploring through play

5.3(c) COGNITIVE DEVELOPMENT

By about nine months of age your baby will be aware that objects are permanent. To develop this, you could hide a toy with a small piece showing. After two or three weeks, you can cover the toy totally and he will search for it.

Once he knows a toy is permanent even when he can't see it, he will begin to experiment. An early way is for him to drop a toy when he is sitting in a pram or high chair to see what happens. When he learns that you will then pick it up and give it back to him, this quickly turns into a very good game to get your attention. By ten months, he will have learnt to throw objects to see what happens. Also at this age he can open a box which gives another hiding place. However, be sure that any item you don't want him to get is kept securely out of his way. He is learning a great deal at this stage, much of it by imitating adults, and can perform tasks that have been demonstrated to him such as ringing a bell when it has been rung for him.

It is during this second half-year that the baby becomes aware of which people are strangers and which are familiar in his life, and at around ten months he can wave 'bye bye'. He may sometimes use this to show he knows someone is a stranger.

Language development

Most babies will imitate speech and sounds such as 'Dada' and 'Mama' from around 7–8 months. They will also respond to being called and, in turn, will shout for your attention. By around 10–12 months, your baby will be very specific about saying Mama and Dada, and will shake her head for 'no'. The remainder of any sentence she attempts will still be babble. She will also be paying attention to the way you speak to her including your tone of voice.

Responding to the individual

Children vary in development. Some may achieve some skills earlier than suggested, but be later in others. What is important is how much time you (or another carer, such as a babyminder) spend with your child encouraging him. If you surround him with toys without showing him what to do, his progress will be slower. Similarly, for his speech development he needs to hear you talking, particularly to him. Many parents find it useful to put the baby in a safe place, such as a baby chair or play pen while they continue with household chores. If he can see you and hear you (for example, if he is just inside the hallway while you are in the kitchen) you can cook the dinner, talking to him as you do so. This will help his progress a great deal.

Equally, the toys do not need to be expensive. You will find at this stage that he will be as interested in the brightly coloured box or paper as the toy itself. It is far more important for you to vary the colour, texture and size and consider his safety than worry about how much you pay for each item.

5.3(d) SOCIAL DEVELOPMENT AND NUTRITION

Because your child will be able to sit up well by 9–10 months, he will appreciate sitting in a high chair at the table with the family. From around eight months you can adjust his weaning diet to fit in with family meal times so he can enjoy this period. Around this time, he will be cutting teeth to enable him to chew; therefore from about nine months, start incorporating a few soft lumps, such as potato or peas, into his diet. Also at this age, he is able to hold a beaker while he has a drink. He will want to do this because he is imitating you. But he will probably still want a bottle or breast feed at night or if he is feeling unwell.

As new food textures and tastes continue to be introduced, you may find he rejects them sometimes. This could be because he is not used to them, or because he is thirsty or tired. Sometimes, he may just want to attract your attention. It is important not to worry unduly, or meals become a battleground and he may use this as he gets older. Try the different foods at another time or give a small

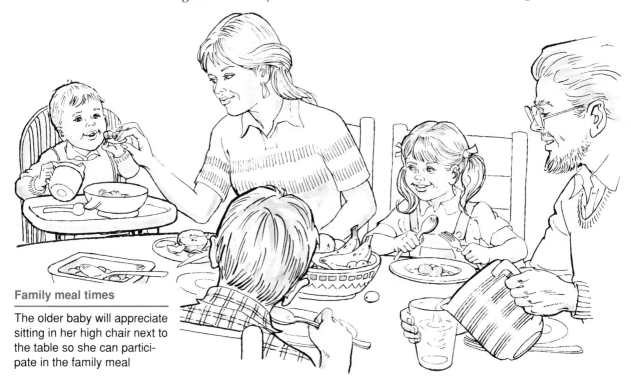

Family meal times

The older baby will appreciate sitting in her high chair next to the table so she can participate in the family meal

amount of fruit juice first. As he approaches his first birthday, he might like to hold a spoon himself, but he will want to use it for play rather than feeding himself. If you guide his hand, however, he will, at least, make an effort.

By the time he is one year old, he should be able to eat the food that the rest of the family is eating, as long as it is not too tough, rich or spicy and is cut up into very small pieces. His diet should contain a balance of protein, fruit and vegetables and cereals. The protein could be in the form of meat or fish, but if your family is vegetarian, it would be useful to discuss your baby's diet with your health visitor to check the balance. If he has adequate milk, cheese, beans and pulses he will probably be getting sufficient protein.

It may also be necessary for you to give him vitamin supplements, but it would be wise to consult your health visitor or family doctor before starting him on a course of these.

You can start the gradual introduction of ordinary pasteurised milk (as delivered by the milkman) from about nine months. The changeover to the same milk as the rest of the family use should be complete by the time he is a year old (or shortly after) provided you are no longer breast feeding. Do be sure though, that the milk you buy is whole milk, not skimmed or semi-skimmed which are unsuitable for small children. It is important too to be careful about hygiene. Your baby should never be given milk from a bottle that has been sitting open in a warm kitchen for any length of time.

5.4 THE TODDLER

5.4(a) DEVELOPMENT

Your child's development will continue throughout his life, but during this stage he will be finding his own personality.

He will start off by experimenting more in all aspects. As he should now be walking well, without understanding danger, you may begin to feel that you need eyes in the back of your head as well as in the front.

During his second year he will improve all aspects of mobility, including going backwards and upstairs – although at the end of this year, he will still often come down on his bottom. He will have learnt to run early in this stage but, without a good understanding of different levels, he may not see objects lying in his way and therefore may trip over them.

As he will be experimenting with independence there is a very real danger of him running away from you, particularly if something catches his interest. This can be particularly hazardous if you are near a road, or water, or in a busy shop.

Towards the end of this stage, he will also learn to jump and pedal a tricycle which will help his independence.

His speech will improve, with simple three word sentences or phrases being used. It is important to remember that he can understand more than he says and that you should continue to talk to him to improve his speech.

He should be able to point to some objects or parts of the body when they are named – but obviously this won't happen if you haven't helped him by using the name in his hearing.

By the time he is three years old, he will be able to say his name on being asked. He will understand requests and will enjoy running errands (for example, if asked to 'fetch mummy the comb'). He will, in fact, imitate you in some activities around the house, such as dusting, and as he reaches two and a half or three years will relish helping you in some jobs.

As part of that imitation, he will at about 16–18 months remove items of clothing and also gradually learn to dress until by two and a half years he should be able to dress himself while you supervise, and at three years old be able to do up his own buttons.

5.4(b)   TANTRUMS

Because she is striving for independence during this time, she becomes very self-centred. She will play alongside other children, but not *with* them until she is about three years old, and gets very frustrated at times, feeling real anger. This causes her to feel frightened and often presents as a temper tantrum. It may be made worse if she is tired or frustrated. If you think about when you last felt 'like screaming' – but didn't because you recognised the feeling and knew how to calm down and deal with the problem – you will have some idea of what a tantrum is like for your child. Unfortunately, she has not yet developed the ability to reason, neither is she able to tell you what the problem is. You can help her by understanding the problem and explaining it so that she will gradually develop the ability to think through it. Above all, you should remember that all children go through this time – often referred to as 'the terrible twos' – and it is an important part of your child's development.

Another way to help is by consistency. If a child is told by one parent when he can or can't do something, he learns the rules. When the other parent, or a grandparent, then says something opposite to this he becomes confused and this adds to his frustration. This problem must be discussed and a common policy agreed. Confusion will also arise if *you* are not consistent. It is easy to state something at one time but, when you are tired or busy, change the rules. If this happens it is important you explain to him, again to help him to learn to think. He will show his desire to learn by always asking 'why?' and 'how?' etc.

5.4(c) INDEPENDENCE

One of the questions parents find most difficult at all stages concerns balancing their child's need to become independent against his safety. On the whole you can be guided by his desire to try something such as coming down a slide, but minimise the danger by making sure the slide is appropriate to his age, or positioning yourself so that you can catch him if he falls. Your child, however, will not develop skills if, in minimising the risks, you never let him experiment. He may wish to walk without holding your hand, even when you walk along a busy road. You can allow him this freedom, while being aware of the danger of him running in front of a vehicle, by the use of reins to give you some control.

Other ways he may demonstrate his growing independence will be in eating and going to bed. He may start to refuse certain foods which he has enjoyed before, or refuse to eat at all occasionally. Equally, he may, quite naturally, have given up a day time sleep after about 18 months (although some still need it up to the age of four) but still not want to go to bed in the evening. Again it is important to be consistent in both cases. Develop a routine for him over bed-time, allowing a period of play in the evening. You might also find it useful to substitute a nutritious sandwich or fruit for a missed meal. It is important that you do not show your anxiety or allow him to feel *he* is gaining control over you. This would only confuse him further.

Another area of great anxiety for parents, and a frequent cause of arguments with grandparents is when to start toilet training. Generally, you will find he will be mature enough around the age of 18–24 months. If he responds to requests to fetch things, and also shows in his face or by gestures when he has dirtied his nappy, he is probably ready. Again, he needs consistency in the words used, and a routine should be decided upon. For example, try sitting him on

Toilet training

The child can start with a standard potty and progress gradually to using the toilet

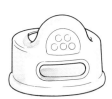

(i) Ordinary potty

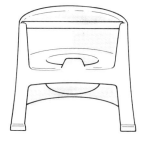

(ii) Built-up potty/chair

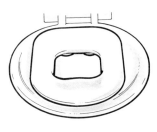

(iii) Trainer seat to fit on the toilet.

the potty first thing in the morning, after each meal and before bed-time. You should praise him whenever he uses the potty, or when he tells you he needs to use it – even if, by the time he gets there, he has used his nappy. You must not punish accidents – just accept them as part of the process. As he gets older, he may prefer to use a special trainer seat on the toilet to show everyone he is 'growing up'. He will still require nappies at night for a short while.

5.4(d)   A NEW ARRIVAL

See also Chapter 4, section 6(d) for more advice on coping with Sibling rivalry

This is a time when parents may consider having another baby. You must prepare him for this by involving him, while again maintaining his routine as near to normal. However, you must expect a cert-tain amount of jealousy. This can be kept to a minimum if you recognise the signs and prepare for it. The vital point is that a new baby will make him feel insecure as to his place, and you must show him he is still loved and wanted.

5.4(e)   WORRIES ABOUT HEALTH

See also section 5.11 below on Looking after a sick child at home and section 5.12 on Common health problems

During this stage, children will be mixing more with other children at mother and toddler groups or when friends get together. As your child will still be building up immunity to infections, you will find she may often have a rise in temperature. This is not a major problem for most children but for some the rise in temperature leads to a small convulsion. You should be aware of the possibility until your child is 6 years old. Always keep a thermometer in the house, and if she shows signs of a temperature, keep her in light cotton clothing, give her plenty of drinks and possibly some paracetamol elixir for children to bring her temperature down.

See also section 5.9 below on The child who needs to visit hospital

If your child should need to go into hospital around this time you will need to put some careful thought into preparing her for the experience, supporting her through it, and coping with the feelings of your other children. More detailed advice on this topic is given later in the chapter.

5.5   THE OLDER PRE-SCHOOL CHILD

When your child reaches the age of three years, he will be ready to socialise and will separate more easily from you. This makes this the ideal age to consider a play group for him. He is more likely now to play *with* others rather than just alongside them. Being in a group of children will also teach him that people's feelings are important and he will begin to understand about sharing and taking turns.

When you are considering which play group or nursery school to send your child to, pay a visit while other children are there and talk to some of the mothers. Ask questions of the play group leader or nursery school teacher – in particular about supervision of play. It is important for children of this age to have some plan for their activity, so ask whether they are encouraged to change from one form of play to another rather than just left to get on with it.

5.5(a) COGNITIVE DEVELOPMENT

At three years of age your child will be able to understand concepts. For example, if he is told that the iron or fire is hot, even though he cannot touch them to feel 'hot', he can understand if he has been told that the sun is hot and you link the two ideas. By the age of four, he will be able to reason this out for himself.

He will also be able to understand ideas of time – but not time as limited by the clock. You will need to link time with his everyday activities to get complete understanding saying, for example, 'to-morrow after breakfast' rather than '10 o'clock tomorrow morning'.

Because of this greater understanding, you will find you are more able to reason with him. Linked to this is the ever-growing vocabulary. By his fourth birthday, he will be able to tell quite long stories, and within a year will be able to define some of the words he uses.

Reading your child story books will help to stimulate his cognitive development

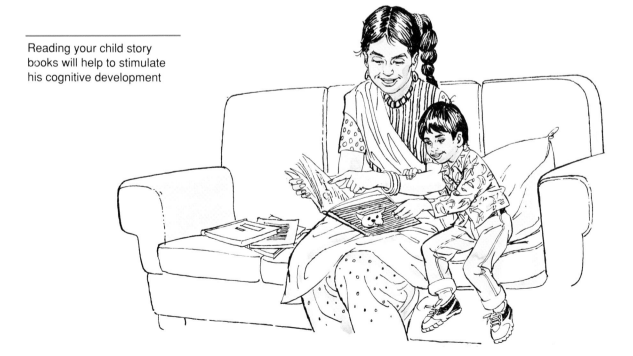

If you wish to help him to develop in this way, you will find it useful to read him story books. Most libraries have sections of books for this age group which will give you a good idea of those suitable. He may even sit with familiar books and appear to be reading them out loud – although the chances are he has remembered the story, or is making one up from the pictures.

Again this is demonstrating his independence which he will also show by being able to dress himself without supervision around the age of three and a half or four years.

Various aspects of play will be developing quickly at this stage. Your child will probably be showing more skill in artistic pursuits such as painting and using plasticine. You will find, however that she enjoys being messy with paint, just as she will love playing with sand and water.

See also section 5.8 below on Learning and exploring through play

She will gradually develop more control over fine skills. After about the age of three, she should be able to do jigsaws of up to six large pieces. This skill will develop until she can do the puzzles with more smaller pieces. You will also find she will enjoy playing musical instruments – particularly those making noises which please her – such as piano and drums.

The more she mixes with others, the more she will learn quite elaborate games. During this stage, she will learn to take part in quite elaborate make-believe, particularly if she has some clothes to dress up in. A group of up to six children around the age of four and a half will be able to take part in this, and you will find you don't need to provide much more than the most minimal of props. By playing in groups like this, children learn that games have rules, but initially they expect the rules to change to suit them.

See also section 5.10 on Keeping your young child safe

When your child can understand concepts, you will be able to discuss such issues as safety with him. You should teach him to repeat his name and address as soon as possible in case he gets lost. He should also be taught never to talk to or go with strangers, and how to cross a road. This should be repeated any time that is applicable but you should expect him to forget it quite frequently. As he will practise all that he observes you doing, it is vital that you are careful to cross roads safely as well.

5.5(b) LOOKING AHEAD

By the time he is three years old, he will have cut all his first set of teeth, therefore you should also teach him at this time how to brush his own teeth and also start regular check-ups at the dentist. You may find it best to take him with you when you go for a check-up, so that he learns it is a natural thing to do.

Towards the end of this time, the increased activity will cause your child to feel quite tired at times. You will find she will be happy to have a period of peace and quiet, preferably before going to bed to help her relax. To help her with this, you could sit with her with a book, talk about what she has done during the day, help her to say her prayers (if this is appropriate in your household) or use the time to teach her a quieter activity.

Before your child reaches his fifth birthday, you will be thinking about a school for him and, just as you will have visited play groups or nurseries, so you should visit and question the school. You should also consider which school his friends are to attend, as moving from play group to school together with an established peer group will help the transition.

5.6 EMOTIONAL AND SOCIAL NEEDS OF BABIES AND YOUNG CHILDREN

All babies are recognisable as unique individuals and are stamped with their own personalities and characteristics from the moment of birth.

Parents will often comment on the temperament differences in their own children even as babies; one may be noisy and rumbustious whilst another is quiet and placid. While there are these differences from one baby to another they all have in common, as developing individuals, certain emotional requirements that need to be met for future well-being.

Just as it is important to meet the infant's basic needs for food, warmth, protection and security, so too it is crucial that the baby is provided with the opportunity to form secure attachments with parents or constant care givers for satisfactory emotional development later in life.

Attachment or bonding

See also Chapter 4, section 7(a), on Getting to know the baby

The process of attachment – also sometimes called bonding – develops throughout infancy and some authorities even believe that it starts with pregnancy. But there is good evidence that the first hour or so immediately after birth is especially important for early attachment to take place. The opportunity for the baby to remain quietly with the parents immediately after delivery enables the new mother and baby to have early close physical contact with one another. The father, too, is often closely involved in this early contact and should also be given the opportunity to have a first cuddle with the new baby.

A few mothers may not immediately want to touch or cuddle their new baby and perhaps will want to wait until the baby is clean. (Some mothers too may have been given a general anaesthetic or may be simply too tired.) Other mothers may feel disappointed at first in the way their baby looks. Such variation in response is quite normal, and parents should be reassured that it is perfectly possible to 'make up for lost time'.

Communication

From this early stage develops a reciprocity of communication in the new partnership, by which the mother and father become sensitive to their babies' signals of communication and able to interpret 'the messages' for the varying cries, babbles or smiles.

Even at a very early age babies respond to a calm voice and a cuddle. The fractious baby is often soothed by close physical contact and may particularly enjoy being rocked gently as well. Gentle handling, together with being spoken to by the parent in a voice that expresses interest and concern will all help to develop mutual feelings of trust, security and confidence.

Social development

While babies' first relationships are usually with mother and father, this slowly begins to extend to others in the family circle.

The baby learns from her early interaction with her mother during the daily routine of feeding, bathing and play time how to initiate contact with others by imitation to elicit responses. At first the newborn baby shows a visual preference for the human face and, as early as one week of age, watches her mother's face intently when she speaks. At the end of about six weeks, the first smiles appear. At this stage the baby begins to show an interest in the environment and in other people.

Play activities

Stimulation is as important for social and emotional growth in the young baby as food is for physical growth. There is a need only for a few well chosen toys, but the baby needs to be 'played with' rather than simply being allowed 'to play'. As the baby enjoys watching his mother's face and being spoken to, nursery rhymes and songs are usually popular.

Suitable toys include rattles, soft toys of a hand-holding size, squeezy toys for the bath, musical toys, nursery mobiles and unbreakable mirrors.

See also section 5.8 below on Learning and exploring through play

Provide stimulation by altering the baby's position so that a different perspective on activities going on around can be obtained. Carry the baby from room to room as different activities are going on in the family. Constantly talk to the alert baby, call her by name repeating any sounds that are made which will aid social and emotional development.

The following are a few suggestions for making babies' lives more exciting.

- Use of the human voice for the baby is fascinating . . . . take every opportunity to use it during daily routines.

- Patterned effects especially geometric shapes are preferred to straight lines just as contrasting colours (e.g. red and white) are preferred. Incorporate this knowledge in the making of mobiles to hang above the cot.

- The baby enjoys variety and tires quickly so remember to change mobiles frequently. Do not put out all the toys in one go but change periodically.

- Auditory toys (such as musical boxes or squeaky teddies) are particularly appreciated.

As the child grows older, she will continue to need love, attention, consistency and stimulation. Particular periods when insecurity may raise its head are:

- Times of any change in routine – e.g. if one parent is away on business for a couple of weeks;

- The period around starting at nursery or school for the first time;

- Whenever the child is ill;

- The arrival of a new baby.

See also Chapter 4, section 6(d) on Sibling rivalry

Parents may need to be particularly sensitive to their child's need for affection around such times. Other people (such as grandparents or close family friends) who have strong relationships with the child may be able to help too.

5.7 BEHAVIOURAL PROBLEMS

We live in a world that is changing at an increasingly rapid rate. The challenges that parents face in order to help their children grow into happy and mature adults are wide-ranging. Parenting is very important, but should not revolve around 'am I doing it right?'. Children need a patient, caring and loving relationship with their parents, in order to grow up liking themselves and being able to relate to other people. Children require appropriate limits. They need encouragement and praise. Parents need to recognise the needs and feelings of their children. Children are very perceptive and parents can unknowingly create problems by expecting too much or too little of their child.

Children's behaviour can also be worsened by fatigue, boredom and hunger. Bored, unhappy children are much more likely to get into trouble than well-occupied and contented ones. Thus by using ingenuity, understanding their needs, having a sense of humour and avoiding conflict, many potential behavioural problems can be avoided. A distraction 'ploy' is so much more effective than 'No's' and 'Don'ts'.

Children have differing personalities and react in differing ways to situations that arise in family life. Ideas on the ways in which to manage children also change with fashion. Parents often become very concerned about the behaviour of their child and can wonder if this naughtiness is related to a physical condition. But many behavioural difficulties are part of normal childhood and when handled appropriately with understanding, consistency and patience can be overcome.

5.7(a) SOME COMMON BEHAVIOURAL PROBLEMS WHICH MAY OCCUR IN CHILDREN UNDER FIVE YEARS OF AGE

Shyness

Children can have phases of shyness, sometimes arising from insecurity. Plenty of contact with other children is helpful, particularly in a structured play situation. Shyness should not be discussed in front of the child and, if it is handled tactfully, will usually disappear.

Fears

It is quite normal for small children to have some fears, due to their lack of experience and understanding. Unfortunately, fearfulness may be suggested by adults. Excessive fears can be prevented by supporting the child with a sense of security and building up his self-confidence. Should fears become excessive then professional advice can be helpful in eliminating this problem. A discussion with the health visitor on her family visit or in the clinic may help to dispel parental concerns.

Jealousy

All children are jealous at times, and this may show itself in many obscure ways. Basically it is due to the fear of the loss of parental affection. Jealousy can manifest itself in stuttering, excessive clinging, asking to be fed by mother (long after the child can feed himself), bed wetting, habit spasms, frequent passing of urine, demanding bottles, being aggressive, destructive, unduly negative and refusing food – among other symptoms. Certainly some children are more jealous than others.

Jealousy is normal and part of the development of the child's personality. Every effort should be made to understand the cause, for example, avoiding changes in the first born's routine when the newborn arrives. Patience and understanding, and time to show the jealous child that he is still truly loved, are important. The opportunities for appropriate play sessions, just with the parent or in a small mother and toddler group, can be very beneficial for a child who has overwhelming feelings of jealousy.

See also Chapter 4, section 6(d), on Sibling rivalry

Resistance and negative behaviour

Parents experience great joy and satisfaction with their growing child, interspersed with exasperation, utter despair and depression. Toddlers can shatter the family peace and can be most difficult to understand. All normal children go through this very troublesome stage, usually between 18–30 months but there can be a broader timespan of 9 months to 3 years. The behaviour of children in this age group fluctuates wildly. This results in an erratic mixture of good, bad and appalling behaviour. They manipulate their parents; are stubborn and attention seeking. As most parents have little idea of normal behaviour, they feel very alone, inadequate and isolated with this toddler. Parents too feel reluctant to discuss their problems as they fear criticism and being made to feel inadequate. These behaviours are normal in the child and there is a degree of variation so that some children may seem to be more difficult than others. Early identification of the problem and firm handling is important. Here the local mother and toddler group with a good play input can be an enormous support for the harrassed mother. Should parents feel their child's behaviour to be excessive, the family doctor or health visitor can advise.

Attention seeking

Another feature of normal child behaviour ranging between 9 months and 3–4 years of age is that of 'attention seeking'. The child delights in anything that causes consternation and anxiety in the house. She may find that refusal to eat, chew, swallow or even to be sick over the table causes a maximum amount of fuss, and her mother a great deal of distress. She may be able to manipulate the entire household regarding what she eats, or how her bowels work. She cries and screams when she receives a trivial knock, and cultivates the habit when rewarded by being picked up or given a sweetie. Parents need to be constantly on their guard against this sort of behaviour; most intelligent children try these 'tricks'.

Most problems are effectively dealt with by ignoring them and distracting the child's attention. The less fuss about the problem

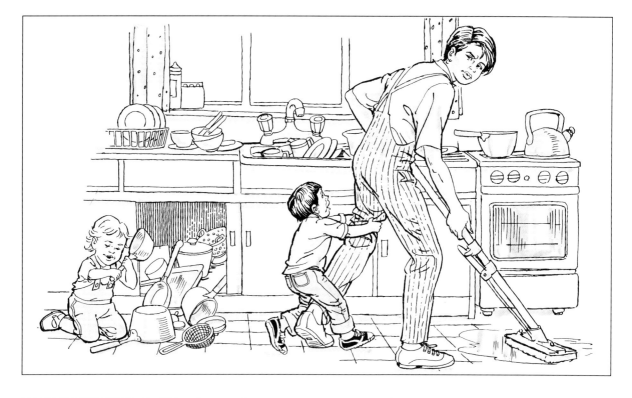

the quicker it goes away. Punishment is rarely effective. Catching the child when being good and giving adequate praise, attention and encouragement is the most effective treatment for almost all behavioural problems. This will help her to develop her self-confidence and the feeling of security.

Temper tantrums

These occur mostly between the ages of 18 months to 3 years. The strong willed and increasingly independent child finds it difficult to conform and not have his own way. Most temper tantrums can be considered normal. They can be increased by jealousy, insecurity, fatigue and hunger. The child has tunnel vision for his own needs. A temper tantrum usually involves hitting, kicking, screaming. Efforts to reason with a child during a tantrum are futile. The best method of coping with a tantrum is by having a complete lack of interest and indifference to the outburst. The tantrum must achieve nothing or it will be repeated. If they do get out of hand, you should seek the advice of your health visitor.

Breath holding attacks

These are not easy to deal with. Here the parent needs to make as little fuss as possible in order that the child does not achieve the result she wants. Yet the parent is concerned that the breath holding attack may turn into a convulsion. Knowing when to intervene is essential – not too soon, not too late. Breath holding attacks are frightening for parents and if they continue a visit to the family doctor should be made for further advice.

Overactivity

There are children who are always 'on the go' and it is very easy for parents to term these children hyperactive. This is rarely the case. Some children are just more active than others and this behaviour can be aggravated by hunger or boredom. It is more common in boys than in girls.

These children should be allowed as much freedom as possible, particularly out of doors with appropriate play material and activities. Only in cases of excessive overactivity will professional advice be needed.

Aggression – hitting and biting

Most normal children are aggressive, particularly around the age of two years. These difficulties again can be increased by fatigue, hunger, boredom, insecurity and jealousy. An effective method of treating these symptoms is through lots of opportunity for play activities – both indoor and outdoor – and sufficient freedom in which to choose play activities, alongside firm disapproval and consistency in dealing with the problem.

Destructiveness

Destructiveness need not be deliberate and may be simply due to a lack of experience in holding an object or childish curiosity. All breakable objects should be removed from the child's vicinity. She should be stopped from throwing objects across a room and any toy which she deliberately tries to break should be put away for a week or two. She will enjoy it when it returns.

Every effort should be made to keep this child occupied with suitable play activities, playmates and opportunities for other outlets for her energies, particularly out of doors.

Bad language

The child does not know the meaning of the words he is using and provided he is not laughed at and the language is not used in the home the most effective treatment is simply to ignore it.

Telling lies/tale telling

There is no need to feel anxiety about untruthfulness in the first five years. Being truthful develops slowly. Normal 3 year olds delight in making up stories – it is part of their normal development and should be encouraged and turned into imaginative play.

Selfishness

Small children are very self-centred and have no idea of taking turns. They have a very normal 'smash and grab' technique. Parents are keen for their child to share toys with visitors but 2–3 year olds do not understand why. The child will gradually learn by imitation and wise guidance, and here again the planned use of toys, playmates or supervised mother and toddler groups can be very supportive.

Crying

Parents can get very confused with the ever changing behaviour of children – particularly toddlers, who may go through phases of crying without apparent cause. Adults can often be cross and irritable when they are tired or hungry; so too will small children cry for similar reasons. The big problem is that the child who cries does not realise how tired her mother can be, and these are the pressures that cause friction. However busy a parent is the toddler or small child demands immediate attention; she cannot wait one minute for the baby to be fed or the telephone to be answered. These rapid changes in behaviour that are seen in a small child can cause considerable confusion to parents who may feel that their child could be ill, or have a 'Jekyll and Hyde' personality. However, such behaviour is usually quite normal.

A child who will not sleep can make life miserable for the parents

Sleep problems

When it comes to bedtime most children cause difficulties. The following points need to be taken into consideration.

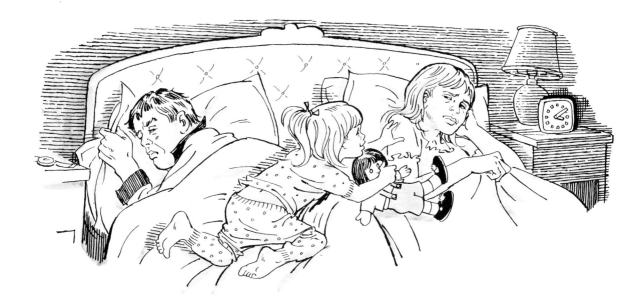

The right bedtime   All children have different needs of sleep, just as adults do. Looking at their needs is essential. How much sleep is necessary during the day should be identified and then a routine can be established.

Calm and routine   It helps to have a bedtime routine and this should follow a regular sequence of events – evening meal, bath, gentle play, drink, story, cuddle and sleep. Calm is as important as consistency. Children need soothing. No delaying tactics should be allowed, and firm handling is paramount for a good result.

Other considerations to take into account are:

- Where should she sleep?

- Is she warm enough?

- Cot or bed?

- Duration of sleep and naps.

The main sleep problems are:

- The child who cries in the middle of the night;

- The child who won't go to bed;

- The child who comes into the parents' bed each night.

See Appendix VII for Addresses of useful organisations and support groups

Parents need to use a very firm, consistent approach when handling sleep problems and seek the advice of the experts if they are worried. Sleep problems often start after an illness or family disruption but, with good firm handling and a consistent bedtime routine, the sleeping pattern should return to normal.

If the situation is really getting you down, you might find a support group, such as Cry-sis, helpful. Your health visitor will also advise you.

Poor appetite or food refusal

Many parents become distraught because they cannot get their child to 'eat enough'. Actually the child has the whole household revolving around what he will or will not eat. He is allowed to develop food fads because of the anxiety he causes. The more fuss that is made over the appetite of a child who refuses food, the more he will refuse. Children's appetites do vary. A poor appetite should be ignored. No well child ever starves.

At the end of the day, should parents feel that the behaviour of their child seems excessive or out of control, then professional help is available through the family doctor or health visitor. But it is good to remember that most problems are part of normal childhood and disappear with time.

LEARNING AND EXPLORING THROUGH PLAY

Playing is one of the most important functions of childhood. Learning happens as a direct consequence. The adult or parent has a very important role in the encouragement of play. It is only through play that a child develops new skills and learns about the world in which he lives.

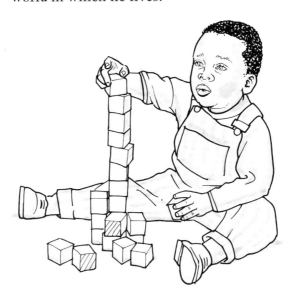

Through play, the child develops new skills and learns about the world he lives in

It is essential to understand the purpose of play, and to recognise the various categories, in order to provide a rich variety of early experiences for the child. Play is not easy, it demands effort and perseverance. Busy parents find it difficult to set aside 'time for play'. However play opportunities can be created alongside the 'household chores'. Children can learn from everything going on around them. By involving the child in all that the parent is doing, giving the child attention from time to time and talking to him about what is happening, you can create an atmosphere in which he can explore, play and learn.

A flexible daily routine will enable you to enjoy being with your child and doing things with him. It also enables you to encourage, through a wide variety of experiences, the normal development of your child.

5.8(a) TYPES OF PLAY

Play can be divided into varying types, each concerned with encouraging differing aspects of development. Play covers a wide range of activities which improves the physical skills, intellectual skills, social skills and communication skills of the child. Play helps to improve the ability to concentrate, and gain a wider knowledge of the world. Although play can be loosely grouped into specific types, many play activities encompass several types of play at the same time.

Energetic play

Physical activities enable a child to master movement, developing from very simple responses to the more complex movements of everyday life. The baby learns to control voluntary movement in order to recover a toy. Physical play increases motor co-ordination as in early attempts at walking. Physical play includes pushing, pulling, climbing, holding, catching and balancing, eventually developing into the precision of gymnastics, dance or football.

Discovery play

A child observes, explores and experiments with various materials and toys. At first he takes objects to his mother to explore and as he matures he learns to use his hands more skilfully, until eventually he handles materials expertly. Through incessant exploration, i.e. trial and error and repeated experimentation with various toys and materials, the child is building up knowledge of the way in which everyday objects work. Discovery or experimental play is 'What does it do?' 'How does it work?' play. Children need a great variety of things to explore, for instance, water, cardboard boxes and paper as well as toys suitable to their age.

Creative play

For young children everything is fresh and new. Creative play is very enjoyable. Creative play takes a long time to set up and pack away but is very rewarding. As wide a range of material as possible should be available. The opportunity to use colour, touch and feel things with their hands and use a variety of materials is very satisfying. Useful materials to have available for creative play with children are:

- Paints, paper, brushes;
- Crayons, felt tips;
- Chalks and blackboard;
- Playdough or plasticine.

Creative play allows the child to gain confidence in himself, knowing he can do things for himself.

5.8(b) HOW TO HELP CHILDREN LEARN AND EXPLORE THROUGH PLAY

Whatever a child learns, it will be more easily learnt and be more meaningful if it is done with enjoyment. Toys are only one of the tools of play. They must fulfil the role of presenting a challenge to the child, yet allowing for a high degree of success. There are many materials available that can also enhance a child's play opportunities other than just toys. Interaction with, and talking to, the child is as important as using toys.

Materials and activities that encourage learning and exploring

Books   Books can be introduced at a very early stage. Books made of cloth or board have pictures of everyday things to name and point out and talk about together. From these the child develops to simple story books with clear pictures and a little writing. Public libraries have children's sections which include picture books for children and the children's libraries can advise about story books for differing ages.

Water   Almost all children enjoy water. Babies enjoy splashing in their bath, toddlers learn from finishing the washing up with a plastic cup and dishmop. Children learn a great deal by playing with objects in water that float or sink as well as pouring from cup to cup. Young children however should never be left on their own to play with water.

Painting and drawing   Children start by scribbling and need to have available fat wax crayons with paper such as old computer paper. As the child progresses, she will enjoy learning to use and experiment with paint. The result pinned up on the wall for all to admire makes her want to do more.

Playdough   Playdough is immensely satisfying and involves all the senses of touch, sound, sight, smell and taste. Three year olds onwards thoroughly enjoy it and find it very satisfying.

Recipe for playdough

> You will need:
>
> - Two cups of plain flour
> - Half a cup of water
> - Half a cup of salt
> - A few drops of edible food colouring
>
> Mix it all up and, when not in use, keep in a damp cloth in the fridge

AGE-APPROPRIATE OPPORTUNITIES FOR PLAY

Young babies	Need to see and hear what is going on around them. They learn by looking, listening and touching. Young babies enjoy company and need the adult to talk, sing, smile and touch them. They are particularly interested in human faces. Mobiles make very good visual toys and can be bought or made at home. Rattles create interesting noises, but must be safe, clean and too big to swallow.
Sitting and crawling babies	Still like company but need a safe environment. Everyday objects can fascinate them. They are into everything and so it is important to cover electrical sockets and lock away cleaning materials and medicines. The child is beginning to use fingers more adeptly. Toys with textures and materials will encourage exploration. Playpens can be very useful as the baby can stay safe, yet be with adults.
12–15 months	This is when baby books, peg boards, posting boxes, inset puzzles, can provide interest but not necessarily be used appropriately.
15–18 months	Push or pull toys become valuable to increase balance and the simple toys are now used in a more recognised way.
18 months to 2 years	The child now begins really to enjoy books, likes playing with water, is able to use construction toys such as Duplo or Stickle bricks and happily tries simple nursery rhymes with the adult.
2 years old	Hand movements are more finely controlled. The child uses a wider range of toys and materials, and is beginning the more complicated hand control activities of threading beads or screw toys. Play with water and sand is valuable to encourage exploration. Children this age spend a lot of energy on running and wandering around.
3 years old	This is the time for wider opportunities for more complex creative play with paints, crayons, paste, etc. Balls become popular around this age, so do toys that encourage 'pretend' play. Construction skills are becoming much more sophisticated. Children in this age group enjoy bicycles, tricycles, pedal cars and climbing frames. They need considerable practice in energetic play and fine hand movements. They can concentrate and settle for longer on a number of different activities and enjoy the company of other children.
4 years old	The child's speech is now very clear and he can play with words. He prefers to play with other children rather than alone and uses toys in inventive ways. He uses more complex jigsaw puzzles, his concentration is much better and he notices shape, colour and quantity. Construction toys can be used which involve detail.

5.8(c)   DEVELOPING SPEECH AND LANGUAGE SKILLS

All play activities should encourage speech. From the first moments of life, parents are anxious to communicate with their child. Children learn to speak by imitating what they hear. Babies soon learn the meaning of various sounds, for example, running water for bathtime. By nurturing the child's natural curiosity and excitement of sound the development of speech is achieved. Children need to be talked to, have stories read to them and learn to tell stories to adults. Learning to speak, to think and to communicate must be a pleasure.

5.8(d)   CO-ORDINATING THE USE OF HANDS AND EYES

For toddlers this may mean balancing bricks. For 3–4 year olds it means threading beads, more complicated jigsaw puzzles or complex floor brick building. It is important to encourage this type of play to increase the skill of thinking and develop reasoning.

5.8(e)   CHOOSING TOYS

There is no need to spend money on buying lots of toys. Good playthings can be found in many household objects. When you do buy toys, however, make sure they are tough, safe to be sucked and easily cleaned. Toys should be chosen for their play value, safety, durability, value for money, versatility and learning potential. A baby has fun knocking down a set of plastic bricks; older children learn to build them up themselves and later on to take them apart.

The age range is put on the packaging of most toys in order to help you choose the toy best suited for your child. There is nothing more frustrating for a child than to be given a toy too challenging for him or not challenging enough.

Many individual toys are recognised as standard developmental aids – for example, shape inset boards, bricks, activity frames and peg puzzles. All these toys provide progressive challenges, with rewards that continue, but above all the important ingredient of enjoyment. Why not stay with the tried and trusted toys in the traditional flavour? They are always new toys to the child. Too many toys can lead to confusion.

Safety and toys

It is important to look for safety marks when buying toys (e.g. the British Standard Kitemark, the Lion Mark). When presents are given to children they should always be checked over for loose buttons, sharp pieces, etc.

5.8(f) EXTENDING PLAY OPPORTUNITIES

Mother and toddler groups

By attending mother and toddler groups the busy parent avoids the isolation of her own home. She learns of the experiences of other parents and sees new ideas for play. The toddler begins to experience the first steps of independence and enjoys playing alongside other children and using the new materials and toys provided.

Playgroups, nurseries, pre-schools

These facilities extend the experiences for the child prior to school. Children are usually enrolled from the age of three onwards. They help to extend development including social behaviour and play. Local clinics, libraries or your health visitor will be able to give further information.

5.9 THE CHILD WHO NEEDS TO VISIT HOSPITAL

5.9(a) GOING TO HOSPITAL

See Appendix VII for Addresses of useful organisations and support groups

Sometimes it becomes necessary for a child to be referred to hospital either for admission or to attend outpatients. Hospitals can seem to be very frightening places, especially for a young child. Try, if possible, to prepare your child beforehand. Most public libraries have available children's story books about going to hospital that you can read to your child, which answer questions simply and honestly without being frightening. NAWCH (The National Association for the Welfare of Children in Hospital) will also provide advice and suggestions for appropriate reading.

If the child needs to be admitted to hospital, most hospitals will encourage parents to stay with their children throughout the day and many offer overnight accommodation. If your child is under seven years old, try to do so. Children of this age need a parent with them as much as possible as the fear of separation may be terrifying. For the older child, base your decision on previous separation experiences, the child's wishes together with other family and home commitments. But always try to visit at least once a day.

5.9(b) DISCHARGE HOME

Familiarity with the care your child has received, and his reactions while in hospital, will help you to prepare for discharge home. Your child will be discharged when he no longer requires the specialised nursing and medical care which can only be provided as an inpatient in hospital. You may be required to continue some additional nursing care at home.

Parents should ensure that they feel confident to care for their child following discharge and that they have been given adequate information to do so. If relevant to your child's care you will require advice about ongoing treatment, for example medicines, instructions relating to diet, restrictions on mobility, return to school and attendance at outpatient clinics.

Some children are diagnosed as having chronic or long term illnesses; as a parent you would then require information about the condition and advice about what action to take if your child develops further symptoms and when to seek medical advice.

If you are anxious about your child following discharge from hospital, you should seek support and advice from your family health visitor or family doctor.

Liaison health visitors work within many children's hospitals and children's wards in local hospitals. Their role is to liaise with your family health visitor, providing relevant information about your child's illness and admission to hospital. Your family health visitor is therefore able to provide continuing support and advice about your child's care at home.

In some areas of the United Kingdom, specialist children's community nurses provide additional care and support for children with chronic illnesses and their families. District nurses are also available to undertake and advise on complex nursing procedures in the home or local health centre.

Many children exhibit altered behaviour when they return home from hospital; often this only lasts for a short time. Small children may be unsettled; they may cry more frequently or become quiet and withdrawn; their normal sleep pattern may also be disturbed. Older children may demonstrate a temporary regression in their behaviour, reverting to thumbsucking or bedwetting. Normally changes in behaviour will resolve spontaneously as the child settles at home and regains a sense of security within the family. Understanding the reasons for your child's altered behaviour will help you, as the parent, to handle it appropriately.

5.10 KEEPING YOUR YOUNG CHILD SAFE

'Prevention is better than cure' should be every parent's motto. Before your baby starts to crawl, take a good look at your house and consider the cheap and effective ways in which you can make it safe for your growing children.

Hundreds and thousands of young children attend Accident and

Hazards	Safety measures
Small objects	All body orifices offer opportunities for young children to push beads, peas, balls of paper etc into them. The observant and watchful parent should spot the toddler doing this sort of thing before any harm is done.
Knives/scissors	All these should be kept out of harm's way. If left lying around they are likely to be misused and dangerous. Playing with them should be forbidden to the very young. When the child is a little older their use should be supervised. The 'first' scissors should have rounded ends and they should not be too sharp.
Safety pins/pin boxes and needle books	If left lying around safety pins should be fastened. If in use they should be inaccessible to the child. On nappies, safety pins should be pinned horizontally.
Matches	Children should be taught to respect matches as dangerous when used by very young people or indiscriminately.
Matchboxes/lighters	Should not be left lying around the house. The same applies to them as to matches.
Fireworks and bonfires	Children should know that both may be enjoyed only while supervised by adults.
Clothing	Flame-proofed materials are obtainable; their advantages greatly outweigh the extra cost.
Mirrors	Should not be fixed over fireplaces. Clothes can easily catch fire as the child leans over the fireplace to look in the mirror.
Guards	Safety guards should be fixed on windows of any rooms in which young children may have to be left alone. Fireguards are particularly important too.
Chairs and step ladders	May invite the child to climb on them and lean out of the window. If unguarded this may have serious results.
Stairs	Where there is a toddler in the house stairs should be made safe by placing safety gates at the top and bottom of flights of stairs.
Disinfectants	Should be kept locked away or out of reach even if the toddler climbs to get at them.
Medicines	Keep all medicines in a locked cupboard out of reach.
Berries	Do not allow children to pick and eat berries as some are poisonous.
Cosmetics	Cosmetics should be kept out of reach of toddlers as some are harmful when taken internally.

Hazards around the home

Emergency Departments every year because of accidents at home. The most common causes of such accidents are falls, burns and taking of poisons. Many accidents in the home can be avoided. The chart above highlights some areas of particular risk, together with advice to help you minimise the dangers.

If your child does have an accident (such as a severe fall, a scald from a boiling saucepan or a few unnoticed minutes with a medicine bottle) you will need to take immediate First Aid measures while waiting for the ambulance to arrive or before driving your child to hospital. Detailed advice is given elsewhere

See Appendix II on First Aid

in this book, and you are advised to read Appendix II at regular intervals. It should be stressed, however, that this is no real substitute for proper instruction by a qualified instructor. Many parents can benefit by attending one of the First Aid courses run by a recognised body such as St John's Ambulance. Their children may benefit too – sometimes with their lives.

It should not be forgotten either that accidents can take place outside the home – particularly if the child is a passenger in a car or a pedestrian in an area where there is traffic. All children should be adequately restrained in the car, with seat belts and an approved model of child car seat. Furthermore, it should be appreciated that it is never too early to introduce children to the principles of sensible crossing of roads – always walking on the pavement, using pedestrian crossings where possible and looking 'both ways' carefully to ensure that no traffic is coming. Children should not be allowed to play unsupervised anywhere near traffic.

It is advisable too, that parents impress upon their children from a very early age, that it is not wise to talk to strangers, to accept sweets or other gifts from such people, or to go anywhere with someone they do not know. This applies to children in older age groups also.

5.11   LOOKING AFTER A SICK CHILD AT HOME

The majority of childhood illnesses can be managed safely at home. The best person to care for a sick child at home is a parent. However, where this is not possible, perhaps because both parents are employed, somebody who is well known to the child will be

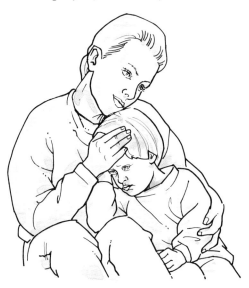

The best person to look after a sick child is the parent

the most appropriate carer. Children are always happiest in their own surroundings, and whenever possible a sick child should be cared for in her own home. A child who is ill at home will need a lot of additional care, attention and reassurance.

It is rarely necessary to confine a sick child to bed. Generally, children will be happier if they are cared for, during the daytime, in the centre of the household; they can easily be tucked up in an armchair or on the settee in the living room. This also reduces the number of times the carer will have to run up and down stairs to attend to the child's requests or needs.

Children may be listless and miserable one moment and running around quite happily the next; unless given specific advice by your doctor, it is not necessary to restrict their activity.

A child who is only mildly ill and spends all day lying on the settee or bed cannot be expected to sleep at night in the normal way, so a different activity or a short session downstairs watching television should be planned prior to the normal bedtime.

The room should be kept warm, not hot; it should be maintained at a comfortable temperature for the rest of the family, i.e. 18°C (65°F) with the usual amount of fresh air.

5.11(a) WHEN TO CONSULT YOUR DOCTOR

Signs of illness are always more worrying in a baby or small child. With an older child, a parent may decide to observe her at home for a while and see whether the signs of illness or pain continue.

As a parent, you always know your own child best, and if you are worried you should contact your family doctor; an important part of the family doctor's role is to relieve family anxiety. The health visitor can provide advice and help parents decide whether their child is really unwell or not, but the family doctor is the only person who can prescribe medicines and treatment for the sick child. Even if the child does not seem really ill in herself, unexplained fever or persistent symptoms such as cough, earache, vomiting or noisy breathing should all be reasons for seeking medical attention.

On the majority of occasions it will not harm a child to be taken to the surgery, and medical attention will be given more quickly. If you are uncertain whether to go to the surgery or request a home visit, telephone and ask the advice of the receptionist or doctor. If you think your child might have an infectious illness, inform the receptionist, as you may be given special instructions about attending the surgery.

If you have your own car it is relatively easy to transport a sick child to the surgery, but if you would have to travel by bus it may not be possible, and you will have to ask the doctor to visit your child at home.

When a child requires urgent medical attention or the parent is seriously worried about her condition, the family doctor should be telephoned day or night. If you do not have a special number for calls outside surgery hours, telephone the usual number and wait for an answer. If the doctor does not answer or cannot travel to the family home quickly enough, you should take your child to the Accident and Emergency department of the nearest hospital with a children's unit.

Parents who think their child's life is in danger, due to illness or an accident, should dial 999 and ask for the ambulance service. You can dial 999 free of charge from a public telephone box.

When you consult a doctor about an episode of illness in your child, he will need to ask a number of questions about the signs and symptoms and when they started. When the diagnosis has been made, he will advise on management and prescribe any necessary medicine or other treatment. If you always have difficulty remembering what you want to ask, write a list in advance of seeing the doctor.

If you have already consulted your doctor but your child's condition appears to get worse, you should not hesitate to telephone your family doctor again.

5.11(b) TAKING YOUR CHILD'S TEMPERATURE

The temperature may be taken using a mercury thermometer, an electronic thermometer or a strip-type thermometer. All are available from a chemist's shop. Electronic thermometers are the most expensive, but quick to use and very safe. Strip-type thermometers, which you hold on your child's forehead, are not as accurate as mercury or electronic thermometers because they show the skin, not the body, temperature. However, they are safe to use and will give an indication of whether or not your child has a raised temperature.

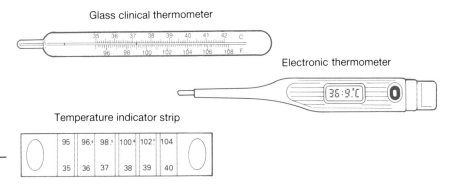

Glass clinical thermometer

Electronic thermometer

Temperature indicator strip

Three types of thermometer

When using a mercury thermometer to take a child's temperature, first shake down the mercury in the glass thermometer. A baby or young child should be held on the parent's knee. The thermometer is placed under the armpit and then the arm held against the child's body, leaving the thermometer in place for three minutes. It helps if the child is amused during this time, perhaps by reading a story or watching television.

From five years of age, many children will safely hold a thermometer under their tongue in the normal way. Hot or cold drinks given shortly before taking the temperature can lead to inaccuracies, so avoid giving them until after the temperature has been taken. You should wipe the thermometer clean after use and never put it into hot water.

Normal body temperature under the arm is 36.4°C (97.4°F). Taken under the tongue, normal body temperature is 37°C (98.4°F).

5.11(c) TEMPERATURE/PYREXIA

In an older child a slight fever is not usually of major concern. The child should be given frequent drinks; cold clear drinks such as fruit squashes or water are best. Even if the child says he is not thirsty, it is important to encourage him to drink little and often to prevent dehydration.

It is important to reduce a raised temperature (pyrexia), both because it will make the child feel more comfortable, and because a continuing high temperature in a small child may cause a fit known as a febrile convulsion.

See section 5.12(e) below for advice on dealing with a febrile convulsion

A child with a raised temperature should not be wrapped up. The clothing should be reduced; younger children may wear a vest and pants or a nappy. Older children may be happier wearing light cotton clothing. The amount of bedding on a child's bed should always be reduced when a child has an illness with a raised temperature; many children will be happy to lie naked under a sheet.

Paracetamol may be given to reduce a child's temperature. Read the label or check with the chemist to ensure that you have an appropriate form of paracetamol for your child's age. Give the medicine as directed on the label, unless instructed otherwise by your doctor. The dose will usually be repeated every 4–6 hours.

See also Chapter 2, section 2(g) for a more detailed description of tepid sponging

If the temperature remains high with the above measures, tepid sponging should be undertaken. This involves sponging the child's face, body, arms and legs with lukewarm water. Do not dry her; let the moisture evaporate and it will assist in cooling the body. A child with a raised temperature should never be immersed in a cold bath. Repeat the tepid sponging, but not for longer than 20 minutes nor more frequently than every two hours.

5.11(d) MEDICINES

A wise policy is to use medicines as little as possible, but sometimes medicine is needed for your child.

It is advisable to give paracetamol to reduce your child's temperature. Preparations containing paracetamol are available from the local pharmacist who will advise you which preparations are suitable for your child's age. Medicine should always be given as stated on the label; do not exceed the dose recommended.

Aspirin should never be given to children under the age of 12. This is because it has been linked with a very rare but dangerous illness called Reyes syndrome.

Antibiotics will not treat viral illnesses, but your doctor will prescribe an antibiotic medicine if your child has an infection caused by bacteria, for example tonsillitis, an ear infection or a urinary tract infection. It is essential to finish a course of antibiotics, which will usually last a minimum of five days. Even if your child seems better, the antibiotics will continue to kill off the hidden bacteria, whereas the illness is more likely to return if you do not finish all the medicine.

When a medicine is prescribed by your family doctor, enquire about possible side-effects, for example will it make your child drowsy or irritable. If your child has a more severe reaction to the prescribed medicine, for example rash or diarrhoea, stop giving the medicine immediately and consult your family doctor.

Always remember the following important principles, for your child's safety.

- Keep all medicines out of the reach of children; if possible they should be stored in a locked cupboard.

- Never leave medicines in a child's bedroom for use at night.

- Always check the date stamp on medicine bottles, and return any medicines or tablets which are out of date to the pharmacist who will destroy them safely.

Getting a child to take medication

Many medicines for young children are in liquid form and may be taken from a spoon or tipped into the child's mouth without protest. Medicine put into the front of the mouth may be spat out, so if the child is reluctant to take it, liquid medicine may be added to a small drink. It is then essential that the child takes all the drink, so add the medicine to a small amount of fluid only.

Almost all medications can be taken with meals and tablet medicines can often be crushed between two spoons and the powder blended with a spoonful of food.

For babies or small children, liquid medicine can be instilled into the back of the mouth using a syringe. If you are having a problem giving medicine to your young child, your health visitor may be able to advise you about different approaches and techniques. Firstly always assume that your child will like the medicine and take it easily. If children refuse to take medication, it is usually either because they do not like the taste or because they are suspicious and frightened of having an adult leaning over them, encouraging them to take something special which they do not understand. Sometimes there is no easy answer to the problem, but parents develop their own tricks for getting their children to take medication.

Many liquid medicines have a sugary base, so it is important that sick children are encouraged to continue regular cleaning of their teeth.

The family medicine cupboard

Suggested items to keep in a family medicine cupboard include:

- A thermometer;

- A 5 ml medicine spoon or a syringe to administer medicine to a baby or small child;

- Paracetamol elixir;

- A supply of sachets which can be made up to provide an electrolyte solution when your child has diarrhoea;

- Calamine lotion for application to rashes or sunburn;

- Antiseptic cream and antiseptic solution for cleansing of grazes and cuts;

- Antihistamine cream for insect bites and stings.

Remember that medicines must always be stored out of the reach of children and preferably in a locked medicine cabinet.

5.11(e)   FOOD AND DRINK

A child who is unwell will often have a reduced appetite but she will need plenty to drink. If a child refuses food during the acute stage of an illness, it does not matter as long as she has been given plenty of fluids. Generally, unless the doctor has advised a special diet, the child may eat whatever she wants and parents will be best guided by what the child fancies. Small portions of favourite food, attractively served, at whatever time the child wants it, are the most tempting. Milk drinks are nutritious and help to provide energy for recovery; if your child does not like milk, try flavouring the drink.

Children who have been vomiting or had diarrhoea will need extra fluid and initially should be given watery drinks in frequent small amounts. The risk of dehydration is greatly reduced in a child over two years of age. An electrolyte solution, obtainable on prescription from the doctor or from the chemist, is advised for a baby or small child under two years of age who requires plenty of liquid to maintain the fluid balance of the body. A child who is unable to take in fluid by mouth, or is already dehydrated, will require hospital admission to be put on an intravenous drip. Therefore if your child cannot retain fluid, continuing to vomit clear fluids or the electrolyte solution, recontact your family doctor.

Children who have lost weight during an illness will soon regain it following their recovery, when their normal appetite will be restored.

5.11(f) GENERAL HYGIENE

A high standard of hygiene is important in everyday living but particularly so when you are caring for a sick child at home as it will help to prevent the spread of infection. Hands should always be washed before and after giving care to the sick child.

Bedbathing your child

If your child is ill enough to remain in bed, it may be appropriate to give a bed bath. Firstly, you should ensure that all the windows and the door are closed and that the room is warm. Remove the top

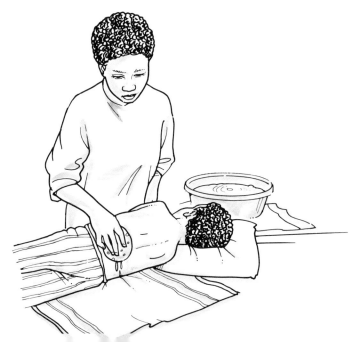

Bedbathing a child

bedclothes and then the child's nightdress or pyjamas. Place a towel beneath a small child, or under each part of the body in turn as you wash, to protect the bed. During the process of washing, the child should be covered with a sheet or blanket as much as possible to prevent excess chilling. Wash each area of the body and then dry it thoroughly. Your child can then be helped into clean night clothes; he should also be helped to brush his hair and clean his teeth.

Food handling

Gastrointestinal illnesses, characterised by the symptoms of vomiting and diarrhoea, are common in children. Generally the illness is caused by a viral illness but it may also be caused by poor hygiene or eating contaminated food. Always ensure that you follow these simple rules:

- Wash your hands before handling food;

- Store food properly at the correct temperature, taking care to separate cooked food from raw food;

- Prepare food hygienically, and cook it in an appropriate manner.

Food which requires reheating must be heated thoroughly at a high temperature before it can be safely used. If you suspect that food is going off, it is safer to discard it.

As soon as they are old enough to do so, children should be taught to wash their hands before meals and after going to the toilet, as this will help to prevent gastrointestinal illnesses.

Isolation – is it necessary?

Isolation is another important way of limiting the spread of infection. Many infections are contagious and spread from person to person in various ways; by coughing, sneezing, direct contact or contact with vomit, urine or faeces. It is usually impractical and inappropriate to isolate your sick child from other members of the family, including siblings. Many infectious illnesses, particularly diseases such as measles and mumps, are passed on during the incubation period, which is the latent period between the time the infection first invades the body and the time of the onset of the symptoms. Therefore siblings will generally have been in contact with the sick child during the incubation period and may already be developing the illness themselves by the time it is diagnosed in the first child.

See also Chapter 6, section 6(b) on Infectious diseases and Appendix IV on Immunisations

Relatives and friends may wish to avoid contact with known infection, so it is courteous to tell them before they enter your home. Your sick child will always enjoy visits from his or her own friends, and most children will develop the main infectious diseases, such as chicken pox or mumps, at some stage unless they have been immunised against them.

Generally a child who is well enough to run around the house and garden is well enough to resume peer group activities. Your health visitor or doctor will be able to give advice about when your child may return to playgroup or school after one of the infectious illnesses.

5.11(g)   KEEPING A SICK CHILD OCCUPIED

Occupying a sick child and providing for her play needs can be a very demanding task. Children who are ill are less able to amuse themselves than when they are well and they are likely to have a shorter attention span, tiring more easily.

When a child is ill, her behaviour may regress, showing play behaviour and skills of an earlier developmental stage, which parents thought she had outgrown.

Play will encourage mobility in a child who is lethargic and generally unwell; it often seems to aid a speedy recovery as well as helping to alleviate any feelings of pain or anxiety.

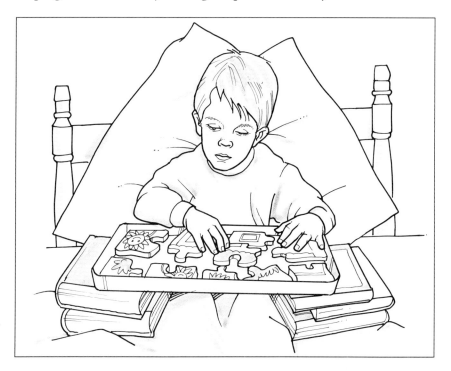

Play will encourage an unwell and lethargic child

A small stock of games and books hidden at home becomes invaluable when you are suddenly faced with amusing and occupying a sick child. Items included in this store may well be extra presents saved from Christmas or birthdays, a colouring book and set of crayons or old birthday cards, magazines and mail order catalogues to cut up and stick in a scrap book. The latter can be bought or made up from scrap paper and cardboard. Older children may be encouraged to write captions and stories about the pictures they stick into the scrap book.

See also section 5.8 above on Learning and exploring through play

A sick child will enjoy story reading; young children will only be able to listen to short stories lasting a few minutes, older children may listen to stories for longer or enjoy serial reading from day to day. Children of all ages like parents to tell them stories, particularly if the stories are from their parents' own childhood. A child who is well enough will enjoy visiting the local library to choose a book, or parents may choose a selection to take home. Children will also enjoy singing or listening to song and story tape cassettes appropriate to their age. Television programmes and videos may also provide occupation.

5.11(h) LOOKING AFTER YOURSELF AS A CARER

Looking after a sick child at home can be exhausting for the main carer. You should make things as easy for yourself as you can, reducing time spent on household chores to a minimum. The carer also requires sufficient rest and sleep so, if at all possible, you should identify somebody to take over from you regularly, enabling you to take a much-needed break. This will be particularly important if the nights are disturbed by your sick child. In a two-parent household, where the mother is the main carer and the father employed outside the home, he may be able to look after the sick child for part of each day, allowing the mother to rest or sleep. In a single parent household the help of a relative or friend may often be enlisted. If there is nobody available to offer help and your child's illness is expected to be prolonged, discuss your need for help with your family health visitor or doctor.

See also Chapter 2, section 6 on Help for the carers

A sick child usually demands constant company and attention from the parent to whom he is most attached. He will want to be cuddled and loved, and it is appropriate to give him extra attention, responding to his needs and allowing him to choose what he would like to eat or play with.

However, once your child has recovered, it is important to return to your normal family routine as soon as possible. During the illness, he will have learnt to expect extra attention and may have become used to getting his own way, so he will naturally expect it to continue.

A child who has previously slept well may have become used to waking at night during the illness and unless you deal with it carefully and appropriately he will continue to expect a parent to come into his bedroom at night and provide a drink or a cuddle whenever he wakes up. Therefore, when the child has recovered, parents should use understanding as they seek to modify their child's behaviour, resuming normal family routines and patterns of care. Your family health visitor can provide advice about particular behavioural problems.

5.12 COMMON HEALTH PROBLEMS IN BABIES AND YOUNG CHILDREN

Following the joy, happiness, worry and anxiety of pregnancy and childbirth you now find yourself in charge of a tiny new member of humanity and generally speaking, once most parents have got over the euphoria of having successfully brought a child into the world, there is a great potential for irrational panic.

No matter how many antenatal classes have been attended, how many baby care books read, or video tapes watched, or how many health visitors, midwives or doctors have been listened to, the slightest problem to affect our child can result in us calling into question our parenting skills. 'My baby is crying – why?' 'Am I feeding her properly?' 'My baby won't sleep – why not?' 'She has wet her nappy five times this morning and my friend next door's baby only did it twice!' 'WHAT AM *I* DOING WRONG?'

The usual answer is absolutely *nothing*. Many problems encountered by babies and infants are perfectly normal and would have occurred no matter what the parents had done or not done. Nevertheless, seeing our children in pain or discomfort can cause us a great deal of distress. This section of the book offers simple explanations for some common childhood problems, and straightforward advice in how to deal with them – exploding some myths and old wives' tales into the bargain.

5.12(a) COLIC

What is colic? A dictionary definition is 'griping belly pain' and unfortunately for baby and parents alike, this belly pain usually shows itself as recurrent, violent and inconsolable fits of crying and screaming. Other definitions have been offered such as a baby crying for more than three hours a day, for more than three days a week, or alternatively, a baby who is 'miserable or crying' for 30 minutes continuously on at least five days a week. Today though it is generally accepted that if your baby is less than three months old, cries inconsolably in the evening and in doing so draws his legs up to his chest – then he is showing signs of 'colic'.

Of course whatever we call it, and no matter how we define it, what we want to know is how to deal with it.

Even though one in ten babies suffer from colic type symptoms nobody has managed to identify the real cause. Spasms in the gut, allergy, an immature nervous system, babies picking up parental anxiety, and wind, have all been offered as possible reasons, but none has been proven. Consequently, the care of the child with colic concentrates on the relief of symptoms rather than attempting to 'cure' it like some form of illness.

What to do

Firstly check out that there is not a specific reason for your baby to be crying in the first place. Is she happy? Is she wet/dirty? Is she cold? Has she been frightened? Is she tired? Or is there an obvious source of pain such as a nappy pin sticking into her? Only after we have been through this sort of check list can we try and deal with the baby's colicky symptoms.

As with any crying baby the first approach should be to try and soothe and comfort the baby. Most babies respond to sound and movement, even from quite unexpected sources such as a washing machine, vacuum cleaner, or even a budgie on its swing. Certainly, rocking your baby in the chair or walking with a 'dancing' movement while talking gently to her will help. Bouncing your baby in your arms or carefully on a bed can also be useful. A ride around the block in a car or out in the pram – even at night – can also help. If you are really brave try holding your baby close to you in a sling and letting her cry while you get on with whatever it is you want to do.

Other possible remedies have been suggested which generally reflect some of the most common theories about the causes of colic. As mentioned above, none of these has been proved to be a definite cause as yet, but you may find some of the following suggestions useful.

If we consider that wind trapped in the baby's gut is a likely cause of colic symptoms, it makes sense to try and help him to get rid of that wind.

Conventional 'burping' is one useful means of helping your baby to clear air from his gut, although it is important not to go over the top with this. In almost all other countries but Britain, routine 'burping' of babies following feeding is viewed with scepticism, yet with a baby showing signs of colic it is well worth a try.

The parent should support the baby on her knee, and rub the back gently in a circular motion, occasionally *gentle* patting may also be used. A successful outcome will be indicated by the production of a 'burp' as the baby expels trapped air. Remember that unless the baby is in discomfort from trapped air it is not necessary

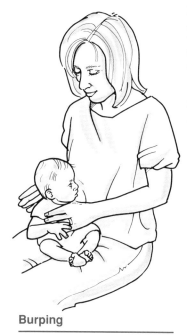

Burping

Support the baby on your knee and gently rub her back in a circular motion to carry out the burping operation after every feed as wind will generally find its own way out of the gut one way or another.

Still looking at ways of encouraging trapped air out of the gut, many manufacturers have quickly realised that parents faced with a squealing baby will try anything, and there are now many liquid-based products on the market. The traditional remedy of 'gripe water' has now been discredited amongst many health workers as, while it may have been effective in some cases, its alcohol content is not ideal for a young baby. More recent additions to the anti-colic range of liquids available use a derivative of silicone called dimethicone to act on the small gas bubbles in the baby's gut, causing them to merge together and be expelled more easily. Infacol is a good example of such a liquid; it has a pleasant orange taste and, when given orally in a dropper before meals, has been shown in trials to reduce colic symptoms. This, and similar products, are not drugs and only act on the air in the baby's gut. They may be worth a try therefore.

A treatment method which seeks to deal with both trapped air and also the theory of anxiety and tension in the baby as a contributor to colic symptoms, is that of massage. As colic attacks tend to follow a set pattern each day for several weeks, it is often possible to predict when your baby will start to cry. Massage treatment is thought to be more effective if done about one hour before your baby normally starts to cry, but not immediately after a meal.

There are several methods and it may take time for you to see which is most effective for your baby. One way is to lie your baby on his back facing you, then with a circular clockwise motion, the

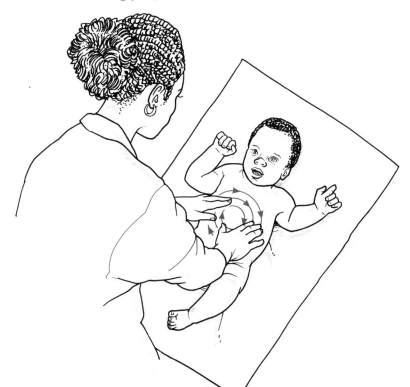

Massaging your baby

Massage should be very gentle and follow a clockwise, circular motion from the navel outwards

See Appendix I, How the body works for more information on the different types of muscle

See Appendix VII for Addresses of useful organisations

belly is massaged softly in larger and larger circles starting from the navel and working outwards. During this massage process, the smooth muscle of the intestine is relaxed and wind should eventually be passed.

Perhaps the newest of treatments advocated for colic symptoms is a chiropractic technique of spine manipulation pioneered in Denmark. The theory is that by gently manipulating the baby's spine the nerves which affect the gut can be stimulated in such a way as to reduce tension and stop painful spasms. This technique should only be carried out by someone who is specifically trained to do so. (A list of qualified chiropractors can be obtained from the British Chiropractic Association.)

Finally, as far as the allergy theory of colic is concerned, while it may be tempting to switch from breast milk to formula milk, or from one brand of formula milk to another in an attempt to rule out the possibility of allergy, research seems to indicate that colic is as common in breast fed infants as it is in formula fed infants. Also, as there are a wide variety of formula milks on the market, it is best to seek the advice of your health visitor or general practitioner before making any changes to your baby's diet.

It is worth noting that in the case of breast fed babies, the diet of mothers may be successfully modified to reduce colic symptoms in their babies. For example, foods such as bananas, oranges, strawberries, coffee and chocolate in the mother's diet are often implicated in leading to an upset stomach in the child. Again, it is best to seek the advice of your health visitor or general practitioner about changes in your diet if you are breast feeding.

In summary, colic is still one of the mysteries of modern medicine, with no agreed causes or guaranteed cures. Whilst it will not resolve the problems, it is reassuring for parents to know that, depending upon the definition used, somewhere between 10–35 per cent of all babies will have colic, and there is nothing to show that it is linked to 'poor parenting'.

An acceptance by parents that it is not their fault, and that they are either supportive of each other or able to find support from a close friend, is often the most crucial factor in management of colic. At the very least it is good to know that colic should disappear after three months, and that apart from the other usual 'ups and downs' the remainder of your child's life should be a lot less stressful to all concerned.

5.12(b) TEETHING

A teething baby can be the cause of some upsetting times for parents. This section examines the process of teething and suggests some ways of minimising problems.

When do teeth appear?

There is considerable variation in the age at which a baby's first tooth may appear. Teeth begin to form while the baby is in the womb so it is not unusual for a baby to be born with at least one tooth. Neither, however, is it abnormal for no teeth to have appeared by the time the child has reached his first birthday.

As a broad generalisation, however, teething usually starts at approximately six months, followed by the majority of the remaining teeth during the first and second years. The order in which the teeth arrive rarely differs between children.

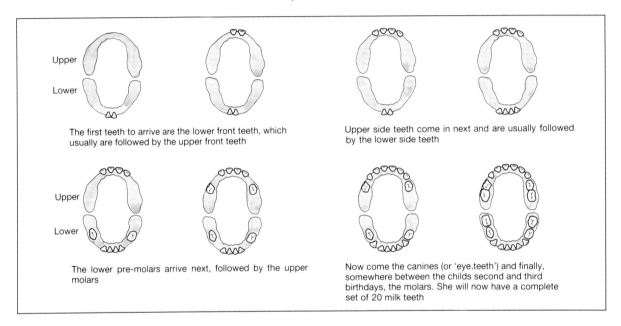

Upper
Lower

The first teeth to arrive are the lower front teeth, which usually are followed by the upper front teeth

Upper side teeth come in next and are usually followed by the lower side teeth

Upper
Lower

The lower pre-molars arrive next, followed by the upper molars

Now come the canines (or 'eye teeth') and finally, somewhere between the childs second and third birthdays, the molars. She will now have a complete set of 20 milk teeth

The usual order of appearance for milk teeth

You can usually tell when your baby's first tooth is about to appear due to the fact that as it begins to push through the gum it forms a small, pale bump. Obviously this process causes some discomfort and the teething baby may be irritable and fretful, but, in addition to an increased amount of dribbling, these are the only symptoms which should be blamed on cutting a tooth. Claims that teething causes vomiting, diarrhoea, convulsions, fever, rashes and even bronchitis, are unfounded. Any disturbances of this sort should be sorted out separately and not put down to 'cutting a tooth', otherwise it is easy to overlook real problems such as symptoms of an ear infection for example. If in doubt do not hesitate to contact your health visitor or doctor for advice.

Responding to problems

As far as easing the discomfort of teething is concerned, there are a number of simple options open to parents as well as a whole range of proprietary products. Firstly, working on the principle that it is best to avoid giving any form of medicament to a child unless absolutely necessary, you can try a number of 'non-chemical' ways of helping to relieve discomfort. The simplest tool to hand – literally – is your little finger! Gently rub your child's gums; the fact you are paying attention will certainly help, at the very least, in addition to providing some local relief of discomfort. The second option is to give the child objects to bite upon. Safety is of course paramount when giving a baby anything to put in her mouth, so things which she may usually chew, such as a raw carrot or sugar free rusk, are ideal choices.

Cold objects also seem to bring the greatest relief, so teething rings which have been kept in the fridge are usual. Make sure that the teething rings you choose are safe and easy to clean, and if they are filled with a 'gel' substance, examine them regularly to ensure that there are no leakages. Care must also be taken that a ring is not so cold as to cause frostbite in a baby – keep them in the lower part of the fridge, NOT the ice compartment or freezer.

Ideally these methods should be sufficient to pacify a child but, as some parents may choose to use proprietary preparations to ease teething discomfort, a brief consideration of these is given here.

The two main groups of products designed to relieve teething discomfort are those which act as local anaesthetics, or alternatively those which act as minor analgesics (pain killers). In the first group, the two local anaesthetics used in proprietary teething preparations are benzocaine and lignocaine. Of the two, lignocaine is the least likely to cause an allergic reaction and therefore preparations which contain lignocaine should be used in preference to those containing benzocaine. The side panels on the containers of proprietary products will show details of the local anaesthetic used. It should be noted however, that some of the products containing lignocaine are also recommended for other uses. It is important therefore to get the dosage right when using such a product on your child. If you read the instructions carefully there should be no problems, but it may well be safer to use a product specifically formulated for teething infants (e.g. Dentinox) in which the concentration of lignocaine has been adjusted accordingly. Even so, follow the instructions carefully; you are doing your baby no favours by using more of the product in a misguided belief that this will get rid of the pain any quicker.

The second group of products, the minor analgesics, contain an active ingredient called choline salicylate which is related to aspirin. Examples of such products are Bonjela and Teejel.

Because of the recent concerns about a possible link between the use of aspirin for children and the rare condition Reyes syndrome, a cautious view suggested by some pharmacists and paediatricians is that preparations containing choline salicylate should be avoided in teething infants. It should be stressed that this goes much further than current Department of Health recommendations and if you are at all unsure about which products to use it is best to discuss the issues with your health visitor or family doctor.

See also Chapter 6, section 2(f) on Dental health

Children should be taught that teeth need to be cleaned and cared for from the earliest days. A child under one year can enjoy having her teeth cleaned with a tiny toothbrush or piece of cotton wool as part of her bedtime routine.

Treatment of teething problems: a summary

- Give the child teething objects to bite. Cold objects seem to give better relief and should be kept in a clean container in the fridge. Hard sugar free rusks are also a useful option.

- If the pain is troublesome use the appropriate dose of a sugar free paracetamol liquid – available from your chemist. This may be given regularly every 4–6 hours.

- If additional pain relief is needed, lignocaine based teething gels (e.g. Dentinox) may be used.

5.12(c) COUGHS AND COLDS

A cough or a cold is one of the first common childhood illnesses that your baby will experience. It is also one of the most upsetting for the parents, especially for 'first timers', as the baby can become quite distressed by the symptoms.

A baby is protected by immunity gained from its mother for approximately the first three months of its life to most of the common contagious illnesses. This period of immunity can be extended if the baby is breast fed as the baby will continue to receive immunity from the breast milk. As this immunity wanes though the child will become susceptible to catching coughs and colds from those around him, and as he builds up his own immunity, he may seem to catch everything going especially if he has older brothers and sisters who go to school, or if he attends a nursery etc. But you cannot wrap your child in cotton wool. The 'average' baby has about eight colds a year. The worst of the symptoms are over after a few days and after the first cold or two you will become experienced at coping with the symptoms which will pose less of a problem to you.

Coughs and colds are caused by viruses, so the doctor cannot cure them with antibiotics and the baby cannot catch them by being outside in the cold. True, babies do catch more colds in the winter but this is probably due to everyone being shut up indoors and in close proximity.

Colds

A baby or young child with a cold will present with a similar picture to that of an adult. She will have a runny nose and may sneeze a lot (but as she cannot blow her nose this is the only way she can clear the mucus). Her breathing may be noisy, her appetite subdued and she may appear to be generally 'under the weather'.

So, what can you do about these symptoms, and when should they give you cause for concern?

The runny nose, sneezing and noisy breathing are caused by mucus in the upper airways and nose. You can be an attentive nose wiper but there is not a lot more you can do. This is the body's own way of removing the virus from your baby's airways. If the baby is having problems sucking the breast or bottle because of her blocked nose the doctor may prescribe nose drops (e.g. Ephedrine) to give before feeds. If the baby is waking up at night and appears very snuffly you may want to try some of the decongestant drops which can be applied to the cot sheet, so that the baby can breathe in the vapours. These drops are usually menthol, pine or eucalyptus based and can be bought from the chemist – your health visitor will advise you on a suitable brand. At night, you can raise the head of the mattress if the child is under one year old, or give a firm pillow to an older child. This will encourage secretions to drain into the stomach and away from the nose.

If your child has a decreased appetite during his cold, this is only to be expected and as long as he is taking fluids there is no need to worry about him. All children lose a little weight when they are ill but soon put it on again when they are better. Offer your child small portions of his favourite foods at mealtimes but don't make a fuss if he doesn't eat. Do, however, offer frequent drinks throughout the day and night. If your child is refusing to eat and drink, then you should consult your doctor – especially if the child's temperature is also raised.

It may help to give your child the recommended dose of paracetamol. This will help to reduce the temperature and also relieve any other cold symptoms, such as a sore throat, which a baby cannot tell you about. Paracetamol elixir, specially formulated for babies and children, is available from your pharmacist and is free on prescription from the doctor. Aspirin preparations are no longer recommended for children.

Coughs

A cough often accompanies a cold and coughs are described as 'chesty' or 'dry'. A 'chesty' cough sounds harsh as if the child is trying to cough up some mucus from the chest. A 'dry' cough sounds less traumatic and could be described as 'tickly' or irritating and is more common at night. There is a wide variety of cough medicines on the market, but before buying them check the age range and the dosage. If you are in any doubt consult your pharmacist or doctor.

Remember that although a cough may sound distressing to you it is actually the body's natural way of removing infection and mucus from the chest and upper airways. Therefore some doctors believe it is better not to give any medicines at all.

If your child has a persistent cough, that is one that does not seem to be improving with time, or if it becomes a 'wheeze', always consult your doctor. A 'wheeze' is a noise that once heard is never forgotten. The breathing becomes very harsh and noisy and the child seems to have more difficulty breathing out than in. This often happens in the middle of the night and is very distressing for the child. If you are concerned and get anxious this will increase the child's anxiety so stay calm and call the doctor.

Croup

Croup is a nasty sounding harsh cough, associated with a cold, which is brought on by the child having an anxiety attack usually in the middle of the night. The child appears to be struggling for breath and may be sweaty and confused. As a parent you must stay calm, cuddle the child and reassure him, offer him a drink and try and 'normalise' the situation. These attacks are usually only short lived and infrequent. If you have central heating or the air seems very dry, you could try to humidify the air by placing bowls of warm water around the bedroom at night.

Coughs and colds: a summary

- Coughs and colds are very common in young children;

- Ensure the child has plenty of fluids;

- Contact the doctor if the child has a fever, a persistent cough, wheezes, refuses fluids or if you are worried;

- If in any doubt check with the pharmacist about the suitability of medicines for young children.;

- Finally, there is no need to stay in the warm – as long as the child is dressed sensibly, you may find that some fresh air will do you both good.

5.12(d) THROAT AND EAR INFECTIONS

Tonsillitis

Tonsillitis is a fairly common illness in young children but occurs most commonly in school-age children. Some years ago the 'cure' for recurrent tonsillitis was to remove the tonsils and there are a great many adults walking around without their tonsils. Today tonsils are seen for what they are, that is, a barrier against infection. Tonsillitis is caused by a bacterium, and the tonsils' function is to destroy the bacteria and prevent the infection spreading. As it is caused by bacteria, tonsillitis can be treated with antibiotics and paracetamol for the raised temperature. As the child may have difficulty in swallowing she should be offered frequent drinks or soft foods, for example, good old 'jelly and ice cream'.

A point to note: tonsillitis is not the same as a sore throat. To check for tonsillitis the doctor will examine the child's throat and look for red, enlarged tonsils which will often be speckled with white pus.

Ear infections

- **Otitis media**
  Infection of the middle ear

As a baby or small child has a very small gap between his ears, nose and throat so ear infections are often diagnosed following a common cold or tonsillitis. Otitis media is caused by bacteria in the middle ear and is treated by antibiotics. Very occasionally, if the infection does not clear with antibiotics, the ear has to be drained surgically.

- **Auriscope**
  A special instrument designed to look in the ear

Ear infections are difficult for parents to diagnose, but the child is usually unwell, has a raised temperature and may suffer some slight hearing loss. The inner ear looks red and inflamed but this may only be seen by the doctor using an auriscope. Paracetamol should be given to reduce the temperature and make the child more comfortable. Lying the child with the infected ear down on a warmed pillow may also provide some relief.

5.12(e) ### FEVER OR RAISED TEMPERATURE

A raised temperature is the body's natural way of demonstrating infection. Your child is likely, therefore, to have a raised temperature when she has a cold, any of the infectious diseases mentioned above or in section 6.6(b), or following vaccination as mild or killed forms of the viruses are used in the injections.

See also Chapter 6, section 6(b) on Infectious diseases of childhood and adolescence

You can tell whether your child has a raised temperature as she will look flushed, her skin will feel hot to touch and she will be generally miserable and unhappy. You may also take her temperature by using a thermometer or one of the commercially available temperature sticks which are held against the skin. It is important to have some idea as to how much above normal her temperature actually is.

See section 5.11(b) above for advice on Taking your child's temperature

Febrile convulsions

The danger of raised temperature in a small child is the likelihood of febrile convulsions or fits. These fits are generally harmless to the child, unless he falls against something, but very distressing to the parents. During a fit, the child will roll his eyes, become quite floppy and then start to twitch and shudder. This only lasts for a few minutes, but may seem longer. The general rule is to make sure the child cannot harm himself by falling or bumping into anything and to turn him on his side so that he doesn't choke on his secretions. Following the fit, the child will be sleepy and then may get upset. Stay calm, reassure the child and then contact the doctor. Febrile convulsions are most common in young children aged six months to three years. It is important to know how to prevent them if possible.

Keeping the child's temperature down

See section 5.11(c) above for a description of 'tepid sponging'.

- Strip the child down to his nappy or pants;

- Sponge the child with lukewarm (not cold) water;

- Encourage the child to drink;

- Give the recommended dose of paracetamol elixir for children;

- If the above doesn't work or the high temperature keeps returning, contact the doctor.

5.12(f) NAPPY RASH

Nappy rash is caused by ammonia accumulating on a baby's sensitive skin, resulting in a red, inflamed area around the genitals and anus, sometimes becoming so bad that open sores develop which can bleed. Ammonia is found in both urine and faeces but a stronger reaction is caused when the two combine. It is therefore important to change your baby's nappy frequently to prevent the build-up of ammonia.

Nappy rash is more common in bottle fed babies than in breast fed babies as cows' milk is less easily digested by the baby resulting in a bulkier stool. Nappy rash is also more commonly found in babies wearing 'terry' nappies rather than disposable ones. This is due to the ammonia not being washed out of the terry nappies properly. To avoid this happening always soak nappies immediately after use, there are special sanitising solutions available, and then wash and rinse them properly. A washing machine will do this most effectively. One-way nappy liners will also help to prevent nappy rash as will careful washing and drying of plastic pants. Disposable nappies contain an absorbent gel which helps to keep the skin dry, but all babies should have periods of being 'nappy-free' whenever possible, not only to allow air to get to the skin but also to allow the baby to exercise his legs without restriction.

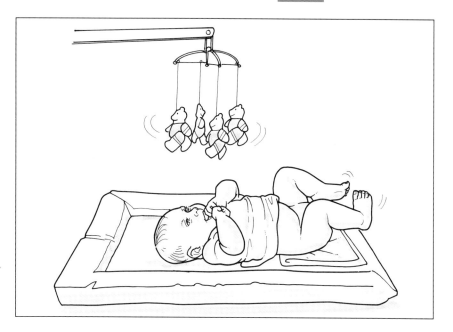

It is important to leave your baby without a nappy on for a short period each day to allow her to exercise her legs while the air circulates around her bottom

To treat nappy rash change the baby's nappy very frequently (this may be ten times a day at first). The nappy area should be washed with warm water and then patted dry, paying particular attention to the skin creases. A barrier lotion should then be applied. If you usually use petroleum jelly you may wish to try an 'antiseptic' barrier cream instead, but don't put too much on. Again, allow the baby to be exposed for as long as possible, much easier in the garden in the summer when the baby can be laid on a towel or mat.

If the nappy rash persists and does not appear to be responding to treatment, do go and see your doctor, in case there is another cause (for example, thrush – see below).

5.12(g) THRUSH

Candida is the name of the yeast-like organism which can cause the infection 'thrush' in babies and infants and sometimes results in infection spreading to and from parents, particularly mothers.

Candida albicans (as it is more correctly known) is spread as airborne spores (in addition to person to person contact) and thrives in many moist areas of the body. The mouth and nappy area are favourite sites in babies, as are the vagina and skin creases in adults.

Candida infection in babies and infants

The Candida organism is a common inhabitant of the gut and, perhaps surprisingly, and contrary to popular belief, newborn babies are more likely to acquire thrush from their mothers as a result of infection from this organism during their birth, rather than from anything else in their environment such as dirty feeding bottles, or any other equipment.

However, unclean feeding equipment, and the common habit of putting an often not too clean finger into a hungry baby's mouth instead of a feed are good ways of passing over the Candida organism, and causing oral thrush.

Oral thrush is exceedingly common and is generally the best known form of Candida infection. It is characterised by creamy white patches in the mouth, on the tongue and inside of the cheeks. It is important not to confuse these with flecks of milk which can easily be wiped off. On the tongue in particular it is often difficult to identify thrush, although coatings of milk are generally finer, white and clearer, while thrush deposits are usually more crusty, coarse, and creamier. If infected particularly heavily, a baby will be less inclined to suck.

At the other end of the baby, the moist covered conditions are ideal for the breeding of Candida and the development of what is known as 'nappy dermatitis' type thrush.

Nappy dermatitis thrush usually appears when the baby is home in the second or third week after birth. The baby with this condition is generally a well cared for breast fed baby – dispelling the myths of poor hygiene when changing nappies etc. The baby with nappy dermatitis thrush does not necessarily have to have oral thrush, and in some cases the Candida organism somehow must have been swallowed whole, and passed out intact to settle in its breeding ground in the moist folds of the groin, insides of the upper thighs, and over the penis or vulva.

As is the case with its orally occurring counterpart, thrush in the nappy area is often wrongly confused with other things. The tell tale signs, however, are a rash of small pin head papules (almost like tiny blisters yet to burst) which may join together, but leave the generalised area of rash with a definite edge to it.

Nappy dermatitis type thrush is commonly and mistakenly put down to nappies not being changed often enough or the nappy area not being cleaned or managed properly – often leading to inappropriate treatment. You need to be aware that home treatments such as the application of zinc and castor oil (as if the rash were just a simple soreness) will actually encourage the growth of Candida and make it much worse. In older babies, thrush commonly invades and makes 'ordinary' nappy rash worse and these will not clear unless the Candida is treated. Here, the same characteristic small round papules can be seen at the edges of the rash and can also be seen across the tummy, at the navel, in the armpits and in the folds of the skin.

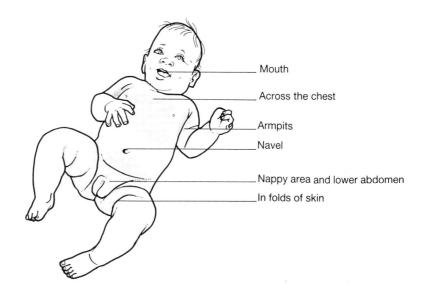

Mouth

Across the chest

Armpits

Navel

Nappy area and lower abdomen

In folds of skin

Possible sites for Candida
infection in babies

- **Areola**
  The darker area around
  the nipple

*See section 5.1(a) above
for more advice on
cleaning and sterilising
feeding equipment*

- **Topical preparations**
  Preparations which are
  applied to the skin

Maternal infection

In addition to the problems which thrush can cause at both ends of
the child, it needs to be recognised that the infection can also
cause the mother problems.

If a child with oral thrush is breast feeding, it is very easy for the
mother's nipples and areola to become infected, particularly if
these areas have been scratched, or are at all sore in any way. Once
an infection is established on a mother's breasts, it is possible to
transfer this back and forth between her and her baby, each continually reinfecting the other.

Prevention and treatment

As mentioned above, a most common cause of thrush in babies is
the transfer of the Candida organism from the mother at birth.
However, unclean feeding equipment, such as bottles and teats,
also rank highly as possible harbourers of Candida, and from these
babies can easily be infected and develop thrush. Such equipment
and all items used for preparing feeds should be scrupulously
cleaned and sterilised.

Both oral and nappy dermatitis thrush respond rapidly to the
application of creams and suspensions containing preparations
specifically formulated to attack the Candida organisms.

Oral thrush is generally treated with topical nystatin (e.g.
Nystan Oral Suspension) or miconazole (e.g. Daktarin Oral Gel),
but whichever is used, it is important to employ the right
technique in order for the treatment to be successful. The solution
or gel must make contact with all the white patches, as its action
depends upon a high surface concentration of the preparation being

in contact with the organisms. For this reason, the treatment should be applied after feeds in order that it is not washed away. Be careful not to confuse the thrush patches with the milk curds left behind after feeding.

Nappy dermatitis type thrush is also effectively treated with topical nystatin (e.g. Nystan or Multilind cream), miconazole (e.g. Daktarin cream), or clotrimazole (e.g. Canesten cream). Which ever cream is used it should be applied lightly at each nappy change, and the treatment continued beyond the time the rash has actually disappeared in order to minimise the risk of reinfection. Such creams can also be used for effective treatment of any maternal infection around the nipple and areola.

When treating a baby either orally or in the napkin area, it is essential that your hands are cleansed thoroughly before and after, and that if more than one child is being treated, or if you are treating yourself, separate tubes of cream are used.

5.12(h) GASTROENTERITIS

Acute gastroenteritis is a combination of signs and symptoms characterised by a sudden onset of diarrhoea and/or vomiting, often accompanied by a rise in temperature and general malaise. It is estimated that, in the United Kingdom, 5 per cent of children under the age of one will develop acute gastroenteritis, although only 10 per cent of these will need to go into hospital. While it is simple to treat, it is easy for a child suffering from this syndrome to become very ill quite quickly unless proper treatment is given.

Acute gastroenteritis is of infective origin, with bacteria, viruses, and protozoa (microscopic animals) all being possible agents of infection. The method of action of all of these is different, yet all essentially produce the same characteristic signs and symptoms. Unlike the other problems discussed in this chapter so far, there is no doubt whatsoever that gastroenteritis is connected with the cleanliness of a child's surroundings, feeding equipment, and purity of the water supply.

Signs and symptoms

A baby suffering from gastroenteritis will invariably begin by passing loose watery stools. Vomiting may or may not occur at the same time. The colour, frequency, and consistency of the stools may vary – remember that a healthy fully breast fed baby may pass up to 10 loose yellowy stools in a day and this must not be confused with the diarrhoea characteristic of gastroenteritis where up to 20 stools in a day may be passed.

The colour of diarrhoea stools also changes from normal brown to watery yellow, and later green. It may contain mucus, blood or pus. (Unsavoury as it may seem, it is useful to know what your baby's normal stools look like as a reference point for any future problems.)

The baby's tummy may also appear bloated, and there may be some signs of dehydration for example:

- The fontanelle may begin to hollow inwards;
- The temperature may be raised;
- The baby may be lethargic.

• **Fontanelle**
The 'soft spot' or gentle dip in the top of a baby's head, where the bones of the skull have not yet closed up

What to do

As with all childhood illnesses, there will be a wide range in the extent to which any single child suffers, but should your child have any of the above symptoms it is important to contact your doctor immediately. Describe the signs and symptoms and, as the cause is infectious, request a home visit.

Treatment

The most important part of modern management of infantile gastroenteritis centres upon appropriate oral rehydration therapy. This means giving the affected baby a special solution orally, which contains all that is needed to replace essential parts of the diet lost in diarrhoea and vomiting. You may hear this referred to as an 'oral glucose electrolyte solution' – a common brand name is Dioralyte.

Babies whose gastroenteritis is not too severe will often be able to stay at home, with their normal milk feed replaced by the rehydration solution for around 24 hours. If the child is breast fed it is usually recommended that this is continued in addition to the oral rehydration therapy.

In the past, in the United Kingdom, it has been usual for the infant's normal milk feed to be gradually reintroduced following oral rehydration therapy, although in recent years this practice has been abandoned for infants over six months of age. Although caution is necessary, there are now new studies which indicate that even in the under six months age group immediate return to normal formula feeds is to be recommended as routine practice.

For some babies, though, the severity of the symptoms of gastroenteritis will warrant their admission to hospital where they can receive specialist care, and while oral rehydration therapy is successful in around 80 per cent of cases, an intravenous infusion (drip) may be necessary for the child who is very ill or who is vomiting persistently.

Gastroenteritis: summary

It is worth remembering that while gastroenteritis, more often than not, can be a self limiting infection of short duration and easily dealt with at home, every case may well be different and it is important to avoid any temptation to treat your child without seeking the appropriate advice. Remember that the simple treatments for gastroenteritis usually have good results, but you may need expert assistance in caring for your child.

It is particularly important to remember that, in the case of medical conditions such as gastroenteritis which have a very rapid onset, reading a passage in a book such as this is *no substitute* for seeking a medical opinion. It is far better to seek advice from an expert such as your general practitioner than to have your baby overcome by a condition which more often than not can so easily be treated.

It should always be remembered that good hygiene precautions and, in particular, careful attention to handwashing, will help to prevent the spread of gastroenteritis.

5.12(i) MORE SERIOUS AND LONG TERM PROBLEMS

- **Pyloric stenosis**
  A condition which occurs in some babies, usually becoming apparent in the second month of life, where the opening between the stomach and the intestine is narrowed resulting in an obstruction

- **Coeliac disease**
  A failure of carbohydrate and fat metabolism apparently caused by a sensitivity to the gluten in wheat

Some babies are unfortunate enough to be born with a condition (such as congenital dislocation of the hip, or cleft lip and palate) which will require treatment, sometimes extensive, to put right. Other babies and young children will go on to develop conditions which may be alarming, long term or life threatening. A condition such as pyloric stenosis (which tends to affect babies in the first few months of life and which is characterised by very forceful vomiting) is now being treated easily by surgery, but the fact that the necessary operation is 'routine' for the hospital staff will not be much consolation to worried parents taking their tiny baby into hospital. Other conditions, for example coeliac disease or epilepsy, may involve radical adaptation on the part of the parents over a long period.

There is not the space in a manual such as this to consider all the more serious and less common health problems that may be encountered by parents with children under the age of five. Coverage would necessarily be far too superficial to be of any real benefit. Some general principles may be suggested, however, to help you find the support and advice you will need if your child becomes really ill.

- Do follow the advice given above (in section 5.2(c)) on when to call the doctor. Most importantly, always consult a health professional if you are worried about your baby or child.

- If your child is referred to hospital for tests or examinations, then ask the staff as many questions as you wish. Do not feel intimidated – you have every right to know what is happening to your baby.

- You may find it useful to prepare a written list of questions to take to the appointment with you as it is easy to forget what you want to ask if you are under stress.

- Many hospitals are sympathetic to parents now and will give you as much information as they can. Some even prepare information sheets or booklets about specific conditions so it is always worth asking whether such information is available.

- If your child has to be admitted to hospital for investigations or treatment, you will almost certainly be able to accompany her and stay overnight – provided of course that your other family commitments allow this.

- Do not be shy to ask friends, neighbours and relatives for practical help and support. Most people are only too happy to be useful in a crisis and you may be surprised at the warmth of the reactions you receive to such requests.

See Appendix VII for Addresses of useful organisations and support groups

- There are numerous national and local agencies and support groups concerned with specific conditions and illnesses. These can often provide a great deal of useful information as well as putting you in touch with other parents who have been through the same experience as you are going through now.

- Another useful organisation is NAWCH (The National Association for the Welfare of Children in Hospital). Any parent whose child needs hospitalisation will find this organisation most helpful. NAWCH also produces a booklist which is regularly updated and which suggests appropriate reading/picture books for young children either preparing for a hospital stay or after admission.

- Local parent groups (for example, many local branches of the National Childbirth Trust) may run 'link' schemes for parents who have had similar experiences.

- Make sure that your local general practitioner and community nurse know if your child has a chronic health problem, or if you have a lengthy period of stressful trips to the hospital while a treatable problem is being sorted out. Your own health and resources are likely to be taxed and it is important that your doctor knows this.

THE OLDER CHILD AND ADOLESCENT

6.1 NORMAL DEVELOPMENT

6.1(a) FIVE TO TWELVE YEARS

Physical development

After the earlier years of rapid growth, the school-aged child experiences a more stable period, during which bodily changes occur more gradually. Height increases about 6.25 cm (2.5 inches) a year and weight gain is approximately 3 kg (7 lbs) a year. The trunk becomes longer, and arms and legs grow rapidly, so that the chubbiness of the younger child disappears. The face becomes longer and the jaw develops a more adult prominence. Around the age of 6–7 years, baby teeth start to be replaced by permanent teeth at a rate of approximately four teeth a year. As these are full size, they can cause the child's mouth to appear very full, but this becomes less obvious as the jaw continues to grow.

Heights and weights for children aged 5–11 years (NB – these are averages only)

Age in years	Boys				Girls			
	Height inches	(cm)	Weight pounds	(kg)	Height inches	(cm)	Weight pounds	(kg)
5	43	(107)	40	(18)	42	(108)	40	(18)
6	45	(112)	44	(20)	45	(112)	44	(20)
7	48	(120)	50	(23)	47	(117)	50	(23)
8	50	(125)	56	(25)	49	(122)	55	(25)
9	52	(130)	60	(28)	51	(127)	62	(28)
10	54	(135)	67	(30)	53	(132)	68	(31)
11	56	(140)	73	(33)	57	(142)	75	(34)

Muscles grow rapidly during middle childhood, particularly in boys, and muscle aches may occur if the child is over using relatively immature and developing muscle. Boys and girls differ very little in size, although boys tend to be very slightly taller and heavier than girls.

Shoes should be bought with growing feet in mind, as badly fitting shoes at this stage could lead to skeletal deformities for the rest of the child's life. Trousers, shirts and skirts which have room for growth will also be advisable, to maximise the use of such items.

The diagrams show the change in shape of the mouth, and the age at which milk teeth are replaced by permanent teeth

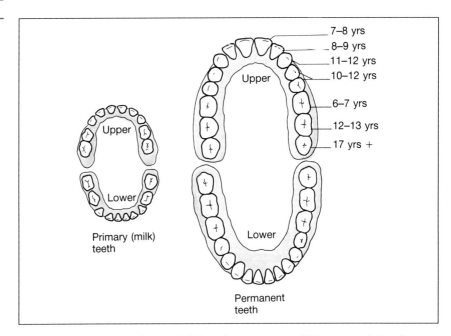

Primary (milk) teeth

Permanent teeth

7–8 yrs
8–9 yrs
11–12 yrs
10–12 yrs
6–7 yrs
12–13 yrs
17 yrs +

The body shape the child develops now will be more like that in adult life; a tall slim child will usually become a tall slim adult.

The eyes are now fully developed and eyesight should be at its maximum potential.

As the body becomes leaner and more muscular, the child is eager to take part in strenuous physical exercise. Activities such as riding a bicycle, skipping, skateboarding and playing football are popular, and although the skills may be fairly limited initially, the child shows increasing stamina in practising and so becomes more proficient. Boys tend to be ahead of girls in throwing, jumping and running, although they do have greater strength and more muscle tissue available for use.

School provides an appropriate environment where children can practise fine motor skills, such as handwriting, sewing, painting and making models. Most children of five years should be able to dress and undress themselves, coping with buttons, zips and shoelaces with minimal assistance.

The manual dexterity required to play a musical instrument develops, and the child can learn to co-ordinate fingers and breathing, for example when playing a recorder. The child should also be able to sing in tune and follow simple harmonies.

Mental development

Going to school marks a broadening of the child's world, at a time when his thinking ability is ready for greater challenges. Children are curious about the use of letters and words to convey meaning, and have the manual dexterity to hold a pen or pencil and begin to write. Together, reading and writing broaden the child's experience,

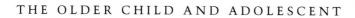
Age (in years)	Co-ordination skills	Mental development
5	Has good control – can climb and jump well Can walk backwards Can wash himself without getting clothes wet Manipulates pencil to write first name	2,000 word vocabulary Talks constantly Knows primary colours – red, blue, yellow Can count to 10 Names days of the week Asks for definitions
6	Balance improves Uses manipulative skills such as cutting and hammering Can draw large letters or figures	Learns to read with understanding Knows some streets in his local neighbourhood Knows difference between morning and afternoon
7	Less active than younger child Can print sentences Muscular skills such as ball throwing improved May develop nervous activities such as nail biting	Begins to show interest in cause and effect Knows the value of coins Gains satisfaction in conclusions and logical endings Understands past, present and future time concepts
8	Develops grace and balance Co-ordination obvious in sports activities Has ability to start joined up writing rather than print	Begins to understand logical reasoning and implications Aware of time, can begin to plan activities for a day Develops understanding of left and right Appreciates degrees of concepts such as light, pain
9	Can use both hands independently Skilled hand/eye co-ordination required for sewing, and sport	Likes to have secrets Can break down difficult skills into manageable component parts Focuses on details
10	Energetic, restless May demonstrate active movements such as foot tapping Works hard to practise skills	Enjoys learning Likes to memorise Identifies facts Concrete and specific thinking
11	Has skilful manipulative movements nearly equal to those of adults	Likes action in learning Concentrates well when working Able to identify and discuss problems
12	Skilled and co-ordinated in all physical activities	Motivated more by inner drive than competition Able to classify, arrange and generalise Can be critical of own work

enabling him to learn more about the world he lives in. His mental ability allows him to understand the symbols of letters and numbers, and by manipulating these, new experiences develop.

The vocabulary of a five year old is now about 2,000 words and, with exposure to new ideas and other children, this will rapidly increase to 50,000 words by the age of eleven years. Although some of the rules that govern the English language are hard to learn, children can use increasingly complex sentences and make fewer grammatical errors as they go through school.

One of the key tasks involved in mental development at this age is logical and consistent thinking. Children learn that mathematical skills, such as counting, can be used to deal with seemingly apparent changes that have taken place.

In the box on the right the rows of buttons appear the same; in the box on the left the lower row looks longer but contains the same number of buttons

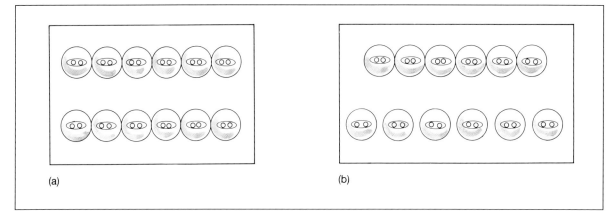

(a) (b)

Those who are unable to count may feel that the lower row of buttons shown in the figure (b) contains more buttons than the one above it as it is longer. Similar skills have to be learnt to deal with apparent differences in weight, volume and mass.

The school-aged child also learns to create more and more sophisticated classification systems – such as the characteristics of reptiles and mammals, or the differences between towns and cities. They often involve these new skills in their play; collecting types of cards or stamps, playing games that require classifications such as Happy Families. Even a seaside walk can be punctuated by frequent stops to collect another type of unusual shell.

Relational concepts such as left and right are tackled during this phase of childhood, although this is difficult for the child to learn. When number skills are developing, concepts such as clock time can be introduced and also the use of money.

Emotional development

During the school years, the child learns much from the peer group. By comparing themselves with others in the class, children can adjust their behaviour to meet society's expectations and gain more insight into themselves. They also learn to identify which situations require co-operation and which are more competitive.

Emotions such as anger and aggression can be seen in a variety of expressions – physical shoving, sullenness, and swearing. Many will be aware of the schoolchild's enjoyment of jokes, and use of humour. School also provides the child with opportunities for self-evaluation, developing self-confidence or doubt. Being picked by other children to join a team game, or being sent to a remedial group for reading, will give the child messages about how others perceive him, which may differ from perceptions at home. It is important for those caring for children that they are aware of the attitudes of others, and offer opportunities to the child to talk about this. Praise means a lot to a child of this age (as it does to most people) and efforts should be made to recognise each child's special attributes.

Moral development should have occurred to the level that the child is able to obey rules set by adults. Children tend to demonstrate obedience in order to avoid punishment and to earn rewards. Rules need to be stated and children also need to know why such rules have been made and what the consequences are for failing to follow them.

At home, many children spend between two and three hours a day watching television. Research has been undertaken to identify the effects of such viewing and it would appear that children tend to play more aggressively having watched violent incidents. But there are positive outcomes as well – television can increase language development and broaden experience. This is particularly apparent where adults talk with the children about the programmes they have been watching.

Although friends at school and teachers are an important influence on the child at this age, the family continues to be the major

SUMMARY OF THE MAJOR DEVELOPMENTAL TASKS

For the 5–12 year old	1. Decreasing dependence on the family and developing relationships with other adults and children 2. Becoming an active, contributing member of the family 3. Learning how to deal with strong feelings appropriately 4. Learning how to reason and solve problems logically 5. Developing understanding of concepts such as number, time and money 6. Adjusting to changing body image and coming to terms with sex role identity
For the adolescent	1. Developing a satisfactory body image after puberty 2. Establishing a firm, positive identity 3. Establishing sexual identity and intimate relationships 4. Achieving independence from parents 5. Demonstration of commitment to educational and occupational goals

source of support. Parents may find it frustrating that the child seems eager to get out of the house to meet friends or pursue other activities. However, under pressure, or at stressful times such as hospitalisation, the child wants his parents with him, and will appear to be very dependent on them.

6.1(b) PUBERTY, PHYSIOLOGICAL CHANGES

Puberty is the name given to the biological changes that take place between childhood and adulthood. Most people think of the development of sexual characteristics, but almost all parts of the body are affected during puberty.

Rapid changes in weight and height take place. A growth spurt begins in girls (9–11 years) and in boys (11–16 years) and the most rapid rate affects the legs, giving a leggy, gangly appearance. By the age of 17, most girls have reached their adult height, boys by 21 years.

Heights and weights for adolescents aged 12–18 years (NB – these are averages only)

Age in years	Boys				Girls			
	Height		Weight		Height		Weight	
	inches	(cm)	pounds	(kg)	inches	(cm)	pounds	(kg)
12	56	(140)	80	(36)	59	(147)	90	(41)
13	58	(145)	90	(41)	62	(155)	105	(48)
14	60	(150)	108	(49)	63	(157)	118	(53)
15	63	(157)	125	(57)	64	(160)	122	(55)
16	66	(165)	134	(61)	64	(160)	125	(57)
17	68	(170)	138	(63)	64	(160)	125	(57)
18	69	(173)	140	(64)	64	(160)	125	(57)

The weight changes are due to increased size of organs, skeleton, muscles and body fat. Sex differences occur in the fat distribution – girls develop fat in the pelvis, breast, upper back and upper arms, giving rounded contours.

Sexual development occurs in predictable stages. For girls, the first sign will be the beginnings of breast development. The uterus and vagina also develop at this time, and mucus is produced from the vagina. Pubic hair and hair under the arms develops shortly afterwards.

The first menstrual period normally occurs between 10 and 16 years of age, usually between 12–14 years. This means that the uterus has reached mature development but not necessarily that the girl is fertile – a process which may take another year. The menstrual cycle may be irregular for the first year, but usually settles down to a regular cycle of around 28 days.

Sequence of female development at puberty	Average age (years)	
	8–13	Nipples protrude slightly and surrounding tissue enlarges External genitalia become more prominent Pubic hair appears Pelvis starts to grow
	9–14	First menstrual period Nipples and surrounding breast tissue enlarge further
	12–15	Breasts continue to enlarge Menstrual cycle becomes more regular Hair in armpits becomes obvious
	12–17	Breasts assume globular shape Hair in pubic area may spread to thighs Facial hair increases

Sequence of male development at puberty	Average age (years)	
	10–14	Increasing size of testes and penis Pubic hair appears at the base of the penis
	11–15	Nocturnal emissions (wet dreams) begin Testes and penis continue to grow in size, and scrotal skin becomes darker Hair in armpits appears Voice changes as voice box begins to grow
	12–16	Testes and penis continue to grow Facial hair increases over lip and cheeks Voice deepens
	13–17	Pubic hair now thick and curly, and extends to thighs Increase of body hair on chest, legs and arms Adult voice achieved

Male sexual development is characterised first by an increase in size of the testes, usually around 12 years. The penis, scrotum and testes continue to grow at varying rates until mature development is achieved. Pubic hair begins to appear and approximately two years later, facial and underarm hair appear. Some boys develop sore nipples and should be reassured that this is quite normal.

The production of mature sperm occurs at about 15 years. Most boys are first made aware of this by nocturnal emissions (the ejaculation of semen during sleep). Chest hair, which is a late characteristic, continues growing into adulthood.

Other major changes include increased activity of sweat glands and the voice breaking, caused by the lengthening vocal chords.

Both males and females experience sweat gland development, particularly under the arms. Excessive sweating may embarrass the adolescent, and care needs to be taken with hygiene. This may well be the time to start using a deodorant or an antiperspirant.

Acne is the most common skin problem of adolescents, and is caused by grease production of the sebaceous glands. Blackheads appear, which are due to partial blockage of the pores, and red spots can be seen. For the majority of teenagers regular washing is all that is needed, but if the young person is very troubled by the problem, treatment can be prescribed by the family doctor or a skin specialist.

See section 6.3(f) below for advice on coping with acne

As with all aspects of development, it should be noted that the rate at which bodily changes occur is unique for each child. However, at this stage, perhaps more than at any other, the young person strives to be like his friends and very late development can be a source of extreme anxiety. Those caring for adolescents need to be sensitive to this, and willing to understand the psychological effect that late development can cause. Generally, developing earlier than the peer group causes little upset, in fact it may be advantageous, especially among males.

6.1(c) MENTAL AND EMOTIONAL DEVELOPMENT

Adolescence has been characterised as a time of storm and stress but, as with many other topics, it is only the bad news which hits the headlines. Many young people make the transition from child to adult with relative ease and with little trauma either to themselves or to their parents.

See also section 6.7 below on Behavioural and emotional problems

It is not surprising that, while their bodies are so rapidly changing, youngsters become quite preoccupied with themselves and wonder what they will become. Girls may see the first period as a positive achievement towards adulthood, or a dreadful event which signifies the end of childhood. Boys fear to speak as their voice breaks, or delight as the facial hair becomes obviously present. The attitudes displayed will often reflect the attitudes and values held by those closest to them, the family or the peer group.

Friendships with peers become increasingly close during adolescence as the young person seeks acceptance and also has friends with whom to share the new feelings and experiences. Peer groups offer necessary security as the youngster tries to loosen the ties to his parents. Friends can also provide a forum where the adolescent can try out new values and attitudes, in order to help clarify his new identity.

Adolescents tend to conform closely to peer group norms in order to gain acceptance. They pay particular attention to the style of dress, length of hair and popular activities. Some peer groups even have their own language and particular words and phrases to signify group membership and gain acceptance.

Adolescents also begin to experiment with sexual behaviour. It has been suggested that this is as a result of hormonal influences although the social factors are equally important. Young people have a variety of reasons for engaging in sexual behaviour. These may include reinforcing a sense of identity and attractiveness to others, challenging parental authority, and as an escape from loneliness or other pressures.

Thinking skills continue to develop into adolescence as problem solving becomes more sophisticated. The adolescent can hypothesise – think about potential situations and their likely outcomes. This type of thinking is brought into use when debating moral or ethical issues as the young person tries to clarify his own values and beliefs about a whole range of situations.

School continues to provide opportunities for rapid expansion of knowledge and skills. Teaching relating to practical skills such as cooking and woodwork is available. Adolescents may select subjects to be undertaken, which have direct links to future work. Career guidance and adequate information is required to help them select appropriately.

Homework is often provided from secondary schools and the adolescent needs appropriate space in which to carry out the work required – a table and a quiet environment if possible. If provision of these is not available at home, schools or libraries may provide this facility.

During this time, crushes on school teachers are common and the young person will often work exceedingly hard to earn the respect of the particular teacher. Other members of staff are not admired, and adolescent pupils can make their views known very clearly – sometimes by truanting or being disruptive. It is important that schools are flexible but firm in the rules they set for this age group, and consistent in their dealing with those who break the rules. Occasional relaxations – for example, a 'no uniform day' – can be used to allow the students to express their identity. Many schools have student councils which allow teenagers the opportunity to express their own ideas on school policy and activities through nominated representatives.

6.2   HEALTH

6.2(a)   DIET

Schoolchildren grow and develop rapidly and expend vast amounts of energy. This calls for a diet which is high in protein, iron and calcium and essential vitamins. Studies have shown that there is a difference in the eating patterns of adults and children. Children tend to want to eat more frequently, at any time of day and prefer foods which they can eat with their hands. Most parents do not favour eating between meals but if this fits in with an active lifestyle and foods eaten are nutritious and energy giving it may be necessary to adapt to a child's needs to some extent.

Eating habits are established early in childhood and in a society where television and advertising play a big part in family life it is difficult for parents to insist that children adhere strictly to a healthy diet. However there are certain guidelines which it is important to follow.

Breakfast

In households where children sleep late or have to get themselves off to school there is a temptation to skip breakfast. If a child is hungry it can affect her concentration level and lead to poor performance at school. Most children like breakfast cereals which can make a valuable contribution to the required dietary intake of fibre, iron, vitamin B and calcium if served with milk. Choose a cereal which the child likes but which also has a high fibre content; many are fortified with vitamins and iron. Avoid sticky sugary cereals as these can contribute to dental caries. If the cereal is accompanied by a glass of pure fruit juice high in vitamin C, this will make a good start to the day.

See also section 6.2(f) below on Dental health

Lunch

Since 1980 the requirement on schools to provide a nutritionally balanced meal at lunchtime has been removed. Schools can provide whatever they wish and charge whatever price they feel appropriate. In order to keep costs low, many authorities provide fast food such as hamburgers and chips as they know these foods are popular with children.

Health promotion departments in many areas are lobbying to improve the nutritional content of school meals and parents can participate in this by being active in parent teacher associations. Children themselves often have health educational projects to complete which may encourage them to change to a healthier diet and parents can co-operate in the process.

Many children do not partake of school meals but take a packed lunch and here parents can have more control over their children's eating habits. Contrary to popular belief, bread is a healthy energy giving food and will not cause overweight unless eaten in excess, but that can be said of most foods. Sandwiches containing savoury spreads such as peanut butter or marmite are a nutritional and healthy basis for the lunch box with the addition of a piece of fruit and a carton of fruit juice. Obviously some treats are necessary but damage limitation can be effected by giving lower fat crisps and low sugar confectionery bars.

Evening meal

Eating is not only necessary for life but is also a social event. If families can sit down to an evening meal together they can share the events of the day and enhance family life. Children who are encouraged to participate in preparing family meals may take more interest in the nutritional content of their diet. A balanced meal consists of a serving of meat or a meat alternative such as fish, eggs, nuts or pulses; a serving from the fruit and vegetable group and, if daily requirements have not been met, a serving from the cereal and milk groups.

Disordered nutrition

Obesity is present in about 10 per cent of schoolchildren and can result in the child feeling miserable and being ridiculed at school. Obesity is best prevented by monitoring weight gain and limiting the intake of too many high calorie foods. Children who are overweight can be encouraged to diet although, if the child is unmotivated, this can be difficult. In adolescence girls particularly are conscious about their body image and weight control may be easier. The family doctor or school nurse can advise and assist in this matter.

See also section 6.7(d) below on Body image and eating habits

Anorexia nervosa, though thankfully not very common, is a condition affecting young people, usually (but not exclusively) girls. Parents need to be on the alert if their child embarks on an intensive slimming programme or drastically alters her eating pattern.

6.2(b) EXERCISE

Young schoolchildren are very active and participate in lots of play which involves physical activity and sport as they get older. It is important to encourage such activity and where possible participate with your children. Walking, swimming and cycling are just some activities which families can do together and thus enhance the quality of family life.

323

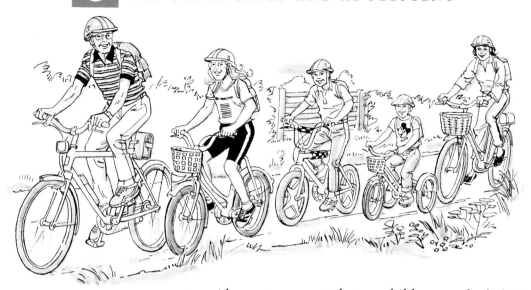

Exercising as a family

Group activities, such as cycling, can enhance the quality of family relationships as well as physical health

See also Appendix VII for Addresses of useful organisations

There is evidence to suggest that as children reach their teens they become less active physically and there have been positive attempts to encourage teenagers to participate in physical activity at their local sports centres. Most areas now have a sports or leisure complex where young people can take part in and try out different sports. There are wide variations in children's abilities to succeed in certain sporting activities. Most children have a competitive spirit and it can be soul destroying for the child who cannot reach the same performance levels as his peers. It is important that parents emphasise that it is not the winning that is important but the taking part. For disabled children or those with special needs there are various organisations that cater for such children and it is worth enquiring at your local leisure centre.

Exercise does not have to be pursued to the point of exhaustion in order to be beneficial. The important factor is that it is regular. In childhood, exercise fosters the development of muscle and bone structures and helps to prevent excessive weight gain. Children should be encouraged to participate in exercises which they enjoy, which make them feel good, which involve minimum expense and which can be done regularly and fitted in easily to their everyday routine.

In the United Kingdom, the Health Education Authority recommends that for all round fitness individuals require *suppleness, strength* and *stamina* – the 'S-factors'.

Suppleness   is the ability of joints to move through a full range of movement.

Strength   is important for lifting and undertaking physical tasks, which demand strong shoulder, trunk and leg muscles.

Stamina   is necessary for staying power and the ability to keep going without gasping for breath.

Suppleness and stamina are usually quite high in childhood and strength develops with maturity. However, it is important to maintain and improve these factors into adulthood as one way of reducing the risk of heart disease, which is still the major cause of death in our society.

The table shows the benefits on each of the three S-factors of different types of exercise. For activities to be beneficial they should be undertaken at least three times per week. Parents should ensure their child's safety by ascertaining that activities such as swimming are always adequately supervised, safety precautions are adhered to and children are not exposed to risks of injury. Accidents are the most common cause of death and injury in children and therefore safety is of paramount importance in any physical activity.

The effects of different forms of exercise

Activity	Stamina	Suppleness	Strength
Badminton	★★	★★★	★★
Canoeing	★★★	★★	★★★
Cricket	★	★	★★
Cycling (hard)	★★★★	★★	★★★
Dancing (disco)	★★★	★★★★	★
Football	★★★	★★★	★★★
Gymnastics	★★	★★★★	★★★
Running	★★★★	★★	★★
Judo	★★★★	★★	★★★★
Rowing	★★★★	★★	★★★★
Sailing	★	★★	★★
Squash	★★★	★★★	★★
Swimming (hard)	★★★★	★★★★	★★★★
Tennis	★★	★★★	★★
Walking (briskly)	★★	★	★
Weightlifting	★	★	★★★★

Key ★ No real effect ★★ Beneficial effect
★★★ Very good effect ★★★★ Excellent effect

6.2(c) SLEEP AND REST

Periods of rest and relaxation are necessary for everyone throughout the day and children are no exception. The amount of sleep needed differs from one individual to the next. When a child first starts school, he may come home exhausted at the end of the day. However, energies are soon replenished in healthy children and those who are put to bed too early might wake in the night or early in the morning thus interrupting parents' sleep. It is much better to encourage your child to relax for a time with a favourite game or book or watching television. Eight to ten hours sleep is the average requirement for children depending on their age. As children get older they will require less sleep and parents may find they get little time to themselves. It is therefore important that the child has his own private space where he is encouraged to spend time alone or with his friends.

Lack of sleep causes children to be irritable or perform badly at school as concentration is impaired. Children may suffer from anxieties which can disturb sleep. Talking through these anxieties with parents, friends or teachers may help to resolve any problems. Simple relaxation exercises such as deep breathing or concentrating on relaxing each part of the body in turn may relieve tension and promote sleep. Good sleep patterns can be established by the following:

- Setting and keeping a regular bedtime;

- Establishing a bedtime routine;

- Having a warm drink;

- Being read to or reading a book for a short time before going to sleep.

6.2(d) THE SCHOOL HEALTH SERVICE

In the United Kingdom, legislation gives health authorities an obligation to provide or arrange provision of a school health service for the benefit of all children in schools and their parents. This legislation generally applies to state run schools and arrangements in independent schools may differ.

The aims of the school health service are:

- To make certain that every schoolchild is as fit as possible so that each may obtain maximum benefit from education;

- To teach children about health so that they can make choices about healthy lifestyles;

- To arrange for the identification and treatment of various groups of children with special needs, and to work closely with parents and teachers of these children to make sure they receive education appropriate to their needs.

These aims are achieved in the following ways:

- Surveillance of the physical growth and educational, social and emotional development of all children attending school;

- Identification and regular monitoring of children with physical or mental defects which may affect their ability to learn in the ordinary school situation;

- Advice for teachers to help them understand the educational significance of what doctors might know about particular children;

- Maintenance of immunisation programmes for schoolchildren;

- Advice and participation in health education programmes in schools;

- Provision of an independent listening service for children who are experiencing difficulties in matters relating to their health and well-being;

- Establishing links between home and school and being available to parents or carers who are concerned about any aspect of their child's health.

Schoolchildren, their parents or carers, teachers, doctors and nurses all have a part to play in promoting children's health in school.

Parents
- know their child's health from day to day;
- know what is normal for their child.

Children
- know when they feel happy, sad or unwell.

Teachers
- know how children learn in the classroom;
- observe how children interact with other children and adults.

The family doctor
- has the child's medical history;
- knows the whole family.

School doctors and nurses
- have records on each child from the child health clinic and health visitor;
- carry out health checks;
- are trained to know about child development and childhood illnesses.

It can be seen therefore that an effective school health service requires a team effort between children (depending of course on their age and ability), parents or carers, teachers, doctors and nurses. In some situations the school psychological service, voluntary organisations and social workers may also be involved in handling specific problems.

Every school has a named school doctor and named school nurse. The school nurse spends time each week in the school where she is available to give advice to children, parents and teachers. School nurses and doctors can help with many different problems encountered by school children and their families. Examples are:

- Talking with parents and teachers about how to help a child suffering from a chronic condition such as asthma;

- Working with children who have problems of bedwetting or weight problems;

- Arranging more help for children with speech problems;

- Offering help and support for children with emotional and behavioural problems;

- Helping children with handicaps or learning difficulties.

See also section 6.6(a) below, on Infections and infestations, for more information about treating head lice

School nurses no longer inspect children's heads in school for head lice. The practice of such inspections was found to be ineffective as at best each child could only be inspected once per term and could easily be infested after the inspection from another child attending a different school. Parents are now encouraged to check their own child's hair each week and seek advice and treatment from the clinic or school nurse should they find any nits or lice. School nurses are happy to teach parents how to carry out this procedure. It is important to remember that head lice are still very common and most children become infested at some time during their school career, regardless of the standard of cleanliness maintained. There should be no stigma attached to such incidents and no harm will come to the child or the rest of the family providing advice and treatment are sought early.

6.2(e) SCREENING TESTS

Throughout the first five years of life children are monitored by the health visitor and doctor to ensure that they are growing and developing at the expected rate. By detecting any defects early, treatment and correction can be instigated to correct or ameliorate such defects.

Such monitoring continues throughout the child's school career. Parents should expect to receive a medical questionnaire soon after their child starts full time school. It is important that parents try to attend school medical check-ups but if this is not possible they should write down as much information as possible concerning any worries they have about their child.

Parents or guardians are asked to sign consent for medical examinations in school and also for immunisations to be carried out at school. No examinations or immunisations can be carried out without this consent and new legislation will shortly be implemented which will require the child's consent too provided she is of the appropriate age and maturity.

Typical programme of health checks on schoolchildren carried out in the United Kingdom

Under 5	Children who attend nursery school may have a pre-school entry medical before starting full time school. Alternatively this may be carried out by the family doctor if such a service is offered and it is the parent's wish.
	The health visitor will usually see the child to test vision, hearing, speech development and monitor weight and physical and mental development. In some areas this might be a joint assessment by the health visitor and school nurse to give parents and children an opportunity to meet their school nurse.
	A pre-school immunisation booster of diphtheria, tetanus and polio is offered at this age, often through the family doctor.
First year at primary school (5–6 years)	– Growth, height and weight checked – Eyes tested – General health check and health interview with the school nurse – Hearing tested – Full medical examination by the school doctor
7–9 years	– Growth, height and weight checked – Eyes tested – General health check This is carried out by the school nurse and the child is only seen by the school doctor is there is any problem. Ongoing health surveillance is carried out by the school nurse throughout the primary school years according to the individual needs of each child and family.
At secondary school: 11–13 years	Immunisation against rubella (German measles) is offered for girls and TB immunisation for both boys and girls.
	A senior school health interview will be carried out by the school nurse building on information passed on from the child's previous school.
	Growth, height and weight continues to be monitored where necessary throughout the senior school years. School nurses are available for specific health advice and routinely monitor vision and general health as appropriate according to the individual needs of each child. The wishes of the child in relation to confidentiality of information should also be taken into account.
	The school doctor will see any child where there is a problem.
14–15 years	Immunisation booster of tetanus and polio is recommended, and may be carried out in school or by the family doctor.

Parents may elect to have health surveillance of their children carried out by their family doctor and certain family doctors with the appropriate training may offer this service.

The frequency and nature of health checks during the school years will vary from area to area but on average will follow a similar pattern to that indicated in the table on the previous page.

6.2(f) DENTAL HEALTH

In the United Kingdom the incidence of dental caries among school-aged children remains high in spite of fluoridation policies over the past couple of decades.

Preventing dental caries saves a lot of suffering and discomfort in later life. Children should be encouraged to brush their teeth from an early age using a fluoride based toothpaste. Tooth decay can also be prevented by avoiding snacking on sugary foods between meals as this is the time when sugar can do most damage to the teeth.

To avoid harm to teeth children should be encouraged:

- To cut down on sweets, chocolate, cakes and biscuits and soft sugary drinks;

- Not to have sugar in tea or coffee;

- To have yoghurt or fresh fruit instead of other puddings and desserts;

- To avoid too many soft fizzy drinks as these may eventually cause thinning of the tooth enamel.

Children can be introduced to the dentist at an early age, even before they go to school. More and more dentists are endeavouring to make their services more child centred so that children's anxieties are minimised. Children who accompany a parent to routine appointments can begin to see the dentist as a friend rather than as someone who inflicts pain.

The school dental service aims to inspect each schoolchild's teeth annually but this is dependent on local resources. All dental inspections and treatment are free on the NHS for children under 16 and students in full time education up to the age of 19. It is advisable for children to have a dental inspection every six months. Many preventative treatments are available which can protect against the development of dental caries.

Dentists and dental hygienists can teach children how to brush their teeth correctly and how to use dental floss to clean between the teeth and around the gums. Advice can also be given on types of toothbrush suitable for children. A toothbrush should be replaced at least every two months, or earlier if the bristles become bent and worn.

6.2(g) MENTAL HEALTH AND RELATIONSHIPS

See also section 6.7 below on Behavioural and emotional problems

A survey of teenagers in the late 1980s demonstrated that nearly one in ten felt fed up or depressed every day, over one quarter at least once a week, and only three per cent of girls and seven per cent of boys never felt depressed. The most frequent reasons were boredom and school. Families and family arguments also figured high on the list as did rejection by friends. These findings are quite worrying when one considers that suicide is the third leading cause of death among the 15–34 age group. Another worrying finding is that the incidence of drug abuse among young people has increased during the past two decades.

Promoting good mental health should begin with healthy families who encourage open and frank discussion of relationships and their problems. This is not always easy in a society where family breakdown is on the increase and many children are brought up in families where one parent has the burden of responsibility to provide all the physical and emotional care required. In such circumstances it may be that other relatives, schoolteachers or close family friends can help too.

Young people can often learn to cope with disappointment and feelings of depression if they can first begin to recognise the signs: Depression affects a person's mood making him feel:

- Low, sad ('life has no meaning');

- In despair ('there's no light at the end of the tunnel');

- Helpless ('I've no control over my life');

- Guilty ('I'm to blame');

- Isolated ('no one cares about me');

- Worthless ('I'm no use to anyone');

- Unloved and unwanted ('I have no one to live for').

Depression causes physical symptoms such as:

- Indigestion;

- Reduced or increased appetite;

- Weight loss or weight gain;

- Headaches;

- Sleep problems.

Everyone experiences some of these problems at some time but if a young person has several of these problems, and they persist for more than a month, then he should consult a doctor.

In many cases there may be an underlying reason for the depression such as a recent loss which causes the individual to go through a period of mourning. Such 'losses' may include:

See also Chapter 3, especially section 2 on Adolescence and section 10 on Bereavement and loss

- Losing a treasured object;

- Changing schools;

- Becoming an adolescent and having to leave childhood behind;

- Moving house;

- Parents separating;

- The death of a pet;

- The break up of a relationship with a girlfriend or boyfriend.

In such situations the young person needs to experience a period of mourning which may involve anger, resentment, denial and gradually acceptance of the loss.

A number of suggestions for relieving depression are given in the box below. Organisations which may provide help and support are listed in Appendix VII.

Relieving depression

These suggestions are based on material in the Open University *Health Choices* course. You may find them useful

- Get up – get washed – get dressed
  (staying in bed or sloping around in a dressing gown only worsens depression)
- Set small goals that are easily achievable
  (ring a friend, write a letter)
- Avoid habits which make depression worse
  (e.g. putting yourself down, reading depressing press reports)
- Stop thinking about bad times as they only stir up bad memories
- Don't run yourself down to yourself; avoid conversations in your head in which you criticise yourself and compare yourself unfavourably with people you consider are more successful than you
- Teach yourself new habits; make a list of things that made you happier in the past and use this list each day to choose four or five pleasurable activities – and do them
- Check your diet; avoid unhealthy snacks, cakes and biscuits (weight gain will only increase depression)
- Take regular exercise. There is evidence to suggest that exercise relieves feelings of depression

6.3   CARING FOR AN OLDER CHILD AT HOME

See also Chapter 2, sections 1, 2 and 5(a), also Chapter 5, section 11

Caring for a sick child or adolescent at home will normally have many similarities with caring for other sick family members. A child with a minor illness will usually recover spontaneously with general care at home and the provision of any appropriate medication or treatment from your family doctor.

School-aged children who suffer major acute or chronic illnesses, or who have to spend a period of time in hospital, require special consideration of their needs. Handicapped and chronically ill adolescents need help to come to terms with any real limitations on their lifestyle, so that they can achieve maturity with a level of independence and responsibility for themselves.

6.3(a)   EATING AND DRINKING

See also section 6.2(a) above on Diet, and section 6.7(d) below on Body image and eating habits

The nutritional needs of growing children vary according to their rate of growth at a particular time and will be altered if your child has a chronic or long term illness. The rapid growth period, turbulent emotions and hectic lifestyle of most adolescents make increased demands on their nutritional state and this is often a time when young people experiment with new eating habits.

Young people should be helped to gain nutritional knowledge so that they can develop good eating habits. This is particularly important if your child has a chronic illness involving a special diet. Diabetes and bowel disorders are two conditions which will impose some dietary restrictions on your child. Gradually he should be taught to take control of his own diet.

Some adolescents, who have previously accepted their family's meat containing diet, become vegetarians because of major concerns about animal welfare or environmental issues. If your child seriously wishes to adopt a vegetarian diet you should help him to develop an understanding of nutrition. Without appropriate advice he may have an incomplete diet, which avoids animal products but does not substitute adequate amounts of good quality vegetable protein, such as soya.

If being unwell is putting your child off his food, you may have to tempt him to eat by making a special effort to serve the foods he likes. In such cases, it is important too to ensure that he drinks adequate amounts of fluid.

6.3(b)   ELIMINATING AND VOMITING

As children become older they become modest about their appearance and bodily activities. It is therefore necessary to provide

333

privacy during personal activities such as toileting and bathing. Brothers and sisters should be encouraged to respect this need for privacy, allowing family members to use the bathroom or toilet undisturbed.

Illnesses associated with vomiting, or loss of bowel or bladder control may be distressing and humiliating to school-aged children because they are seen as 'babyish'. Sensitivity to your child's concerns is very important. If brothers and sisters normally share a bedroom it may be possible to reorganise the sleeping arrangements temporarily, thus enabling the sick child to have his own room for a period.

If your child is violently sick several times in succession, or if vomiting is associated with another symptom such as abdominal pain, fever or diarrhoea you should not hesitate to contact your family doctor. Serious loss of fluid from vomiting or diarrhoea may cause dehydration.

Recurrent vomiting may occasionally occur as a reaction to stress or anxiety. Some children react to stress by producing physical symptoms. If your family doctor cannot find a physical cause for your child's symptoms he may suggest that they could be stress related. By looking at events in your child's life in relation to the physical problem you may be able to identify the cause of his anxiety. Offering sympathy and support will generally enable him to overcome the problem. In other cases additional help is available from your family doctor or by referral to the Child and Family Psychiatry Department.

The majority of children achieve bowel and bladder control without any problem but some regress and start wetting or soiling at times of illness or emotional distress. Usually children are ashamed and embarrassed, often attempting to deny that the problem exists. They need general encouragement and support to help them overcome the problem.

6.3(c)   SLEEPING AND RESTING

Children who are ill often have an increased need for sleep and should be encouraged to rest as necessary. Those suffering from a chronic illness or recovering from a severe acute illness may also have an increased sleep requirement.

Children of different ages require different amounts of sleep and this may create a problem where brothers and sisters share a bedroom. Conflict over bedtime is a common problem and it is usually staggered according to age; so that the older children stay up later than their younger brothers and sisters.

Many siblings of different sexes have to share bedrooms and this is generally acceptable until they reach puberty. At this age children usually begin to demand their own bedroom or space to group their possessions and entertain their friends. It may be possible to resolve both problems by putting the beds at opposite ends of the room.

Bad fears, night dreams and true sleeplessness may occur during childhood. They may be associated with illness or follow a period of hospitalisation. Children are often frightened of night time dreams. Reassuring your child that he will not dream may be unwise, but remind him it is only a dream and that he will wake from it. Offer support by telling him that you are there in the night to comfort him and he can share his bad dream with you.

Some children seem unable to get to sleep in spite of the usual sleep inducing remedies such as warm drinks. Illnesses and additional periods of sleep during the day often make this problem worse. There is no specific treatment but, except in the most rare circumstances, such a phase passes. If your child has slept during the day a period of activity or occupation prior to bedtime will help to tire him. Children who have an increased need for sleep following illness may be accommodated by an earlier bedtime or rests during the day. Watching videos, reading, jigsaws, board games, sewing or model making may encourage a child to rest by reducing physical activity.

Sleep walking most often affects children aged 10–14 years. A sleep walker rarely injures himself and the best plan is to take him gently back to bed. It is unnecessary to wake him up unless he is in the middle of a nightmare.

6.3(d)   MOBILITY

If your child is acutely unwell and wants to sleep he will be quite happy to stay in bed. Unless advised to do so by your family doctor or the hospital medical team it is rarely necessary actually to confine a sick person to bed. It is much better to encourage some mobility and your child or adolescent can spend his daytime in the centre of the household, resting when necessary on the settee in the living room.

When your child begins to recover it is important to encourage some activity. Board games, jigsaws, model kits, sewing, watching television and videos will provide interest for most young people.

Some schoolchildren and adolescents are notorious for their inactivity; others pursue physical fitness and active pursuits relentlessly. A change in level of activity enforced by illness is often stressful and frustrating for a young person.

School-aged children who have previously participated readily in sport will resent decreased freedom and mobility, caused by illness or injury. It may also hinder peer group activities as they are unable to participate in team events such as football, hockey or tennis. At such a time it is important to find substitute activities which enable your child to maintain contact with his friends. Perhaps they could be invited to visit and play board games, or you could form a Scrabble club at home.

Swimming provides a gentle form of exercise during rehabilitation. If your child has had an inguinal hernia repair, for example, he will not be able to play strenuous games such as rugby for a while after surgery but once the wound has healed he may channel some of his energy into swimming.

Children who are expected to have long term problems with mobility following surgery or illness may see a physiotherapist or occupational therapist. They can offer useful advice and supply walking aids or wheelchairs enabling the child to regain some independence. The Mobility Allowance is payable to children aged five years and over. It is designed to give those with severe walking difficulties or an inability to walk, the chance to get around.

See also section 6.4 below on The child with a physical handicap and Appendix VI for more information on Benefits

6.3(e)   BODY IMAGE

As children grow up they begin to show an interest in their own body and ask questions about differences in the bodies of boys and girls. You should answer these questions, without embarrassment, in a simple way which your child can easily understand.

Questions about changes in body appearance due to illness or surgery should be answered in a similar way. To your child these questions are no different to others he has asked over the years. Children only absorb information at a level which they can understand. Your answers should be pitched at the same level as your child's questions. Listen to the question and try to tell your child exactly what he wants to know.

If you discourage your child from talking about certain subjects during the early years he will not be open about them later or share his concerns with you. Young children ask their parents everything; if you encourage this you will nurture an environment where your child feels he can say anything and always discuss his problems with you.

See also Chapter 3, section 9 on Sickness and body changes

Children with conditions which alter their appearance may find it difficult to participate in any activity outside the family. This is usually because they are afraid of rejection by their peers, friends of a similar age. Fear may be influenced by a previous experience of teasing at school, or it may arise from your child's own feelings about his appearance. As parents you can help him by encouraging him to participate in youth groups and sporting activities outside school.

Loss of a part of the body is probably the most difficult medical situation for an adolescent to cope with. Whichever part of the body is lost or cosmetically disfigured, your child will require active help and emotional support to become as independent and self-managing as she can. Advice about the use of cosmetic make-up to conceal unsightly birthmarks or scars may increase a teenager's confidence.

Adolescents with congenital disabilities can be particularly perceptive about the way their parents feel about the abnormality or condition. The degree to which the whole family accepts a child's problems has a strong influence on the child's ability to adapt to changing lifestyles during adolescence. Therefore the attitude of the immediate family will encourage or inhibit him from becoming independent with his own identity. If you overprotect your child he may never be emotionally capable of functioning alone, even if physically he could live independently.

Children with chronic illnesses (such as well controlled diabetes or epilepsy) which require the taking of regular medication or compliance with certain dietary restrictions should be able to undertake all the normal activities of adolescence.

6.3(f) KEEPING CLEAN AND WELL GROOMED

See also section 6.2(f) above on Dental health

Cleanliness and hygiene is important throughout life. By 7–8 years of age, children are able to wash and dress themselves, but you will need to give some supervision. At times this will have to be discreet to enable your child to develop independence. Teeth need

Acne — some hints for coping

- There is no completely effective treatment for acne but its development may be limited by cleanliness:
  - wash skin well with soap or a cleanser twice a day
  - do not share facecloths with others
- Do not squeeze blackheads or pustules as this encourages infection
- Ask your pharmacist to recommend a suitable ointment
- In severe cases of acne, your doctor may prescribe a prolonged course of antibiotics
- Some foods appear to contribute to the problem, so it is wise to avoid the following:
  - chocolate
  - nuts
  - fizzy drinks
  - fried food
  - foods with a higher sugar content

careful brushing especially after sweets are enjoyed. Regular dental check-ups should also be planned.

During adolescence, young people should acquire personal responsibility for body hygiene and personal presentation. Children are generally acutely aware of the way other people smell and this can often be used to stimulate discussion about their own body and personal hygiene.

Skin problems are frequently experienced by adolescents, girls suffering more than boys. Almost all teenagers develop some spots of acne on the face. This is a disorder of the sebaceous glands in the skin which normally produce a greasy secretion. In acne the glands become blocked causing blackheads, red raised spots and small pustules. Diet, stress and infection will make acne worse. It is generally not helped by the need to shave the face in boys and the application of make-up in girls.

6.3(g) DRESSING/KEEPING WARM

Girls and boys naturally become more interested in their appearance as they grow older and want to wear fashionable clothing. Schoolchildren are often eager to make their specific likes and dislikes regarding clothes known to their parents. They will require guidance on colour and the importance of keeping warm and wearing suitable clothing in cold weather. Often children are happier to wear several layers of clothing rather than one very thick warm item. Schoolchildren playing outside may become so engrossed in play that they are unaware of the cold. You should ensure that they are adequately dressed to help prevent lowered resistance to infection (particularly coughs and colds) and to aid good circulation.

The ability to wear fashionable clothing will be very important to your older child if she has a chronic illness or disability. She may already feel her disability makes her different to her friends. A sense of belonging to the group is often sought by wearing the same style of clothing.

6.3(h) COMMUNICATION

Families may experience communication difficulties during childhood but they are always present during the adolescent period. Ten year old children are generally sociable and secure, happy to share their experiences with the family, but teenagers seem to be up in the air one moment and down in the depths the next. They lack tact, frequently criticising and saying things which should not

See also section 6.2(g) above on Mental health and relationships, and section 6.7(e) below on Anxiety

have been said. This is quite natural for young people who are unsure of themselves and searching out a new identity.

Adolescent children need a lot of understanding. It often helps to meet together as a family to discuss their problems and the difficulties experienced. Making time to talk is important although some rows with parents are inevitable. Adolescents desire to be independent and go their own way but need parents to rely on when experimentation goes wrong. Frequently one parent is viewed as the favourite and always used to request special favours. This may lead to one parent being played off against the other but an awareness of this problem will avoid family arguments.

It is difficult for parents to achieve the correct balance of permitting independence while providing support, particularly if your child is diagnosed as having a chronic illness during her teenage years. A natural reaction is to become overprotective and undertake tasks which she is quite capable of doing herself.

If you feel you have a major problem communicating over a specific issue you may be able to enlist the help of another person to talk to your child. A well known adult, teacher, school nurse or youth group leader may act as counsellor. Families experiencing multiple problems may request referral, through the family doctor or the child's teacher, to the Child and Family Psychiatry Unit.

Parents often feel their guidance is ignored but the stability of a secure and loving family background will help the child through the upheaval of adolescence.

6.3(i) THE PEER GROUP

The most influential groups are friends and idols. A schoolchild relates to different peer groups but is not totally influenced by them. During the adolescent period, however, the influence of peer groups often overrules parental guidance. There is a need to belong to a peer group and this becomes particularly important if your adolescent child feels threatened by a condition which influences appearance or limits mobility. Adolescents frequently use acceptance by the peer group as a test of their own normality.

A child also needs to participate in different peer groups in and out of school. Membership of clubs undertaking sporting activities and youth groups such as scouts and guides is important. If your child has a disability it is particularly important to encourage contact with different people; it will help him with relationships, social interaction and employment at a later stage.

Your child may need assistance to approach a new club or activity. Initial contact with the relevant organiser and an explanation about the disability often eases his introduction to the group.

group. Parents should encourage contact with friends and promote understanding of their child's illness or handicapping condition. With the appropriate understanding, friends are generally willing to provide support and specific assistance with mobility problems.

Many hospitals and voluntary support groups promote meetings and recreational activities for children with conditions such as cystic fibrosis and diabetes. They provide an opportunity for adolescents to share problems and anxieties in a social setting.

6.3(j)   SCHOOL AND WORK

School is a child's workplace. In addition to learning academic and practical skills, children have the opportunity to form constructive relationships with their peer group and teaching staff. They have to survive, apart from their family, in a less protective environment.

School should continue to play an important part during adolescence. Most adolescents enjoy the opportunity to widen their knowledge and develop a competitive approach to school work, promoted by sporting activities and examinations. Schooling is important in providing the adolescent with a direction and goal towards the future. Those who miss out on secondary education or play truant at school may experience difficulty in finding a job. Occasional truancy, taking time off school, is common during adolescence. If it becomes regular or persistent the problem will need handling tactfully but firmly. It may indicate underlying problems such as anxiety or stress associated with school or home.

See also section 6.7 below on Behavioural and emotional problems

Children must receive suitable education between the ages of 5–16. The 1981 Education Act makes arrangements for the education of children with 'special educational needs' due to a learning difficulty. Not all such children attend special schools; with extra support they may attend their usual local school. Others benefit from facilities at special schools or special units attached to local schools, where staff are trained to support children with learning difficulties and there are regular opportunities for therapy of various kinds such as speech therapy or physiotherapy. A small number of children who need very special facilities, such as severe epileptics or asthmatics, may attend residential schools.

See also section 6.5 below for more information about The child with a learning disability

School phobia is a state of anxiety in a child, induced either by going to school or because of fear of leaving home. Symptoms such as headaches, abdominal pain, nausea or feeling faint may occur. Parents can usually handle minor problems with the co-operation of school staff, but more severe school phobia may require assistance from a child psychiatrist.

Older children, who are undertaking a programme of study towards exams, may become very anxious about any interruption in school progress caused by long periods of sickness. Early contact with your child's teaching staff will facilitate continuing structured home study. Helping your child to set aside time to study at home will enable him to keep up with his school work.

Many hospitals have their own schools where teachers aim to provide an education appropriate to each child's needs. They also offer support to long stay patients after they leave hospital so that there is a smooth return to the child's own school.

Parents should be aware of the dangers of overwork when their child is striving to achieve academic success. Children need encouragement and support, but it is also important that they take regular breaks from study and enjoy periods of relaxation.

6.3(k)   AVOIDING DANGER

Adolescence is generally described as a difficult period in life. Young people are exposed to various dangers in society including drinking alcohol, smoking, teenage pregnancy, drugs and solvent abuse. A more detailed discussion of these problems, and some suggestions for dealing with them, are given in section 6.7 below.

6.4   THE CHILD WITH A PHYSICAL HANDICAP

Physically handicapped children suffer from a variety of conditions and diseases, all with their own characteristics and prognoses. In general, the child who walks with crutches and the child who is totally dependent upon help and an electric wheelchair will be grouped together as 'physically handicapped' or 'disabled', despite their very different needs and abilities. Therefore the following section takes into consideration the multitude of disabilities, and offers ideas and pointers for parents and carers to pursue, in seeking what they consider best for their child whatever his strengths or weaknesses.

See also Chapter 4, section 8(c) for more information about The handicapped baby

Recognition of the child actually being handicapped is traumatic and difficult, but it is the starting point to helping her develop to her full potential. To understand as a family the changes and emotional strains this may have upon a marriage, siblings, friends and relatives is one of the first steps towards the future. Support and help for the whole family is required from an early stage, and this can be sought from the many professionals and charitable organisations available. Contact with people in similar circumstances is a source of great support to many families, and there is an agency associated with almost every disability, however rare.

See Appendix VII for Addresses of useful organisations and support groups

Regular visits to or from medical and nursing teams soon

become familiar to the parents and to the handicapped child. Often, however, information and awareness of professional help available through hospitals, special schools and social services is lacking. Preconceived ideas of what they can or cannot offer should be rejected until contact has been made with the local physiotherapist, occupational therapist, speech therapist and social worker, all of whom have important roles to play in meeting the child's physical, functional, communication and emotional needs.

6.4(a) THE HOME ENVIRONMENT

Every house is different, and space is a precious resource in any home with children. It is often the use of specialised equipment that enables the child with physical difficulties to reach his full potential, yet equipment necessitates space for use and storage.

If the family does not intend to move, an extension that will serve as a playroom, study-bedroom and ultimately a bedsit type arrangement should be considered as early as possible. The additional space will house the extra toys, equipment, computers and wheelchairs that the disabled child might use, and that are so difficult to accommodate in many homes. The inclusion of a bathroom is essential, as the handicapped person often spends a lot of time attending to personal needs and could cause stress to a busy family queueing for the bathroom.

Help and advice, both with finance and with design, can be sought from the Social Services Department, either through your social worker or occupational therapist. Guidance will be given about the type of equipment available and the layout of rooms, particularly as circulating and manoeuvring space is important.

6.4(b) DAILY LIVING

Standard furniture and fitments in the house may be easy to use with the handicapped child. However, in certain situations, specialised equipment may be required, for the following reasons:

- To maintain a good posture for the child;

- To encourage functional activity;

- To be independent with a task;

- To help the carer help the child;

- To help the carer 'care';

- To ensure the carer is not put under excessive physical strain.

See also Chapter 2, section 4 for more advice on Lifting and transfers

Lifting and transfers

As the child grows, the difficulty of moving a person who cannot transfer herself from chair to chair (etc.) becomes an increasing problem. Instruction from a physiotherapist, or attendance at a 'how to lift' lecture, is invaluable to a parent or carer, to ensure that they maintain their own fitness. The basic rule to remember when lifting anyone or anything is to keep your back straight and lift using your leg muscles.

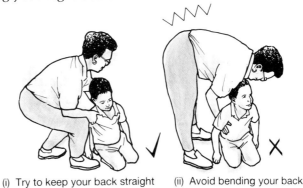

(i) Try to keep your back straight when lifting – use your leg muscles.

(ii) Avoid bending your back when lifting.

Correct and incorrect ways of lifting

For the heavier child, the helper with a 'weak' back or the pregnant mother, using a hoist is a quick and simple method of transfer. The technique, particularly of fitting the slings, requires a little practice to gain confidence, but is worth pursuing.

Stairs may present a problem and the installation of a through-ceiling lift or a stairlift track can be a solution.

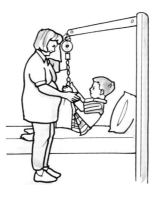

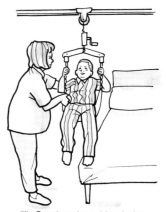

Two examples of different types of hoist available. Both ensure safe and easy transfers

(i) Mobile floor hoist.

(ii) Overhead tracking hoist.

Personal care

The bathroom is probably the main area where special equipment will be necessary. Use of either a shower or a bath is, to a certain extent, personal preference; however, consideration is also given to manoeuvring space and the type of help required.

There are many types of bath aid available as well as adaptations for the shower. Visiting a Health Authority Disabled Living Centre, where there is a therapist to advise and the items can be seen and tested, would be useful.

Use of the toilet is a basic requirement and, where possible, toilet training should be developed in the normal way. A child may be physically handicapped but the aim should be for him to:

- Communicate his need;

- Control the bladder/bowel;

- Allow sufficient time to get organised to use the toilet.

Difficulty in achieving continence may well be due to a problem with time if the toileting procedure involves difficult manoeuvres and/or particular seating. One child may need total support to enable him to feel relaxed and happy on the toilet, yet another child may require only the security of a grab rail to give him confidence. Special equipment, therefore, can have an important role to play in his daily toilet programme.

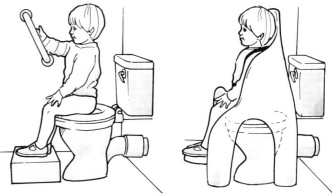

Different types of toilet equipment

(i) Using a wall fixed grab bar, and a suitable height footbox increases stability when sitting on the toilet.

(ii) A totally supportive seat, with a harness, may be required for the child to use the toilet confidently.

See also Chapter 4, section 8(c) on The handicapped baby

Eating and drinking

Independent eating and drinking skills are often one of the primary areas to be aimed for with the disabled child. Following the 'normal' patterns of development, finger food is the first eating goal to set. Likewise drinking, either using one of various trainer beakers or through a straw, is a first step — but note, a straw is not always recommended for children who have difficulty controlling the movements of their mouth or tongue. A speech therapist will give advice about this.

There is a wide range of special cutlery available, but generally standard children's trainer cutlery is a good starting point, as much of the adapted cutlery comes only in adult sizes. Alternatively, sloped or deepened plates, or the use of a plate guard (a clip-on plastic ring to push food against) can help develop the movement patterns required to eat successfully.

The child who has a degenerative type condition, who is used to being able to feed himself, is likely to have problems adjusting to using alternatives and will, therefore, need careful introduction. Often the solutions to maintaining independent feeding, such as long handled or lightweight implements, are rejected when first presented. Using them privately, or alternatively in a situation where other children with similar difficulties are already using the items, can build up confidence.

Sitting appropriately is also a consideration for learning to eat or drink successfully. If, due to size or use of a wheelchair, the child is prevented from sitting correctly at the table, then alternative seating should be investigated. This is to ensure that she is given the best opportunity to feed herself and participate in family meals.

Mobility

Standard wheelchairs and mobility aids are available from your doctor or therapist. Generally, the appearance of this type of equipment is uninspiring to the young person, but with a little imagination, and the use of stickers, fluorescent strip or fabric, these items can be made more pleasing.

See Appendix VII for Addresses of useful organisations

A growing range of privately manufactured wheelchairs that have a more ergonomic design and use bright colours on the paintwork and upholstery is now available. These types of wheelchair are generally easier to manoeuvre and can open up more opportunities to the child, but they can be prohibitively expensive. Investigation for funding from local and national charities is suggested, as there is a great willingness and understanding

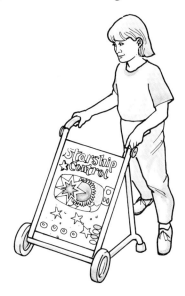

Tying a colourful fabric picture to a walking frame makes it more fun for the child to use

concerning the purchase of a suitable wheelchair to help improve the quality of life for a disabled youngster.

Mobility is probably the most emotive subject for parents and carers to deal with concerning the physically handicapped child. Issues of walking and use of a wheelchair are frequent worries. Despite consultation and advice from professionals, parents often have the final decision to make about mobility, and want to be sure that they are making the best choice for their child. Therefore, careful consideration of every aspect of the child's life is encouraged. Facing the difficulties ahead is also important, and, as the child approaches adolescence, many ideals have to alter, due to both physical and emotional changes. The following points should be debated.

- The use of a 'Major Buggy' pushchair rather than a wheelchair belies the child's age and develops a poor posture.

- Learning to walk must have a realistic aim such as:
  - two or three steps to enable independent transfer;
  - indoor walking;
  - walking at all times;
  - walking with or without equipment.

- Use of either a manual or electric wheelchair increases social and peer interaction, motivation and self-confidence.

- Lack of opportunity to use a wheelchair for the deteriorating walking child causes distress and frustration.

The most important factor is to know *why* and *where* you are aiming with your child's mobility.

Recreation and play

During 'normal' development, a child learns to explore and experience the world around him. He develops his skills and perceptions through simple everyday experiences such as washing up, climbing stairs, flushing the toilet, opening and closing doors etc. The child who is handicapped is prevented, by physical limitations, from experiencing many of the formative encounters generally taken for granted. Therefore the familiarity of daily living, along with other childhood activities, should be structured for the child. It may take time and imagination to organise and prepare activities that are a traditional part of childhood, for example, pastry-making, water play and painting but, by allowing the child to follow as normal a pattern as possible, you will help him to develop his own self-confidence and personality, as well as his physical activity.

Using recreation time well is perhaps one of the greatest problems for the growing disabled child and one of the frustrations for

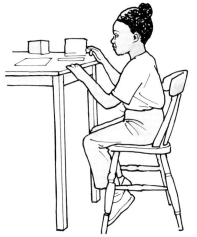

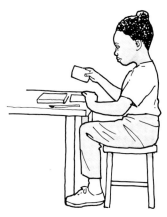

Alternative positioning 1

Furniture at an appropriate height will facilitate play opportunities and improve posture

(i) Adult size furniture can disadvantage the handicapped child who cannot adapt herself to the size.

(ii) An appropriate size table and chair will give the child the opportunity to function at her best.

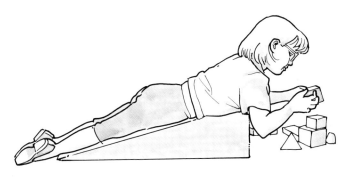

Alternative positioning 2

A foam wedge may enable a child to play independently

parents seeking new ideas. The familiar 'What can I do now?' is a greater challenge than normal to the parents and carers of a child with physical and, possibly, associated perceptual difficulties. For babies and young children, the normal range of toys and books can satisfy their needs; however, positioning and facilitating the child actually to play with toys may take more thought. It should be remembered that an able child will quickly adapt himself to adult-sized furniture, yet the child who is physically disadvantaged will require his environment tailored to suit his needs. A table of suitable height or a simple foam wedge may enable the child to attempt playing with toys previously thought impossible.

Toy Libraries are found in many towns and the local branch address can be sought from the national organisation. An increasing number of special-needs toy libraries can offer large or specialised equipment suitable for all sorts of handicapped children. For example, an adapted tricycle can be ridden by many children who cannot walk independently, and this can open up a certain amount of freedom and peer equality. Your physiotherapist must assess first and will then give more advice on this aspect.

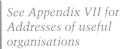

See Appendix VII for Addresses of useful organisations

Pastimes

As your child grows older, he will want to widen his play into hobbies and pastimes. Modern video and computer games, remote-control cars and electronic music keyboards are easy to use and can broaden the experience of a physically handicapped child. Traditional hobbies, however, should not be dismissed as being too difficult, as the suggestions below indicate.

- Paint, glue and collage can be cheap and fun. The tactile experience and increased spatial awareness derived from these activities is essential for normal development and should therefore be experienced by the handicapped child.

- The use of lightweight or small tools, raised flower beds and indoor miniature gardens are all ways of giving the disabled child an opportunity to develop horticultural interests.

- 'Write Away' is an organisation encouraging penfriendships between children with special needs, or their siblings.

- The use of non-slip mats, thicker-handled spoons and lipped spreading boards can enable a child to try basic cooking. The severely handicapped child will also benefit from stirring, spooning and rolling, even if his hands are constantly guided.

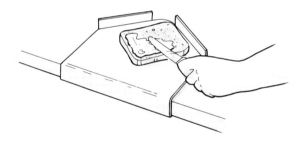

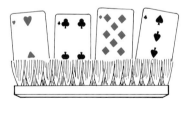

- Organisations such as the Girl Guides or Boy Scouts will welcome handicapped youngsters, and there are also many 'Phab' (Physically Handicapped and Able-bodied) Clubs. Your Social Services Department can give information about local swimming or Riding for the Disabled and any special play schemes available. Advice concerning outdoor pursuits can be sought from a number of other organisations.

• Spatial awareness
Understanding depth and movement of objects

See Appendix VII for Addresses of useful organisations

Learning to cook

Use of a thicker handled knife and a lipped spreading board can increase the child's ability to prepare food

Practical tip

Ordinary household objects can be used in imaginative contexts – for example an upturned scrubbing brush will hold playing cards upright

Practical hints

It is sometimes small and irritating things that prevent a child from participating in family or friends' games and hobbies. Some of these simple ideas may help

Playing cards:	If they are difficult to hold, stand them in the bristles of a scrubbing brush
	Large easy-to-see cards are available in some toyshops
Board games:	Large foam, plastic or home-made cardboard-box dice can be knocked or kicked rather than thrown
	Painted jam jar lids, bottle tops or large buttons can make counters which are easier to handle
	Non-slip mats under the board increase stability
Scissors:	Spring loaded ('squeezy'), battery operated, left-handed and other alternative scissors are available from both specialist companies and general stationers

6.4(c) IDENTITY AND SEXUALITY

See Appendix VII for Addresses of useful organisations

As puberty approaches, children with physical disabilities will have exactly the same preoccupations with identity and developing sexuality as other members of their age group. Parents are therefore advised to read section 6.7 below which deals with these and the other sensitive issues of adolescence. Both parents and the young people themselves may find it useful to contact an organisation such as the Brook Advisory Centre or SPOD (the Society to aid Personal and Sexual Relationships of Disabled People) for information or advice if sexual issues become a worry for them.

6.5 THE CHILD WITH A LEARNING DISABILITY

See also Chapter 2, section 5(d) People with a learning disability, and Chapter 4, section 8(c) The handicapped baby

This section is concerned with the special needs of children with learning disabilities, and their parents. It emphasises the importance of developing consistent routines within the family, with the aim of balancing the pattern of family life to meet the needs of all of its members.

The presence of a child with special needs does not necessarily indicate the need for a major disturbance to family life. Sharing the care with friends, other family members and professional support staff may reduce the impact that longer term care may cause.

Children require regular and consistent stimulation (both cognitively and emotionally) and during the formative years of childhood the pattern of future developmental potential is established. Children with learning disabilities grow up to become adults and by carefully responding to their earlier needs, many of their obvious handicaps may be reduced or overcome completely as positive learning experiences are provided within the context of a caring and loving family.

6.5(a)   MEETING FAMILY NEEDS

The majority of families cope well and settle to accept their child within the balance of ordinary life. Many will require the support of their relatives, friends and professional advisers, as well as other people in the same position. The establishment and discovery of a support network may assist in breaking down some of the isolation that parents may feel after coming to terms with their child's special needs, and the opportunity to revitalise 'ordinary' family life will be a key to this goal.

See Appendix VII for Addresses of useful organisations and support groups

Parents are generally considered to provide the best possible therapy for their children in their own homes. The consistency of their care and love may reduce the need for inconvenient (and often irregular) visits to hospital, development centres and clinics and may reinforce the importance of home-based training programmes.

Portage

One such approach is the Portage method. This is a carefully struc-tured system designed for teaching children with learning difficul-ties new skills. The method involves regular home visits by a home teacher or adviser with the specific aim of assisting parents to help their children learn new skills. It is based on the principle of 'goal planning' which breaks down skills into easily managed and taught steps or sequences. Parents are actively involved in setting target dates and in developing teaching plans which are administered regularly. They are assisted in this task through the provision of 'teaching cards' which provides ideas for day by day and week by week training ideas and methods. For more informa-tion about Portage, talk to your community mental handicap nurse.

This sense of achievement may be further enhanced by working within the family to establish balanced routines which allow each family member to receive the benefits of home life. A family with a handicapped member does *not* need to develop into a 'handicapped family'.

Other family members

The dynamics of family life demand that attention is shared equally between its members and by virtue of the additional needs of a child with a learning disability, this balance needs constant evaluation. The pattern of needs will, of course, be unique to each family and child, and will vary over time as needs change.

The family as a whole will have the same needs as any other family and it may be helpful to consider these to be of primary importance. The social needs of each family member may vary and time should be taken to assess the demands that each person makes on the family's resources. Some time, for example, should be given each day to other children in the family and this may reduce the possible emergence of jealousy or 'sibling rivalry'. If you are a parent, don't forget that there will be limits to your energy, and 'no points are scored' for being a martyr to the cause.

We all need our personal space and diversions from the chores of everyday living. Sharing and caring therefore go hand in hand and the demonstration of a willingness to involve each family member in the care of the one with a handicap may encourage more understanding of the tasks involved day by day which, in turn, may reinforce balance within the family circle.

In order to meet these objectives the family may need to reserve certain times when the priority of caring for their child with special needs takes second place. Trips to the theatre, cinema, to a restaurant for a family meal or to another social function should not be met with feelings of guilt but should be considered diversionary and healthy for all family members. There may be a 'home-sitting' service in your area which can give you some respite, knowing that your child is being well cared for for a few hours. Ask your social worker or community mental handicap nurse for any relevant information.

As parents, you may also need:

- Emotional support – to be listened to, to have someone share your needs, and acknowledge your experiences, anxieties and accomplishments;

- Practical assistance – written information about your child's needs, financial assistance to meet additional heating, clothing and mobility requirements, aids and adaptations to assist with mobility, professional advice, and access to respite care facilities;

- Spiritual advice to help you come to terms with the difficulties you and your family may face.

6.5(b)   SPECIALIST SUPPORT SERVICES

There is a wide variety of experience and advice on offer to families. Some of these are listed in the box on page 353. Many of these services are available in each area. Access may be obtained

See also Chapter 4 section 6(d) on Sibling rivalry

through your family doctor or through local teams which co-ordinate professional services. The concept of the District Handicap Team or Child Development Centre has been particularly helpful in the co-ordination of services and simplifies access arrangements for parents. The role of teams and centres is to ensure that children with special needs, and their parents, receive responsive services.

6.5(c) PHYSICAL CONDITIONS AND ADMISSION TO HOSPITAL

Children with a learning disability may have additional needs which require that they attend hospital from time to time for assessment or corrective treatment. Some of the more common specific conditions may be:

See also section 6.4 above on The child with a physical handicap, and Chapter 5, section 9 The child who needs to visit hospital

• Stabilisation of epilepsy;

• Operations to reduce spasticity and to improve muscle tone;

• Investigations and surgery for respiratory and heart conditions.

Some of these conditions may be directly related to the learning disability, while others may emerge as secondary illnesses later in childhood or the teenage years. There are excellent treatment facilities now available which suggest that the majority of children with learning disabilities can live to enjoy the same life span as other members of our population.

Admission to hospital for any child represents a period of intense insecurity and for a child who has limited comprehension and communication skills these feelings may be enhanced. It is now common practice for parents to be present with their children throughout the admission period and when this is possible the problems associated with new care régimes are minimised. When this is not possible it is helpful to:

• Provide a full, written account of the child's likes and dislikes;

• Outline the child's communication system (e.g. gestures and mannerisms) if speech is absent;

• Provide 'comforters' from home territory to encourage security;

• Provide documentation of the child's daily routine.

There are very few actual clinical conditions associated with mental handicap that require special attention or treatment and the provision of a stimulating environment may be more important therefore. Highly developed levels of communication,

Some of the professionals you may meet

Audiologist assesses hearing abilities and provides advice on aids to minimise sensory loss

Speech therapist assesses language and comprehension and advises on programmes to develop language and communication skills; may also offer advice on feeding programmes

Occupational therapist assesses aspects of daily living and self-help skills; advises on aids and appliances at home

Clinical medical officer assesses development, medical screening and health education; often acts as a co-ordinator to professional services and advises on health matters to schools

Educational psychologist assesses developmental performance and skills; advises on appropriate school placement

Clinical psychologist identifies specific learning difficulties, assesses behaviour patterns and assists in the delivery of teaching/training programmes; advises on sleep problems

Physiotherapist assesses mobility needs and ability; advises on exercises to enhance mobility potential and co-ordination; advises on the reduction of handicapping conditions such as athetosis and cerebral palsy (spasticity); advises on correct positioning, sitting and mobility techniques/aids

Paediatrician assesses medical and causative factors, undertakes neurological investigations; provides genetic counselling and monitoring of epilepsy

Child psychiatrist advises on behavioural needs and difficulties, and appropriate interventions related to severe psychological stress and psychiatric illness

Social worker advises on family support and dynamics; co-ordinates access to social service facilities (e.g. respite care) and benefits

Community mental handicap nurse provides practical advice and nursing skills to families; advises on the management of continence, communication, behaviour, self-help skill training and family support and counselling

Health visitor aspires to promote a healthy family and advises on health promotion; assesses child development; liaises on behalf of child health services as a point of contact/access to wider health care resources.

observation and listening skills will be needed by hospital staff to interpret the needs of their patients.

No matter how well we prepare our children for hospital admission there is no substitute for parental care. It is for this reason that more and more care is being transferred to the home setting, thus reducing stress for all family members.

COMMON HEALTH PROBLEMS IN CHILDHOOD

6.6(a)   INFECTIONS AND INFESTATIONS

Infection occurs when the body is invaded by harmful organisms commonly known as germs. These organisms are commonly viruses or bacteria. In general terms, bacterial infections are usually treated by your doctor with antibiotics. Antibiotics have no action against viruses and are therefore not prescribed unless a viral infection such as the common cold is also accompanied by a bacterial infection such as a chest infection.

• The first and most vital principle to remember is that thorough handwashing is the most important means of preventing the spread of infection.

Some common signs lead us to suspect the presence of infection:

• A raised temperature;

• Green sputum coughed up from the lungs or green nasal discharge;

• Swelling and redness;

• Pain;

• The infected place may be hot to the touch;

• There may be green discharge or pus from a cut or scratch;

• Vomiting and/or diarrhoea.

Not all of the above signs will be present in every case and there may be other signs which indicate that the child is developing an infection. For example, she may be unwilling to eat or drink, her skin may be irritated and a rash may develop, she may be generally irritable, tired and lethargic and her sleep patterns may be disturbed. A vital piece of equipment is a reliable, accurate thermometer which can be purchased from all good pharmacists.

See Chapter 5, section 11(b) for advice on taking a child's temperature

Colds

The common cold is the most likely infection to occur. Colds are caused by viruses of which there are thousands of different types. Treatment should aim to prevent the spread of the cold to others so it is advisable for the child to remain at home while she is feverish and sneezing a great deal. This phase usually lasts about 48 hours. Keep the child warm with plenty of refreshing drinks and do not worry if she is not eating her usual meals. Vitamin C in the form of drinks or capsules is said to help relieve the symptoms. Sometimes a cold worsens, a cough develops and the child may cough up green

See also Chapter 5, section 12 on Common health problems in babies and young children

sputum. This will need treatment from your general practitioner. Dry, tickly coughs usually improve after a few days with plenty of fruit drinks. Earaches sometimes complicate a cold, needing expert advice from your doctor.

Vomiting and diarrhoea

It is important to establish the cause of the infection. Where several members of the family, or perhaps the class or peer group, develop either of these symptoms together then it is possibly due to an outbreak of viral diarrhoea and vomiting which occurs from time to time with no real rhyme or reason. Keep the child at home until he has been completely clear of symptoms for 24 hours and notify the school. Inform your general practitioner who may decide to visit the child or, in times of large outbreaks where she is certain of the diagnosis, may advise you to give the child fluids only for a full 24 hours to try to empty the bowel of the infection. Do not give any medication without the consent and advice of the general practitioner.

See Chapter 2, section 2(d) for advice on collecting specimens

Children who develop vomiting or diarrhoea for no apparent reason, or who have severe pain, must be seen by the doctor. She will examine the child and may decide to send a specimen of stool (faeces) to the laboratory for analysis. Sometimes contaminated or badly cooked food may be the cause and this is diagnosed by the presence of specific bacteria such as Salmonella in the stools. Other members of the family who have shared the same food may be similarly affected.

Good handwashing by the affected persons and the carers is vital to prevent the spread of diarrhoea and vomiting.

Skin rashes including scabies

Skin rashes may occur for a variety of reasons. The majority of rashes in children are a specific reaction to an irritant substance such as the detergents used to wash clothing. Many children also develop eczema, their skin is very sensitive to many substances and situations. Diagnosis and treatment by your doctor is vital to decide the cause of the rash and the appropriate treatment. The doctor may refer the child to a skin specialist or dermatologist if the problem is likely to become a long term one.

Infectious skin rashes are uncommon but do occur, and a likely cause of such rashes is scabies. Scabies mites are small animals which burrow into the skin and cause are great deal of irritation. These are neither bacteria nor viruses but are known as parasites. They are passed from person to person by close contact usually within the family. Treatment is with a lotion applied over the total body surface. It is left on for 12 hours (overnight is best) and then bathed or showered off the next day. This treatment is highly

Common parasites

The left hand picture shows a scabies mite and the right hand one shows thread-worms. Both are greatly magnified

effective and the child can resume school immediately afterwards. It is usual to repeat the treatment after one week to make sure. The whole family should be treated at the same time. After treatment all the family must put on clean clothes and remake all the beds with clean linen. The washing must be done at as high a temperature as the fabric will allow. Tumble drying until the items are completely dry, drying in strong sunlight or hot ironing will ensure that any mites surviving in the bedding will be killed.

Worms

Threadworms, which are also parasites, are a common problem in school-age children and are not solely related to poor hygiene. They can be picked up from unwashed fruit and vegetables, from the soil so the hands should always be washed before eating, or from other people suffering from threadworms. They rarely cause long term damage although they are embarrassing and distressing. They are commonly discovered when a child's appendix is removed as they can block the appendix completely, as well as some of the bowel, causing pain.

The worms lay their eggs aound the anus. These hatch at night, causing the child to be irritated and restless. Severe scratching of the anal area may cause some bleeding which will be found on the sheets. Children may suffer from threadworms without showing signs of irritation, but their motions show threadlike worms. The child should be seen by the doctor who will prescribe some medication, usually in tablet form. Just one dose will kill the parasites which will then be passed in the stools. All the family must be treated at once. It is vital that everyone should learn to wash their hands thoroughly after visiting the toilet. As threadworms can be transferred from anus to mouth by dirty hands, sufferers may continually reinfect themselves and possibly others.

Headlice

Headlice are very common in school-age children and are *not* connected with poor hygiene or dirty hair. Some children may have headlice several times, as they are easily transferred from head to head when children play closely together. They are treated with a lotion which is applied to the hair and allowed to dry. This is shampooed off after 12 hours and usually repeated in one week. There is no need to keep children away from school. A good pharmacist will advise which lotion to purchase, or ask your health visitor, school nurse or general practitioner.

Infected cuts or scratches

Most cuts and scratches will heal quickly if washed with soap and water when they occur. Mild skin disinfectants can be used but the first priority is to remove any dirt from the wound. If a cut or scratch does not heal but begins to discharge pus, becoming painful and swollen then your doctor must be consulted. She may prescribe antibiotics and/or specific dressings. The practice nurse may be asked to dress the wound or a prescription supplied for the appropriate materials.

<table>
<tr><td>6.6(b)</td><td>

INFECTIOUS DISEASES OF CHILDHOOD AND ADOLESCENCE
</td></tr>
</table>

6.6(b)

INFECTIOUS DISEASES OF CHILDHOOD AND ADOLESCENCE

Infectious diseases in childhood are not the scourge they were in former years thanks to the effectiveness of immunisation programmes. Very soon after the birth of a child the family doctor and health visitor will ensure that the parents are aware of the need and the appropriate time for the immunisation programme to begin. Many parents still have concerns about the side effects that some vaccinations have had in the past, but it is wise to consider how many thousands of children receive vaccination without damaging side effects and are thus protected from a distressing illness which in itself may present considerable long term risks. Talk to your doctor or health visitor if you are worried: they will be able to reassure you.

See Appendix IV for details of Immunisation schedules

Chicken pox (varicella)

Chicken pox is a viral infection for which vaccination is not available. Neither are antibiotics effective when the disease develops. The illness is usually mild in children and the child is most infectious before the development of the spots. Typically the child does not feel unduly unwell and therefore continues to attend school and play with friends. Thus the disease is spread freely, commonly occurring in epidemics. Tiredness, sore throat and headache may precede the spots which occur in crops. They begin as small, round, white spots, slightly raised above the level of the skin. They blister and break, oozing a clear fluid. The spot then dries and becomes red and hard, eventually disappearing altogether. The rash is very irritating and the child will find it extremely difficult not to scratch. Applications of calamine cream, or lotion, may soothe the irritation. Encourage the child to drink plenty of fluids but do not worry if she is not eating the usual amount of food. Although the child is highly infectious at first, particularly before the spots develop and while they exude fluid, when all the spots are dry and she feels well she can return to school. Usually this will be after about seven clear days.

See also Chapter 7, section 11(n) on Viral illnesses

Complications of chicken pox are rare but if the child's condition appears to worsen with the development of a chest infection, vomiting and headache, irritability and confusion then seek urgent medical attention.

Measles

This viral illness is now included in the vaccination programme. It usually begins 10–14 days after contact with an infected child. Immunisation dramatically reduces the effects of the disease and the child may feel unwell for only a day or two. Initially the child appears to have a severe cold and small white patches may appear in the mouth. After four or five days a bright red rash appears beginning behind the ears and spreading down the arms, trunk and legs. After this the temperature falls slowly and the child recovers.

Treatment is to relieve the symptoms. Mild painkillers, soothing drinks and cool washes usually help.

Occasionally the child develops an ear infection which will need medical treatment as will any chest infection which may arise. Antibiotics may be prescribed but they have no action against the measles virus.

Meningitis

Meningitis simply means inflammation of the membranes which surround the brain. The cause can be bacterial or viral. The infection causes swelling of the membranes thus causing severe headache, stiffness in the neck and may go on to cause vomiting and confusion. Urgent medical advice is needed.

Viral meningitis is the most common variety and patients usually recover in four or five days without any lasting damage. They may feel weak and tired for some time.

Bacterial meningitis is much less common but, unfortunately, sensational reporting in the media has caused undue panic. Small epidemics do occur but prompt treatment and isolation of affected individuals usually halts the spread. Treatment is with antibiotics in hospital. One form of bacterial meningitis may mean that all members of the family and very close contacts will need preventative antibiotics but it must be remembered that this is a comparatively uncommon disease. Recovery is usually complete but may be slow.

Mumps (parotitis)

This viral illness is so called because the parotid glands, situated just below and in front of the ears over the angles of the jaw, become swollen when affected by the virus. No rash appears. Children are now immunised against mumps.

Parents may worry about male children believing that a long term effect is sterility. Only very few males, all above the age of puberty, have been affected in this way.

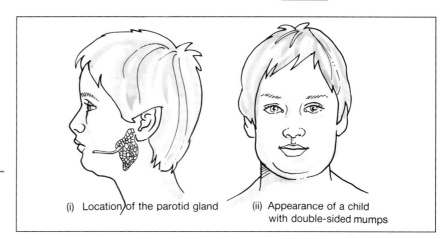

(i) Location of the parotid gland

(ii) Appearance of a child with double-sided mumps

Mumps or parotitis

Swelling of the parotid glands causes pain and affects the appearance of the child's whole face

Treatment is aimed at relieving the symptoms with drinks, mouthwashes and mild painkillers. The infection is spread by coughing and the child should be kept at home until the swelling of the glands resolves.

Rubella (German measles)

Despite its similar name the virus that causes rubella is quite different from the measles virus. Protection is provided by the immunisation programme. The illness is not as severe as measles but may begin similarly with the appearance of what seems to be a cold. Sore throat and a red rash usually occur and treatment is with a mild painkiller.

See also Chapter 4, section 4 on Antenatal care

The most important aspect of this condition is that the child must not come into contact with a pregnant woman particularly during the first 16 weeks of pregnancy as contact with the disease may have disastrous consequences for her unborn child causing major abnormalities. Children are infectious from the time they develop first signs of catarrh not just when the rash appears. They must be kept at home. If a mother of the affected child is pregnant then she should take advice from her family doctor who, in any case, will have screened her for rubella. Any contact with a child infected with rubella must be reported to the doctor.

Whooping cough

Whooping cough (or pertussis) is caused by a bacterial infection affecting the respiratory organs. It causes long periods of coughing followed by a characteristic 'whoop'. The child becomes distressed and exhausted and may turn blue and vomit after an attack. The cough can persist for up to three months and immunisation is strongly advised to protect the child against this illness. Whooping cough can have serious complications such as pneumonia and brain haemorrhage. The child is infectious for up to two weeks after the cough begins.

The doctor must be consulted and antibiotics may be prescribed to combat the infection and prevent more serious lung infections. Cough linctuses may be prescribed too, but some have a sedative effect and may also be constipating.

Babies are frequently admitted to hospital if they develop whooping cough as they may be unable to feed. Sucking may trigger an attack of coughing so nutrition is provided by other means.

Glandular fever

Epstein-Barr virus is the causative agent of infectious mononucleosis (glandular fever). Glandular fever is a disease of children and young adults and not infrequently affects teenagers. Although the exact mechanism for its spread is not fully understood, the virus is present in saliva which has earned glandular fever the label 'the kissing disease'.

Common symptoms are sort throat, enlarged lymph nodes, extreme fatigue, malaise and fever. There is no specific treatment (apart from plenty of rest) but antibiotics may be given if a secondary bacterial infection of the throat occurs. The illness usually lasts between one and two weeks and may then be followed by a period of variable length during which the young person is tired, weak and depressed.

The debilitating effects of glandular fever can be particularly trying for the older child or teenager for whom life outside the home is gaining an increasing importance. This is also the time when commitments and pressures such as examinations, responsibilities in the school hierarchy and intense social relationships may be particularly evident, and the young person may become anxious about his lack of ability to do very much. Parents will need to be patient and supportive. Talking to the school may help and short visits from friends can be encouraged provided they understand that the patient must not be overtired.

See Appendix VII for Addresses of useful organisations

The youngster can be reassured that, in time, he will feel perfectly well again. Some individuals have found reflexology beneficial in restoring usual levels of energy but, as with any alternative treatments, it is important to ensure that the practitioner you consult is reputable. A sensible precaution is to contact the relevant professional body first.

6.6(c)   ASTHMA

Asthma is a common condition which affects approximately one in every four children in the United Kingdom. It affects the respiratory tract or airways which lead to the lungs and is characterised by a wheezing noise when the sufferer breaths out. In some children asthma begins with prolonged episodes of coughing at night or wheezing when taking exercise. Good medical management is the key to ensuring that the child leads a normal life and is not regarded by himself or his family as delicate or frail. Most children eventually grow out of asthma before adulthood.

What happens during an asthma attack?

The air passages narrow and become constricted making it difficult to breathe out which makes the sufferer breathless and anxious.

What causes asthma and what makes an attack happen?

Children differ in the course and nature of their condition. All or only some of the factors listed in the box may apply, but it is a good idea to take them into consideration and observe the child so that you have a good idea what his particular triggers are.

Treatment

Management of allergy   Try to keep the house as dust free as possible by regular vacuum cleaning, preferably with a cleaner that is

POSSIBLE CAUSES OF ASTHMA	
Allergy	Allergy to certain well known substances is common. The house dust mite is the usual culprit and this is almost impossible to eradicate from modern houses where the mite is found in large numbers in soft furnishings and fitted carpets. Pollens, animal hair and feathers are also very common irritants. Unfortunately, children affected by these substances may also suffer from hay fever and eczema.
Coughs and colds	The initial responses to viruses may be complicated in asthmatic children by a subsequent bacterial infection affecting the chest. Chest infection is a common trigger to an asthma attack.
Exercise	If exercise causes an attack, it may then be referred to as *exertion asthma*.
Environmental pollution	Many experts are studying the effects of industrial pollution on asthmatics but common substances are well known to upset some sufferers. Cigarette smoke and petrol fumes are two of these but some people have a reaction to essentially clean but very cold air.
Emotional factors	Although much has been written about emotional upsets in regard to asthma the evidence is still unclear. Parents should not think that an asthmatic child cannot be disciplined in the same way as a non-asthmatic child. One would run the risk of the child becoming very spoilt and unmanageable. It is essential that a normal life should be strived for. An asthma attack is very upsetting and the child may very well be irritable and difficult during an attack – as would any of us who are having trouble getting our breath. It should not be assumed that only grumpy, difficult or otherwise emotionally unstable children have asthma.

fitted with a good filter. Use a damp cloth to dust and do this when the child is not in the room. Roller blinds, synthetic fibre filled duvets and pillows, and non-fluffy carpets in the child's bedroom are better at resisting the dust mite.

It is rather hard on children to deprive them of family pets and riding lessons etc. – so only do this on the advice of your general practitioner or the paediatrician who will confirm whether the child appears to be allergic to all animals or only some.

Medication prescribed by the doctor will help to control pollen allergy in season – but cut the lawn and sweep up the cuttings when the child is out for the day.

Early treatment of coughs and colds The asthmatic child should be seen by the doctor early in the course of a cough or cold as he may decide it is prudent to prescribe antibiotics to ward off secondary bacterial infection.

Exercise All children need regular exercise but some forms may be better for the asthmatic child than others. Swimming is often cited as a very tolerable and enjoyable activity for such children. Good medical management will allow the child to pursue such sports as he feels able. Good supervision is essential; long distance running may mean the child is unsupervised for some time in unpopulated areas and this may be unwise therefore. The child will soon realise:

- What his limits are;

- The importance of taking any prescribed medication before beginning exercise;

- That he must rest if wheezy.

Environmental pollution This is surely a good reason for any smokers in the house to give up the habit. Ask visitors not to smoke in the house and take advantage of all non-smoking public areas when on outings.

Wrap the child up well if he has to go out in very cold air. A scarf around the lower half of the face is very comforting and will filter cold air.

Emotion Try to aim for normality. Don't tiptoe around the child – the usual family interactions will not upset him.

Medication

The drug usually used is Ventolin (salbutamol) which is a bronchodilator. This means that the drug allows the constricted airways to open up again and allow the child to breathe normally. The

*See Appendix III for
more information about
Drugs and medicines*

drug is available as tablets, syrups and inhalers but the latter are
the most commonly and effectively used as these penetrate
directly into the airways. Correct use of the inhaler is vital and the
technique is a little tricky to master but once the child gets the
hang of it there should be no problem. The doctor and health visitor will undoubtedly help.

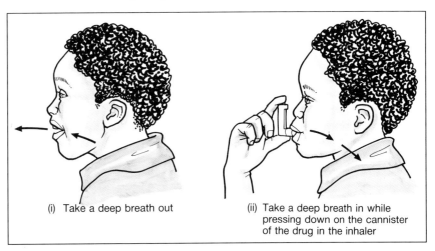

(i) Take a deep breath out

(ii) Take a deep breath in while
pressing down on the cannister
of the drug in the inhaler

Using an inhaler to treat an
asthma attack

Another drug which may be used in inhaler form is a corticos-
teroid known as Becotide (beclamethasone) which helps to reduce
any inflammation in the airways but does not have the more serious side effects associated with steroids taken in tablet form which
affect the whole body. Unfortunately these may be have to be used
if the asthma attack is very severe and needs admission to hospital.
Here they would be very carefully used and discontinued as soon
as possible.

Intal (sodium cromoglycate) is another inhaler which is used to
prevent attacks occurring in the first place.

These three drugs used correctly as prescribed help most asthmatics to avoid attacks altogether.

Nebulisers are used by some asthmatics at home to deliver
higher concentrations of Ventolin during an attack. This would
only be done on the advice of the paediatrician or the child's
general practitioner.

- Always call the doctor immediately if the child's condition fails
  to respond to usual treatment, or if his condition worsens, to
  prevent a more serious attack.

Alternative medicine

Many people are turning to alternative therapies to treat many illnesses and while some of the treatments may be of some value it
would be foolhardy to ignore the advice and treatment of conventional medicine in the treatment of asthma. However, dietary

modifications such as reducing the amount of fast food eaten in favour of more wholesome high fibre, low fat foods will benefit most children. It is important to ensure that a good mixed diet is taken which provides all the protein, carbohydrates, fats, vitamins and minerals in the recommended quantities.

6.6(d) ACCIDENTS

In the year 1988–9, there were 14,000 accidental deaths in the United Kingdom and 7,000,000 other cases requiring hospital treatment. An unquantifiable number of accident injuries are also treated by general practitioners, first aiders and other persons notably parents.

See also Chapter 5, section 10 on Keeping your young child safe, and Chapter 7, section 7 on Safety at home and outside

Accidents are unfortunately part of a child's life. Few children will escape without the occasional grazed finger or cut knee. However, many, many children have more frequent and more serious accidents, some of which could be prevented. The key word is prevention, so this section aims to establish some common causes of accidents and what can be done to prevent them.

The Royal Society for the Prevention of Accidents (RoSPA), is a charitable organisation dedicated to the prevention of accidents via education and training.

A staggering 5,100 deaths in the United Kingdom in 1988–9 were caused by accidents in the home and a further 2,400,000 persons needed hospital treatment after having an accident at home. Falls accounted for the major number of fatalities. The first preventative measure is to identify the potential risks and hazards in the home environment. Not all safety measures are expensive and may simply mean a little reorganisation. Good housekeeping, that is tidiness, will go a long way to preventing accidents.

Some equipment is essential and may cost a little money. Smoke detectors and fire extinguishers are vital and the benefits far outweigh the cost. The Fire Prevention Officer from the Fire and Rescue service will advise on the purchase, placement and use of these items.

Treatment

A First Aid kit is essential in the home. These can be purchased from good pharmacists but you can assemble a kit by purchasing the relevant items and storing these in a secure container. The kit should be easily accessible to adults but out of reach of children.

See Appendix II on First Aid

The Red Cross and St. John Ambulance offer very good courses in first aid in which parents would be wise to enrol – particularly those who are involved in play groups or leisure activities for groups of people.

Road safety

Road safety should be taught from a very early age. Before allowing the child to cross the roads unattended by an adult, you must ensure that the child is competent to do so. The child should not be allowed on the roads on a bicycle until effective training has taken place. Most schools run a Cycling Proficiency course in conjunction with the local constabulary and this excellent course is invaluable in the area of accident prevention. In Great Britain alone in 1988, 226 cyclists and 1,753 pedestrians lost their lives on the roads. A large proportion of these were children.

Seat belts should always be worn by passengers in the car.

Water and leisure safety

Children should learn to swim as soon as possible. They should be taught in safe surroundings by a competent instructor. The local municipal pool will normally offer reasonably priced tuition in safe and hygienic surroundings. In 1988 there were 571 drowning accidents in Great Britain, two of which occurred in garden ponds.

Leisure activities

Leisure activities can be highly dangerous if not properly planned and supervised. If introducing a child to an outdoor leisure pursuit such as climbing, sailing, go-carting, windsurfing etc. do not cut corners on the purchase of safety equipment. Buy the equipment from a reputable dealer and make sure that the child will receive effective instruction from a credited source.

Educational material

See Appendix VII for Addresses of useful organisations and Appendix VIII for suggested Further reading

RoSPA have developed a series of booklets, videos and educational material on all aspects of safety management, and can be consulted for advice and support by all members of the general public.

See Appendix VII for Addresses of useful organisations and Appendix VIII for suggested Further reading

6.7 BEHAVIOURAL AND EMOTIONAL PROBLEMS

See also Chapter 3, section 2 on Adolescence

Adolescence is the time in a person's life when the change from childhood to adulthood occurs. For the majority of youngsters, this process is a gradual one of adaptation which they pass through relatively happily and successfully. For some youngsters, however, their past, their background or their physical condition causes them emotional problems which are reflected in their behaviour. This not only has an effect on the youngster's personal life, but may also have quite serious consequences for his family.

6.7(a) THE FAMILY

The family is a social organisation providing a structure within which individuals can feel safe and from which they can engage with society at large. Members of the family use family rules to guide their behaviour while finding within these rules the space to express and realise themselves as individuals. This structure provides a fixed and stable view of 'the way things are' that members of a family can rely upon while supporting its individual members in times of trouble or illness.

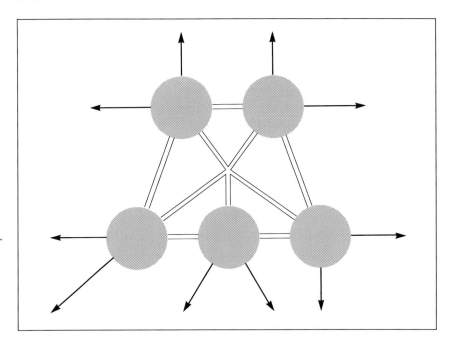

A healthy family is bound together by mutual support and a framework of family rules – from which base each individual can relate to others in the outside world

Where family boundaries either do not exist or are too strict, it is likely that the family organisation will cease to work for the people within it. The family will become fragmented and unable to meet both parents' and youngsters' needs for stability, support, care and love.

Rectifying such a situation is not easy. It requires a willingness on the part of both the young person and his parents to:

- Want to do something about the problems they are experiencing;

- Consider whether circumstances are so serious that the help of outside agencies is required.

See Appendix VII for Addresses of useful organisations

Such help would in all probability aim at improving communications between the members of the family. Improved communications enable the youngster to come to an understanding of the difficulties faced by her parents, while parents can begin to appreciate the problems being experienced by their youngster in the transformation into adulthood.

Of course by no means all family groups are constructed in the same way: one or both parents may be absent, grandparents or other adults may be particularly significant or children of different natural parents may live together as siblings within one family unit. It can generally be accepted however that all young people need loving and consistent support from at least one reliable adult.

6.7(b)   ADOLESCENCE AND FAMILY LIFE

Perhaps the main concern for all adolescents is independence. Though not yet adults, they wish to be treated as such. When they are not, a burning indignation at the injustice of the world can often be seen. What this means for parents is that treating their child as a young adult, with the accompanying duties and responsibilities that adulthood brings, has a pay off for all the family. In essence, this is to say that treating the young adult *as* a young adult goes a long way to ensuring that he will behave accordingly. It is important that parents communicate a wish to trust him in his growing independence and to demonstrate this. Equally, it is important for parents to realise that doing this will be anxiety provoking for them. In this manner, trust and responsibility can be experienced in action.

Parents also need to recognise that their own wishes and expectations for the next generation will, in all likelihood, differ from those of their youngsters. Here, there is always a possibility that parents will seek to realise their own frustrated ambitions through their children. When made obvious, this pressure is often resisted by the young person, if not directly rebelled against. When pressure to conform to parents' wishes is applied in less obvious ways, perhaps when parents are not aware that they are trying to influence their youngster, the young person often recognises this and reacts against it. Within this context, it is valuable if adults seek to recognise their own hidden agendas for their children and, where relevant, to share these with them.

Perhaps the best solution in this situation – and in many other situations of difference between parents and youngster – is 'synthesis'. Where parents can make clear their wishes for their child, while at the same time accepting and taking into account the young person's own wishes, this provides for a situation of mutual understanding and responsibility. If an adolescent can accept her parents' expectations of her, and balance these against her own requirements, there arises the possibility of a satisfactory and agreed outcome. This is particularly important since it allows the youngster to express her individuality; a necessary development in the move from being a child who is conventionally not allowed opinions, to being an adult who is.

The relationship between an adolescent and her brothers or sisters is a particularly difficult area. Rivalries and disputes both within and between gender groups are extremely common. It is one way for an adolescent to mark out her individuality in relation to a sibling, but also may be an inappropriate strategy the youngster adopts to get her own way. Regarding herself as equal to an older sibling, for example, may result in a young person demanding that she be treated accordingly even though this would not be appropriate according to her age.

Where parents and youngster have to deal with difficult issues it is important to establish clear and fair family boundaries if these do not already exist. Such boundaries are important not only because of what they do – ensuring a young person comes home by a certain time, for example – but because they express parental concern for the youngster *to* the youngster. Boundaries show that parents care.

For an adult to take control and resolve a youngster's problem should be seen as a last resort, but one which may have to be faced. For an action that resolves or changes a problematic situation to come from the young person is a confirmation of personal effectiveness and is, therefore, preferable. Any route involving self-determined action on the part of the youngster should be supported, so that if all else fails, at least the attempt has been made.

Confrontation should be resisted. Parents offer youngsters most when they listen, provide information and show interest by asking general rather than personal questions. Recognising and responding when a youngster does something well is not as easy as being extremely critical of someone whose dress and interests may be at variance with the parent's own. However it is far more productive, as is being prepared to be personally honest even when this means presenting oneself in a less than desirable way.

It is a perfectly normal and expected parental reaction to get anxious when an adolescent son or daughter is perceived as facing a risky or threatening world. Responses born of this anxiety, however, may generate more difficulties than they resolve. This is especially the case when parents relate their own experiences as if they were those of their child.

In this manner, the youngster may conclude that his parents do not understand him. Similar blocks to communication arise if parents do not take the trouble to find out about their son or daughter's interests. If instead, parents adopt stereotypical views or beliefs about what young people actually do, whether these be to do with drugs, sexuality, violence or any of the aspects of life that we see as personally threatening, this may lead to confrontations between the youngster and parents that are potentially extremely damaging to their relationship.

6.7(c) SEXUALITY

In many ways, adolescence *means* sexuality. It is the time of puberty when sexual maturity is reached. In biological terms, the child has become an adult. A girl has become a young woman who can have a child and a boy has become a young man who can father children. Because the adolescent has reached biological maturity, however, does not mean that he has reached emotional maturity.

Sexual identity

Having sexual identity, becoming a woman or a man, is a time of excitement, experiment and anxiety for all adolescents. It is also the time when the events of childhood may become problematic. A youngster possessing a sexual identity on the one hand, feeling emotionally uncertain about her sexuality on the other, may try to resolve feelings derived from the past through sexual behaviour. Alternatively, the events of childhood may make it difficult for a youngster to make sense of what is happening to him in adolescence leading to problems associated with sexual behaviour.

Physically, sexual maturity confers on youngsters certain biological changes. Females have the ability to ovulate and menstruate and develop breasts. Males have the ability to produce sperm and develop facial hair and deeper voices. Both sexes develop body hair and experiment with masturbation. In terms of accommodating

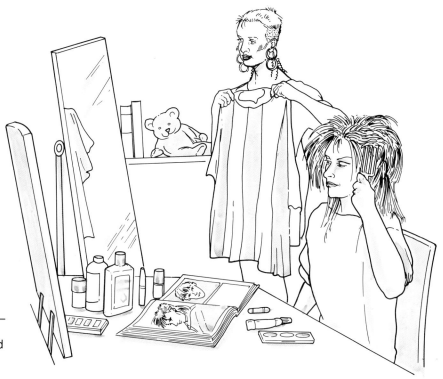

Adolescence is a time for experimenting with image and appearance

369

these changes and developing a sexual identity, both sexes tend to institute certain changes themselves. They may dress differently and become aware of 'teenage fashion'. Females may use a lot of make-up to accentuate their adulthood and may attempt to dress older than their years. Males may seek to present themselves as 'macho' and tough. Romantic attachments to members of the opposite or the same sex will occur. Adolescents will flirt and talk with one another about sex, often covering up their embarrassment and lack of knowledge with jokes and crudities. Both sexes may develop a fairly extended social life and begin to make quite challenging demands of parents and others within the family – to be allowed privacy, to be allowed to make decisions for themselves, to be allowed more money for their personal use, etc.

Parents have to meet these demands as they occur and in relation to their particular set of circumstances. However, it is important to remember that adolescents are in the process of becoming independent from them, sexually, socially and emotionally, and require help to do this. Because of this, it is important to get the balance right between supporting the youngsters and allowing them to be responsible for what they do.

Too much support on the one hand, or excessive constraint on the other, may foster dependence or provoke rejection. As a result, the youngster's right to make decisions about himself may be either eroded or non-existent. Giving the adolescent too much responsibility for what he does – allowing him a 'free rein' – may result in a myriad of problems and be interpreted as 'not caring' by the youngster and become problematic in itself. Getting this balance right is important for every aspect of adolescence. It is particularly important in relation to a youngster's sexuality, since the problems which may be encountered during this time may be particularly traumatic and emotionally damaging. With the emergence of HIV, they are also potentially life-threatening.

Where youngsters have feelings towards members of the same sex, they may feel imprisoned by these homosexual or lesbian feelings because of possible parental reactions and the values and constraints society imposes on individuals who are 'different'. In order to feel fulfilled, lead a happy and healthy life and feel good about herself, a youngster needs to be empowered to make informed decisions about the form of sexual life she leads. This principle applies to all the problematic issues of adolescence.

Male values

From cultural and group values, adolescent males are under pressure to 'act like men' and 'prove' themselves. It thus becomes confirmation of adulthood and identity to make sexual conquests.

Failure to make such conquests, or the extent of their nature, is likely to remain unreported and become instead a matter of myth, such is the power of the pressure to 'act like a man'. Because of this, the adolescent male may choose to conform. He hides any sexual ignorance he has and puts aside any finer feelings or notions of responsibility towards female adolescents, since to display either would be to open himself up for ridicule by other youngsters. It would also be to admit to himself and to others that he is not who he claims to be: a strong, well-informed adult male.

Due to this complicated system of cultural values and pressure and counter pressure, both within groups of the same sex and between groups of a different sex, the focus of sexual activity and any resulting problems tends to be on the adolescent female.

Sex and the adolescent girl

Occasionally promiscuity by the adolescent female may be a problem. Not only is she likely to become stigmatised by the double standards of peers and adults alike for her sexual activities, but she may also be in danger of contracting a sexually transmitted disease or becoming pregnant.

When a child has been sexually abused, this early sexualisation may bring about promiscuity in adolescence due to such issues as feelings of low self-worth and self-esteem. Feeling as though she is totally worthless, the sexually abused adolescent may have no inhibitions against promiscuity because she feels she is not worth anything. At the same time, sexual activity provides for her the pretence of emotional bonding and being cared for. For the same reason, an adolescent female who feels unloved and uncared for at home may seek this affection elsewhere, even to the point of wanting a child as a means of attaining a meaningful and dependent relationship, so that she may provide the child with the love she feels she did not receive.

The equation of sexual activity with abuse may be equally likely to lead to frigidity and a fear of any sexual relationship.

It should also be pointed out that young males who have been on the receiving end of sexual abuse are also likely to demonstrate disorders of sexual feeling and an inability to form satisfactory relationships.

Since such reasons for establishing a relationship with a member of the opposite sex are reactions to both past and present situations, without thought for self-control and responsibility, such a relationship is likely to be brief and possibly damaging in itself. Impermanence tends to confirm for her the reason she began the relationships in the first place: that she is not worth very much.

Where an adolescent's biography, socialisation process and emotional state predisposes her towards promiscuity, it is also likely that there will be attendant behavioural problems. Being out all night or running away from home for lengthy periods may occur. As a result of this, the youngster may put herself at risk because of the places she frequents (e.g. public houses, bus and railway stations) and by associating with much older males. The development of such potentially dangerous activities may also occur where a family has a loose structure, without boundaries or rules, such that a youngster is permitted to act like this. The consequences for adolescent males acting in this way may not be so serious, though this is not necessarily the case.

Educating teenagers

The dilemma for parents and all educators about contraception and 'safer sex' is that talk of it may be seen as encouraging the youngster to engage in sexual activity. However, by doing and saying nothing, we as parents and responsible adults are leaving things to ignorance; the young person is left to learn about sex by chance and experimentation. The dangers of pregnancy and disease here are obvious.

Where parents themselves feel uncomfortable or inhibited speaking about sexual matters, this may be transmitted to their youngster. Such inhibition may in this way be reflected in the youngster's behaviour or reacted against, possibly in a promiscuous manner. One possible strategy here is for parents to use family meetings for serious discussion of general topics related to sex, including teenage pregnancy, abortion and AIDS.

How parents approach this is a matter, ultimately, for their consciences. They have to bear in mind the possible consequences of imposing their views upon their youngster when they decide either for or against sex education or agreeing with or prohibiting contraception. Here there are no right answers, only outcomes which may or may not be extremely damaging to all concerned.

6.7(d) BODY IMAGE AND EATING HABITS

A sense of identity is what makes an individual who she 'is'. In terms of adolescence, gaining a separate, adult identity is a youngster's central aim. It also constitutes a problem to be overcome. For youngsters, the development of identity consists of establishing their independence from and difference to others, while assuring themselves of their normality and consistency with others. The focus of such development and assurance, more or less inseparable at this time from identity, is body image. Physical attractiveness, influenced by films, television and fashion, is extremely important to youngsters. Where a youngster experiences the way he looks as being unsatisfactory, he may try and do something about this. Attention is likely to fall on eating habits and food. Such attention is likely to have behavioural consequences.

Behaviours associated with food can range from the relatively simple, such as a youngster wanting to go on a diet, to the extremely complex and serious conditions of anorexia nervosa and bulimia nervosa. In between these two extremes are to be found such problematic issues for parents as compulsive eating and obesity.

As youngsters reach adolescence with the onset of puberty, they experience great uncertainty about who they are, what they will become and what they want to become. Within this perfectly normal and expected situation, necessary for the attainment of maturity, it is extremely common for youngsters to want to signal to their parents and others that they have control over themselves. One way this can be done is for the youngster to go on a diet.

Such attempts at dieting are usually temporary developments as the adolescent enjoys for himself for perhaps the first time his newly experienced independence. The impetus to diet on the other hand, may be because the youngster feels under pressure from other youngsters at school or in the near neighbourhood. This could be in terms of bullying or teasing about his appearance, because he wants to be like a friend or someone he respects or simply because of fashion.

Interactions between the parents and teenager

As the young person grows up and gains independence, the interaction will change from that of parent to child to something closer to the interaction of adults. This will be reversed, however, if the teenager behaves in a way the parents find unacceptable

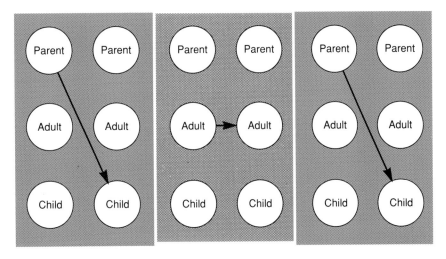

Whatever the reason a youngster has for going on a diet, it is important for his parents to respect his views and not to reinstate the parent-child relationship, where the parent takes all the decisions. Providing the conditions for support and understanding are important here, since making the youngster feel accepted as an adolescent also provides the conditions for an important exchange of information about other adolescent issues.

Eating disorders

Compulsive eating   Where it is extremely common for adolescents to want to go on diets and have control over how they look, sometimes a youngster's anxiety about his body image will result in him becoming a compulsive eater. This may be related to a strong feeling of insecurity. Rather than sometimes diet or eat normally, such a youngster will eat and eat until he puts on a gross amount of weight which hinders his movements and actions and puts his health at threat. Compulsive eating and obesity are unlikely to be simply indicative of the passing phase of adolescence and will not, by themselves, go away.

Anorexia and bulimia nervosa   Whereas in dieting there are attempts, successful or unsuccessful, to resist food, in anorexia nervosa a young person – usually but not exclusively an adolescent female – demonstrates an iron will, a deception of others and an increasing preoccupation on controlling food intake beyond that which is necessary for survival. Denial of the problem, disguise via clothing, exercise and secrecy, all dominate. As well as obsessive control of intake, getting rid of food ingested by self-induced vomiting and the use of non-nourishing foods are all seen, as is the use of laxatives.

Where a youngster binges on food and then purges herself by self-induced vomiting, the problem is identified as bulimia which, like anorexia, is potentially life-threatening.

Both these problems require the intervention of professional help which may have to be sought by parents, despite the probable protestations from their daughter or son. Delay may result in the young person being admitted to hospital as a consequence of infection or extreme malnutrition or collapse. This may bring the severity of the problem to light for the first time. In the case of the young person who vomits persistently, it may be a visit for dental treatment that indicates the severity of the problem as the acid in vomit attacks the teeth.

This preoccupation with limiting food intake may express a variety of concerns. Many factors contribute to it which are not specific to it, for example:

- Anxiety about identity;

- Wanting control;

- Worries about the future.

What formulates the exact nature of anorexia is the way these factors come together. This leads to the feelings and behaviour that are specific to the condition: poor body image and avoidance of normal body weight.

In treatment terms, causing a profound shift in an anorexic young person's behaviour is extremely difficult and may necessitate the provision of a potentially therapeutic environment in which the youngster can experience personal and emotional growth. It must be noted though that such is the nature of anorexia, the young person so affected will probably be strongly resistant to any treatment. Just as the anorexic youngster needs help, so too does her family need support and the opportunity to develop their resources for coping.

6.7(e) ANXIETY

Most people commonly experience uncertainty and doubt when considering some course of action or making an important decision. In adolescence, the feelings of uncertainty and doubt are important to the experience of growing up. A youngster has to try and discover and accept who she is while contemplating the future. 'Who she is' and 'what she will become' are two of the central themes of adolescence. Within this process, doubt and uncertainty in conjunction with self-control, allow the youngster to make considered judgements about herself, those around her and what she is going to make of her life.

See also Chapter 7, section 10(b) on Depression and anxiety

For some youngsters, however, anxiety may become an overwhelming experience which comes to rule and disrupt their lives. Where, because of the effects of a traumatic childhood for example, a person is unable to reconcile who he feels himself to be in relation to who he wants to be, he may begin to feel there is no future for him at all. When a youngster is in such an emotional state, daily events and experiences may further provoke his anxiety. Painful memories about the past may be evoked making him feel worse. Trapped within this bleak situation the adolescent is likely to become depressed and, in an attempt to make real the emotional pain he is feeling, may attempt to harm himself.

6.7(f) ALCOHOL, TOBACCO AND OTHER SUBSTANCES

For the adolescent, experimenting with life is a fundamental characteristic. It is how he learns about the new world he is entering. One aspect of learning to be an adult is acting in the way adults act. Groups of friends may get together and, instead of playing pretend games as they did as children, do things that adults do – as they see it – for real. In this way, the smoking of tobacco and the drinking of alcohol confers upon the adolescent, he feels, the significance of adulthood.

When the adolescent's smoking or drinking is 'found out' by parents or other adults, they are likely to forbid such behaviour and possibly punish it. This re-establishes the youngster's previous position as a child, a position he thought he had left, and kindles in him a sense of injustice. His parents may smoke and drink. Other adults certainly do. So why not him?

Well-established and maintained family patterns of communication also enable the transmission of valuable information and facts from parents to youngster that the youngster may not know (e.g. about the effect some behaviour can have on health) and vice versa (e.g. the feelings that the youngster has when he wants to do something he may know he should not do). However, because identity, independence and separation from parents are such important issues for the youngster, they exert a powerful sway over him. Having such feelings in common with friends and schoolmates who are in like situations means that the youngster's peer group is likely to have considerable sway over what he subsequently does.

This is particularly relevant in the case of youngsters who use cannabis and abuse solvents. Both are social and cultural activities which the newly adolescent youngster may learn from other youngsters. When a youngster has become well versed in the use of cannabis or solvents, more solitary use of such substances may take place and may be found to occur in the home. The possession of cannabis is an offence in law. Possessing and sniffing glue, aerosols, typewriter correction fluid and a wide range of other substances is not an offence in law.

Cannabis smoking has a particularly strong in-group identity which may be particularly attractive to the adolescent in search of who he is. Regular users of cannabis have a form of language particular to them which marks out those who are 'in' and those who are 'out' (particularly parents and other adults) which focuses attention on use of the drug. Activities centre around the purchasing of cannabis, rolling it into 'joints' or 'spliffs' and smoking these, often in the company of others.

The youngster who engages in the abuse of solvents is a particular worry to his parents. This form of behaviour is both life-threatening and may be an expression of great sadness and hopelessness. Carried out both with others and alone at times of stress, solvent abuse involves the inhalation of gas from aerosols or the fumes of glue or correction fluid from plastic bags. The practice may leave the young person with physical symptoms such as those described in the box.

Solvent abuse and cannabis use are both learned group activities which give youngsters some sense of identity. By engaging in these activities, youngsters both place themselves outside conventional society (in this way, the activity *belongs* to them) and affirm their

Signs of solvent abuse

> • Abuser appears giggly or 'high'
> • Red, watery eyes
> • Dilated pupils
> • Runny nose
> • (In long term abusers) sores around the nose or mouth

independence and ability to make decisions for themselves. Because part of youngsters' grievance against wider society is that they have nothing provided for them in terms of something to do and somewhere to go, use of cannabis and solvents provides them with a focus around which they can organise social activity.

Where adults may go to a public house, adolescents may well use a particular place in the neighbourhood where they sniff solvents or smoke cannabis. The dangerous or rebellious element in such activities may be another attractive element to a youngster. It places her, as she sees it, outside the bounds of 'normal' society; a rebel willing to take risks adults would not dare take.

When a secretive activity begins to take predominance over other adolescent activities, when the youngster turns to solvent or drug use before or rather than anything else, this tends to be indicative of something problematic in the youngster's life. It may be to do with the past, the present, the future or a combination of all three. In this sense, the use of solvents or drugs is not *the* problem, but rather an expression of the problem.

It is unlikely that the use of solvents, cannabis or other drugs will be the only response to the feelings that troubled adolescents may be having. They may smoke and drink alcohol, while there may well be difficulties with behaviour at home and at school or work. School attendance may also be problematic. Running away from home or staying away from home for long periods may also occur. All are indications that the youngster is possibly attempting to stave off a crisis to do with her emotions. Because of this, such behaviour can be seen as the young person attempting to communicate with her parents the way she feels. Such communication may take more radical forms, where the youngster both attempts to make the pain she is feeling real for herself and convey this to those around her, for example by self-harm or attempted suicide.

6.7(g) SELF-INJURY AND ATTEMPTED SUICIDE

Self-injury such as biting, burning, hair pulling, head banging and cutting is an expression of anguish. Harm to the wrists or forearms, for example, may begin initially as scratches, but progress to more severe cutting by the use of knives, pieces of glass or razor blades. There tends to be little or no suicidal intention associated with occasions of self-injury. Rather it is an expression of adolescent despair in order that the youngster may experience physically the pain she is experiencing internally and make herself feel better.

Commonly, self-injury follows some traumatic event such as a family argument or the awakening of a painful memory (e.g. the anniversary of the death of a family member or knowledge about being adopted). Difficult social relationships between friends, particularly boy and girlfriends, may result in self-injury. This may be an expression of anxiety by the youngster, when he is pinning all his hopes for the future and the resolution of his emotional difficulties on one person.

Serious self-injury, such as the cutting of the throat and neck, jumping from buildings and attempts at self-strangulation are examples of serious suicidal intent and require immediate medical and psychiatric intervention. It is more likely to be adolescent males who attempt suicide by such methods.

Deliberate self-poisoning is usually but not exclusively carried out by adolescent females. Overdoses are usually of drugs commonly available in the home taken impulsively with only a few minutes thought beforehand. A common drug such as paracetamol, harmless in the usual doses, can have permanent and devastating side-effects if taken to excess.

Like deliberate self-injury, an overdose may be a response to a traumatic or emotionally upsetting event.

Where a youngster has a particularly disrupted and painful family background, she may not engage in self-injury or attempt suicide at all. However, something that appears quite trivial to others (such as splitting up with a boyfriend) on top of the more serious and long-standing problems may result in the forces acting towards suicidal behaviour being stronger than the constraints against self-harm which usually operate.

The reasons given by young people for attempting to harm themselves are likely to revolve around the theme of 'wanting to die'. Yet, what the youngster may mean is that at the time of the attempt he felt as if he wanted to die. That is, the suicide attempt can be viewed as a communication of the strength of feeling the young person was having at the time he made the suicide attempt.

It is extremely important to remember however, that the intention behind an attempt may well be serious. As such, professional help should be sought in ALL cases of attempted suicide. Indeed, all cases of behaviour that can be described as harmful to the youngster need intervention and treatment.

6.7(h) AGGRESSION AND BULLYING

An angry youngster is likely to be a lonely youngster. Because she conducts her relationships in an aggressive manner, others will respond to her in a fearful way. Thus, wanting relationships but not being able to sustain them, it is tempting for a young person to try and force others to go along with her and do what she wants to do. Lacking control of herself she seeks to control others. By doing so, and perhaps without realising it, the youngster has become a bully.

In a wider sense, bullying is an expression of power relationships between youngsters and as such may be a reflection of how adolescents see their relationships with adults. The bully of one youngster is quite likely to be being bullied himself by another. In terms of the form and extent of the bullying that occurs, in schools for example, this may very much depend upon environment. Bullying in a rural community is likely to contrast starkly to that which occurs in inner cities. Because of the high density of population and the breadth of available experience in the city, bullying may quite normally involve extortion or violent assault.

A youngster who is being bullied at school is likely to experience an extremely difficult and unhappy time. One reaction to this situation is for the youngster to absent herself from school. The first parents may know of this is when they are informed by the school. Alternatively, she may develop minor illnesses and ailments as a way of remaining at home and so escape being bullied. The dilemma for parents in such a situation is great and can only be resolved in relation to the individual circumstances that apply in a particular case.

Some involvement of the school authorities will almost certainly be needed. Possibly the police will have to be informed if an offence has been committed. With respect to the adolescent who is being bullied, it may be found to be helpful for parents to discuss the situation with their child. Such a discussion should not only address what has happened, but also attempt to examine and evaluate why some youngsters feel a need to bully others.

In this way the bullied youngster may be able to come to understand why he is in the situation he is in – that in all probability, he is not to blame for what is happening to him but is having to undergo the irresponsibility of others. Doing this will not stop him from being bullied, but should buoy up his self-respect and enable him to view and handle what happens in the future in some more appropriate way than truanting from school.

Should an aggressive youngster become involved with the police and court procedures, the process of justice may well officially confirm for him something he may have long suspected – that he is 'a bad person'. He may come to feel that being aggressive, having few friends and getting into trouble with the police is his lot in life. It is what he was born to do. Further, having had experience of the penal system, the youngster may come to lose all fear of it.

In such a situation, with the involvement of the police, probation officers and possibly social work agencies, the youngster and his family may be offered help with the problematic situation they find themselves in. There is, however, no easy solution as the difficulties between parents and youngster which have resulted in serious misunderstandings may well go back for years.

The future for youngsters who have problems with controlling their aggression is far from certain, especially if their behaviour results in them becoming involved with the police and courts. In order to alleviate the genuine despair that these youngsters and their families undergo, specialised help is likely to be needed which, ideally, would involve all the family. The purpose of such therapeutic work would be to assist the youngster and his parents with setting personal objectives, self-education, problem solving, using appropriate means for attaining specific ends and promoting other methods used for internally controlling impetuous thoughts and emotions.

6.7(i) IDENTITY

For a troubled youngster to come to terms with herself, to know who she is, to have a positive identity, she has to face up to possibly daunting feelings about her increasing emotional independence, the values she is to believe in and how she is to act in terms of her sexuality and friendships. Decisions also have to be made about employment and the future. During this process of identity building, adults may further complicate matters by responding to the youngster in ways which appear ambiguous, sometimes demanding compliance of her as a child, at other times expecting her to act in a mature and adult manner.

In coping with all these elements of change, where past experience meets anxieties about the future, a youngster with emotional problems is likely to become uncertain about her ability to cope, with both the transitional period of adolescence and adulthood. As a result of having negative feelings about herself, she may experience difficulties in forming relationships. The possibility of getting close to someone may be viewed as threatening, since to do so might destroy the thin veneer of behaviour the young person has constructed to protect herself both from the intrusions of others and her negative feelings. In this situation, the youngster has become isolated and perhaps only engages with people in

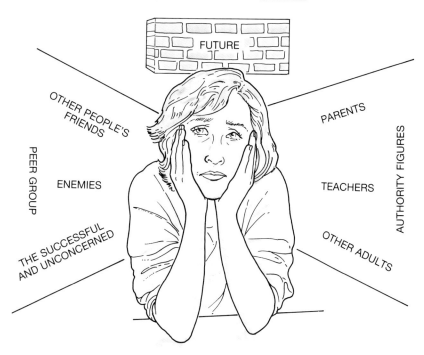

FUTURE

OTHER PEOPLE'S FRIENDS

PARENTS

PEER GROUP

AUTHORITY FIGURES

ENEMIES

TEACHERS

THE SUCCESSFUL AND UNCONCERNED

OTHER ADULTS

A troubled youngster may find relating to other people difficult, seeing them as stereotypes only, while the future may seem bleak or impossible

stereotypical relationships – as parents, teachers, potential threats – rather than in personal terms as individuals. As a result, thoughts about the future for such a youngster are out of the question. Caught up in the present, the concept of a future may not exist for a youngster, certainly not in terms of her becoming an adult. There may be further fears about what will be expected of her if and when she does become an adult.

Adulthood and having a positive identity may confront a troubled youngster as something insurmountable, a task he cannot possibly achieve. What this amounts to is that the youngster experiences adolescence while anticipating that he will fail in the process. This may be viewed as a defence, brought about by the gravity of the task. As a result a youngster may become totally confused by what he is supposed to do as an adolescent, how he is supposed to act.

In the search for a positive identity, young people with emotional problems have to battle against the idea of themselves as worthless, hopeless individuals – a self-conception derived perhaps from the experiences of childhood – while conducting their day to day activities. Here, where low esteem meets interaction with others, the troubled youngster is more likely to encounter failure than success.

Culture and identity

It is while trying to create a sense of their own identity that young people may appear to reject the cultural norms or religious beliefs held dear by their parents. This may be particularly likely if many members of the peer group come from different backgrounds. Such rejection can cause parents great anxiety and even pain, but it may pass in time – especially if the parents make some effort to respect and understand their child rather than merely confronting her. Young people themselves should also be encouraged to be sensitive to the fact that some of their friends may have been brought up with different values, beliefs and expectations from their own which it may not be appropriate to challenge.

Chronic conditions and identity

Youngsters who have medical or physical conditions have to face a similar dilemma with regard to identity. Where a youngster has diabetes, psoriasis or a deformity for example, he has not only to attempt successful negotiation of all aspects of adolescence, but also to assimilate into that process the personal feelings and possible social reactions occasioned by his medical or physical condition. In this situation it is highly likely that the individual and his family will adopt specific strategies and ways of behaving which seek to normalise the youngster's sense of identity within the family.

In the case of diabetes, for example, this condition imposes on a young person and the other members of his family a daily routine which results in the family world being re-ordered. In this way, that which is different about the youngster from other youngsters intrudes into the life of those close to him. They respond by accommodating this difference. Such a response forms the basis of the familiar daily routine. It becomes the norm. When family and friends make these reactive adjustments, the condition fades into the background and out of mind. Alternatively, where a condition has no immediate remedy or there is nothing practical that can be done to alleviate a youngster's day-to-day existence, such as in the case of a deformity for example, the family may simply choose to act as though there is nothing 'different' about their member in an attempt to deny that difference.

As well as ordering the family's daily activities, this process of normalising a person's medical or physical condition also serves to protect the youngster's identity from painful or distressing encounters outside the family. It is a perfectly understandable response from caring parents to want to protect their children from possible hurt, but there may be problems associated with such a protective approach.

When an adolescent with severe psoriasis or a deformity, for example, who has come to have a self-conception of herself as 'normal' within the family has to mix with other people she does not know, reactions to her as being 'abnormal' can be extremely hurtful. Where a youngster's medical condition is not readily apparent, there still exists the potential for emotional damage.

With diabetes, for example, because of the need to take insulin injections and regulate diet, a person may have to make a decision whether or not to tell those people he socialises with about his condition. Should he decide to do this, he must be prepared for the consequences, which are likely to focus in some way upon him being 'different'. Otherwise, only when a situation occurs which ignores, overlooks or points the diabetes out (perhaps a moment of thoughtlessness such as telling a diabetic youngster that a meal has been ordered for a certain time and then allowing the time to be changed without informing him) does evidence of the abnormality and associated feelings come flooding back.

How a young person reacts to situations such as these will largely be defined by the extent to which he has been prepared to meet them, something that the normalising, protective stance may not have done. Overly protecting young people may in fact encourage them to remain childlike, since behaving in such a way ensures protective treatment. In terms of the effects on a youngster who experiences negative feelings about herself, possibly feeling herself to be 'abnormal' despite all the efforts of her family to the contrary, these are likely to be similar to those of other youngsters who, for emotional reasons, feel socially isolated. School avoidance might become a problem, for example. The youngster might attempt to harm herself while relationships with peers who she might envy, and parents who she might blame for her medical condition, may be difficult.

Positive and negative feelings

For troubled youngsters, encountering the different aspects of adolescence is predominantly about seeking to discover who they are; an enquiry in search of a positive identity but which, because of features in their backgrounds and experience of everyday living, serves only to confirm the features of a negative identity. Things the young person does and says, every aspect of adolescence, revolves around this critical theme of positive-negative identity.

Identity is usually and routinely found in the way people look, what they say and what they do. With respect to the relationship between troubled adolescents and adults however, a youngster's identity generally means adults taking what he does wrong as synonymous with himself. This perspective results in problems of communication.

What a young person does is indicative of his identity at a particular time when the behaviour occurs, but if this is taken literally rather than interpretatively it becomes impossible to understand what the individual is experiencing. If instead, an adolescent's behaviour is regarded as an expression of what he is *feeling* (rather than of what he *is*), then the possibility exists for parents and others to establish a dialogue with him through which he might be able to resolve his troubled feelings. In attempting this extremely difficult task parents need to encourage their youngster to respect and accept himself as he is, rather than as how he might have been.

THE ADULT YEARS (20–60)

7.1 ## INTRODUCTION

The adult years comprise the greater part of most people's life. They certainly make up the period in which more is expected of individuals, both by themselves and by others. It is during adulthood that most people:

- Choose and develop a career or occupation;

- Find a partner and raise a family;

- Have responsibility for the health and welfare of others;

- Are able to make choices about health, activities and lifestyle to a greater extent than at other periods.

People in this age group are less likely than young children or elderly people to develop complications as a result of common illnesses such as colds or influenza. If an adult with dependent children or elders becomes seriously ill, however, the whole family may be profoundly affected. It should be remembered too that a healthy lifestyle during these years is likely to prolong quality of life and contribute to many years of happy retirement. The pressures of daily living, demands of family and workplace, should not cause us to ignore the importance of good eating habits, sensible exercise, and a balance between work and recreation.

See Chapter 1 for advice on maintaining and promoting health

This chapter is concerned firstly with the well adult, the responsible adult, the adult as carer, and considers ways of maximising the potential of such individuals. It then moves on to consider adults who are not not well or who have some specific difficulty. Ways of helping and supporting are explored and readers are referred to the appropriate professionals or agencies where necessary.

7.2 ## MAKING A WILL

'Why should I make a will? I'm not going to die yet!'
'I don't have much to leave so what's the point of making a will?'
'Why should I bother? I won't be around.'

These are some very common reactions when the topic of making a will is discussed. This section aims to show why it is advisable to make a will, how to plan your will, how a will should be drawn up and what to do if you wish to make changes.

Reasons for making a will

It is easy to underestimate the value of your property. With the increase in home and car ownership, the value of a person's financial worth has increased dramatically over recent years. Add to that the value of personal property, jewellery, a few shares and an insurance policy and the total may be surprising.

In the United Kingdom, when the value of a person's estate reaches a certain figure (£140,000 for 1991/92) then Inheritance Tax becomes payable. If a will is made it may be possible to find ways of leaving your valuables to avoid the payment of this tax.

Finally a will may make life a greater deal easier for your nearest and dearest who might not necessarily benefit in the same way if there is no will. For example, a surviving spouse does not necessarily receive all of the estate and a common law spouse or step-children may not benefit at all.

Who can make a will?

- Anyone who is 18 years or over. However if a person of under 18 years is on active service in Her Majesty's Armed Forces, he can make a valid will.

- A person of sound mind. If there is the likelihood that this might be challenged it is important to have medical evidence. Eccentricity or even some degree of mental illness does not necessarily equate with an unsound mind.

7.2(a)   PRACTICAL STEPS TO TAKE IN PLANNING A WILL

First of all, draw up a list of everything you possess. Remember to itemise property (less mortgage owing), money and insurances as well as personal effects. Next decide who you want to benefit – this might include some charities as well as relatives and friends. You will then be in the position to decide who is to have what. A difficulty is always trying to predict the future value of a gift in the will. Really the only answer is to re-examine the will at intervals and if necessary to remake it.

You also need to decide whether to include in the will any requests regarding burial, cremation or organ donation and what you want to happen to your remains.

It is important to name an executor in your will. This person will have the duty to see that your wishes are carried out in accordance with the will. These duties are quite onerous and therefore it is not unusual to appoint several executors. You need to ask the person whether he is willing to act in this capacity. If no executor is named, an administrator will be appointed by the Probate Registry. Quite often family members or a firm of solicitors will take on these roles.

7.2(b) REQUIREMENTS FOR A VALID WILL

A will must be clearly worded (see the boxed feature below for some frequently used words). In many circumstances it is possible for the individual to draw up a will without legal advice by using the checklist given overleaf and one of the commercially available will forms. However in certain circumstances it is wiser to take legal advice if the will involves trusts, residency or property in another country, a business or farm, or complex family situations (e.g. separation). If the estate is large, legal advice can also help to reduce the effects of Inheritance Tax but it is worth noting that this is not payable on property passing to a spouse, a charity or a recognised main political party.

It is important that for the will to be valid it must be properly witnessed. It is best for the testator and the two witnesses all to sign and witness each other's signatures together. Each witness should also give his full current address. Neither a spouse nor a beneficiary should witness the will as any gift is then forfeit.

Some definitions of words frequently used

Assets – possessions

Beneficiary – a person who inherits (benefits) under a will or under intestacy law

Bequest – a gift of estate

Children – legitimate, illegitimate and legally adopted children (not step-children)

Devise and bequeath – to give a gift

Estate – whatever you own

Infant or minor – a person under 18 years old who cannot hold possessions from an estate

Joint tenant – two or more people jointly owning property (dead person's share passes to the survivor)

Legacy – gift of money or property other than house or land

Life interest – right to enjoy the benefit for life of any property

Pecuniary legacy – specific gift of money

Residue – remainder of an estate after all legacies and bequests have been given and all debts, taxes and expenses paid

Testator – person making a will

Possible format of a will

1. 'This is the last will and testament of . . .
2. Full name
3. Full current address
4. Date the will is made
5. 'I hereby revoke all former wills, codicils or other testamentary provisions at any time made by me and declare this to be my last will'
6. Appointment of executor and any payments to be made to him
7. Any wishes regarding funeral, etc.
8. 'All gifts are subject to the payment of my just debts, funeral and testamentary expenses and all taxes and duties payable'
9. Legacies:
   'I give and bequeath (full details of gift) to (full name and address)'
10. Clause disposing of residue of estate
11. Attestation clause
    'Signed by the said testator in the presence of us present at the same time and by us in his/her presence'

If the will is long, the testator and witnesses should sign at the bottom of each page to help prevent forgery and also draw a line through any blank page and initial this. Numbering the pages will also reduce the risk of fraud.

The above paragraphs relate to the situation in England. The witnessing of wills is different in Scotland. The two witnesses need not be present together and a witness will not lose a legacy although the gift could be challenged. A holograph is also a legal will in Scotland. This is a will written by the testator's own hand and signed at the end without a witness. If a holograph is typed, the testator can write in his own hand 'adopted as holograph' above his signature.

Changing or altering a will

Situations change and it may be necessary to alter a previous will.

Both marriage and divorce invalidate a will (not in Scotland) and a new one will have to be made. Other changes in family circumstances may also make it advisable to write a new will.

If a simple alteration only is required, this could be done by means of a codicil. This must be signed and witnessed as for a will and must refer by date to the previous will.

Where to keep the will

The will should be kept in a secure place and the executor informed of its whereabouts. If it is in a safe or locked drawer, the executor should have the combination and duplicate key. If a solicitor or bank is named as executor, they can keep the will for you.

WORK AND OCCUPATIONAL HEALTH

Hard work never hurt anyone. How many times have you heard that? The fact is that the work you do can be an important influence on the state of your health. Work related illness ranges from minor musculo-skeletal disorders, caused by lifting or repetitive movements, right through to chronic and irreversible disease caused by exposure to toxic chemicals.

Occupational illness is probably more common than you think. The trouble is that it is not always easy to establish a cause. The clinical effects of most work-related diseases are indistinguishable from those of non-occupational ailments so your occupational history could be just as important to your doctor as your medical records when it comes to assessing the effects of work on health.

Take bronchitis, for example. There is a long list of industrial materials which are known to cause bronchial problems – from oil mists and fibreglass to wood dust and isocyanates in paints. But smoking is also a common cause. A persistent cough in a non-smoker exposed to such materials at work might arouse a doctor's suspicions; its appearance in a smoker in the same workplace setting could be dismissed as being due to his habit.

Asthma can be brought on by exposure to certain fumes, dusts or chemicals in the workplace. But asthma is also very common in the general population and some doctors now believe that the occupational causes may have been underestimated.

Certain groups of workers have long been recognised as being 'at risk'. Miners suffered pneumoconiosis, a debilitating lung disease caused by inhaling coal dust. Workers in the rubber industry were found to have a greater risk of bladder cancer while some asbestos workers contracted fibrosis and cancer of the lung. Doctors and nurses employed by industry have been able to recognise and treat a large number of work-related illnesses. Establishing cause and effect has often required painstaking detective work and a detailed knowledge of the working environment. It is only relatively recently that family doctors have begun to ask patients about their work; yet a person in full-time employment spends roughly a third of his life at work where he may be exposed to a whole range of physical, chemical or biological hazards.

He may be expected to handle heavy or awkward loads. He may work in hot or dusty conditions alongside noisy machinery and he could even be exposed to hazards which he cannot see or hear. Some industrial chemicals are dangerous at very low concentrations detectable only by using sophisticated monitoring equipment. Some commonly used chemicals are toxic or irritant, others can cause cancer. By the time the hazard has been identified the damage may have already been done.

See also section 7.10(d) below on Occupational disorders

There are very few jobs which do not carry some risk. Even those in 'safe' occupations like retailing or office work are not immune – but the good news is that occupational diseases can be prevented. The acceptance that work can be harmful to your health is the first step towards prevention. Next comes an understanding of the hazards present in the workplace. Once identified, occupational hazards can be controlled or removed.

Every employee should feel confident that the conditions in his place of work are not going to damage his health. In European Economic Community countries, among others, every employer is obliged by law to protect the health of his workers. New regulations in the United Kingdom stipulate that employers must make a thorough assessment of the possible impact of harmful or dangerous substances. That means looking at the workplace in detail and asking questions about chemicals used at work or produced as byproducts. It means identifying and measuring contaminant vapours and gases. It also means assessing the health risks from dusts and fibres in the air and it even extends to everyday items like bleaches, disinfectants, detergents and paints used at work. What are the dangerous substances, how and where are they used and what are the risks to health?

There are strict legal limits governing workers' exposure to chemicals known to be toxic, irritant or cancer-causing. These limits (which are usually expressed as maximum permitted doses during a working shift) are set well below the levels known to cause clinical effects.

Where potential health risks are identified managers have a duty to control exposure either by substituting a safer alternative, by enclosing risky production areas or (as a last resort) by providing protective clothing and equipment. They must keep a check on their controls by regular monitoring which may include air sampling or even periodic blood or urine testing.

These are the basic principles of occupational hygiene and it is fair to say that leading British companies have been putting them into practice for years. Good managers have an interest in keeping employees healthy. Occupational illness means absence from work and lost production and no firm, large or small, can afford to lose trained staff. To make sure this does not happen many companies employ medical officers or nurses specially trained in the recognition of work-related illness. Most of them are firmly committed to preventive medicine and provide regular health checks aimed at making sure that employees are fit to do the job and are not being affected by it.

Company health schemes are now seen as something of a perk. The Post Office and Marks and Spencer, for example, have recently introduced cervical smear tests and checks for breast cancer. This is not strictly occupational health, more an extension of the preventive medicine approach which has been pioneered by industrial occupational health services.

Occupational health cover is patchy in many countries. In the United Kingdom, for example, at least half the workforce has no regular access to a company doctor or nurse. The general practitioner may be the only source of advice on work-related illness and this, of course, will be only a small part of her total workload.

If you suspect that your job is affecting your health tell your doctor exactly what the work entails. Tell her what conditions are like and what materials you use. Your employer may be unaware that he has a problem and you might just discover that your work does not agree with you.

MENTAL HEALTH

Caring for mental health is very much like caring for physical health. People who do not care for themselves physically may find they begin to feel unwell or tired and listless. Similarly, mental health is about caring for your emotional well-being and being aware of the amount of stress under which you are placing yourself.

Many people think that having emotional problems is like becoming mentally ill; however, much is now known about the connection between the mind and body and how one can be affected by problems caused by the other. A good example of this is ulcers caused by increased gastric flow due to anxiety.

The stress that is placed on people in early adult life is quite considerable. This is the time of our lives when the greatest changes, both physical and mental, are taking place. Career choices, exams, decisions about leaving home, and/or starting a family all occur around the same time and this places individuals under a lot of stress. Research has shown that this is the time when the majority of men with long term mental illness will become ill for the first time. Women, on the other hand, tend to experience mental health problems later in life, usually in their mid to late twenties. This is thought to be because they do not leave home as early as men and face different types of stresses.

Thinking of mental health in terms of how individuals feel about themselves and their relationships with other people is a good starting point. Mental health is about individuals being generally happy with who they are and achieving their hopes and wishes to the best of their ability. It is not, however, about feeling inadequate or second best to others. All of us are different, and have different strengths and weaknesses, and one person's unique strengths may be admired by others. Family and other close relationships can provide much of the love, warmth and affection which all people need, but if these relationships make someone feel stressed or unhappy, this can begin to have serious effects on that person's mental health. Sometimes the solution is to begin to examine how to change or confront these issues. It is worth remembering at this point that individuals can only change their own behaviour, no one else's. For example, how other people behave can make you very unhappy, but it is unlikely that they will change overnight. If this is the case, perhaps it is better to examine the basis and nature of the relationship rather than responding to the immediate stress.

Most people will feel stressed by events at some point in their lives. Work pressure, financial worries, and relationship problems are probably the most common causes of stress, but it is important to remember that some of these stresses can be removed or reduced if recognised and changes are made to a person's lifestyle or attitude. Excessive alcohol consumption, smoking, and sometimes drug or medication abuse are methods which people use to deal with stress. However, these themselves can lead to mental and physical health problems. If you suspect that someone close is relying too heavily on these kind of 'props', try not to judge them but help them to seek advice or support to stop.

Maintaining a balance between activity and rest is an excellent method of combatting stress. Physical exercise or simply walking regularly instead of driving can help burn up excessive tension and make people feel more relaxed. Setting aside a short period of time each day to read, spend time on a favourite hobby, or just to unwind, are positive ways to combat stress. To people caring for young children this may seem difficult, but it is not impossible. Enlisting the help of partners, friends or relatives to take the children out so that you can go shopping or even for a brisk walk can make a great deal of difference.

Taking regular short breaks or holidays is another method of dealing with tension at work and provides leisure time to be with family and friends. Attempting to resolve the underlying cause of the problem, however, will be of greater benefit in the long term.

If you are feeling stressed or unhappy about your life, it may be worth seeking professional therapy or counselling. Counselling can take many forms, for example individual or group therapy, and many different approaches are now used. When deciding to enter this form of treatment, it is worth asking other people or health professionals if they know of any recommended counsellors, or enquiring at your place of work whether they employ a counsellor for staff.

The relationship that is built with any therapist is very important, but a useful rule of thumb is that you should not feel at all

See also section 7.10(k) below on Problems associated with tobacco, alcohol and other drugs

See also Chapter 1 for advice about maintaining a healthy lifestyle

See also Appendix VII for Addresses of useful organisations

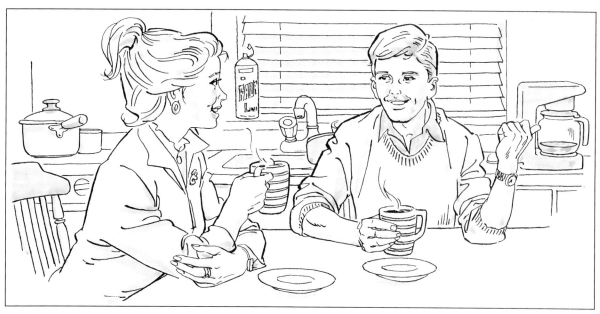

It is important to remember that talking through feelings with family members or a good friend can be very helpful

See also section 7.6 below for advice on Counselling skills

uncomfortable with your counsellor. If you do, it may be wiser to look further and find someone else.

Professional counselling is not something that everyone feels comfortable taking part in, however, so it is important to remember that talking through feelings with family or perhaps a good friend can also be very helpful. This may help you to look at your feelings and behaviour in a more objective way. This, in turn, may help you to make clearer decisions about your life and issues which concern you. If you find yourself in the role of 'listener', then giving someone time, space and showing concern for their well-being will help them feel they can discuss their fears and anxieties with you without being judged or criticised.

Finally, do remember that laughter is a wonderful way of reducing stress and trying to look at issues positively and constructively can help you to retain mental well-being and good health.

7.5 CARING FOR OTHERS AND ITS EFFECTS ON HEALTH

Caring for someone is both easy and difficult. It demands something of you and it also gives you something.

When you care for someone you are affected, both physically and emotionally, by this care. The way in which you are affected physically is often seen in terms of restrictions:

- You are tied to the house;

- You are with just one person;

- You may lose friends and any social life.

Your physical health may suffer because of the following:

- Lack of exercise;

- Lack of sleep;

- Frequent lifting of a heavy person which can lead to back pain.

All these points will vary depending on your circumstances. The problems of a mother with a young baby are very different from those of a mother or father with a teenager at home with a bad cold, or those who care for an elderly sick or confused person.

If you care for someone only for a short time, and you know that the end is in sight, you may be able to cope with broken nights, being tied to the house, and having your social life disrupted. Many people welcome an opportunity to care for someone intensively for a while for the rewards this can bring in terms of close contact with the patient, and the satisfaction of being of help.

The situation is very different when you care for someone on a long term basis. Again, it will depend on the circumstances. A major difficulty in caring for a physically ill or handicapped person is the heavy lifting that may be involved, from bed to chair, to bath, and back again. If you are in this situation it would be wise to have instructions on lifting procedures and to consider the use of hoists and other lifting aids. You should ask your doctor for referral to a physiotherapist and a community nurse who can help with equipment.

See also Chapter 2, section 6 on Help for the carers, and Appendix VII for Addresses of useful organisations

If you feel that you suffer from strain due to heavy lifting, or stress due to lack of sleep or exercise, you should consult your doctor sooner rather than later. Any such problem is easier to tackle when it has not yet become chronic.

The way in which caring for someone can affect you emotionally is also very varied. Some of the main problems often are:

- The relationship with the person becomes strained;

- Feelings of resentment, being used, taken for granted etc. can arise;

- You may have had to give up a job and now regret this;

- You may have lost your friends and feel out of touch with 'the outside world';

- You may be tied to the person and the telephone but with little to do and become bored.

Such feelings, when they cannot be brought into the open, can lead you to be irritable, short tempered or moody. Your temperament may change and instead of being kind and caring you become uncaring and help only grudgingly. This in turn can lead to guilt and worry. It is then often only a short step to either eating too much or too little, and to drowning your sorrows with alcohol. Instead of caring for someone, you are now also sick.

These are some of the difficult aspects of caring, and in order not to let them get on top of you you need to maintain your own emotional and mental health as well as your physical health. This is often not easy because it feels 'selfish'. It may not be that however, but rather a more realistic awareness of your own limits and needs.

Caring is never just done 'to' someone. Carer and patient depend on each other, give to each other, receive from each other, and fulfil each other.

Because of the very close relationship with the person you care for, the health of you both depends on the openness between you. This is obviously not possible with a confused or mentally ill person, but if you are at all able to talk with the person you care for then it will always be better to air any grievances. Much pain and misunderstanding is actually based on assumptions. Talking openly about what you see or feel to be happening will invariably help to get the air cleared, and both of you will get on better. You are not just caring for the other person as a body, but by making the relationship between you a healthy one, you are caring for the whole of that person – and consequently for yourself. This type of care is often the most difficult and delicate, but therefore actually the most enriching. You owe it to yourself to care for yourself. By doing that you help the person you care for – and he or she is then free to care for you in turn.

7.6 COUNSELLING SKILLS

The word 'counselling' is used a great deal today, and often quite wrongly. Counselling is frequently confused with giving information, advice, or guidance. These are all aspects of helping which can lead to counselling, but are not counselling in themselves.

Counselling is helping someone to look at a problem in such a way that he can explore it, and thereby discover ways and means of living more resourcefully and with greater satisfaction. At the end of such a 'helping talk' the other person is in a better position, emotionally, than at the beginning. Counselling is therefore talking with a purpose, with a goal; it is not just letting off steam. It is that, but more. Letting off steam produces a lot of energy, and if this energy can be directed into more positive action and attitudes, then counselling will have taken place.

The main elements of counselling can be divided into the following:

- The *attitudes* which you as the helper bring;
- The *model* (or process or sequence) which you use;
- The *skills* which are essential if helping is to take place.

7.6(a) ATTITUDES

In order to enable counselling to happen, it is first necessary to give the other person your full *attention*. This means being there in body and in spirit. In this way a trust will be created between you and the person you are helping which is imperative if any real work is to be done. You show your attention by the way that you listen. What matters is that you hear the other person rather than yourself.

You can really only hear the other person when your attitude is *non-judgmental*. Rather than making assumptions, you let the person tell his own story. You don't decide that he is such-and-such a person; you are with him as a unique individual.

Helping someone means being a person of *hope*. This is more than optimism. Hope is a kind of stubbornness that the person with you can do 'it', is worth it, has it in him. It means encouraging what is not always obvious and believing – despite what the person thinks – that he is good, beautiful, lovable.

7.6(b) MODEL

The main things to listen for in a helping conversation are the *feelings*. The person presents you with a problem: not getting well, not having confidence, not getting on with a manager. Rather than concentrate on the problem and look for a solution, concentrate on the *person herself* and on *her feelings now*. For example:

- She is not getting well – she is *frustrated*;
- He has lost his confidence – he *feels inadequate*;
- She does not get on with her manager – *she feels let down*.

The problem is not often presented in terms of feelings. Therefore ask: 'How do you feel about . . . ?' You often have to ask it several times before someone really takes this question in.

A feeling has a *reason* to exist. Someone is angry because of . . . , or happy because of . . . . As you search for the main feeling you hear a story. The person who asks you to listen wants to tell you a story, because there is a story to tell. It is often in the talking that a person can come to understand what is going on.

A reason is often something external: 'he did it . . . it went wrong . . . .' As you are with the person, try to help her to see if there is any *purpose* or *meaning*. Try to help her to see that it is not really a question of 'he made me angry', but of 'I am angry'. What does anger mean? In what other situations does she get angry?

When you have helped the other to 'personalise' the problem, then it is time to look for a *goal*. It is not usually a solution, but a goal to strive for. You can often not change a situation, but you can change yourself and how you live with that situation.

7.6(c) SKILLS

The most basic skill in all forms of helping is that of *listening*. This means *really hearing* what is said. Most of the time you listen selectively and only absorb what interests you. When you listen to someone's story you have to listen to all of it.

In order to show that you have listened well, you need to respond. This is often done by *reflecting*.

Simple reflection means repeating some of the words said:

> – I am really not feeling well today.
> – You're not feeling well?

This shows that you are 'with' the person, not judging and not jumping ahead, but wanting to hear more.

A more advanced form of reflection is often called empathy:

> – I am really not feeling well today.
> – You said that with a hint of despair in your voice.

This shows that you are acknowledging the whole person, hearing also what is not said, but implied.

An important skill is *challenging*. With empathy and care try to challenge any blind spots, any unwillingness to see reality. But this has to be done with care, and always with the positive aim of reaching a goal.

Goal setting is the skill needed when the conversation is moving on. You focus the talking, shaping it towards a main point.

Helpers often feel that they should or would like to have the (right) answers. But it is the person who is helped who has to give himself or herself an answer. It may be more useful for the helper to ask the right questions. Some of these, following the steps outlined above, are listed below.

• What is happening?

- What is the meaning of it?

- What is your goal?

- What are you doing about it?

7.7   **SAFETY AT HOME AND OUTSIDE**

7.7(a)   A SAFER HOME ENVIRONMENT

Most people have an image of home as protective, warm and secure but home can be an extremely dangerous place.

- Around one third of accidents requiring hospital treatment occur at home and most of these could be prevented.

You and your family can increase home safety in numerous ways, for example by fitting smoke alarms, and by developing an increased awareness of potential hazards such as faulty electrical wiring.

See also Chapter 5, section 10 for advice on Keeping your young child safe

First aid

A useful addition to any home is a well equipped first aid box/kit. This should be kept in a place accessible to adults but out of the reach of young children. There are several types of first aid box available; these can be obtained from most high street chemists and from organisations such as St John Ambulance, or you can make up your own, as described in Appendix II.

See Appendix II for more information about First aid

You and members of the family could also consider learning more about first aid techniques. Courses in basic first aid are offered by associations such as the Red Cross or various Ambulance Associations. The purchase of a first aid manual for use at home will be helpful, but always ensure that you buy the latest edition of an authorised version.

See Appendices VII and VIII for Addresses of useful organisations and Suggested further reading

Fire

House fires and smoke account for many injuries and deaths each year. The numerous measures which can be taken to protect your home and family include:

- Care with cigarettes and matches;

- Fire guards;

- Smoke alarms;

- General purpose extinguisher for small contained fires;

- Furniture of approved safety standard;

- Checks on electrical wiring with updating as required;

- Fire blanket for kitchen to smother chip pan fires or similar;

- Knowing how to get the family out in a hurry or protect them until help arrives.

Services

It is very important to know the location of the main switch/tap of the various services (e.g. electricity, gas, water and oil) and be able to turn them off in an emergency. A vital part of the electrical circuits in your home is an earth leakage circuit breaker which should be installed to prevent electric shocks. You should also know how to contact the various companies in the event of an emergency (e.g. British Gas or its equivalent for gas leaks).

Security

Feeling secure in the home is important to everyone but certain individuals may feel especially vulnerable. This will include older people and those living alone. The police (crime prevention department) are always happy to advise on matters of home security. You can certainly improve security by fitting adequate door and window locks, bolts, door chain, door viewer and a door phone where appropriate. Other measures which may be appropriate are alarm systems and outside lighting. You should always 'lock up' whenever you leave the house and consider leaving lights on when the house is empty after dark.

If you are away from home ask a neighbour to check your home periodically and move any post. Also be sure to cancel deliveries of milk and newspapers.

An area of concern, especially for older people, is a caller at the door who may pose as an official to gain entry. *All* unknown callers who claim to belong to an organisation *should be asked for identification* and where doubt exists the organisation should be telephoned for verification. Large sums of money are best not kept at home and cheque books, credit cards and the like should be kept in separate places.

The measures to keep intruders out are certainly important but you should not overlook the fact that *you* might need to escape in a fire. For example, could you open patio doors quickly?

Household chemicals

A quick examination of the house, garden and garage will reveal a considerable collection of potentially dangerous chemicals. The list is endless and includes: bleach, toilet cleaners, cosmetics, over the counter medicines, paint stripper, white spirit, poisonous plants, weedkiller, antifreeze, and battery acid. Obviously there is a need for many of these substances to be in the house but, with sensible precautions, you can minimise the risks.

- Only keep small stocks of essential chemicals.

- Dispose of those chemicals not needed; many local authorities provide a disposal service.

- Follow manufacturers' directions regarding protective clothing, dilutions and use.

- Consider removing poisonous plants from the garden.

- Keep chemicals in their original containers; many children have been poisoned by drinking chemicals stored in soft drink bottles.

- Where possible keep sheds and garages locked (this is also good security).

- Keep household chemicals in locked cupboards or, where appropriate, fit 'childproof' catches to kitchen cupboards.

Medicines/drugs

Most homes have a variety of prescribed and non-prescribed medicines which represent a real threat to safety. Obviously all medicines should be kept safely out of reach of children whose ability to climb and open cupboards should never be underestimated. Preparations such as brightly coloured iron tablets are commonly mistaken for sweets by children.

Medicines should always be taken as directed and only by the person for whom they were prescribed. Small stocks are advisable and medicines not needed or out of date should be disposed of safely. It is a very unsafe practice to store medicines in anything other than their original container.

Older people often need to take a number of different medicines and to minimise the risk of mistakes they should be discouraged from hoarding 'old' medicines.

See also Chapter 8, section 7(a) on Polymedication

Falls

Accidents involving falls in the home are extremely common. It is worth remembering that it is not just older people who are injured in falls. Preventing falls and injuries is very much a question of common sense.

- Use safety glass in doors and large windows.

- Make patio and other glass doors easily visible, e.g. with eye level stickers.

- Ensure there are no trailing wires.

- Lighting should be adequate, particularly on stairs.

- Carpets and rugs should be fixed and in good condition.

Kitchen hazards and food hygiene

Numerous opportunities exist for minimising kitchen hazards and maintaining food safety. These include the following.

- Care should be taken with hot pans – handles should always be turned inwards.

- Deep frying can be extremely hazardous so always have a lid/fire blanket available in case the fat catches fire.

- Store sharp knives in a rack or block.

- Electric kettles should have short or coiled leads.

- Wash your hands and work surfaces before preparing food.

- Use different utensils for cooked and uncooked food.

- Use only food which is in date and in good condition.

- Store food according to instructions.

- Defrost food adequately, especially poultry.

- Follow cooking instructions.

Ideally, you should never handle food if you have a septic lesion on your hands nor if you have gastroenteritis. In practice, this will not be possible for many people with families to cook for so alternative precautions must be taken. Any sores or lesions should be completely covered with a waterproof dressing. People with gastroenteritis must be especially vigilant about hand washing. Wearing rubber gloves to prepare food is a sensible extra precaution.

Pets

Many families derive great pleasure from keeping pets but they can present problems. Animals need separate bowls and utensils, and should be excluded from food preparation areas. Always wash your hands after handling pets or litter trays. Removing dog faeces from the garden makes sense aesthetically apart from the risk of *Toxocara canis* infestation to small children. Further to this it is a good idea to worm cats and dogs at regular intervals. Your veterinary surgeon will advise you on worming and other pet health issues.

Home maintenance (DIY)

Home maintenance can certainly present hazards for the unwary and many accidents can be prevented by:

- Using proper equipment, e.g. a stepladder rather than chairs for climbing on;

- Never using ladders when alone;

- **Gastroenteritis**
  An infection of the gastrointestinal tract resulting in diarrhoea and vomiting

- *Toxocara canis* **infestation**
  Infestation with the larvae of *Toxocara canis* (a small worm that lives in the intestines of domestic animals) can cause fever (occasionally leading to pneumonia or seizures) and loss of sight

- Reading instructions for decorating products, e.g. ventilation required during painting;

- Calling in an expert for work requiring special skills such as electrical wiring;

- Working in a tidy environment;

- Maintaining electrical tools in a safe condition;

- Minimising time spent in the sun (see the section below on Travel for precautions).

7.7(b) SAFETY OUTSIDE THE HOME

The list of potential hazards outside the home is endless and it is impossible to mention every risk. This part of the manual offers a few suggestions for precautions which will help to keep you safe.

Travel

Keeping a first aid box/kit in the car is a sensible measure. A few dressings and mild pain killers can also be carried in handbag or pocket. Stress and other hazards associated with travel can be reduced by the following measures:

- Careful planning;

- Allowing sufficient time;

- Checking timetables, weather, road works and other factors which may affect the journey;

- Wearing seat belts and protective helmets and clothing as appropriate (these are legally enforceable precautions in many countries now);

- Making regular stops during long car journeys for refreshment and relaxation.

If you are travelling by car, make some checks before you set out, and ensure that you have the following:

- Petrol, oil, water, correct tyre pressures, clean lights, full windscreen washer reservoirs;

- Spare petrol can and de-icer;

- Tools for changing a wheel;

- Spare tyre at the correct pressure;

- Maps;

- A torch;

- Coat and shoes suitable for a walk should it be necessary;

- Change for telephone and phonecard if appropriate;

- Membership documents/telephone numbers etc. for an organisation such as the AA or RAC to contact if your car breaks down.

Winter travel presents extra problems and it is sensible to undertake only essential journeys in extreme weather conditions. If you *do* need to travel in bad weather, however, the following additional items should be in the car:

- A blanket;

- Coat, gloves, hat, boots etc.;

- A spade and a piece of carpet in case you become stuck in snow;

- Flask of hot drink or soup;

- High energy food such as chocolate (only for an emergency).

Travel in hot summer weather can also be a problem especially if you are faced with long delays in an extremely hot car. Remember to pack your sunglasses to reduce glare and take plenty of water and non-alcoholic drinks to prevent dehydration. You will need to protect your skin from the sun if you are travelling with open windows or in an open car. Animals and people (especially children) should never be left in an unventilated car – not even for a few minutes. In such circumstances heat and lack of air can kill.

Travel abroad

Travel abroad is increasingly common both for business and for holidays. It is worth remembering a few simple precautions which will ensure that the trip is without problems. Fairly minor incidents, easily dealt with at home, can become exaggerated when you are abroad especially if you are unable to communicate effectively in the language of the country concerned.

See Appendix IV for more information about Immunisations

Well before the journey you should check which immunisations are required and if it is necessary to take anti-malaria medication.

Air travel is particularly stressful but this can be minimised by allowing plenty of time for the journey to the airport and the 'check in' procedures. Long flights can certainly cause physical effects such as 'jet lag'. You can help prevent these unpleasant effects by: wearing loose comfortable clothing, taking plenty of non-alcoholic drinks to prevent dehydration, eating moderately and moving around the aircraft at intervals.

Other health risks are considered overleaf.

Excessive exposure to the sun and high temperatures The risks associated with sunbathing and high environmental temperatures include:

- Sunburn;
- Heatstroke;
- Dehydration;
- Premature skin ageing;
- Heat exhaustion;
- Skin malignancy (e.g. melanoma).

Although this topic is discussed within the context of travel it is worth remembering that all the information applies to *any* exposure to sun. It is essential that you take the following precautions:

- Limit time outside (don't forget that this includes any time outside not just time spent sunbathing);
- Use a sunscreen which provides a high sun protection factor (SPF);
- Wear a hat and sunglasses;
- Restrict alcohol intake (alcohol dehydrates);
- Take adequate amounts of other fluid;
- Don't over exert yourself when environmental temperatures are very high.

N.B. Remember that sunburn can occur on a cloudy day. Wind and salt water both increase sunburn. Snow reflects the sun's rays and may cause severe sunburn and eye damage.

- **Gastroenteritis**
  An infection of the gastrointestinal tract resulting in diarrhoea and vomiting

Gastroenteritis/food poisoning This common occurrence can be prevented by sensible precautions. Eating unaccustomed foods, such as highly spiced or rich dishes, can cause an upset. It is wise, therefore, to limit your intake. In many regions it is advisable to drink only bottled water – remember that this also applies to water used for teeth cleaning. Always wash fruit and vegetables before use and avoid salads which may be contaminated. Do not have drinks with ice cubes which may be made from unsafe water. Resist the temptation to consume large quantities of inexpensive wine, especially the red which may cause diarrhoea. You might consider packing an antidiarrhoeal medicine to take if required. If you are affected by diarrhoea try to take plenty of non-alcoholic fluids and stop eating until the diarrhoea ceases.

Insurance Adequate insurance is essential for any travel abroad. It is important that you take expert advice to obtain insurance which covers medical care, transport home in the event of illness or accident, your property and other appropriate areas.

Personal security

Violent crimes against people are a worrying feature of our society but it is worth remembering that the vast majority of families are never affected. Women and older people may feel at particular risk from personal attack but there are several 'self-help' measures which can be considered. Some common sense measures which can help prevent incidents include:

- Avoiding certain districts and isolated areas (especially after dark);

- Not accepting or offering lifts;

- Not travelling alone;

- Carrying limited amounts of cash etc.;

- Attending personal safety courses such those organised by many women's groups;

- Carrying personal alarms;

- Arranging to be met at the bus stop or station.

Sport/leisure activities and exercise

See also Chapter 1, section 2 on Exercise

Many injuries occurring during sport and leisure activities could be avoided by proper preparation. Always consult your family doctor before commencing exercise, if you have a medical condition such as high blood pressure or consider yourself to be unfit. The following ideas should ensure that you gain maximum benefit from the exercise or activity without the risk of injury:

- Join a club or class to learn the correct techniques;

- Build up gradually; don't attempt too much too quickly;

- Wear correct clothing, e.g. properly fitting running shoes, gardening gloves to prevent blisters from digging;

- Never exercise if you are ill and stop if you feel unwell;

- Always start and finish gradually;

- Make sure you can be seen by traffic if you are jogging.

7.8   MID-LIFE

Mid-life is not easy to define, every publication you read uses slightly different criteria. For the purposes of this manual the period 40–60 years will be considered. It is important to remember that mid-life, in common with all other stages of life, should be a

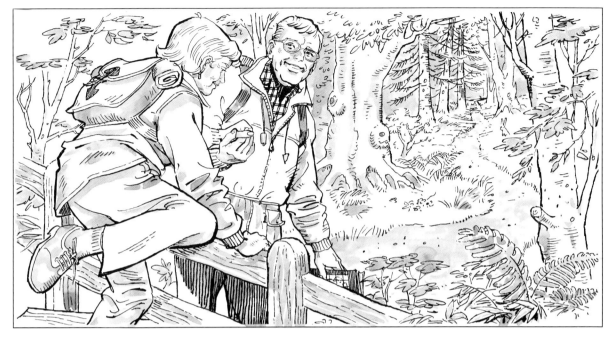

Mid-life, like all other stages of life, should be a positive and fulfilling time

positive and fulfilling experience. You will probably cope better with mid-life if you are aware of, and understand, the changes occurring in your body.

During mid-life you start to notice physical changes and possibly some decline in body functions. However, there are many 'self-help' measures which you can implement to maximise health. Care taken during mid-life often helps ensure that you enjoy a healthy and active retirement.

7.8(a)   PHYSICAL CHANGES COMMON TO WOMEN AND MEN

As you reach the fifth decade there are definite physical changes occurring which herald the events of normal ageing. The gradual decline in body function is normal but remember that it takes many years to occur. It is also worth noting that all individuals age at different rates and that the process is irreversible; there are no magic remedies for advancing age.

The ageing of certain body cells, although predetermined, is accelerated by physical and chemical factors such as radiation from the sun, alcohol, chemicals in cigarette smoke and bacterial toxins. Many of the diseases mentioned as part of physical changes are discussed in more depth in section 7.10 below and the appropriate paragraphs should also be consulted. The cells, tissues and organ systems of the body change, from mid-life onwards, in ways that include the following.

See section 7.10 below on Health problems also Appendix I on How the body works

- The skin becomes thinner and less well lubricated. It is more vulnerable to injury and wounds heal more slowly. Loss of elastic tissue leads to the development of wrinkles. There is a decrease in the amount of fatty tissue insulation under the skin and you feel the cold more. The hair thins in both sexes and loss of pigment results in greying.

N.B.   Skin ages more quickly when exposed to sun and wind.

- Muscle mass and physical strength start to decrease.

Osteoporosis is discussed in more detail in section 7.10(i) below

- Bone density declines (osteoporosis) in both sexes but in women it is most marked in the postmenopausal years. Lack of exercise is an important factor in the development of osteoporosis.

- Joint problems, such as rheumatoid arthritis and osteoarthritis, are increasingly common as mid-life progresses.

- The intervertebral discs (pads of cartilage between the vertebrae) start to shrink and by the mid fifties overall height has started to decrease.

- The nervous system is at peak efficiency during young adulthood. The gradual loss of nerve cells (neurones), which occurs from mid-life, is hardly significant until after the age of 60. However, you may notice a decline in reaction time, ability to learn new skills, decision making and memory. The effect of this decline is largely compensated for by the vast store of experience which you have accumulated over the years. Sensory function may also show some changes; taste and smell become less acute (especially if you smoke) and the ability to hear high pitched sounds is lost by the age of 60. This hearing loss may occur earlier in individuals subjected to high noise levels – at work for example.

Urinary problems associated with the menopause and enlarged prostate are discussed separately in sections 7.8(c) and 7.8(d) below

- Bladder capacity is reduced and you may find it necessary to pass urine more often and many individuals need to get up at night. Cystitis (inflammation of the bladder) continues to be a common problem for women.

- **Autoimmune diseases** Diseases where the immune system malfunctions to destroy the body's own cells

- A general decline in the immune system probably accounts for the increased incidence of malignant and autoimmune diseases from mid-life onwards.

- **Diverticular disease** Pouches in the walls of the colon

- The digestive system slows down and you may have problems with indigestion and constipation for the first time. Appetite may change as taste and smell decline. Conditions such as peptic ulcer (certain types), gallstones and diverticular disease all become more common.

- **Metabolic rate** The rate at which cells consume energy

- The metabolic rate falls during mid-life. This means that, in the absence of vigorous exercise, you will need less energy from

- **Glucose tolerance**
  The ability to absorb and use glucose efficiently

See section 7.10(c) below on Diabetes

See section 7.10(g) below on Diseases affecting the chest

- **Cilia**
  Microscopic hairs lining the air passages

See sections 7.10(e) and 7.10(f) below on Blood pressure problems and Coronary heart disease

- **Peripheral vascular disease**
  Narrowing of blood vessels in the limbs restricting the flow of blood and causing pain and injury to tissues

food (measured in kilocalories or kcal) to maintain stable body weight. Another change is a decrease in glucose tolerance. This change is reflected in the increased incidence of diabetes (usually of the type which is controlled with tablets and/or diet) during mid-life.

- The lungs become less efficient in exchanging gases and their capacity decreases. This is due in part to loss of elastic recoil in the lungs and increasing rigidity of the chest wall. If you smoke there are additional abnormal changes, e.g. loss of mucus clearance as cilia are destroyed.

- The heart and circulation function less efficiently. Unless you exercise regularly the heart does not respond well to sudden or sustained demands such as may occur if you run for a train. In our affluent society blood pressure tends to rise (hypertension) during mid-life. If this is uncontrolled, it may lead to arterial disease. The serious effects of hypertension and arterial disease (also linked to smoking, high fat intake, lack of exercise and stress) include strokes (cerebrovascular accidents) affecting the brain, heart attacks and peripheral vascular disease with gangrene and the possibility of leg amputation.

7.8(b)   SEXUALITY IN MID-LIFE

The need to express sexuality continues throughout life but the emphasis may change as you enter mid-life. Many individuals will be in a stable relationship and others may be single parents. Some people will now be alone: through choice, or following the death of their partner or the breakdown of their marriage or relationship.

- **Climacteric**
  The period of several years during which reproductive function declines. It is often mistakenly called the menopause which is actually the last menstrual period

The frequency of ovulation declines in women during early mid-life and finally ceases during the climacteric. Men, however, continue to be fertile well into old age.

The need for contraception continues until about one or two years after the menopause but individual women should consult their doctor. Couples who have completed their family may decide upon sterilisation (vasectomy or tubal ligation) as contraception. Older women, for whom oestrogen containing pills can be unsuitable, may find that the progesterone only pill will meet their contraceptive needs. Many couples continue to use barrier methods during this time. Problems with natural family planning methods occur if the woman has an irregular menstrual cycle during mid-life.

See also Chapter 4, section 1(a) on Family planning

- **Libido**
  Sex drive

Libido is unaffected for many individuals but for others there will be changes associated with mid-life. Physical illness, tiredness or anxiety can cause a decrease in libido in both men and women.

Some women notice that their interest in sex decreases during the climacteric but an equal number have increased sexual needs.

The physical aspects of sexual relationships may change. During and after the climacteric, women may have vaginal dryness which can make intercourse painful. This difficulty may be relieved by using one of the readily available lubricating jellies (e.g. KY Jelly) or oestrogen creams prescribed by the doctor. Men will find that the refractory or latent phase increases after the age of 50.

Impotence can occur at any age but it may become a problem during mid-life. Causes of impotence include:

- Anxiety;

- Tiredness;

- Illness;

- Excessive alcohol intake;

- Fear of 'failing' sexually;

- Certain prescribed drugs (e.g. those for hypertension).

In common with most other problems those affecting sexuality are more likely to be solved if you and your partner are able to talk about sexual needs and expectations. An informed and understanding partner will usually contribute to a solution. If you feel that expert help is needed with the problem it is a good idea to talk with your doctor.

- **Refractory phase**
  The time interval following orgasm during which further erection is impossible

- **Impotence**
  Failure to achieve and maintain erection

7.8(c)   WOMEN

Specific physical changes

The climacteric (a period of some years), which you probably know as the 'change of life', usually occurs between the ages of 45 and 55. It covers the physical and emotional changes associated with declining reproductive function and includes the menopause (most women have their last period by the age of 50). During the climacteric the ovaries shrink and become less responsive to the sex hormones. The menstrual cycles are often anovulatory, erratic and shorter but for some women menstruation ceases abruptly.

- **Anovulatory cycle**
  A menstrual cycle in which no egg is released

Changes to the uterus and ovaries

During the climacteric, the uterus and ovaries start to decrease in size. The surface of the ovaries will have lost its smoothness due to the release over the years of so many eggs

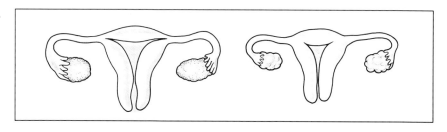

- It is important to realise that, for many women, these events cause little or no disruption to their lives.

The reproductive organs become smaller and fatty tissue is lost from the breasts. After the menopause, prolapse of the womb becomes more common and may be accompanied by urinary problems (e.g. stress incontinence when you cough or laugh). If this becomes a problem, you should seek the advice of your general practitioner, a nurse specially trained as a continence adviser, or the Association for Continence Advice.

The decline in oestrogen levels has two other important effects.

1. Postmenopausal women develop the same risk of heart attacks as men in that age group.

2. Bone mass is lost rapidly and osteoporosis is common in older women, who have a particularly high risk of hip fractures.

Some women are troubled by the following:

- Vaginal dryness, infection and painful intercourse;

- 'Hot flushes' and night sweats;

- Backache and joint pains;

- Insomnia and depression;

- Feeling unattractive;

- Loss of confidence.

Helpful measures

There are simple measures which may help such as wearing several layers of clothes which can be removed if a hot flush occurs and remembering that hot flushes are not usually noticed by other people. Many women find that wearing cotton night clothes helps to minimise the effects of night sweats.

Hormone replacement therapy (HRT) with oestrogens and progesterone can be prescribed to help women cope with some of these problems. HRT also has the benefit of slowing bone loss. It will not make you young again and it may possibly increase the risks of cancer in the endometrium or breast.

You should also be aware that vaginal bleeding will occur during the tablet free week (each course is 21 tablets followed by a seven day break) even if your periods had stopped. Women approaching mid-life should take the opportunity to discuss all aspects of the climacteric (including HRT) at the Well Women's clinic, with their doctor or at a women's self-help group.

Good health and a positive approach to the climacteric will help you to cope with this period in your life.

See also Chapter 2, section 2(d) on Eliminating, Chapter 8, section 6(b) on Urinary and bowel related problems, and Appendix VII for Addresses of useful organisations

- **Endometrium**
  The lining of the womb

See section 8.2(b) below for advice on maximising health in later life

7.8(d) MEN

Specific physical changes

The 'male pattern' baldness occurs in addition to the hair thinning which affects both sexes. Male baldness, probably due to the activation of a delayed action gene, is linked with the secretion of testosterone (male sex hormone) from the testes.

• **Testosterone**
The male sex hormone

Men have no physiological event which corresponds to the female climacteric and menopause. The levels of testosterone decline but fertility is not greatly affected. If men are able to achieve erection and ejaculation they remain capable of fathering a child.

Enlargement of the prostate gland (benign prostatic hypertrophy) is very common after the age of 50. The prostate is a walnut sized gland surrounding the bladder neck and urethra. It produces a small amount of fluid which, forming about a third of the volume of semen, helps to activate sperm. As you can imagine, any prostatic enlargement will cause problems with passing urine.

Urinary problems

The enlarged prostate may suddenly obstruct the flow of urine to cause acute retention of urine which requires immediate relief with catheterisation. The catheter may be passed into the bladder either via the penis or through an incision made in the lower abdominal wall which is known as suprapubic catheterisation.

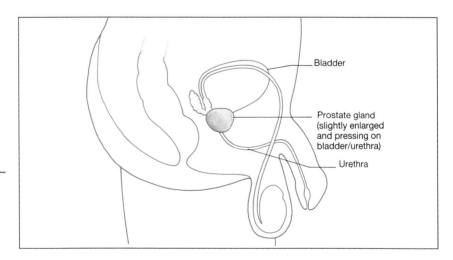

The prostate gland

If the prostate becomes enlarged the bladder and urethra are likely to be affected causing urinary problems

Less dramatic are the distressing urinary problems which include the following:

• Poor urinary stream (reduced force);

• Hesitancy in starting to pass urine;

• Dribbling of urine;

- Frequent need to pass urine;

- Passing urine at night;

- Pain on passing urine;

- Cloudy, offensive smelling or bloodstained urine.

- Ureters
  Tubes connecting the
  bladder and kidneys

It is important that you seek medical help as soon as you notice any urinary problems. An enlarged prostate leads to some urine being retained in the bladder. This static pool of urine increases the risk of urinary infection which is generally unusual in men. The infection may spread up the ureters to cause kidney infection which may damage the kidneys. Another serious problem is the backing up of urine in the urinary tract which, if unrelieved, will eventually cause kidney damage.

Prostate surgery

The treatment for benign prostatic hypertrophy is surgical removal. In many cases (depends on prostate size) it is possible to remove the obstructing tissue via the urethra (transurethral resection of prostate – TURP). This is obviously preferable to having a formal operation which involves an incision in the lower abdomen but sometimes this is necessary.

- Libido
  Sex drive

Libido and the ability to achieve erection should not be affected by prostate surgery if they were satisfactory before the surgery. However, the tendency for semen to be ejaculated into the bladder will clearly affect a man's ability to father a child.

Prostatic enlargement due to malignant tumours is rare below the age of 50 but increasingly common in older men (60+) where they account for around 10 per cent of all cancers.

7.8(e) MEASURES TO MAXIMISE HEALTH (WOMEN AND MEN)

Nutrition

Good nutritional principles for mid-life include the following:

*See also Chapter 1,
section 1 on Diet*

- Avoid obesity;

- Make sure you eat the correct nutrients in the form of a 'healthy' mixed diet;

- Reduce saturated fats and refined sugar;

- Increase your intake of unrefined carbohydrate and fibre;

- Include adequate vitamins and minerals as part of the mixed diet.

N.B.   Taking extra calcium appears to have little effect on preventing osteoporosis in menopausal women.

*See also Chapter 1,
section 2 on Exercise*

Benefits of exercise

Sensible, regular exercise has the following advantages:

- It is important in delaying the development of osteoporosis in both sexes;

- It will improve fitness and the function of your heart and circulation;

- It helps to prevent constipation;

- It improves muscle tone and posture;

- It gives the performer a sense of achievement;

- It reduces stress;

- And it widens social contacts.

Smoking, alcohol and drugs

*See also section 7.10(k)
on Problems associated
with tobacco, alcohol
and other drugs*

If you have not reviewed your intake of these substances recently, now is a good time to do so.

Health screening

This is an important aspect of health care and you should consider attending a Well Women's or Well Men's clinic run by your family doctor. Invitations to attend for individual screening tests, e.g. cervical smear, offer an opportunity to detect disease at an early stage when treatment usually results in cure. Screening tests and self-awareness measures recommended during mid-life include:

*See section 7.10(a) for
advice on breast self-
examination*

- Breast self-examination;

- Breast x-ray or mammography (in Britain this is offered to women aged 50–64);

- Cervical smear test (most experts recommend a smear every three years);

- Pelvic examination;

- General physical examination;

- Testicular self-examination is a sensible precaution although most tumours occur in men under 40;

- Weight;

- Blood pressure monitoring;

- Urine test for protein and glucose;

- Eye testing;

- Blood lipids including cholesterol;

• ECG (electrocardiogram).

Dental health

It is advisable to visit your dentist every six months. It is important, too, to pay particular attention to gum health as most teeth are lost through gum disease.

Recreation

Now is a good time to develop an interest, join a club or society, or to embark on a course such as an Open University course.

Rest, sleep and relaxation

It is important not to allow the concerns of work and everyday life to take you over.

See also Chapter 1, especially section 3 on Sleep, section 4 on Work and recreation, and section 5 on Stress

• Plan adequate periods of rest and sleep.

• Plan your work carefully, avoid long days and delegate tasks that do not need to be done by you.

• Plan breaks from work and proper holidays.

7.8(f) SOCIAL AND EMOTIONAL ASPECTS OF MID-LIFE

The most important points include: change of role (especially for women when children leave home), relationship changes, loss of occupation or early retirement, coping with bereavement, loss and relocation.

See also Chapter 3 on Normal life crises

See Chapter 8, section 4 on Caring for an elderly person at home

See Chapter 6 on The older child and adolescent

If you are caring for an elderly relative the information in Chapter 8, section 4 will be very useful.

People with adolescent children should consult sections 6.1(b), 6.1(c) and 6.7 which cover puberty and development plus areas such as behavioural problems and substance abuse.

7.9 **THE SICK ADULT**

The practical aspects of caring for a sick person are addressed in some detail in Chapter 2 of this manual. Organising a sick room, helping the sick person with the activities of daily living, suggestions on coping with pain and advice on moving and lifting the patient without injuring oneself are all topics well covered in this earlier chapter. There are, however, some particular considerations which apply to people in the 'adult' age group, as listed here.

See also Chapter 2, Caring at home and Chapter 3, section 9 on Sickness and body changes

- Most adults are unused to being dependent on others and many, therefore, will adapt badly to 'the sick role'.

- People in this age group usually hold key positions in the family unit (either as 'breadwinner' or as primary carer/home manager) so illness of any duration can have major repercussions on the whole family group.

- Short term and less serious illnesses are unlikely to be complicated in the way that is common in the very old or very young. Conversely, however, major illness or sudden disability is rarely anticipated so many families thus afflicted have no contingency plans to fall back on.

- Children expect their parents to be strong and unchanging. Severe illness, or even death, of a parent can have a profound effect on children which they must be given the opportunity to express. It is important, too, to be honest with children.

- Illness or disability on the part of one member of a couple, and the necessity for the other to take on the role of total carer, can severely disrupt the marital relationship.

See also Chapter 2, section 1, Introduction to Caring at home and section 7.5 above on Caring for others and its effects on health

7.9(a) THE SICK ROLE

An 'ideal' patient is one who obeys instructions, keeps cheerful, says 'thank you' and gets better. He must be co-operative, grateful and, preferably, not ill for too long. If you are caring for someone for a week or two, and can arrange for friends and other relatives to pop in to sit with the patient or listen to your frustrations, you will probably find that the situation does not get you down too much. You may be able to cope happily with someone whose temper is not always at its best, and who does not necessarily show you gratitude, without becoming at all depressed, run down or 'burnt out'. If, however, you find yourself becoming a full time carer for months on end, you will be an unusual person if your physical and emotional health is not threatened. Many people in this position find that it is made worse by the fact that the person for whom they are caring, and who is the direct or indirect cause of stress, is the very one to whom, in other circumstances, they would be turning for advice and support. Certainly, the sick role can sometimes be combined with that of the loving supporter, but more often this is not the case. Carers who feel they do not have adequate support should speak to their doctor or community nurse, or contact one of the appropriate agencies before the situation deteriorates unduly.

See also Chapter 2, section 6 on Help for the carers

7.9(b) WHEN THE BREADWINNER CANNOT EARN

See also Chapter 1, section 4 on Work and recreation and Chapter 3, section 7 on Retirement

A person who has to leave his job on account of illness or sudden disability is likely to experience a major crisis of self-esteem. This has been discussed elsewhere but a further problem accompanying such a situation is the effect that loss of employment or prolonged sick leave can have on the financial state of the whole family.

If a person's health is bad enough for him to lose his job, but not so poor that he needs full time care, then his partner may be able to continue or resume her career though childcare arrangements can be expensive. In some cases, the family's standard of living may suffer little, if at all. It is a sad fact, however, that women usually earn less than their partner, particularly if they have taken a career break to raise a family.

In most cases, an employee needing to take time off work because of ill health will be eligible for sick pay (for a period at least). The table gives details of sick pay entitlements currently applicable in the United Kingdom. Some employers make available more generous allowances and some people take out insurance policies specifically against loss of livelihood on account of injury or illness. Advice on other benefits which may be available in specific circumstances can be obtained from your social worker, your local Citizens' Advice Bureau or one of the appropriate specialist organisations.

See Appendix VI for more information about Benefits

Payments while you are sick

Statutory sick pay (SSP)	Sickness benefit
This, or an equivalent amount, is available to most employees in the United Kingdom who are sick for more than four days in a row (including at weekends), and who pay National Insurance contributions. SSP is payable for periods of up to 28 weeks. The April 1991 rates were £52.50 per week or £43.50 per week, depending on your level of earnings.	Certain people are not eligible for SSP. These include self-employed people, people whose SSP has stopped, members of the armed forces, people under the age of 16 or over retirement age, and certain other special categories of people. If you are not eligible for SSP but have paid sufficient National Insurance payments you may be eligible for weekly sickness benefit payments of £39.60, or £49.90 if you are over pension age (April 1990 rates).
See DSS leaflet NI244 for entitlement and leaflet NI196 for rates	See DSS leaflet NI16 for entitlement and leaflet NI196 for rates

You, or your family, may be entitled to other benefits. Check with your local Citizens' Advice Bureau and see Appendix VI in this manual. See also DSS leaflet FB28.

7.9(c) CARING FOR THE PRIMARY CARER

If the person responsible for the day-to-day running of the household becomes ill, the family is no less disrupted than it is by the loss of an active breadwinner. Often, indeed, the incapacity of the primary carer will force the breadwinner back into the home. Someone has to bath the baby, take the children to school, prepare the meals. If there is a fully supportive extended family network, or if an outsider can be paid to take on the household tasks, then a large proportion of the other partner's life will remain unaffected. In the event, though, of the breadwinner having to give up his job to look after a sick spouse, dependent children and the house, the problems of role change and radically altered family income will have to be faced – as in section 7.9(b) above.

See Appendix VII for Addresses of useful organisations and support groups

In many cases, where the primary carer is not acutely ill and where children are not too young, a family will manage to 'get by' with support from friends, neighbours and local services. Home helps may be available in some areas (ask your social worker or community nurse) and local voluntary groups may also have something to offer. Furthermore, some sympathetic employers may consider allowing the working partner to reduce his hours or perhaps introduce more flexibility.

However the family manages to reorganise its life, there is no doubt that quality of life will be adversely affected, to some degree at least, by the long term illness of one of its key members. Perhaps couples who take out insurance on the life and health of the major earner should consider placing equal financial value on the life and health of the partner whose work goes largely unrecognised.

7.9(d) SHORT TERM ILLNESS OR CONVALESCENCE

Fortunately, most of the readers of a manual such as this will find themselves caring for a sick adult for short periods only. Acute illness can be alarming, however, and you should receive full support from your family doctor. You will certainly be tired after a brief period of intense caring and, if your partner or relative has made a full recovery, he might enjoy the chance to take care of you for a few days. If this is not possible, try to be especially nice to yourself for a day or two as soon as you are able.

Short term acute illness, or a period of recovery following discharge from hospital, means that you as a carer are likely to need to consult specific sections and subsections of Chapter 2 (and various other parts of this book). The chart overleaf is designed to guide you, letting you know at a glance which sections will make useful additional reading in which circumstances.

If the person you are looking after is:	
Feverish	See Chapter 2, section 2(g), Keeping warm/cool.
Temporarily or permanently disabled	See Chapter 2, section 2(n), Improvising equipment, section 4 on Lifting and transfers and section 5(e) on People with long term disability. Also Chapter 7, section 12 on The adult with a physical disability.
Bedridden	See Chapter 2, section 1, Introduction, section 2(h) on Keeping clean and well groomed and section 4 on Lifting and transfers.
Troubled with nausea/vomiting	See Chapter 2, sections 2(c) on Eating and drinking, and 2(d) on Eliminating and vomiting.
Troubled with constipation or diarrhoea	See Chapter 2, sections 2(c) on Eating and drinking, and 2(d) on Eliminating and vomiting.
Having difficulty with breathing	See Chapter 1, section 5(c) on Breathing as a response to stress. Also Chapter 2, section 2(b) on Breathing.
Confused or suffering from a degree of mental disability	See Chapter 2, section 2(j) on Communicating and expressing needs and section 5(b) on People with a learning disability. Also Chapter 8, section 4(c) on The confused elderly person.
Recently discharged hospital following surgery	See Chapter 2, section 1, Introduction, section 2 on Helping the sick person at home with the activities of daily living, and section 3 on Coping with pain.
Depressed, withdrawn, anxious or unhappy	See Chapter 2, section 5(c) on The emotionally ill. Also Chapter 7, section 4 on Mental health, section 6 on Counselling skills, and section 10(b) on Depression and anxiety.
Prone to insomnia	See Chapter 1, section 3 on Sleep. Also Chapter 2, section 2(e) on Sleeping and resting.
In a lot of pain	See Chapter 2, section 3 on Coping with pain.
Terminally ill	See Chapter 2, section 5(h) on The dying. Chapter 3, section 10 on Bereavement and loss. Also Chapter 8, section 5 on Dying and death.

7.9(e)   THE SPECIAL NEEDS OF CHILDREN

Children of any age may be profoundly affected by witnessing any of the following:

- A parent in obvious pain;

- A gradual change in personality due to the illness itself or an unhappy response to it;

- The physical degeneration of a formerly strong, active parent.

Older children are particularly sensitive to social and peer group pressures and find it hard to cope with being different in any way. The child who cannot invite friends to his home for fear of disturbing a sick parent will undoubtedly suffer.

See also Chapter 3, section 10 on Bereavement and loss

A bereavement response is likely whether the child finds himself losing a parent as he knows her or whether it is merely his lifestyle that is changing. Sensitivity to children's needs is important. They should be given the opportunity to talk about their feelings and any questions should be answered as honestly as possible. Adults should try to pitch their answers at the same level as the child's questions.

This is an area where grandparents and friends can be invaluable as the well parent may be too preoccupied or exhausted to be able to meet children's emotional needs fully in this difficult situation.

It should also be remembered that children might find visiting a parent in hospital distressing, particularly if she is surrounded by drips and other equipment, or if she looks very ill, or is still suffering from the after-effects of anaesthesia or other drugs. Every attempt should be made to prepare children for the way a hospitalised parent may look, without frightening them unduly. Simple but reassuring explanations might help, for example, 'Mummy might be rather sleepy when you see her today because of some medicine the doctor gave her. You mustn't worry though, she will be more chatty again tomorrow'. Ask the ward staff for advice on what to say to children in specific circumstances.

Some children may show severe behavioural problems in response to a parent's illness. If this happens, your general practitioner may refer the child to a psychologist, or the whole family for family therapy.

7.9(f)   ILLNESS AND INTIMATE RELATIONSHIPS

The relationship with a spouse is the most important relationship for many adults. Usually, this will be the person to whom they turn in times of stress, distress or trouble. Such emotions will be compounded, therefore, if the partner is the one person to whom

See also section 7.5 above on Caring for others and its effects on health

the carer cannot turn because he is perceived as being the source of the problem.

Most good marriages or partnerships are based on mutual respect, trust and a knowledge of where the boundaries are. If one partner becomes seriously ill and needs a high level of practical care from the other, everything – traditional roles, power balance, all the familiar staked out emotional territory – changes. Some couples can adapt and refashion their relationship. Others will not be able to and the pain and grief that follow any break up will inevitably be deepened by feelings of anger, guilt and recrimination.

If one partner is acutely ill, chronically ill or disabled, sexual relationships are bound to suffer or even cease altogether. If two people can continue to talk and laugh together, and are able to find other ways of demonstrating their affection, their relationship may survive or even be enhanced. Many couples, though, will benefit from talking to a counsellor from one of the specialist organisations (such as Relate or SPOD) about the changes in their relationship. Seeking outside help is not a sign of weakness or failure. It requires strength and commitment to take such a step.

See Appendix VII for Addresses of useful organisations and support groups

7.9(g) PRECAUTIONS AND SPECIAL PROHIBITIONS

If the person for whom you are caring:

- Has recently been discharged from hospital following major surgery;

- Has a condition which can be controlled or exacerbated by lifestyle factors such as diet;

- Is taking any kind of prescribed medication;

then it is likely that the doctor responsible for him will have issued certain specific instructions. Such instructions will differ in each individual case but topics that may be covered include:

- How soon exercise/other activities may be resumed after surgery;

- Whether it is safe to drink alcohol or drive a car while the patient is taking a particular course of medication;

- Whether certain foods should be avoided, and if so why?

It is important to follow the advice given by health professionals in such circumstances but, equally, it is important that you understand the advice itself, and why it is being given. If there is anything you do not understand, or if you feel you are not being given

See Appendix VII for Addresses of useful organisations and support groups

enough information, then don't be afraid to ask questions. Many hospitals and clinics now give their patients information leaflets which can be taken away and digested at leisure, and some doctors are now using audiotapes in the same way. Other useful sources of information are the relevant society or support group and, for questions relating to medication, your local pharmacist.

7.10 HEALTH PROBLEMS

7.10(a) WOMEN'S HEALTH PROBLEMS

Menstruation

The complex functions of the female reproductive system are governed by a series of hormones, some secreted by the ovaries, others by the tiny pituitary gland situated beneath the brain, which operates as a master control. Every month from puberty until the last menstrual period the pituitary gland stimulates the ovary to release a hormone, *oestrogen*. This in turn causes a number of follicles near the surface of the ovary to mature until, near the middle of the cycle, one, further developed than the rest, releases an egg (ovulation). The empty follicle then begins to secrete a second hormone called *progesterone*, which stimulates the uterus to prepare for pregnancy. Unless the egg is fertilised levels of oestrogen and progesterone begin to wane as, under pituitary control, the cycle moves towards its conclusion. As progesterone levels in the blood fall the thickened, highly vascular lining of the uterus (womb) is shed as menstruation.

A 'typical' menstrual cycle takes approximately 28 days, with ovulation occurring around day 13 or 14 when the first day of bleeding is regarded as the first day of the cycle. Menstruation generally continues for about five days. There is a variable degree of pelvic pain, breast tenderness and often mood changes just before menstruation begins. However, all women are individuals and what is usual for one may differ for another. Thus, some women experience cycles considerably longer or shorter than 28 days, some bleed more heavily than others and the amount of pain and mood change vary.

In view of this complicated hormonal control, it is not surprising that at some stage during the reproductive years many women should experience problems or worrying changes in the amount or character of menstruation.

If you go to your doctor with a problem related to menstruation it is likely that you will be asked the age at which you started to menstruate, the length of your cycle, whether you experience pain, breast tenderness, moodiness or depression which appear to be related to menstruation, the number of days your period lasts and whether loss is heavy, with clots. You will also be asked about any pregnancies you have had. Knowing in advance the type of questions you are likely to be asked is helpful, as it enables you to think carefully about your symptoms, especially any recent departures from what is normal for you and how long ago change occurred. If you have just had a baby or recently changed your method of contraception compare what you feel like now to before. It may be useful to quantify the amount of loss by estimating the number of towels or tampons used.

The uterus contracts at the onset of menstruation, explaining why pain so often occurs at the beginning of a period. Some women lose more blood on the first day, while for others bleeding begins slowly, becoming heaviest on the second or third day. Sometimes fragments of tissue are shed from the uterine lining and this is normal. Large clots, especially when associated with dark blood, usually indicate heavy flow.

Painful periods Most women have period pains at some time, but the degree of discomfort and the extent to which normal routines are disrupted vary. The technical term for painful periods is *dysmenorrhoea.* There are two types, primary and secondary.

Primary dysmenorrhoea is most often a problem in a young women, before the arrival of a first baby. The usual complaint is of colicky pain in the pelvic area which can spread down the thighs, often accompanied by low backache. For many years no cause was known. Individuals seeking medical advice tended to be dismissed with reassurance that all would be well once they had had a baby. Today it is believed that powerful uterine contractions associated with primary dysmenorrhoea are caused by a group of chemicals known as prostaglandins. Medically these locally acting hormones are of interest because they are released by tissues following injury and inflammation. Anti-inflammatory drugs counteract the pain they cause. The simplest drug in this group is aspirin.

See also Chapter 2, section 3 on Coping with pain

If you suffer from painful periods you can help yourself by keeping a strict record of when your period is likely to begin and at the first sign, before pain is established, take one or two tablets in anticipation. Aspirin can act as a gastric irritant, or increase bleeding so paracetamol is usually recommended as the analgesic of choice. You may need to ask your doctor for a stronger analgesic if paracetamol is not successful. If pain becomes severe, then rest with local warmth such as a hot water bottle. A warm bath can be comforting.

- **Fibroids**
  Benign growths arising from the wall of the womb

Secondary dysmenorrhoea usually occurs in women from the late twenties onwards and is so named because it is usually associated with some other gynaecological problem such as fibroids or

SUN	16	
MON	17	✗ Day ① Headache Pains
TUE	18	✗ Day ② Pains
WED	19	✗ Day ③
THU	20	✗ Day ④
FRI	21	✗ Day ⑤
SAT	22	Day ⑥

SUN	23	Day ⑦
MON	24	Day ⑧
TUE	25	Day ⑨
WED	26	Day ⑩
THU	27	Day ⑪
FRI	28	Day ⑫
SAT	29	Day ⑬

SUN	30	Day ⑭
MON	1	Day ⑮
TUE	2	Day ⑯
WED	3	Day ⑰ Breasts slightly tender
THU	4	Day ⑱ Very tired
FRI	5	Day ⑲ Moody / tired
SAT	6	Day ⑳ Very moody

SUN	7	Day ㉑ Better
MON	8	Day ㉒ Moody again
TUE	9	Day ㉓ Tearful
WED	10	Day ㉔ Moody
THU	11	Day ㉕ Very moody
FRI	12	Day ㉖ ⎫ Moody + headache
SAT	13	Day ㉗ ⎭ + sore breasts

SUN	14	Day ㉘ Less moody. Headache, sore breasts
MON	15	✗ Day ① Headache Pains
TUE	16	✗ Day ② Pains
WED	17	✗ Day ③ Pains
THU	18	✗ Day ④ Feeling better
FRI	19	✗ Day ⑤
SAT	20	Day ⑥

SUN	21	Day ⑦
MON	22	Day ⑧
TUE	23	Day ⑨
WED	24	Day ⑩
THU	25	Day ⑪
FRI	26	Day ⑫
SAT	27	Day ⑬

Menstruation diary

sometimes occurs after an intrauterine contraceptive device has been fitted. Medical advice is necessary, because alleviating the pain depends on diagnosing and relieving its cause.

Heavy periods Heavy bleeding (menorrhagia) is another very common problem which can be painful, although this is not inevitable. Often the cause is fibroids or a hormone imbalance called dysfunctional uterine bleeding for which doctors have found no organic cause.

Menorrhagia is investigated by performing dilatation and curettage (D and C). The woman is admitted to hospital as this procedure usually involves a light general anaesthetic. The cervix is dilated gradually with a surgical instrument until it is possible for the doctor to investigate the size and condition of the uterine cavity, where fibroids, if present, are likely to be situated. A biopsy of the lining of the womb is obtained for laboratory examination. The woman is usually well enough to go home the same evening or the next day. A few weeks later she will return to the out-patient

• **Uterine cavity**
The inside of the womb

See Chapter 4, sections 3(a) and 3(b) for advice on recovering after a D and C .

- **Hysterectomy**
  Removal of the womb while leaving the ovaries to continue hormone production

- **Polyps**
  Small fleshy growths

clinic to discuss treatment options with the doctor. If her family is complete a hysterectomy may be suggested. Fibroids can sometimes be removed individually, but this is not always successful as they tend to recur. If the woman does not wish to have a hysterectomy she can be reassured that after her menopause the fibroids will regress and cause no further problems. There is no risk of them becoming malignant. For dysfunctional uterine bleeding hormone treatment is an option.

Women sometimes believe mistakenly that D and C is meant to cure their bleeding as well as to investigate its cause, but any relief is usually temporary.

Abnormal bleeding   Bleeding between menstrual periods or after the menopause is not normal and must always be investigated without delay. In most cases the cause is easily diagnosed and treated. The cervix is a common site for polyps which are easily traumatised and caused to bleed, especially during intercourse. They can be removed surgically and never become malignant.

Cancer of the cervix has been given wide publicity in recent years and can be a source of anxiety. In fact cervical cancer is by no means a common malignancy and today, providing premalignant changes are caught early, is entirely preventable. From the time she first becomes sexually active every woman should have a cervical smear performed at regular intervals. This service is provided by your general practitioner, family planning clinic, many Well Women clinics and increasingly by occupational health departments. If abnormal cells are found they will be removed, often by a simple procedure performed in the outpatient department.

Premenstrual tension syndrome (PMS)   This is the name given to the cyclical appearance of a cluster of symptoms before each period. Although first described over 50 years ago in the United States, most work has been conducted by the British doctor, Katharina Dalton, who painstakingly documented the physical and emotional symptoms appearing during the twelve or so days preceding menstruation. Her findings are summarised below.

PMS is now believed to affect up to 50 per cent of women at some time in their lives. Occasionally dramatic reports appear in the press and there have even been one or two cases in which a

Symptoms of premenstrual tension

• Headaches	• Depression
• Backaches	• Tearfulness
• Abdominal pains ('cramps')	• Irritability
• Breast tenderness	• Mood swings
• Fluid retention	

charge of murder has been comminuted to manslaughter because the woman pleaded that she was a victim of PMS at the time. However, surveys show that most sufferers endure more mundane yet trying symptoms: anxiety, irritability and depression rather than spectacular loss of temper associated with violent outbursts likely to result in crime. Age of onset is usually around 35 years, but some women suffer from their teens. PMS is uncommon among those taking oral contraceptives.

No single cause of PMS has ever been discovered, although hormonal and dietary factors have been implicated. There is certainly no magic cure, but women can do much to help themselves. The starting point seems to be recognising that a problem exists, accompanied by willingness to acknowledge it. Keeping a diary like the one two pages back will help to show what form the symptoms take and the days on which they appear. Discussions with partners, friends and members of a self-help group are beneficial, not necessarily at a time when PMS is actually being experienced. Self-awareness will enable you to understand your own behaviour and point out to those people important in your life that you do not set out to be deliberately wilful or difficult to live with. It is possible to find relief through crying, exercise or learning relaxation techniques. Anger can be worked off constructively by a variety of tasks, especially rhythmic ones (e.g rolling pastry, digging, kneading bread). Because of the possible link between nutrition and PMS a good diet containing adequate vitamins and minerals is sensible. Vitamin B supplements and a compound called gamma linoleic acid (which is found in evening primrose oil and marketed by health food stores as Efamol) have found popularity among women prone to PMS. Prescriptions are not necessary, but if you are in such discomfort that you feel the need to take tablets every month it would be wise to seek an opinion from your doctor. Sometimes mild tranquillisers can help and a diuretic may reduce the discomfort of fluid retention.

Vaginal discharge

Vaginal discharge, like menstrual disorders, is a symptom rather than a disease in itself. It can range from a mild, embarrassing condition to one both painful and intensely worrying. Sometimes there is a simple explanation. Could you be allergic to creams, bubble bath or soap you have not used before? Allergies to rubber (condoms), spermicides and even to washing powders from inadequately rinsed clothing all occur frequently.

Thrush (candidiasis)   The most common infection likely to result in vaginal discharge is thrush, caused by a fungus called Candida, which often assumes a characteristic appearance and has a yeasty

See also Chapter 4, section 4(c) on Minor disorders of pregnancy for more information about coping with Candida infection

odour. Some women remain prone to Candida infections all their lives. They learn to expect it whenever they feel generally run down. Those particularly at risk include women who are pregnant or menopausal and those taking oral contraceptives or antibiotics. Treatment with appropriate creams and vaginal pessaries (as prescribed by your doctor) is usually effective, especially if combined with self-help measures. Good hygiene and hand washing are essential and it may be preferable to wear cotton underclothes which can withstand laundering at a high temperature. Scented soaps and creams are best avoided as there is likely to be local soreness. Patting dry rather than rubbing helps reduce irritation, as will the application of a bland lotion such as baby oil.

Although medication is available without prescription it is expensive and, as one type of infection is often accompanied by another, it is wise to seek medical opinion. If you do not wish to consult your own family doctor, you could go to a Special Clinic where staff have particular expertise in the treatment of genito-urinary and sexually transmitted infections. You can telephone to make your own appointment and may even find that an appointments system does not operate, with people seen in turn as they arrive. The service is completely confidential and many people find it more convenient and efficient than seeing their own doctor, as the cause of the problem can often be identified during the first visit and treatment started straight away. Remember that your partner may need treatment too.

Urinary tract infections

See also Chapter 8, section 6(b) on Urinary and bowel related problems

Urinary tract infections are another common source of distress and again, some women find them a recurrent problem. You will be in no doubt about the symptoms: need to pass urine frequently, accompanied by burning and sometimes pelvic discomfort. You may notice that your urine appears cloudy, even bloodstained and that it has an odour. You must increase your fluid intake to at least three and a half litres in every 24 hours, drinking clear fluids rather than tea or coffee. Unless symptoms disappear swiftly, if your urine is discoloured or if attacks recur you must visit your doctor to be prescribed an appropriate antibiotic. Urinary tract infections are particularly common during pregnancy when hormones cause the tissues to relax, allowing bacteria to travel more easily up the urethra into the bladder. Sexual activity has also been identified as a cause because it encourages bacterial passage upwards into the bladder.

Valuable self-help measures between attacks include drinking at least two litres of fluid every day and emptying the bladder frequently, as bacteria will multiply rapidly in residual urine.

Breast disease

Breast cancer is the most common form of malignancy affecting women in Western society, so it is very likely that most people will either know or know of somebody who has developed this serious condition. The word 'cancer' itself engenders fear among the most stout-hearted members of the public and this has often caused women to deny the existence of breast lumps or delay seeking medical advice because they fear the worst. However, the majority of lumps turn out to be non-malignant (i.e. they do not spread and will never lead to life-threatening disease). Health educationists are keen for women to report abnormalities as soon as they are detected. Early diagnosis is the key to effective treatment if cancer is present and if the lump is benign, the woman and her family will be spared much worry. For this reason, women (especially those in their middle years) are advised to be aware of the normal shape and texture of their breasts. Breast self-examination (illustrated below) may also be sensible.

How to examine your breasts

Reproduced with kind permission of Edward Arnold (Publishers) from *Nursing Practice and Health Care* (edited by S Hinchliff, S Norman and J Schober), page 335

The breasts are best examined after menstruation when they are least likely to be affected by hormonal fluctuations

(1) Start the examination in the bath or shower, as the hands glide most easily over the skin when it is wet. Use the undersides of the fingers – they are the most sensitive. Move them gently over every part of the breast, checking for any hard lumps or irregularities. Use the right hand for the left breast.

(2) Much information can be gained just by looking. Inspect your breasts with your arms by your sides. Next raise your arms above your head and look for any changes in the contour of each breast, especially swellings, nipple changes or dimpling (when the skin takes the appearance of orange peel). Breasts are rarely symmetrical or the same size.

(3) Lying down with a pillow beneath the shoulder, explore each breast with the tips of the fingers in a circular motion. It is important to develop a system so that no part of the breast escapes examination. Finally, squeeze the nipple gently between index finger and thumb – discharge is abnormal except during lactation.

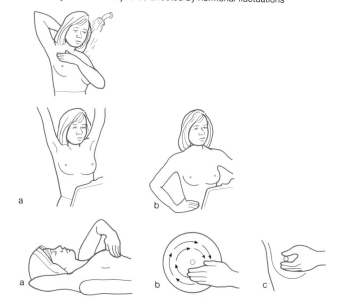

Remember that most lumps turn out to be non-malignant

See also section 7.11 below on *The adult with cancer*

Treatment for breast cancer has not received a very good press as it traditionally took the form of radical mastectomy – involving removal not only of all breast tissue but also the underlying muscle and lymph ducts as well. Much work has been done in this area however and a more usual approach today involves removal of a minimum amount of tissue followed in some cases by radio-therapy. The result is much less disfiguring and appears to halt the disease for an appreciable number of years. During this time the woman and her family can enjoy a good quality of life.

Regular screening does mean that the apparent number of cancers among younger women has increased but it is important to remember that breast cancer, like malignancy in general, can also affect older age groups. Older women who perform regular self-examination, undergo mammography in the event of discovering a lump and receive prompt treatment for any that are malignant may continue to live for many years – and indeed may well die of unrelated disease. In the United Kingdom, women over 50 are encouraged to undergo routine mammography which can be arranged through their general practitioner or local health centre.

DEPRESSION AND ANXIETY

Depression

Most of us could say that we have been made unhappy by events in our lives at some time. Sadness is a natural emotion, like happiness or fear. Sometimes, however, this same emotion can begin to affect our behaviour and the way we live our life.

The term depression is often used to describe a severe form of sadness which can occur either with an obvious cause or without any clear reason.

See also Chapter 3 on Normal life crises

Reactive depression   A depression which is related to an event in someone's life is sometimes called a reactive depression. This can occur following such an event as the loss of someone close, a divorce or separation, or redundancy. The accompanying feelings of grief and loss can make individuals feel unable to cope with aspects of their daily life and emotionally flat or empty. It is important to remember, however, that all such events involve a loss of some sort and the natural process of grieving should be allowed to take place.

Grief can take many forms. The person may feel close to tears much of the time, or feel angry and hurt, unable to concentrate on the smallest things. These feelings may last for days or weeks – it often depends on the individual – but gradually the initial pain will dull and, instead of focusing constantly on the loss, the person will begin to carry on with her life again. This does not mean that she will forget what has passed, simply that her feelings become easier to live with.

During the first stages of this process, it is vital that individuals continue to look after themselves even when they are feeling at their lowest. Simple tasks, like eating well, bathing, changing clothes and regular hair washing are worth the effort as they can make people feel better and enhance their self-esteem.

Clinical depression   Sometimes people appear depressed when others can see no obvious reason or cause. This form of depression is often referred to as clinical depression. Feelings of low self-esteem and worthlessness, inability to sleep or waking in the early hours of the morning are common, and if this becomes severe or prolonged a person may experience depressive thoughts which in turn can lead to suicidal ideas. In very severe cases, these ideas of suicide may be acted upon.

See Chapter 4, section 6(f) on Emotional and psychological problems after childbirth

Some new mothers may experience postnatal depression, which can be very severe. It will often be the woman's partner who first becomes aware of the signs.

Caring for someone who feels this depressed can be very demanding, and quite distressing. It is often difficult to appreciate the depth and severity of the person's feelings, but it is important to remember to remain loving yet slightly firm to encourage him to do as much as he can for himself.

In severe cases of depression, people often talk about harming themselves in some way as they feel it is too painful to carry on with their lives. Caring for someone who feels like this is stressful, but allowing him to talk without feeling guilty is very important. In this way you will retain his trust while showing that you still care for him and want to help. On a practical level, you can remove tablets and other medicines from obvious places, giving only the stated dose of any prescribed medication at the correct time. Above all, be honest with the person you are caring for, as he might think you are turning against him and feel more guilty or hurt. It is sometimes useful to say that you are removing these things as you realise how he is feeling but you do care for him and do not want to allow him to hurt himself. Explain that things may change in the future and you are trying to help at this time by making him feel safe.

People who feel severely depressed often say that the early hours of the morning is the worst time, when their feelings and thoughts are bleakest. This is something to consider if you are caring for someone at home.

Anxiety

Anxiety itself is a natural part of our lives. It is our body's way of alerting us to dangerous or frightening situations and preparing us for 'fight or flight'. However, when people are constantly anxious, they can feel so ill or tense that it begins to interfere with their everyday life and activities.

When caring for someone who is anxious or agitated, you may find it useful to try and teach her to relax. Pre-recorded tapes are now available which guide the listener through deep breathing exercises and help them imagine restful or relaxing situations. You should ask at your local library or health centre whether such tapes are available.

If someone becomes very agitated, and seems to panic, there are ways in which you can encourage her to become calmer again.

- First, remain calm yourself and talk quietly but firmly to the person.

- Encourage her to breathe slowly and deeply, counting to five at each breath in and each breath out.

- Do not allow her to move around the room but get her to sit quietly, or take her to a room which is quiet and away from noise or stress.

- Encourage her to sit like this until her breathing has returned to normal and she feels more in control again.

Responding to depression and anxiety

If someone close to you is feeling this depressed or anxious, it is important to seek help, as she may become physically ill by not eating and drinking, or wish to harm herself. In the past, treatment for depression consisted mainly of anti-depressant medication. This is still the first line of treatment, but now on a short-term basis. There are many other forms of treatment available now, including different types of therapy or counselling, which can be given on an outpatient basis or at home. You should ask the doctor or nurse for further details.

Many of the drugs used for treating depression are now prescribed in quite a different way to the way they were used some years ago. Although they can be very helpful in short term treatment, it has been found that they are not suitable for longer term use. If someone has been taking such medication over a long period, it is important that she seeks help to reduce her dose gradually as the original symptoms may reappear (the rebound effect) or she may experience other distressing side-effects.

You should ask a doctor or pharmacist to explain more about particular forms or types of medication if you are concerned that this may be occurring to the person you are caring for. Sometimes, the original problem which caused the drugs to be prescribed is still present, for example in cases of agoraphobia (fear of open spaces). If this is so, other treatments such as behavioural therapy are now available, and should be discussed with the doctor or community psychiatric nurse.

Following a depressive episode, people often need time to regain their self-esteem and you can help by giving appropriate praise for things they have achieved (however small), and helping them begin to regain their interests or hobbies. Sometimes longer term treatment may be offered, in the form of group or individual therapy to help resolve the underlying causes of the depression.

7.10(c)   DIABETES

It has been estimated that at least 2 per cent of the population suffers from the disease known as 'diabetes mellitus' or 'diabetes'.

What is diabetes?

Diabetes is a medical disorder in which the hormone insulin, which is normally made in the pancreas, either cannot be produced in the body at all, or is produced in insufficient amounts relative to the body's needs. This lack of insulin means that food cannot be used properly or efficiently by your body. In serious cases, the diabetes which results can be potentially life threatening. Part of the role that this hormone plays is shown in the diagram below.

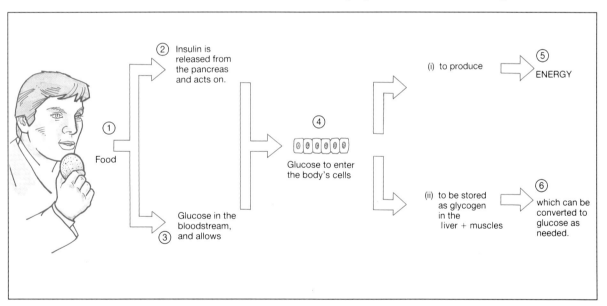

Part of the role that insulin plays in the body

Many things happen inside your body if you have untreated diabetes. Due to a lack of insulin, glucose (the simplest form of sugar) from digested food cannot be relied upon to provide you with energy since it cannot be transported from your blood to your cells. The level of glucose in your bloodstream becomes so high that some spills over via your kidneys into your urine. Since large volumes of water are lost at the same time you will notice that your

See section 7.10(a) above for more information about thrush

urine becomes very dilute, and you may have to go to the toilet far more frequently than normal. Because of this, you are likely to feel thirsty and you tend to drink plenty of fluids. You may also be prone to fungal infections, like thrush, which can cause soreness and itching. A common site for this in women is around the vulval area. Bacterial infections of the skin can often lead to boils or abscesses. If the diabetes has not been diagnosed at this stage, you may experience further symptoms. You will lose weight, because your body will produce energy by breaking down fat and muscle protein. When fat is broken down incompletely chemicals called ketone bodies are produced. These cause problems with your blood chemistry, and your breath may smell of 'pear drops'. Ketones will also be excreted in your urine. You are likely to feel weak and tired. Any cuts or abrasions tend to heal more slowly and are more likely to become infected. You may find that your eyesight deteriorates, and you experience 'pins and needles' in your fingers and toes.

The clinical features described above tend to be more acute in younger people, who will almost certainly require treatment with insulin injections for the rest of their lives. Older people, especially those who are overweight, present with more insidious symptoms. They may be diagnosed as suffering from 'non-insulin dependent diabetes' or, as the condition was previously known, 'maturity onset diabetes'. If your diabetes is of this type, you may not need insulin. If you are overweight it is important to eat a reducing diet. Tablets, oral hypoglycaemics such as glibenclamide, are often prescribed to lower your blood glucose level.

Diagnosing diabetes

If you are suspected of having diabetes, various investigations will be undertaken. A urine test will reveal the presence of glucose or ketones. A drop of blood can be obtained by pricking your finger or earlobe, and this drop is placed on a strip impregnated with a chemical reagent. The nature and degree of the colour change on the strip is analysed. If the reagent strip is inserted into an appropriate machine, your blood glucose level will be displayed. (Many diabetics keep this equipment at home.) If the reading obtained is higher than normal, you may be referred to your local hospital for further tests or treatment either as an outpatient, or as an inpatient for a short time. One test that is often performed is a glucose tolerance test (GTT). For this test, you are advised not to eat or drink from midnight of the morning of the test. A blood specimen and a urine sample are obtained immediately prior to being given a very sweet drink which contains a measured amount of glucose. At one, two and three hour intervals, further blood and urine samples are obtained. If your pancreas does not produce enough insulin in response to the drink, the analysed samples will be abnormal, and

See also Chapter 4, section 4(b) for more information about testing for diabetes during pregnancy

you will be diagnosed as having diabetes. Occasionally, abnormal urine test results are found in pregnant women due to changes in the way their kidneys work. This problem tends to settle down after delivery.

Treatment

If insulin is needed, it has to be administered by injection. This is because it is a protein, and as such, would be destroyed in the stomach. Most people are alarmed at the thought of injecting themselves but with practice (sometimes by injecting an orange at first) the procedure becomes second nature. You will learn how to store insulin and how to dispose of used needles and syringes safely. These syringes are provided free of charge. You will also be taught about the need to rotate the injection sites used, in order to prevent tissue damage. There are different types of insulin available, which may take different lengths of time to act, some then lasting for longer than others. For example, soluble insulin when injected subcutaneously starts to act half to one hour later, and reaches its peak of action after two to four hours.

- **Subcutaneously**
  Under the skin

Before discharge from hospital you will learn how to test your urine and blood. If you are unable to give your own insulin, arrangements will be made for the district nurse to help you at home. A consultation will be arranged with a dietitian and Diabetic Liaison Sister.

It is vital that food is taken after the injection, because otherwise your blood glucose level drops, and you are at risk of suffering a hypoglycaemic attack in which your brain is deprived of the glucose it needs to function properly. If you, or those around you notice any of the symptoms listed in the box, it is wise to take glucose in some form. Carrying glucose tablets or chocolate is helpful as if immediate steps are not taken to remedy your state, you may become unconscious.

See Appendix II, section i, for instructions on how to cope with someone who is unconscious

• Hunger	• Sweating
• Anxiety	• Altered or aggressive behaviour
• Faintness	• Blurred vision
• Palpitations	• Headaches
• Rapid pulse rate	• Unco-ordinated movements

Symptoms of hypoglycaemia

Once an ambulance has arrived and medical help is available, an injection of 50 per cent glucose solution directly into a vein will restore someone who is having a hypoglycaemic attack to consciousness almost immediately. Therefore, if you have diabetes, it is important to carry information with details of your treatment with you. An association such as the British Diabetic Association will advise you about this.

See Appendix VII for Addresses of useful organisations and support groups

If you find that you become unwell, for example if your temperature is raised, it is important to continue taking your medication and then have carbohydrates in a form that can be tolerated, such as orange juice. Contact your general practitioner because your need for insulin may increase with illness. Infection can lead to your diabetes becoming unstable and your blood sugar level rising dangerously (hyperglycaemia). This may necessitate hospital treatment which includes the replacement of fluids and body salts via an intravenous drip.

Controlling diabetes

The basis of good diabetic control is to balance diet, medication and exercise.

An appropriate diet will be arranged by the hospital or community dietitian. The number of grams of carbohydrate to be consumed in a day will depend on your weight, age and usual level of physical activity. It is a good idea to eat carbohydrates which will release energy in a slow and sustained way (e.g. wholemeal bread, pasta, potatoes and beans). There is evidence to show that eating high fibre foods reduces fluctuations in blood glucose levels. To prevent heart and circulatory disease a diet low in animal fats is recommended. Your diet should include adequate amounts of protein.

Associated complications

There are some complications that can occur in diabetics. These include kidney disease and heart disease. Eye problems such as cataract, glaucoma and disease of the retina can interfere with vision, and thus regular examinations by an ophthalmologist are important. Because circulation and feeling can be impaired, it is important to care for your feet. Daily inspections, maintaining cleanliness, cutting toenails straight across and covering any abrasions in order to prevent infection should be done. It is also sensible to wear comfortable shoes and avoid going barefoot out of doors. Chiropodists give priority to diabetic patients. It is thought that good diabetic control can minimise these complications.

There is no reason why you cannot live a normal life if you have diabetes. For example, if you enjoy exercise, a carbohydrate snack can be eaten beforehand to prevent a 'hypo'. You can carry insulin in the form of a 'pen' so that you can inject yourself before dining at a restaurant. Alcohol should not be taken on an empty stomach but is permitted in moderation. Smoking should be avoided because of its effects on the heart and circulation. If you wish to start a family your doctor may refer you for genetic counselling, due to the increased risk of your children developing diabetes. During pregnancy your insulin requirements will fluctuate and

See also Chapter 4, section 1(c) on Genetic counselling

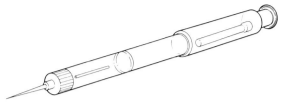

Insulin pen

need careful monitoring. Babies tend to be larger than usual but possibly less mature for their size.

7.10(d) OCCUPATIONAL DISORDERS

There are no reliable figures on the true extent of occupational illness. Workers can be exposed to a battery of industrial hazards from metal fumes to organic solvents, from mineral dusts to man-made textile fibres. There are physical hazards such as heat, cold, noise and vibration while work related stress can lead to psychiatric disorders and hypertension.

The list of harmful agents and associated occupational diseases is long enough to fill a whole book. All this short section can hope to do is to highlight some of the more common classes of work related disorders.

Lung disease

Most workplace toxins enter the body through the respiratory tract. Inhaling dusts, fumes, gases and vapours can cause lung disease and irritation or inflammation of the airways.

Workers often complain of eye, nose and throat irritation following exposure to dust and fumes. In many cases the symptoms disappear within hours of leaving work and the condition can be overlooked until an unmistakable pattern is recognised. Occupational asthma may also go undiagnosed. Some patients suffer an initial acute or severe attack but more typically they develop gradual symptoms (a recurring cough, for example). The list of sensitising agents is steadily growing and includes metal fumes and salts, a range of organic chemicals including dyes and epoxy resins and drugs like antibiotics. Wood dust and grain can also cause asthma.

The key to diagnosis is a history of regular recurrence of symptoms (coughs, tightness of the chest and breathing difficulty) with improvement at weekends and holiday times.

Pneumonitis Some organic dusts cause acute hypersensitivity reactions in the lining of the lungs, resulting in fever, coughs and difficulty in breathing. The symptoms resemble the effects of infectious diseases like flu. Pneumonitis is an immune response and includes conditions like Farmer's lung – a reaction to mouldy hay or grain. Irritant gases like ammonia and chlorine, and metals like cadmium and nickel, cause similar conditions which may lead to damage of the lining of the lung and airways.

Bronchitis Chronic bronchitis (persistent cough with sputum production) is common and often attributed to smoking but it can also be linked to occupation. Coal dust is a known cause. Epoxy resins and acrylic plastics have also been implicated. Some patients stop coughing when removed from the cause, at least in the early stages of the disease, so early diagnosis is likely to improve the chances of recovery.

Pneumoconiosis Long term exposure to certain dusts can lead to chronic lung disease where the lining of the lung undergoes permanent physical damage with thickening or scarring known as fibrosis. The changes show up on x-rays and the symptoms are progressively worsening breathing difficulties leading to an inability to work normally and eventual incapacitation.

The causes include asbestos, coal dust, silica (from rocks including flint and quartz), glass wool and china clay. Improvement in the control of workplace dust hazards, particularly in mining where pneumoconiosis was common, has led to a gradual reduction in the numbers of cases. But the serious nature of the disease underlines the importance of preventing exposure to all dusts.

Skin disease

Probably the most common type of work-related disorder is occupational dermatitis. Skin conditions affect many thousands of workers each year and the vast number of potential causes can sometimes make diagnosis difficult.

Chemical agents are responsible for most skin problems in industry. Many chemicals are irritants, producing lesions at the site of contact. Alkalis seem to produce the most problems but the list of skin irritants is very long and includes most acids, metals, salt and solvents like turpentine.

Other chemicals cause a type of hypersensitivity reaction (allergic contact dermatitis). The sensitising chemical passes through the outer layer of the skin and sets up an immunological response and the production of antibodies. A skin reaction will then occur whenever the sufferer comes into contact with the sensitiser and rashes can form away from the site of initial contact. Sensitisers include dyes, photographic developers, insecticides, oils and synthetic resins like vinyl and polyester.

Whether a skin rash is caused by an irritant or a sensitiser, the effect is much the same. Redness and inflammation of the skin is followed by the formation of small blisters called vesicles which burst to form a weeping wound. A crust may form over the area as the condition begins to heal.

It is not just industrial chemicals which cause dermatitis. Natural plant compounds are a common cause of skin conditions in farmers, gardeners and florists. Tulip and daffodil pickers suffer painful blisters around and under the finger nails. Some types of wood dust can cause dermatitis in carpenters, machinists and cabinet makers.

There are physical causes of skin disease too. Friction and pressure can produce abnormal hardening of the skin called callosities. Cuts and abrasions can become infected and may allow harmful chemicals through the skin. Heat and prolonged sweating can cause skin rashes while cold causes chilblains. Exposure to sunlight can lead to ageing of the skin and even skin cancer.

Occupational cancers

Work-related cancers can attack a number of different sites including the bladder, stomach, liver and lungs. What makes these tumours difficult to prevent is the long period between initial contact or exposure to the cancer-causing agent and the appearance of the disease. It might be 20 or even 30 years before the cancer is identified and proving an occupational link after all that time is very difficult. The cancer risk from a new material could go unnoticed until a generation of workers have been exposed to it.

- **Carcinogens**
  Cancer-causing substances

Nevertheless, a number of chemicals have been shown to cause tumours and many others are under suspicion. Known carcinogens include β-naphthalene which was found to cause bladder cancer and was banned in 1949. Vinyl chloride was found to cause liver cancer while nickel and asbestos have been implicated in cancer of the lung. Ionising radiation (from x-rays, plutonium and nuclear power production) is a cause of leukaemia. Mineral oils have been shown to induce skin cancers.

Suspected carcinogens can be tested on laboratory animals. Positive results will at least give an indication that the material could cause cancer in humans and should be treated with extreme care. Substances with a similar chemical structure to known carcinogens may also be suspected and marked up for investigation.

Reproductive disorders

The increasing number of women going out to work has highlighted a very sensitive area of occupational health – the risk of damage to the reproductive system and any unborn child. Women employed in the chemical and pharmaceutical industries may be particularly at risk. Miscarriage, fetal abnormalities and low birth weight have all been linked to chemical agents. Several studies have shown an association between waste anaesthetic gases and stillbirths. Organic solvents are thought to cause fetal abnormalities such as cleft palate and disorders of the nervous system. Handling cytotoxic drugs could cause miscarriage.

Clearly, it is important for women in the early stages of pregnancy, or planning to become pregnant, to seek counselling on occupational risks. A job transfer for the duration of the pregnancy might be advisable. Failing that, very careful control of exposure to chemicals might be needed.

It is not just women who can suffer reproductive disorders. Some chemicals are known to affect male fertility either by lowering sperm counts or by inducing abnormal development of the sperm. Carbon disulphide, lead and cytotoxic drugs all produce lower sperm counts. Heat and radiation can have the same effect.

Cancer in childhood has been linked with parental exposure to workplace chemicals.

Poisons

Industrial poisons are too numerous to list here but there are three main types:

- Metals (e.g. lead, cadmium, nickel and zinc);

- Carbon compounds (e.g. benzene, carbon tetrachloride and tetrachloroethylene);

- Gases like hydrogen sulphide, chlorine and sulphur dioxide.

Different poisons affect different sites – stomach, lungs, liver, kidney or even the brain. The symptoms range from vomiting, dizziness and headaches to asphyxiation, kidney failure, nervous disorders and death.

Musculo-skeletal disorders

Much attention in recent years has been paid to aches and pains caused by repetitive movements of the muscles and joints, particularly elbows, wrists and shoulders. There is a group of related conditions which have been termed repetitive strain injuries (RSI). They are not new but there has been a blaze of publicity surrounding computer and word processor keyboards with many operators complaining of pain and stiffness of the wrists (tenosynovitis), new technology's answer to writer's cramp. Improved keyboard design and regular work breaks can reduce the problem. Supermarket checkout operators are also prone to RSI.

See also section 7.10(j) below for more information about back pain

Far more serious in terms of lost working days and long-term disability is back pain. Injury caused by lifting heavy or awkward loads is all too common and is nearly always avoidable. Delivery men and storemen are at risk but so too are nurses. Many have been forced to leave nursing because of back injuries caused by lifting patients.

Stress

See also Chapter 1, section 4 on Work and recreation and section 5 on Stress

Finally a few words on stress, the scourge of modern living. Work related stress is very often mixed up with worrying events at home – illness, bereavement, divorce or financial worries. But too much responsibility at work can lead to depression or anxiety. Fear of being unable to keep up with the demands of the job can be a potent stressor. Some people thrive on a challenge, others feel unable to cope and work performance and health can suffer.

Stress can be caused by failure to relate to colleagues or the inability to delegate responsiblity to others. Some workers are unsure of the aims of the job or may find conflicting demands within it. Lack of participation in decision making and lack of job security can also lead to stress.

7.10(e)   BLOOD PRESSURE PROBLEMS

Every time your heart beats, blood is ejected from it and is pushed into the major arteries of the body. The force of blood against the walls of these blood vessels is known as the blood pressure. Maintaining a normal blood pressure is vital, chiefly in order to ensure that your brain, as well as other important organs of your body, is supplied with blood.

A person's blood pressure is checked by the use of a stethoscope and a sphygmomanometer. For convenience, blood pressure is measured in millimetres of mercury (mmHg). The procedure for having this test undertaken is shown in the accompanying illustrated box.

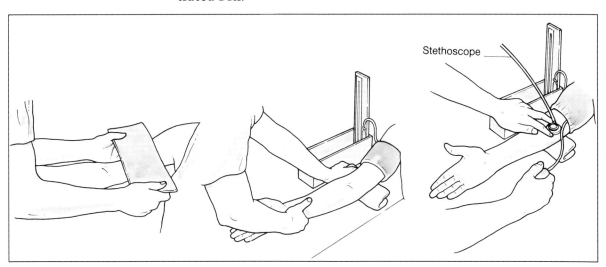

Stethoscope

Medical opinions vary, but a person's blood pressure can be considered to be within normal limits if the systolic reading is 140 mmHg or lower, and the diastolic reading is 90 mmHg or less. If your blood pressure is found to be slightly elevated, your doctor will arrange for further measurements to be made over a period of weeks or months. This is because factors such as exercise and anxiety can affect each reading and may give a falsely elevated result. It is only when a person's blood pressure is consistently high that an accurate diagnosis of high blood pressure (hypertension) is made. If, however, a very high reading is obtained, investigations and treatment are likely to be commenced without delay.

The effects of high blood pressure on health

Generally speaking, a person who has high blood pressure will not complain of any symptoms. This is a potentially dangerous situation because undetected, and consequently untreated, high blood pressure has been shown to be linked to a reduction in life expectancy. A person's health can be adversely affected by high blood pressure in many ways. Firstly, the heart muscle enlarges in order to try to cope with its excessive workload, and heart failure may result in the long term. High blood pressure is a contributory factor in the formation of rough atheromata in the linings of blood vessels. These can restrict blood flow to an organ. The roughened blood vessels are also potential sites for the unwanted formation of blood clots. One example of this occurs when the coronary arteries which supply blood to the heart muscle become narrowed, causing angina, or become blocked when a clot lodges in one of them. In this case, the heart muscle beyond the blockage dies. This is what happens during a heart attack.

A person who has high blood pressure has an increased risk of suffering a stroke, which may lead to disability on one side of the body and possible speech problems. This can happen if any of the arteries which supply the brain become narrowed and blocked, causing damage and death of the brain cells beyond the point of blockage. This is usually caused by a blood clot which may have formed at the site of a roughened lining of a blood vessel or, more rarely, by the breaking off of a portion of a clot situated in another part of the body, such as the heart wall after a heart attack. High blood pressure can also cause a person to suffer a stroke by increasing the chance of bursting a wall of a weakened blood vessel within the brain. If you have a family history of stroke it is helpful to undergo regular blood pressure checks, so that potential problems can be anticipated and prevented.

In the long term, high blood pressure is likely to result in kidney failure. Damage to the blood vessels of the eyes can also occur due to high blood pressure.

- **Atheromata**
  Fatty plaques

See section 7.10(f) below on Coronary heart disease

Treatment

If your blood pressure has been found to be consistently raised, three steps are likely to be taken in order to deal effectively with this situation.

Investigations   The first of these is to investigate any medical problem underlying the high blood pressure. The doctor will examine the blood vessels at the back of your eyes using an instrument called an ophthalmoscope. The state of these tiny vessels give an indication of the state of other blood vessels in other areas of your body, which cannot be observed directly.

There is a rare form of high blood pressure (malignant hypertension) in which damage to these blood vessels is severe and, together with other clinical features, can lead to a poor outcome for a patient, despite treatment.

An ECG may reveal enlargement of the heart due to the effect of high blood pressure, or evidence of angina, or evidence of a previous heart attack.

- **ECG**
  An electrocardiogram or heart tracing

Since many medical causes of high blood pressure are linked to disorders of the kidneys, several investigations may be undertaken in this area. They can be done on an outpatient basis at your local hospital, or you may be admitted for a short time. A sample of urine is tested to exclude the presence of protein, because kidney damage may cause protein to leak out into the urine. Blood tests will also help in establishing a diagnosis. You may be asked to save your urine for periods of 24 hours. This again assesses how well your kidneys are working. A 24 hour urine collection can exclude the possibility of your having a rare benign tumour of the adrenal glands which secretes excessive amounts of a hormone which raises blood pressure, causing headache, palpitations and sweating. Kidney x-rays and scans may also be undertaken to aid diagnosis.

In over 90 per cent of people suffering from high blood pressure, however, no cause is found for the condition. This is known as 'essential hypertension'.

Modifications to lifestyle   The second step in dealing with high blood pressure is to ensure that your lifestyle does not predispose to its occurrence. For example, being overweight makes your heart work harder in order to pump out blood against an increased pressure. Reducing your weight will help to lower your blood pressure. For a person with high blood pressure, risks to health can increase if you smoke, or eat foods high in saturated fats (as found in butter, many types of cheese and red meat). Excessive alcohol intake will contribute to health problems.

Although stress in moderation enhances a person's performance, excessive stress may cause a rise in blood pressure. Many people find that using relaxation techniques and meditation is of use in combatting this excessive stress. The need to exclude salt from your diet in reducing high blood pressure is not proven, but it may be a good idea to reduce the amount you use. A diet rich in fresh fruits and vegetables has a high potassium content and this may play a role in keeping your blood pressure within normal limits. Undertaking moderate amounts of exercise is important in toning up the efficiency of your heart and circulation.

If you are expecting a baby your blood pressure may rise towards the end of pregnancy. If this is accompanied by ankle swelling and protein in the urine, labour may be induced, or the baby delivered by a caesarean operation.

See also Chapter 4, section 4(d) on Complications of pregnancy

Medication Tablets can be prescribed to treat high blood pressure. They are generally required on a long term basis, although the dosage is often reduced with advancing age. You may be prescribed diuretics, or 'water tablets', such as frusemide. This increases the excretion of excess water and salt from the body, hence reducing your blood pressure. Potassium supplements may be needed with some diuretics.

See also Appendix III for more information about Drugs and medicines

Another type of drug used in the treatment of high blood pressure comes from the group called beta-blockers, which includes propranolol. This works by reducing the effect of adrenaline on the heart and small blood vessels. It should not be taken if you suffer from asthma. Similar drugs called alpha-blockers, such as prazosin, may be combined with other treatments. Some people may initially feel a little light headed on starting treatment with blood pressure tablets. If this happens, it is helpful to stand or sit up gradually to prevent faintness. Checks of your blood pressure may be made in both lying and standing positions if this happens, and treatment may be modified. Sexual problems, such as loss of erection, can occur, but the problem resolves with a change in treatment.

Many other types of tablets can be prescribed. They include drugs such as ACE inhibitors and calcium antagonists.

It is useful to keep a record of your treatment. Other drugs may interfere with the effects of the blood pressure tablets. These include MAOI drugs used to treat depression, NSAIDs for arthritic problems, and 'over the counter' cold remedies.

7.10(f)   CORONARY HEART DISEASE

Coronary heart disease kills more people in the United Kingdom than any other disease. It causes far more deaths than road traffic accidents, cancer and other diseases such as AIDS. The death rate from coronary heart disease is now said to be in excess of 300,000 people each year; truly an epidemic. Recent figures seem to suggest growing public awareness of the risk factors which predispose to coronary heart disease and that the death rate figures may have reached a peak and are decreasing slightly.

The structure and function of the heart is described in some detail elsewhere in this book. Readers may find it useful to refer to the relevant pages before continuing with this section.

Arteriosclerosis is thickening and hardening of the artery walls with a build up of fatty-like deposits on the inner lining. This can reduce blood supply to the myocardium (ischaemia), causing the chest pain of angina. A clot or thrombus may form on this narrowed area in one or more of the coronary arteries (coronary thrombosis), blocking the artery and resulting in a total deprivation of blood to the myocardium. This causes the death of the myocardium, known as 'myocardial infarction' or heart attack.

Risk factors

Arteriosclerosis can happen in any artery in the body. When it happens in the heart's arteries, it is called coronary heart disease. Certain factors predispose to the development of arteriosclerosis and some of these factors cannot be changed. These include age, sex (gender), diabetes and family history. Other risk factors can be altered – for example, smoking, high blood pressure, hyperlipidaemia, stress and obesity.

Epidemiology studies

Epidemiologists have shown in various studies that the chance of coronary heart disease is increased even more when the risk factors are combined. So if you are an overweight smoker with high blood pressure, your life expectancy is far less than someone who has only one risk factor. The more risk factors you eliminate, the longer you will live.

Social class   Coronary heart disease has always seemed a disease of the middle-aged, reasonably wealthy male executive. This stereotype is now being exposed as false. Coronary heart disease is now more prevalent among manual workers, people on low incomes, those who are unemployed or from the lower levels of the social structure.

There has been a definite drop in the death rate among wealthy people and those from higher social classes. This could partly be due to being better informed and educated about health, and not just because of better opportunities to enjoy a healthier lifestyle.

See Appendix I, How the body works, section viii on Blood and the circulatory system

- **Myocardium**
  Heart muscle

- **Hyperlipidaemia**
  High levels of serum fats

RISK FACTORS FOR HEART DISEASE

Age	The older you become, the greater the risk of developing heart disease, partly because arteriosclerosis occurs as a part of the ageing process and partly because you have been exposed to other risk factors for longer.
Sex (gender)	Men are more likely to suffer from heart disease than women, although the risks even out as women reach the menopause and apparently lose hormonal protection.
Family history	If your mother or father has died from coronary heart disease, you are at much greater risk of getting the disease yourself than if your parents lived a long, healthy life. If you know that one of your parents died at a young age from heart disease, make sure that you have a thorough health check. A proper health screening will help you to identify and reduce your own risk factors and could extend your life.
Diabetes	Due to the nature of diabetes, diabetics run a two to three times higher risk of developing coronary heart disease than non-diabetics.
Smoking	Smoking is believed to be the major single risk factor, whether self-inflicted or inflicted on others through passive smoking, which if eliminated would lead to increased life expectancy. The nicotine in cigarettes can cause spasm of the coronary arteries; the carbon monoxide produced by tobacco acts on the blood by reducing its capacity to carry oxygen.
Hypertension	Hypertension (high blood pressure) increases the workload of the heart muscle because the heart has to fight to force out blood against a higher resistance. If left untreated hypertension will quickly lead to coronary heart disease. The causes of hypertension are not fully understood but certain factors such as obesity, stress, and hereditary factors may have a part to play. A high salt intake can lead to hypertension – change to a low sodium salt.
Hyperlipidaemia	High levels of serum fats (cholesterol and triglycerides) lead to coronary heart disease. The main reason for high serum fat levels seems to be hereditary. Changing the diet, for example by reducing the amount of fat, will have some effect, but only very little, in reducing the serum levels. The main option for treatment is drug therapy.
Stress	In itself stress may not be a factor that predisposes to coronary heart disease. However, in combination with other predisposing risk factors, it may increase the likelihood of coronary heart disease. So reducing your stress levels could also help to keep your blood pressure down and could potentially increase your life expectancy. Stress certainly does lead to coronary artery spasm.
Obesity	The fact of being fat is not necessarily a risk factor but it may lead on to other risk factors, for example hyperlipidaemia or hypertension. Therefore keeping your weight down by eating a balanced diet and taking regular exercise leads to a healthier body and increases life expectancy.

How do you know you've got heart disease?

For many people, the first indication that they have coronary heart disease comes with the first heart attack. For other people, there may be warning signs of the encroaching disease before the heart attack occurs. The main warning sign is the pain of angina. Anybody approaching middle age who experiences chest pain should immediately seek medical help so the pain can be investigated.

The box below is intended as a reminder only. It is not a substitute for reading Appendix II on First aid or, better still, attending an authorised course on First aid techniques.

What to do if you find somebody in a state of collapse

Based on a Resuscitation Council poster by kind permission of The Resuscitation Council (UK) and Laerdal

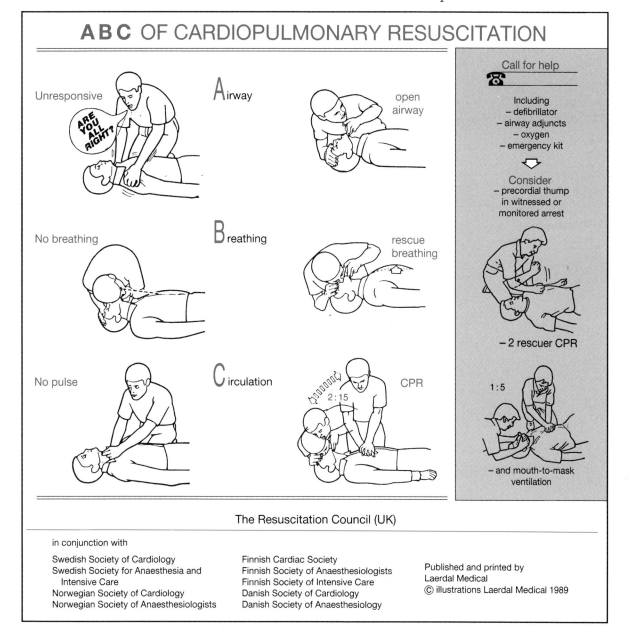

A B C OF CARDIOPULMONARY RESUSCITATION

Unresponsive — ARE YOU ALL RIGHT?

Airway — open airway

No breathing — **B**reathing — rescue breathing

No pulse — **C**irculation — 2:15 — CPR

Call for help

Including
– defibrillator
– airway adjuncts
– oxygen
– emergency kit

Consider
– precordial thump in witnessed or monitored arrest

– 2 rescuer CPR

1:5

– and mouth-to-mask ventilation

The Resuscitation Council (UK)

in conjunction with

Swedish Society of Cardiology
Swedish Society for Anaesthesia and Intensive Care
Norwegian Society of Cardiology
Norwegian Society of Anaesthesiologists

Finnish Cardiac Society
Finnish Society of Anaesthesiologists
Finnish Society of Intensive Care
Danish Society of Cardiology
Danish Society of Anaesthesiology

Published and printed by
Laerdal Medical
© illustrations Laerdal Medical 1989

Initial investigations   These investigations may be carried out by your general practitioner following a full medical examination to record your blood pressure, pulse, respiration, and listen to your heart sounds. He will ask you about the type of pain you are experiencing:

- Is it a central chest pain (as angina often is)?

- Does it come on during exercise?

- Is it relieved by glyceryl trinitrate tablets?

- **ECG**
  An electrocardiogram or heart tracing

He may then request a chest x-ray, blood tests, and an ECG.

Further investigations   If your doctor believes that you have angina, he may feel that further investigations should be carried out by a cardiologist and will refer you to the outpatients' department at your local hospital. At the hospital, further investigations may include ECGs to see whether there are any cardiac arrhythmias or evidence of former heart attacks. A chest x-ray may be carried out to show the size of the heart.

- **Cardiac arrhythmias**
  Irregularities in the heart rhythm

To identify angina positively or to see how much exercise you can tolerate before an angina attack starts, an electrocardiogram may be recorded while you are given increased exercise on a treadmill. This is called an exercise or stress test and is carried out under strict electrocardiogram control.

If there is any suspicion from listening to the heart sound with a stethoscope that there are heart valve problems or heart defects, an echocardiograph is performed where the heart can be seen in action by using ultrasound waves (using colour flow Doppler, an ultrasound probe can actually visualise the blood flowing through the heart). This procedure is completely painless.

- **Catheter**
  A fine tube

Finally, it may be deemed necessary to outline the coronary anatomy and the true level of coronary heart disease by carrying out coronary arteriography which will usually involve an overnight stay in hospital. A catheter is passed under x-ray control from an artery at the top of the leg or arm to the heart. A special dye which can be seen on the x-ray screen is then injected into the catheter, outlining the heart's anatomy and showing any coronary heart disease. The tube is removed and the patient is kept immobile in bed for around six hours before going home. This procedure is uncomfortable at times but not painful and takes about 30 minutes.

Treatment

Following coronary arteriography, a clear diagnosis can be made as to the presence and extent of coronary heart disease. The hospital cardiologist and cardiothoracic surgeon together can now make a decision as to the best mode of treatment. This could be any one of the following:

- Medical therapy (drugs);

- Coronary angioplasty (balloon treatment);

- Coronary artery bypass grafting (surgical operation).

See also Appendix III on Drugs and medicines, especially section iv

Medical therapy (drug treatment)   There are varying drugs that may be used to treat coronary heart disease:

- Diuretics ('water tablets' e.g. frusemide) – these help to excrete excessive fluids from the body in heart failure when heart muscle is weakened and cannot pump fluid around the body so fluid accumulates in lungs and ankles;

- Vasodilators (e.g. nitrates such as glyceryl trinitrate or GTN, calcium antagonists such as Adalat) widen blood vessels;

- Beta-blockers (e.g. atenolol, metoprolol, timolol) help to ease angina pain during exercise by reducing the heart's workload; they also lower blood pressure in hypertension and may help to correct abnormal heart rhythms;

- Anti-arrhythmic drugs (e.g. digoxin, verapamil) may be used if the heartbeat is irregular or too fast, often due to some form of failure in the heart's electrical conduction system;

- Anticoagulants (e.g. warfarin, heparin) stop clots from forming in the arteries. These drugs need to be taken over a long period. Regular blood tests will be needed to ensure the blood clotting time is not too prolonged. Aspirin enhances the effect of warfarin and should not therefore be taken.

- 'Clot busters' (e.g. steptokinase) – at the time of myocardial infarction, a clot may have formed in the narrowed coronary artery and blocked it. A drug such as streptokinase can be given which will have the effect of dissolving that clot.

Coronary angioplasty   The purpose of a coronary angioplasty is to clear narrowings or blockages in the heart's arteries. Under x-ray control, a small tube (guide catheter) is passed up the leg to the opening of the affected coronary artery. A tiny balloon on a fine guidewire is passed up through this guide catheter across the narrowing or blockage. The balloon is inflated to help to dilate and stretch the narrowing or blockage. The balloon and the catheter are then removed. The patient may need to stay in hospital for a day or two only.

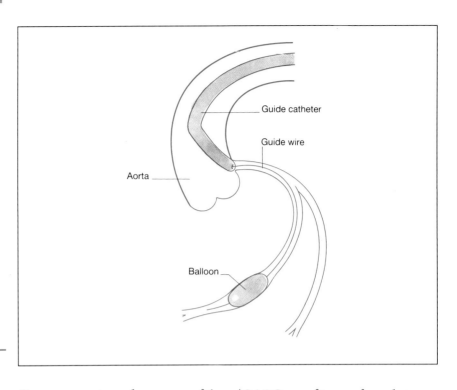

Coronary angioplasty

Coronary artery bypass grafting (CABG – often referred to as 'CABBAGE') Not all coronary artery disease is suitable for angioplasty so in some circumstances it may be decided by the surgeon and cardiologist that the best form of treatment would be a bypass operation under a general anaesthetic. The patient's heart is stopped and the function of the heart and lungs is taken over by a machine while the operation is carried out. Small veins from the legs are removed and stitched from the aorta to below the diseased area in the coronary artery. In addition, mammary arteries may be moved from the breasts and stitched below the diseased area of the coronary artery. Mammary arteries tend not to block as quickly as vein grafts. The result is improved blood flow through the coronary arteries to the heart. The patient will stay in hospital for about 10–14 days.

7.10(g)   DISEASES AFFECTING THE CHEST

Diseases which affect the chest are often distressing because the symptoms that they cause include coughing, pain and breathlessness, together with attendant wheeziness, fear, tiredness and a degree of loss of independence.

The lungs are normally protected from infection by several defence mechanisms. The air passages are lined with mucus and tiny hairs which can trap and waft debris – such as dust, bacteria

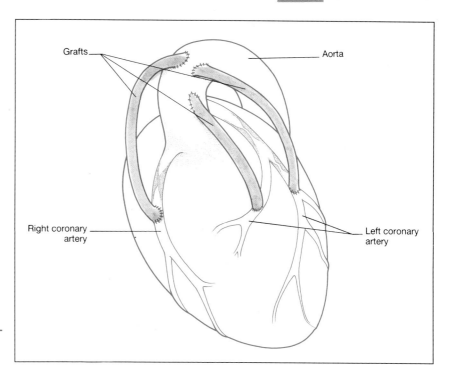

Coronary artery bypass grafting

and smoke particles – away from the delicate lung structures. The reflex action of coughing also serves to protect the lungs from infection. The body's immune system assists in preventing diseases taking a hold in the lungs. However, these defences will be impaired if a person is a smoker and/or is debilitated by other health problems.

Pneumonia   Infection and subsequent inflammation of the lung tissue is known as pneumonia. The infection is often caused by bacteria, but occasionally viral pneumonia can occur. The type of pneumonia is classified according to the site in which it is found from chest x-rays, and from clinical examinations. For example, infection in a lobe of the lung is known as 'lobar pneumonia', whereas 'bronchopneumonia' affects the smaller air passages within the lungs. If a person suffers from pneumonia, he may need hospital treatment. The doctor will prescribe strong pain-relieving tablets to alleviate the chest pain caused when breathing and coughing, or by pleurisy. A physiotherapist may help the patient with expectoration of sputum, which may appear rust coloured. If the person is hospitalised, antibiotics will be administered via an intravenous infusion ('drip'), so that the desired level is achieved promptly. Oxygen is often administered via a mask or fine bore tubing passing into the nostrils. This will help make breathing easier, and ensures enough oxygen reaches the tissues. Regular recordings of the person's temperature and pulse rate are under-

- **Pleurisy**
  Inflammation of the membranes covering the lungs

449

taken. Observations of breathing are made, so that improvement or deterioration is detected promptly. Blood tests will be made to determine the levels of oxygen and carbon dioxide in the bloodstream, and also to diagnose whether disease-producing bacteria are present. A raised temperature will mean that the sufferer is likely to feel alternately hot and cold. Shivering fits can occur which are followed by profuse sweating.

Many nursing measures can be undertaken in order to promote comfort. Pleuritic chest pain can sometimes be helped by the application of an electric heated pad, wrapped in a pillow case, and placed between the sufferer's chest and bottom sheet. Care must be taken if the patient is restless, immobile or confused if local heat is to be used. Cotton bedlinen and night attire is often appreciated when the patient has a temperature, together with washes and talc applications as required. Toothbrushing, giving mouthwashes, cleaning dentures (if worn) and sucking ice cubes are also likely to make the patient feel better. It is important to offer drinks regularly due to the increase in fluid loss associated with the patient's high temperature. It is not too important that food is taken when the sufferer is acutely ill, since it is likely he will resume eating when he feels better. When the acute chest infection is under control, antibiotics will be prescribed in tablet form. It is important to ensure that the course of treatment is completed in order to prevent complications occurring.

It will take a number of weeks before the individual feels completely recovered, although the exact time varies from person to person. A bout of depression may be experienced by some sufferers whilst convalescing.

The nursing measures described above may also be employed during an attack of acute bronchitis.

Chronic obstructive airways disease Many people who have problems with breathing are diagnosed as suffering from chronic obstructive airways disease – a term which includes asthma, chronic bronchitis and emphysema. An individual experiencing any of these illnesses is likely to be distressed because there is interference with the normal flow of air in and out of his lungs.

Chronic bronchitis is predisposed to by exposure to irritants such as cigarette smoke, industrial and air pollution, together with the suffering of repeated chest infections over a number of years. Gradually, the alveoli become distended and damaged. This leads to emphysema, as increasing areas of lung tissue are no longer able to play a role in transferring oxygen from the lungs to the bloodstream.

In Britain and other Northern countries, acute attacks of chronic bronchitis are more likely to occur in the winter months. For most

• **Alveoli**
The air sacs of the lungs

people, it is unrealistic to expect to spend the winter abroad in a sunny and warm climate. However, other measures may be taken in order to minimise or reduce the effects of this health problem on an individual's lifestyle.

Firstly, if the sufferer is a smoker, he should endeavour to stop this habit. If he is motivated to do this, he will receive help and support from his practice nurse or general practitioner. Members of the sufferer's family who share the same accommodation need to be aware that if they smoke, they may be contributing to the poor health of the affected individual.

The individual will need to adapt his lifestyle to his present capabilities. If a person overdoes activities, his breathlessness may well increase to the point where he cannot catch his breath, and feels that he is choking and about to die. Quite understandably, these feelings are accompanied by a sense of panic which adds further to the breathlessness.

There are various ways in which a person with long standing chest disease may be assisted in maintaining a degree of control and independence within his life. For example, many people find that taking showers causes less breathlessness than having baths. If you are unable to install a shower, it is likely that your local social services department will help to arrange this for you.

If you go out for a walk, it is wise to bear in mind the length of your return journey, so that excessive shortness of breath can be avoided. It is advisable to stay indoors during very cold weather, as

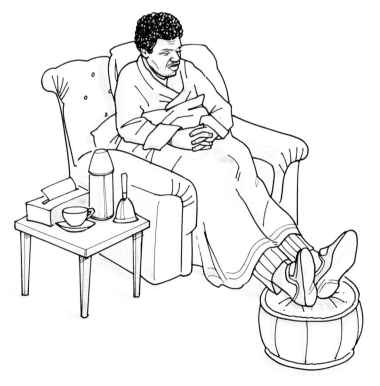

The sufferer from chronic obstructive airways disease may be more comfortable sleeping in a chair than in bed

breathing in cold air can cause the muscle layer of the small air passages to constrict, leading to difficulty in breathing. If you must go out, it is helpful to wrap a scarf over your nose and mouth.

Sleeping is often affected where an individual suffers from a chronic chest disorder. Taking 'catnaps' during the day may be helpful. At night, it may be easier to sleep in a comfortable chair with your feet elevated on a stool. Keeping a box of tissues and a drink nearby is useful for ease of access in the mornings, since many people find their productive cough is at its worst on waking.

It is important that at least two litres of fluid is taken in, not only to reduce the dryness of your mouth, but also to assist in liquefying the tenacious sputum that is produced. Some people find that having a thermos of a hot, steamy drink on a table next to their armchair will ensure an adequate fluid intake, as well as minimising any breathlessness caused by making several trips to the kitchen.

If you notice that the sputum that you produce changes to a yellow, green or grey colour, and is offensive in nature, you are almost certainly developing a chest infection and should contact your doctor immediately.

A wide range of drugs can be utilised in order to help a person who has a chronic breathing disorder. Oxygen can be supplied to your home, usually in cylinders. It is important that the correct percentage of oxygen is used with air, as in some cases too high a concentration can cause slowing and depression of your breathing. Because of the risk of fire, smoking and lighted matches should be banned. If you have given up smoking and you require oxygen for approximately 15 hours a day or longer, an oxygen concentrator (a device which removes nitrogen from room air and provides oxygen) may be recommended.

See Appendix III on Drugs and medicines, especially section v

Drugs are available which relax the muscles of the small air passages, thus easing the flow of air in and out of the lungs. These drugs, (bronchodilators) include salbutamol and its derivatives. The most effective route of administration is by inhalation, either by pressurised aerosol inhaler or, in more severe attacks via a nebulised solution (tiny droplets carried in air or oxygen to the lungs). It is important to be able to use an aerosol inhaler correctly for it to be fully effective. Firstly, shake the container. Sit upright in a comfortable position so that you can expand your chest fully. Exhale, and place the mouthpiece to your lips, making a tight seal. Inhale slowly and deeply, whilst pressing the container to release the drug at the same time. Hold your breath for ten seconds after inhalation. Take the number of puffs that have been prescribed for you, and no more. Side-effects that you may experience include a fine tremor of your hands, headache, and anxiety. If you cannot use this type of inhaler, for example if you have rheumatoid arthritis, dry powder

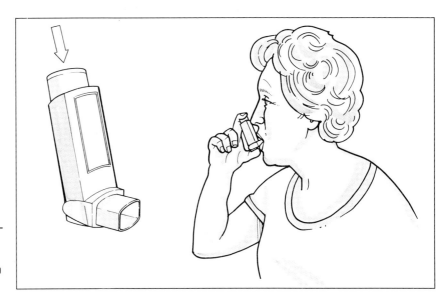

Aerosol inhaler

The picture on the left shows the inhaler in detail, the picture on the right shows it in use

inhalers can be dispensed, which are easier to use. A 'spacing device' can also help improve the effectiveness of the inhaled drug.

Steroid treatment, using drugs such as prednisolone, is of help in reducing inflammation of the airways. After long term use, steroids must be stopped by taking gradually reducing doses under medical supervision.

If your symptoms are not being controlled, further medical advice should be sought. Many people keep a device which measures their 'peak expiratory flow' in litres of air per minute. Signs that an individual is in urgent need of medical attention are as follows:

- The peak flow is so low that it is unrecordable;
- The person is wheezy;
- No relief is being gained from an inhaler;
- The person cannot complete a simple sentence;
- His fingernails and lips may be turning blue or purple;
- He may be agitated, confused or drowsy.

In this situation, call an ambulance, and help the patient sit upright, preferably near a source of fresh air. Loosen tight clothing and stay with the patient until help arrives.

Chronic chest conditions can be rather wearing, both for the sufferer and the carer, but the measures suggested above should help to maintain a reasonable quality of life. Furthermore, it is worth remembering that acute episodes are likely to become less frequent when retirement relieves the sufferer of the need to go out in all weathers.

- **Notifiable disease**
  A medical condition that must, by law, be reported by the patient's doctor to the local health authority

Tuberculosis Finally, one other chest disease, tuberculosis, can affect those people who have no immunity to the disease. It is a notifiable infectious disease, spread by droplet infection, chiefly through coughing. Treatment of tuberculosis is by a combination of drugs taken over six to nine months.

7.10(h) VARICOSE VEINS

It is not known exactly how many people have varicose veins, as many people choose to wait until the condition worsens and complications arise before going to the doctor. It is advisable, however, to consult your doctor sooner rather than later if you have any sign of varicose veins.

Varicose veins – what are they?

The word varicose means permanently swollen and dilated, so the term varicose vein refers to the superficial veins in the leg that have become swollen and dilated. The reason for this will be explained later. Other words which may be used to describe varicose veins include distended, elongated and tortuous. One of the earliest signs that veins are becoming varicose occurs when the individual is standing. Superficial veins of the lower leg or foot may be seen to be distended and swollen.

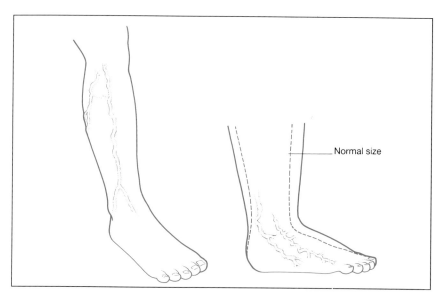

Normal size

Varicose veins

The superficial veins of the leg or foot may appear distorted or swollen

Why do the veins become varicose?

It is the function of the veins in the body to return blood back to the heart. Unfortunately the mechanism for returning blood from the lower limbs is not very efficient. Indeed some would say that varicose veins are the price human beings have to pay for assuming an upright posture; the delicate veins of the leg being unable to cope with the pressure resulting from gravity.

Blood from the veins in the lower limbs is pumped back to the heart by compression of the muscles and fibrous sheath surrounding the veins. When walking the leg muscles contract and squeeze the veins pumping the blood forward towards the heart. Blood is prevented from flowing backwards by the presence of valves at intervals along the inside of the veins. A network of veins consists of both superficial and deep vessels connected to each other either directly or by communicating veins. During exercise blood is pushed towards the heart by the pumping action of the leg muscles squeezing the deep veins. This action creates what is called a negative pressure within the deep veins, which acts as a suction pump drawing blood from the superficial veins through the communicating veins into the deep veins. Respiration can also assist the return of blood to the heart, deep breathing creates a negative pressure in the chest, which also helps draw blood back to the heart. Lying down with the legs slightly elevated enables gravity to aid the return of blood from the lower limbs. Varicose veins occur when one or more of the valves fail to function properly which leads to an increase of pressure within the vessel. If the high pressure is not relieved the vessel wall will, over a period of time, lose its elasticity. The vein will then swell and become dilated due to a backflow of blood. If left untreated the condition worsens and an increasing number of valves are damaged.

The function of valves in the network of veins

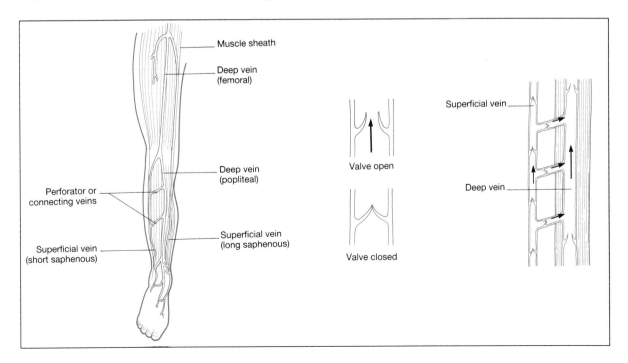

Muscle sheath

Deep vein (femoral)

Deep vein (popliteal)

Perforator or connecting veins

Superficial vein (long saphenous)

Superficial vein (short saphenous)

Valve open

Valve closed

Superficial vein

Deep vein

Clinical signs

In addition to the superficial veins being swollen and dilated other signs may include pain caused by the high pressure within the veins, and swelling or oedema of the surrounding tissues if the tissue fluid is not drained away by the veins and lymphatic system. Sometimes the skin develops a brown colour stain, caused by blood leaking from the damaged vessels. If left without medical attention the surrounding tissues can become starved of essential nutrients and begin to break down causing a varicose ulcer, or eczema to develop. Other complications may include spontaneous haemorrhage due to the vein walls rupturing and thrombophlebitis which is very painful and caused by acute inflammatory changes within the vein.

Factors which may affect varicose veins

Hormones   The hormone oestrogen is known to cause the walls of the veins to relax and expand. This may be why women are more prone to varicose veins than men. However, this does not necessarily mean that women who have varicose veins should not take contraceptive pills or receive hormone replacement therapy. It merely highlights the importance of regular medical screening to ensure the veins are not deteriorating or complications arising. Any aches or cramp-like symptoms in the calf muscle for example must be reported to the doctor at once.

Pregnant women frequently develop varicose veins or find existing ones worsening. This is usually due to a combination of factors, firstly the high levels of oestrogen in the blood; secondly, the increasing size of the womb causing pressure on the pelvic veins which results in stagnation of the blood flow, increased pressure within the veins of the leg; thirdly the blood volume tends to increase during pregnancy. The wearing of support stockings combined with keeping the legs elevated when sitting or resting does seem to help reduce the discomfort experienced by many pregnant women. Exercising the calf muscles also helps.

Some women report too that their varicose veins are worse immediately before they start to menstruate again. This is due to hormonal changes.

Exercise   Many people spend a large proportion of their day sitting or standing. Lack of activity can cause high venous pressure, slowing down of the blood flow, and an increased risk of thrombosis or clotting of the blood. Ideally, exercise should form part of everyone's daily lives. Even when you have very limited mobility, it is usually possible to learn how to improve your health by doing exercise within the limits of your disability.

Exercises that can be done lying down

- Lie either on the floor or on the bed, point both toes and feet down then up towards the head, repeat the exercise, commencing five times gradually increasing to twenty times
- Straighten one leg, raise it and lower again. Begin slowly, gradually increasing to twenty times
- Circle the feet clockwise then anti-clockwise between 15–20 times in each direction
- Pretend cycling is also a very effective method of improving the circulation

These exercises can be repeated as many times as your lifestyle permits each day

It is important that exercise is regular and that you avoid standing or sitting for long periods. Walking, swimming and cycling are three very effective exercises which people should be encouraged to do.

Clothing The wearing of tight garments like corsets, garters or high boots do not in themselves cause varicose veins, but they can severely restrict the flow of blood in people who already have damaged valves. It is always advisable to avoid wearing any garment that constricts the limb. It is helpful to wear comfortable well fitting shoes, and support stockings or tights can alleviate tired aching legs.

Environment People who live or work in environments that are warm and humid may find this aggravates their varicose veins causing oedema or swelling of the tissues. Underfloor heating seems to be more of a problem for some people.

See also Chapter 1, section 1 on Diet

Diet The diet enjoyed over recent years by most Westerners has been made up primarily of highly refined foods containing little fibre. A low fibre diet has a tendency to encourage constipation; the presence of a full bowel increases the pressure inside the abdomen and on the surrounding veins. This results in reducing the blood flow back to the heart and causes stagnation and back-flow. Straining to pass the constipated stools increases the pressure and can lead to valves being ruptured.

If your diet lacks fibre, then try introducing foods which contain more fibre and have at least one portion of fresh fruit every day.

Obesity Not only does the body have to support the additional weight, varicose veins are more awkward to treat in an obese person because they are often difficult to find. Fatty deposits also tend to build up around the blood vessels, reducing their efficiency and increasing the risk of thrombosis. If you are overweight then consult with your doctor or nurse on how you may best reduce your weight.

Heredity   There is some evidence to suggest that varicose veins may be a hereditary condition. Several studies demonstrate that more than one family member has varicose veins. One theory suggests that a congenital weakness in the walls of the vessels may be hereditary.

Treatment

Conservative treatment   The first stage in the treatment of varicose veins when there are no complications present often consists of exercise, elevation and the wearing of properly measured and fitted support stockings. Exercise must be regular and active. The legs should be elevated above the height of the waist. The support stockings must be of the right size for the patient to ensure an even distribution of pressure. The stockings compress the swollen and dilated veins helping to push the blood into the deep veins where it can be pumped back up to the heart. There are a wide variety of support stockings available, hence the importance of correct selection if the stockings are to be of value. Stockings should always be put on first thing in the morning, before getting out of bed, and only removed at night once you are back in bed. Ideally you should sleep with your legs elevated to aid blood flow back to the heart.

Always follow carefully the advice you have been given by your doctor or nurse; and remember the life of your stockings can be greatly increased if you follow the manufacturer's instructions on how to care for them.

Compression sclerotherapy or injection technique   Another method of treating varicose veins is to inject them with a sclerosing agent which causes the walls of the damaged vessel to adhere or stick together, thereby preventing the vein from becoming swollen and dilated with blood.

Before carrying out this technique the doctor examines the leg while you are standing upright. The varicose veins are then marked with an indelible pen. You will be asked to lie on a couch with your leg elevated. This causes the veins to empty. The doctor then examines your leg, places a finger over the area of weakness, and asks you to stand up. The doctor observes the varicose vein to see if it refills when you are standing. If the vein remains empty he knows he has located the correct area and will then inject the sclerosing agent. A pad is placed over the injection site and the limb bandaged using a graduated compression bandage; you will usually be expected to wear a support stocking on top of the bandage. Sometimes several sites have to be injected if the leg has numerous varices. It is quite usual to see patients the following week for an examination and assessment of the results.

For many patients it is the after care which causes the most difficulty. Having a leg bandaged from top to toe for about six weeks does require a little ingenuity when it comes to bathing or taking a shower. A brisk walk of 5 km (3 miles) once a day is an essential part of the treatment and must be done. Patients are usually given a list of instructions by the doctor and it is essential for the success of the treatment that they be followed.

Occasionally some patients experience pain following the injection (or injections) and may require a mild analgesic; it is still necessary however to walk. On no account should you stand still or sit with your legs down. If sitting you must have your legs elevated above the level of your waist. Should the bandage become too tight always contact the doctor or nurse; never take the bandage next to the skin off yourself unless specifically asked to do so by your doctor or nurse.

Surgical treatment A minority of patients do have to have an operation to treat their varicose veins. This is usually when the varicosities extend up the thigh, or when injection therapy has failed or the patient after consultation prefers surgery to injection treatment. There are two main methods that can be used. The first of these is the stripping out of the vein using a long wire instrument. The second is treatment by ligation of the incompetent communicating vein. The effects of ligation are shown in the figure below.

The patient who has had her vein stripped out comes back from the operating theatre wearing a compression bandage, and with strict instructions to keep the limb elevated for about 12 hours.

- **Ligation**
  Tying off

Ligation of a varicose vein

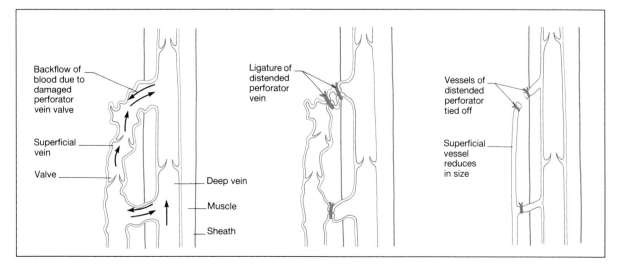

This helps to reduce the swelling and bruising that may occur following this type of operation.

The patient who is having his varices treated by ligation may have the operation done as a day patient. Whatever type of operation, the aftercare is very similar and requires the patient to be committed to following the post-operative instructions carefully.

The leg will have a compression bandage on it which will need to be worn for several weeks. A support stocking may be applied over the top of the bandage. The bandage is removed after approximately 5–7 days for removal of sutures, unless absorbable ones have been used. The limb is then rebandaged. Instructions on how to care for the limb and what to do if the bandage requires changing are usually written out and given to the patient.

Both surgical procedures can cause some patients to feel pain or discomfort; this is normally controlled by the administration of a mild analgesic.

Exercise is of paramount importance to the success of the operation. Patients should commence walking immediately after surgery (the day after if the veins have been stripped). The distance walked should be in the region of 5 km (3 miles) a day. If necessary increase your distance daily until you achieve 5 km. It is important to walk correctly, otherwise the leg muscles will not function efficiently. The initial experience of pain or discomfort felt by some patients quickly disappears with each post-operative day and a mild analgesic may help. Other exercises to improve venous return can be done when sitting or lying (see, for example, the exercise box featured three pages earlier). If you are sitting down or sleeping, your legs should be propped up on a pillow or stool.

Some doctors advise patients not to drive until the wound has healed, because sudden use of the brake pedal can be very painful as well as difficult, and may cause an accident. Support stockings should be put on in the morning before getting out of bed and removed at night once in bed. Bathing or taking a shower with one or both legs covered in bandages can be difficult, but not impossible. The use of a large plastic bin liner secured at the top of the leg can enable you to bathe or shower. Some patients prefer to wash thoroughly instead, rather than risk getting the bandages wet.

Complications

Unfortunately varicose veins can recur, albeit in a few patients. If you suspect you are developing varicose veins again it is important to see your doctor straight away so that he can ensure you get the right advice and treatment to prevent them getting worse.

Sometimes patients with long established varicose veins develop a varicose ulcer due to the tissues in the lower leg receiving inadequate nourishment and becoming thin, pigmented and prone to damage. If you have varicose veins and sustain an injury it is important to see the doctor as soon as possible so that she can prescribe a dressing and compression bandage which will help the ulcer to heal quickly.

7.10(i) ORTHOPAEDIC PROBLEMS

Problems involving bones, joints, muscles, tendons and associated nerves are orthopaedic problems. The first part of this section deals with some orthopaedic conditions which affect more than one area of the body, and the later part deals with common orthopaedic conditions listed under the area of the body affected.

Arthritis

The term arthritis means an inflamed joint. Several diseases can cause it – the two most common being:

• Osteoarthritis (or osteoarthrosis);

• Rheumatoid arthritis.

Healthy joint surfaces are smooth and shiny. When these surfaces begin to wear out the joint becomes painful and stiff (degenerative or osteoarthritis). The joints affected are usually weight-bearing ones – the hip and the knee. There is a nagging aching pain in the joint which becomes worse when the joint is being used and is relieved by resting. However, pain at night is often severe and disturbs sleep.

Treatment for osteoarthritis includes the following measures:

• Pain killing drugs to relieve the pain;

• Exercising your leg gently to help maintain movement and increase muscle strength;

• Using a walking stick to help to distribute your weight when walking;

• Avoiding standing or walking for long periods of time;

• If you are overweight, losing some weight will lighten the load on your joints;

• Severe joint damage may require surgery.

Rheumatoid arthritis is a generalised illness with hot, swollen and painful joints and increasing deformity. If affects more women than men and can occur at any age. There may be a family history of rheumatoid arthritis. The disease has patterns of flare-ups and remissions. The hands and feet are frequently affected and there is a feeling of being generally unwell. The joints are usually very stiff in the morning.

Treatment for rheumatoid arthritis includes the following measures:

- Rest the painful joint to ease the pain;

- Local heat will also help but great care must be taken not to burn the skin which is very fragile;

- Pain killing drugs are important in controlling the severe pain;

- It is important to visit your doctor.

Bursitis

A bursa is a small fluid-filled sac found near a joint. Repeated friction or pressure on an area over a bursa can result in the fluid increasing. A large swelling will then occur near to a joint.

Examples of bursitis include:

- Housemaid's knee;

- Clergyman's knee;

- Student's elbow.

Treatment includes avoiding the position which causes the condition, applying a firm crepe bandage and resting the joint until the swelling subsides.

If the swelling is hot, tense and remains painful, it is important that you see your doctor.

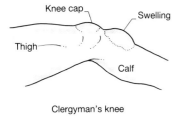

Clergyman's knee

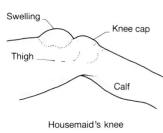

Housemaid's knee

Types of bursitis of the knee

Fibrositis

Fibrositis usually describes a stiff and aching back or shoulder. Treatment consists of pain killing drugs, rest and warmth to help reduce the pain. See your doctor if the pain persists.

Gout

Once considered to be a rich man's disease associated with too much port, gout is, in fact, due to a failure in the waste disposal system of the body causing a build up of uric acid salts especially in joints. The most common joint affected is the big toe. The joint remains extremely painful, red, hot and swollen and can remain so for up to two weeks.

Treatment includes the following measures:

- Rest the joint;

- Raise your foot on a footstool;

- Take pain killing drugs to ease the pain;

- Warmth and gentle massage may help;
- Visit a doctor.

Osteoporosis

As we grow older the bones in our body lose some of their strength, in a process described as 'thinning'. The most common cause of osteoporosis is old age. It is more common in women, especially those who have passed the menopause.

Minor falls can then result in broken bones especially at the hip and wrist. The back bone is also affected with a nagging aching backache and sometimes an increasing round-shouldered appearance (popularly known as Dowager's hump).

Prevention A good diet when young is important and regular exercise should be encouraged.

Hormone replacement therapy during and after the menopause may be prescribed by your doctor.

Care must be taken to avoid falls. Safety in the home, good footwear and care in wet or icy weather are all important.

Tenosynovitis

Tendons run inside smooth shiny sheaths. If this sheath becomes inflamed and damaged during excessive repetitive movements the result is pain and swelling over the tendon involved. This commonly affects the tendons of the hand.

The second part of this section deals with conditions affecting specific areas of the body.

Arm

Frozen shoulder The shoulder gradually becomes extremely painful. The pain may extend into the arm and all movements of the shoulder cause pain. The pain is severe enough to disturb sleep.

There may be no definite injury other than a trivial strain. The pain and stiffness may last for as much as six months or a year, and there may be permanent loss of movement.

Treatment involves supporting the arm in a sling and pain-killing drugs should be taken. Move your arm if possible, and try to use the elbow and hand normally.

You should visit your doctor as other causes of the pain must be excluded.

Elbow

Golfer's elbow Continuous repetitive movements cause injury to a tendon which goes from the elbow to the hand. Pain is felt in the elbow joint in an area just below the joint on the inside of the arm.

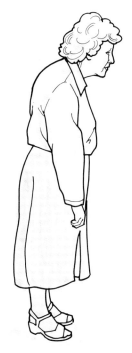

Dowager's hump

One of the results of osteoporosis

Treatment involves resting the arm and avoiding repetition of the movements which cause pain. Warmth applied to the painful area may help.

Once the pain has settled, you can gradually return to using your arm normally.

Tennis elbow   This is similar to golfer's elbow but involves a different tendon so the pain is felt on the outside of the arm just below the joint.

Treatment is as for golfer's elbow above.

Student's elbow (olecranon bursitis)   The swelling is at the point of the elbow. A similar swelling may occur with rheumatoid arthritis.

For details of treatment, see the section on Bursitis, above.

Hand and wrist

Carpal tunnel syndrome   Numbness, tingling and pain are felt in the thumb, index, middle and part of the ring finger in one or both hands. This pain is worse at night often disturbing sleep. There may be weakness of these fingers. It happens more often to women and may occur in pregnancy or after the menopause.

Carpal tunnel syndrome is caused in the following way. One of the nerves and some tendons which go to the fingers pass under a tunnel of tissue on the palm side of the wrist joint. If this tissue becomes swollen and thickened, pressure occurs on the nerve causing pain.

Treatment involves the following measures:

- Avoid excessive use of your wrist;

- At night hang your arm over the edge of the bed and shake your hand gently;

- If the pain regularly disturbs sleep, visit your doctor.

De Quervain's tenosynovitis   Pain is felt at the base of the thumb on the side of the wrist. The pain occurs more often in women and comes on after some repetitive activity such as pruning the roses.

Treatment involves resting your hand and avoiding the activity which causes you pain. Once the pain has subsided you can begin gradually to use your hand normally again.

Dupuytren's contracture   This condition starts with a lump in the palm of the hand. Over a long period of time this area gradually thickens and pulls down the ring and little finger. These fingers curl into the palm of the hand. There is rarely any pain but the

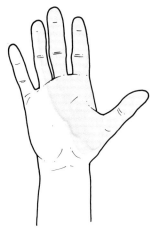

View of the palm of the hand

The shaded area denotes the area of pain and tingling in carpal tunnel syndrome fingers get in the way when using the hand. Dupuytren's contracture affects one or both hands and is common in men.

The condition is progressive so it is important to keep your fingers active for as long as possible. The skin in the palm of the hand should be kept clean and dry and the nails short to prevent soreness developing in the palm.

Knee

For conditions such as clergyman's knee and housemaid's knee, see the section on Bursitis above.

Torn cartilage   The two half-moon shaped pads (semilunar cartilages) within the knee joint can be torn in a twisting injury. A small flap can then catch between the bone ends causing pain and preventing movement (locking). This usually happens as a result of an incident involving twisting the bent knee while it is carrying the body weight. Sportsmen and women are most at risk of such an injury.

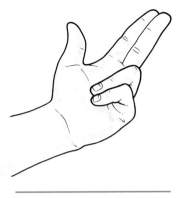

Dupuytren's contracture

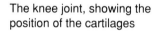

The knee joint, showing the position of the cartilages

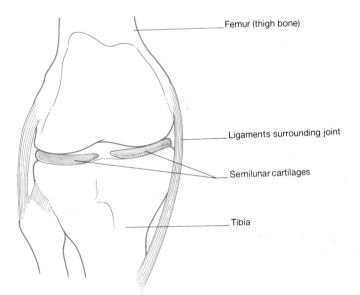

Femur (thigh bone)

Ligaments surrounding joint

Semilunar cartilages

Tibia

A sharp pain is felt on one side of the knee joint. The knee may give way or lock into a slightly bent position. The knee will usually swell slowly (probably overnight) and be painful and stiff.

Treatment involves the following measures:

- Support your knee by applying a firm crepe bandage;

- Rest your leg;

- The pain and swelling should subside after a few days. If there are frequent reccurences of pain, locking or giving way, you should visit your doctor.

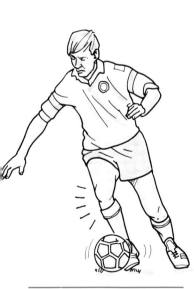

Twisting injury causes a torn cartilage

465

- If the knee joint swells quickly after an injury or becomes hot and tense, it is important that you visit the accident department of your nearest hospital.

Foot

Bunion (bursitis of a deformed big toe joint) A red painful swelling occurs on the side of the foot over the deformed big toe joint. The big toe joint is deformed so that the toe points inwards and the joint is prominent. Pressure from tight pointed shoes increases the deformity and friction over the joint produces an inflamed and swollen joint.

You can do much to prevent the formation of bunions by avoiding the wearing of socks or tights that are too small, and tight, pointed shoes.

Treatment involves the following measures:

- A small soft pad placed between the big toe and the next toe to relieve the pain;

- Exercising your foot to strengthen the muscles;

- Removing the cause of the pressure until the swelling subsides;

- Surgery to correct the deformed joint if the doctor advises.

Ingrowing toenail   The edge of the toenail grows into the side of the toe causing the flesh to grow over the nail. The gully that is produced becomes infected. A red swollen inflamed area appears alongside the toenail, usually on the big toe. The area may discharge fluid or pus and become crusty.

To help prevent ingrowing toenails, always cut your toenails straight across. Never curve the corners as this encourages the nail to grow into the flesh. Avoid wearing tight shoes, socks and stockings, and always keep your feet and footwear dry and clean.

Treatment includes the following measures:

- Cleaning the area with a mild antiseptic in warm water;

- Drying well and covering with a dry gauze;

- If the infection persists, visit your doctor.

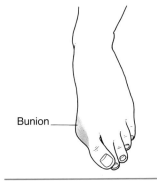

Bunion

Bunion (Hallux valgus deformity)

7.10(j) BACK PAIN IN ADULTHOOD

Back pain is a cause of a great amount of worry and disruption for about 80 per cent of people at some stage in their lives. It affects the young as well as the elderly men and women.

Back pain with its resulting disability causes considerable loss to industry, 26 million working days lost each year, disruption of family life, and there is an enormous cost to the social security benefit system.

Back pain in itself is not a fatal condition, but it can be a symptom of an underlying problem which will need either conservative management or vigorous and early investigation and treatment. Fortunately, the vast majority of cases clear up spontaneously or after treatment – 40 per cent in a week, 56 per cent in a month – while 80–90 per cent will have recovered in about six weeks. Most people cope with their back pain by making various adaptations to their daily living style in the expectation that it will resolve spontaneously.

Onset of symptoms and history of back pain   The onset of back pain may be gradual or sudden. The pain may have occurred during a particular activity (e.g. while lifting a heavy or even very light load) or the pain may have no specific origin. It may be diffuse radiating over a wide area or pinpointed in one particular spot.

The character and nature of the pain is important. The pain may radiate from the lower back down to the buttock, the outer thigh and even cause pins and needles sensation in the toes. The pain may be aggravated by movement such as bending or twisting.

Back pain may occur suddenly associated with the performance of a physically demanding activity. After a spell of heavy and unaccustomed digging in the garden the onset of back pain may not occur until the following day when it may be difficult or impossible to get out of bed.

The back pain may cause severe muscle spasm so that any movement is torture especially trying to sit or stand up.

The onset of significant back pain will need to be carefully assessed by the general practitioner in the first instance. The doctor will need to know how the pain started and the nature of the pain, so that a plan of action can be decided. For this reason it is best to see your doctor at the time of the onset of back pain, especially if it occurs without apparent cause among older people or the very young.

Prevention of back pain   Care of the back is important if further back trouble is to be avoided. There are well accepted principles or rules for people who want to avoid back trouble in the first place or having suffered back trouble want to avoid a recurrence.

Posture   Poor posture can cause backache. It is essential to sit in a firm chair to avoid slouching. A lumbar support in the lower back is a great boon to those who have to sit for any length of time – office workers and car drivers. Some modern car seats have built in

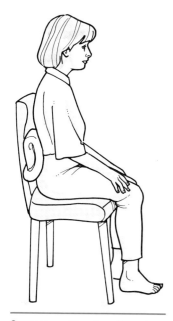

Correct position for sitting in a chair – buttocks well back on the seat and a pillow or cushion in the small of the back

lumbar supports. The buttocks should be pushed as far back into the chair seat as possible.

An erect 'head up, shoulders back' stance should be adopted.

The correct stance when carrying out lifting or other tasks, especially those which require the same stooped posture to be held for some time, is important.

See also Chapter 2, section 4 on Lifting and transfers

Study the chart below and follow the principles of correct posture and manual handling and you stand a good chance of avoiding back problems.

Rules to follow when lifting loads	Postural stress
1 Hold the load close to your body 2 Lift from the floor only between the knees 3 Get help with loads too heavy for you, or use mechanical devices 4 Squat down to bend at the knees not the back 5 Avoid prolonged carrying of heavy loads 6 Do not twist your trunk when lifting loads	Avoid postural stress in these situations – always kneel to the task or rise to the task so that bending is eliminated. Bed making Bathing children Gardening Hairdressing Looking after small children Carry weights in each hand equally

The management and treatment of back pain Management and treatment can take many forms; much will depend on whether the back pain is acute or chronic.

Acute back pain is immediately incapacitating which greatly restricts movement. Often it is impossible to go to work, drive a car or even get out of bed. During this phase the only remedy is to rest and take analgesics to relieve the pain.

Bedrest may be beneficial for the first week, but prolonged bedrest is not advised as this does not always result in a rapid cure and can indeed be harmful.

When lying in bed a firm mattress is required. Some spring interior mattresses are very firm offering support to the reclining body to avoid a slouching posture. If the mattress is not firm, a board under the mattress will achieve the same result. It is thought that by lying down the pressure on the intervertebral disc is reduced.

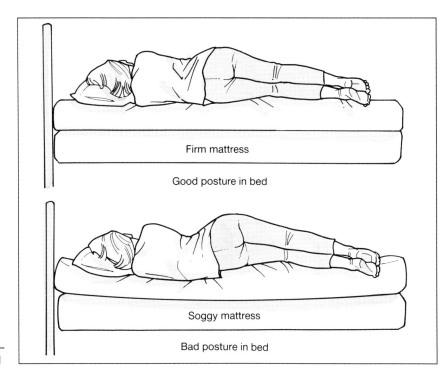

Firm mattress

Good posture in bed

Soggy mattress

Bad posture in bed

Good and bad posture in bed

There are many approaches to treatment of back pain. Conservative medicine relies mainly on rest and analgesics. Other sufferers seek help from the remedial professions – osteopaths, chiropractors and physiotherapists. Your doctor may refer you to such professional practitioners for treatment which can take a variety of forms. A recent study has shown that the remedial professions have a high success rate in the treatment of back pain which can explain the popularity of this approach. However, a word of caution, only approach registered fully trained persons who hold a qualification awarded by their professional institution. Contact the relevant institution if you are at all unsure.

See Appendix VII for Addresses of useful organisations

The osteopath or chiropractor will approach the patient in the following general manner:

- Take a careful history;

- Make a thorough examination;

- Diagnose the possible cause;

- Either treat or refer to a doctor;

- If treatment is decided the practitioner will relieve the condition with manipulation of joints and tissues, after relaxing the muscles in the affected area;

- Exercises may be recommended;

• Treatment may last one session or be repeated as necessary over a long time.

Surgery   Only about one per cent of patients benefit from surgery to relieve pressure on a nerve root. This pressure is usually the result of a prolapsed intervertebral disc pressing on the nerve root which despite treatment may not resolve itself.

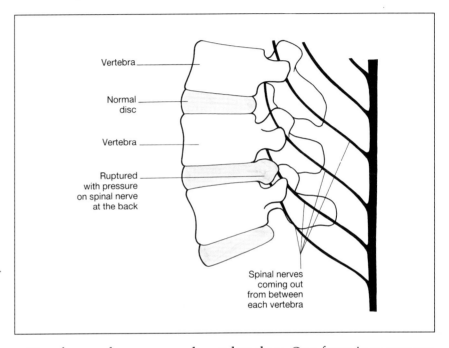

Vertebra

Normal disc

Vertebra

Ruptured with pressure on spinal nerve at the back

Spinal nerves coming out from between each vertebra

A normal and abnormal disc space illustrating how spinal nerve root pressure and resulting pain is caused

Two forms of surgery can be undertaken. One form is to remove the damaged intervertebral disc and relieve the pressure. The other is to fuse the vertebrae together so that they become a fixed joint.

Activity and rehabilitation   Activity should be encouraged as soon as possible. It is more beneficial to be active than passive, providing activities are avoided which are likely to increase the chances of making the pain worse or starting it up again.

Gentle mobilisation such as walking and exercises can nurture the spinal discs and cartilages. It can improve general well-being, both mental as well as physical, and may decrease pain.

Exercise – does it have a value?   There is general agreement that exercise is beneficial. Exercise can strengthen the extensor muscles of the back; other exercises mobilise the spine and open up the disc spaces thus improving nutrition to the disc and relieving pressure on nerve roots. Other types of exercise, such as sit ups and leg raising when lying on the back, improve the tone of stomach muscles.

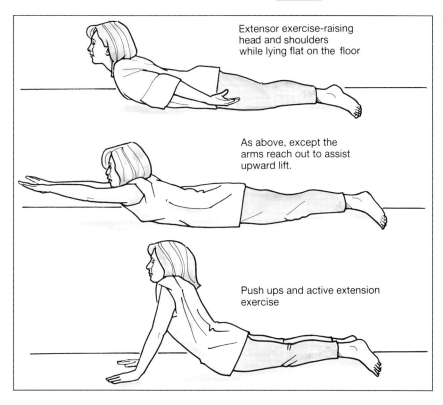

Extensor exercise-raising head and shoulders while lying flat on the floor

As above, except the arms reach out to assist upward lift.

Push ups and active extension exercise

Exercises for strengthening the spinal muscles

Individual approaches   The guidance in this section is of a general nature. The cause, severity and treatment of back pain can vary widely in each person and the problem needs to be assessed and treatment arranged in each case on an individual basis.

For the chronic back pain sufferer who despite all possible avenues of treatment still suffers from back pain, the *Back School* approach can be of benefit. These schools are organised in various parts of the United Kingdom. The programme tries to create a positive attitude among the sufferers, encouraging normal daily living activities, and helping patients recognise their limitations and abilities.

7.10(k)   PROBLEMS ASSOCIATED WITH TOBACCO, ALCOHOL AND OTHER DRUGS

The kind of drugs described in this section are 'psychoactive' or mind-altering drugs. These are substances that have an effect on people's mental state. They can be divided into four groups:

- Tobacco;
- Alcohol;
- Prescribed drugs such as tranquillisers and antidepressants;
- Illegal drugs such as cannabis, heroin, cocaine and LSD.

The great majority of people who use drugs use them for pleasure or social reasons and suffer no obvious harm thereby. Sadly when ever drugs are widely available and popular some people use them in an excessive, harmful or inappropriate way. 'Drug problems' encompass a broad range of illnesses, accidents, social, economic and public order problems as well as drug-related deaths.

Smoking

Most dependent smokers believe that tobacco is soothing on the nerves. In fact tobacco is a stimulant, increasing heart rate and raising blood pressure. Evidence suggests that tobacco smoking carries a high risk of developing cancers of various types. It is the greatest single known cause of cancer of the lung, but also carries a high risk of damage to the heart. Smokers can also affect the people with whom the smoker lives and works. The smoke from cigarettes and tobacco products inhaled by others has been shown to have adverse effects. Children of smokers are more likely to suffer from chest complaints when they are young. People who already suffer from chest complaints such as asthma may notice an increase in breathing difficulties when they are near someone who is smoking.

See also sections 7.10(e), 7.10(f) and 7.10(g) above

Giving up smoking is therefore the best advice possible. Most of the unpleasant withdrawal effects associated with stopping smoking are psychological rather than physical. However the difficulty in stopping must not be underestimated. Help is available in the form of booklets or, in cases of extreme difficulty, your family doctor may be able to advise. Millions of people have given up smoking successfully.

Alcohol

People often do not view alcohol as a 'drug', mainly because 'drugs' are thought of as only illegal substances like heroin.

Most people in the United Kingdom do drink alcohol. Because of this fact alone far more people in this country experience alcohol problems than problems related to illegal drugs. Alcohol, a depressant, typically makes the drinker feel more relaxed and, possibly, less inhibited or tense. Alcohol consumption is *associated* with all manner of behaviours, including harmful or criminal activities. Even so drinking in itself is not the *cause* of such behaviours.

People are often surprised to find they have an 'alcohol-related' problem. Drinking is so much a part of our lives that it is not questioned. It is important for you to be aware of the amount of alcohol you are drinking; this allows you to compare your consumption with the 'low risk' levels suggested by the experts. A simple way of doing this is by using the 'units' system. As you can see from the illustration there is the same amount of alcohol in each of these

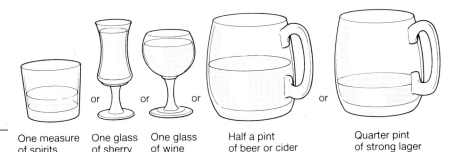

Units of alcohol

| One measure of spirits | One glass of sherry | One glass of wine | Half a pint of beer or cider | Quarter pint of strong lager |

Sensible drinking levels (weekly consumption in units)

Level of Risk	Women	Men
Low	below 14 units	below 21 units
Intermediate	15–20 units	22–35 units
High	over 20 units	over 35 units

drinks, that is one unit. These are 'pub' measures. Home measures may contain two to three times these quantities. 'Strong' lagers may be two to three times stronger than ordinary lager. Thus one pint of strong lager may have the equivalent alcohol content of five single whiskies or five glasses of wine.

Using this system count up how much you drink in an ordinary week. Once you have counted up your week's consumption you can compare it with the table above. You can now decide whether or not your drinking is a cause for concern.

PROBLEMS ASSOCIATED WITH ALCOHOL ABUSE

Short term problems	Drunkenness
	Road traffic accidents
	Hangovers
	Unsafe sex practices with risk of sexually transmitted diseases (including HIV infection)

Mid-term problems	Arguments at home
	Inefficiency or absenteeism from work
	Stomach problems
	Obesity (overweight)
	Infertility

Long term problems	Financial problems
	Breakdown in relationships
	Divorce
	Brain damage (such as memory impairment)
	Liver damage
	Muscle damage – the most important muscle in the body is the heart; people who drink heavily have an increased risk of suffering a heart attack

Some suggestions for
sensible drinking

- Drink less over a long period
- Avoid drinking on an empty stomach by restricting your drinking to mealtimes or when food is available
- Use a proper measure when drinking at home. Don't try to estimate the amount from the level in the glass
- Dilute spirits with at least as much water or something non-fizzy to slow absorption
- Sip your drink slowly, put the glass down between sips
- Don't rush your drink to catch up, drink at your own speed, wait until your glass is empty and then consider whether you want any more
- Rounds and kitties can induce you to drink more than you want during a drinking session
- Avoid habit drinking at lunchtime or on the way home from work
- Don't use alcohol to try to solve emotional problems
- Avoid drinking as a means of unwinding, look for alternatives that are effective: favourite music, a good book, a warm bath
- Avoid alcohol as a nightcap; again look for alternatives that are effective such as a warm milk drink
- Monitor your consumption using a drinking diary; be alert to signs of increase
- Practise saying 'no'

Source: Scottish Council on Alcoholism, 1977

Women and men have different levels of risk. This is because women are more sensitive to alcohol than are men. There are a number of reasons for this, such as, women are usually lighter in weight than men. The harmful effects of alcohol depend on the length of time the person has been drinking heavily. You may now wish to reduce your consumption to a less risky level. If so, a number of tips are given in the table above. The sooner a difficulty is acknowledged the better the chances of success. Help can be sought from a number of sources including your family doctor, specialist hospital clinics and support groups.

Prescribed drugs

See Appendix III for more information on Drugs and medicines and Appendix VII for Addresses of useful organisations and support groups

The fact that a drug is legal (i.e. prescribed by your doctor or bought over the counter in chemist shops) does not mean it carries no risk.

The vast majority of prescribed psycho-active drugs can be of great benefit if used as prescribed *over short periods of time.* These drugs are prescribed by doctors for such problems as anxiety or depression.

Any medication should be taken exactly as recommended with no increase in dosage unless this is checked and agreed on by your family doctor or pharmacist. However even correct doses of drugs such as tranquillisers or barbiturates, if taken over long periods of time, can cause problems. A great many women and a lesser number of men in this country are now dependent on such tranquillisers as Ativan, Valium and Temazepam. One of the major problems in trying to 'break the habit' of these substances is that withdrawal symptoms will often replicate the original anxiety for which the drug was prescribed. This mistakenly makes the person feel that the drug is still necessary. Withdrawal from these drugs is a long term process. Anyone trying to stop taking them must do so by gradually reducing the dosage under the supervision of a qualified practitioner.

Illegal drugs

The media attention paid to use of illegal drugs in this country far outweighs the number of people affected by these substances. Many young people indulge in the limited use of such drugs as cannabis with little or no ill effects. Often what attracts people into using illegal drugs is the accompanying lifestyle which many parents find strange and worrying. Sadly a minority of people who use illicit drugs experience adverse consequences, some of which are fatal. Overdoses, accidents, 'bad trips' are chronic drug-related problems. In some localities many, even most, of those who are HIV infected are intravenous drug users exposed to the virus by sharing infected injecting equipment.

7.10(I) VISUAL AND HEARING PROBLEMS

It is difficult for those of us with unimpaired sight and hearing to imagine what tremendous problems are faced by people who are blind or deaf, and how we can help them to overcome their difficulties. Yet there is one very simple first step: wear a blindfold or a pair of ear plugs for a day, and experience what daily living is like for someone deprived of sight or hearing.

Loss of sight

Nearly a million people in Britain are either blind or partially sighted, according to the Royal National Institute for the Blind. The onset of sight loss can be sudden, as in an accident, or gradual, as a result of disease. The most common causes are cataract, glaucoma, and macular degeneration, which occur most frequently in older people, and diseased or detached retina, which is fairly common among diabetics. Blindness can also result from certain infectious diseases. A degree of sight may remain, perhaps in the centre or perhaps on the periphery of the field of vision, or there may be an ability to recognise colours although vision is otherwise blurred. Whatever the cause, loss of sight is very hard to accept, and depression is, understandably, one of the blind person's greatest problems. The last thing blind people want, however, is pity; they need quiet sympathy and understanding, practical help, and above all to be treated like a normal human being.

Far too many people either ignore a blind person and talk about him as though he were not present, or embarrass him with over-sentimental condolences. The best approach is a matter-of-fact one which shows you regard him as an ordinary person with a particular problem with which you would like to help in a practical way when he is in difficulty. Too much help may deprive him of independence or make him lazy; sometimes it is best to leave him to muddle through on his own.

A blind person has to develop the other senses to compensate for loss of sight, in particular hearing and touch. He can become aware of large objects or buildings near him through changes in the way they reflect sound waves – just as noise changes its quality and tone when a train goes from the open into a tunnel. He can detect changes in floor or road surfaces with his feet, and not only his fingers but also his hands, wrists, and elbows can be used to feel objects near him. His memory becomes more acute in storing telephone numbers, for instance, which he cannot write down. Once a blind person has familiarised himself with a room, or a house, or a garden, or a street, he will not forget it; surroundings which were familiar before the loss of sight are, of course, much easier to memorise and get about in. It is extremely important for people living with and caring for the blind *not* to move any pieces of furniture or other objects from their usual places, and to be sure that there is 'a place for everything and everything in its place' in the home. After washing up, for example, cups, saucers, plates, glasses and cutlery should all be put back in the same position in the drawer or cupboard where they are always kept. Doors should *never* be left half open, because running into them can give a nasty knock: they should either be wide open or shut.

Washing and dressing can be made easier by little practical tricks, such as squeezing the toothpaste into the mouth instead of on to the toothbrush, and putting a safety pin into a certain part of a garment (at the back of the neck or under the arm) to signify its colour. Eating too can be made easier by arranging food on the plate in a fixed 'clock' pattern, so that the blind person knows that the meat will be at 6 o'clock, the potatoes at 9 o'clock, the other vegetables at 12 o'clock, and so on. If fish is on the menu, it is obviously a good idea for someone else to take the bones out before it is served.

It is very important always to announce your presence to a blind person when you enter a room, and to tell him what you are doing

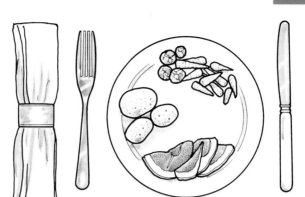

Eating can be made easier by arranging the food on the plate in a fixed pattern

and where you are going to sit. Be sure you don't forget to let him know when you get up and go, even if there is someone else in the room; it could be very embarrassing for him to find he was addressing thin air instead of you. It is equally important when you go to help a blind person in the street who is, perhaps, hesitating at a pedestrian crossing, to say who you are and to touch him, so that he has the reassurance of personal contact. Then the best way to lead him across the road is to ask him to hold your arm (just above the elbow) and to walk slightly ahead of him, warning him of any obstacles.

Organisations which exist to help those who have lost their sight and those who care for them are listed at the back of this book. The aim of the largest such organisation in the United Kingdom, the Royal National Institute for the Blind (RNIB), is to improve the quality of life for visually handicapped people, and to do this it provides a comprehensive range of services:

See Appendix VII for Addresses of useful organisations and support groups

- Schools for children of different ages and abilities;

- A vocational college and a college of further education;

- A school of physiotherapy;

- An employment service;

- Two employment rehabilitation centres;

- Three resource centres.

It also publishes special editions of books and magazines in Braille and Moon, and also on tape; provides an information and advice service; and offers the Talking Book Service, which has more than 6,500 popular books recorded unabridged on loan.

A register of blind and partially sighted people living in the area is kept by every county council, metropolitan district council, and London borough. Registration is voluntary, but it is necessary in order to qualify for the services and financial benefits available.

Eye specialists usually recommend registration to patients whose sight is badly affected; enquiries can also be made about the procedure for registration at local Social Service offices.

Loss of hearing

There are about 10 million people in this country with some degree of hearing loss. Some may have been born deaf, some may have gone deaf suddenly as the result of a blow or a violent explosion, but for many the onset will have been gradual as a result of the ageing process. Some diseases, such as measles, can cause deafness, as can some drugs. Exposure to very loud noises, such as road drills and 'pop' music, can also damage the hearing.

See also Appendix I, How the body works, section 1.xii on The ear

The ear is one of the most delicate parts of the body and can be easily damaged. It has three parts: the outer ear and the canal going down to the ear drum; the middle ear, on the other side of the ear drum, containing three tiny bones which move as the ear drum moves in response to sound waves; and the inner ear, which sorts out the different sounds and conveys them to the brain. Damage to any part of the ear can cause deafness. Hearing is often affected by wax obstructing the external canal; it is dangerous to try and remove the wax yourself, as the ear is so delicate, and you should ask your doctor to do this.

Another common condition affecting the hearing is tinnitus, or loud noises in the head, often like a sustained musical note or the sound of escaping steam. It cannot be cured, but if it is very troublesome it can sometimes be relieved by a small device like a hearing aid called a 'tinnitus masker'.

There are various operations to correct conditions causing deafness, which are done by ear, nose, and throat (ENT) specialists, but if surgery or other treatment is not possible, there is a wide variety of hearing aids available which amplify speech and other sounds. They do not restore normal hearing, and they may not help all deaf people, but they do make hearing easier. There are two main types – those worn behind the ear, and those worn on the body. Patients who will benefit are referred by the ENT consultant treating them to the local hearing aid department, where the aids are selected and fitted to suit the patients' degree and type of hearing loss.

Profoundly deaf people have to learn new ways of communicating, such as sign language and lip reading, but it is helpful for a partially deaf person to be able to lip read in addition. One of the worst aspects of deafness is the loneliness caused by being cut off from normal converse with others, so it is extremely important for relatives and friends and, indeed, anyone meeting a deaf person *not* to avoid talking to him or her, but to make an effort to overcome embarrassment and enter into normal conversation. The one thing

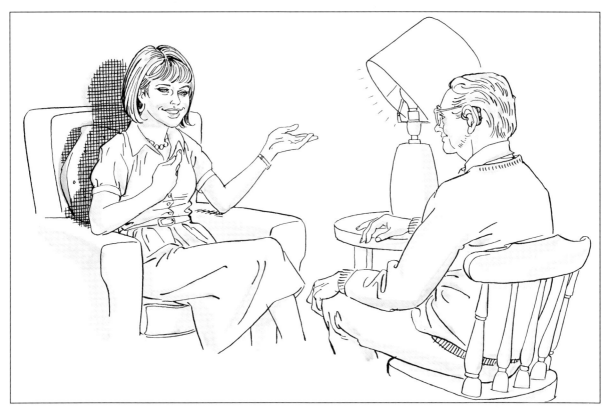

When talking to someone who has difficulty hearing, sit so that he has a good view of your face and form your words carefully

to avoid at all costs is shouting at deaf people, as it contorts the face and makes them feel very uncomfortable. It is best to speak clearly, with a normal rhythm, and a little more loudly and slowly than usual. To make reading your lips easier, you should sit facing the light so that your mouth can easily be seen, and form your words carefully but not in an exaggerated way. Don't sit too close – about five or six feet away is best – and don't turn your head away. Attract the deaf person's attention before starting to speak, and try to use whole sentences rather than single words, as they are easier to lip read.

There is a wide range of aids to daily living for deaf people, to enable them to use the telephone, watch television, and know when the doorbell rings, for example, and details of these can be obtained from the Royal National Institute for the Deaf (RNID). Like the RNIB, the RNID is a voluntary organisation which exists to represent the interests of the deaf, the deaf-blind, and the hard of hearing, and to help them and those caring for them in every way it can. Its library contains the largest collection of information relating to deafness in Britain, and it offers an enquiry service and a reference and lending service. The RNID:

See Appendix VII for Addresses of useful organisations and support groups

- Provides training courses in language and communication for deaf people and professional workers;

- Carries out research in medical aspects of hearing impairment;

- Offers residential care services for the deaf and disabled;

- And its regional offices and centres are an invaluable source of information and advice, particularly about technical equipment.

7.10(m) THE ADULT WHO IS HIV POSITIVE

HIV (human immunodeficiency virus) is, at the time of writing, still the subject of considerable misunderstanding and fear, both in those who have the virus and in the people who care for them. This text is intended to provide clear, practical information for people caring for an adult with the virus.

What HIV and AIDS mean

It is commonly assumed that having HIV is the same as having AIDS. *This is not true.*

With HIV, a sample of your blood is tested to see whether your immune system has reacted to the presence of HIV by producing cells called antibodies. If antibodies are present, you are then called 'HIV' antibody positive, often just referred to as HIV positive. People who are HIV positive often look and feel fine.

HIV is the virus which can lead to AIDS – acquired immune deficiency syndrome. This is a disease which attacks certain parts of the body's immune system. Some illnesses that the body would normally fight off become a serious problem. Doctors diagnose AIDS when they find certain specific diseases in a person with HIV. It can take several years for any sign of the disease to appear – indeed it may never do so.

How HIV is transmitted

You can get the virus in a number of ways:

- Having sex with someone who has the virus (this includes anal and vaginal sex – there is also a small risk with oral sex – otherwise most sexual activities are safe);

- Using or sharing needles and syringes with someone who has the virus (because small amounts of blood are also shared);

- People with haemophilia and others have been infected by receiving blood and blood products – since 1985 however blood banks have adopted strict screening guidelines and now all blood donated in Europe and the USA is thoroughly checked for HIV;

- There is a chance that a woman who has HIV might pass the virus to her baby during pregnancy or birth.

How HIV is spread

HIV is only spread by

- Blood to blood contact
- Sexual contact
- Breast milk (rarely)

You CANNOT get HIV from

- Insects

- Breathing the same air as
- Sharing a bathroom, toilet or shower with
- Touching, kissing, hugging or simply being near } A PERSON WITH HIV
- Sharing the same crockery, furniture etc as

Children and adults can share the same social, living and working environment as a person with HIV

Being HIV positive is not a death warrant. Many people with HIV remain well and have no apparent physical symptoms of illness. The majority of HIV positive individuals may not progress to AIDS for many years, if ever.

For many people, the worst thing about having the virus is feeling abandoned and shunned by the rest of the world. You can help in a number of ways, for example:

- Running errands;

- Preparing meals;

- Providing transport;

- Talking;

- Listening;

- Making telephone calls;

- Helping sorting bills.

Perhaps the most important thing to remember is that you *cannot* catch HIV through ordinary social contact. Helping people with HIV *does not* put you at risk of infection.

Providing emotional support

See also Chapter 3, section 9 on Sickness and body changes

Having HIV means making dramatic changes, and people with HIV experience strong feelings of loss, pain, anger and frustration. Having someone to talk to can make all the difference. All adults like to feel that they have some control over their lives, and this is no different for people with HIV. Encourage the person to become actively involved in his own care, make plans, and take decisions whenever possible. These actions will foster a sense of control and independence. Discuss how much help he needs from you, and how much you are realistically able to give. Decide together how you would like to spend time together. Your company can be just as important as your conversation. Just having you there while reading or watching television may be appreciated.

Caring for someone who has HIV is as individual as the person concerned – there are no strict rules. Don't be afraid to ask the person about the virus or how he is feeling, because often people with HIV want to talk about what is happening to them. However, this is not true of everyone and be aware that some individuals will not feel comfortable discussing it. While it's not always possible, it can be helpful to get to know the person's doctor, nurse, or other care providers that may be involved; they may be able to give you written instructions about medications and procedures. Do not be afraid to contact them if you are concerned about changes in the person's health and behaviour. For example, a persistent cough, fever, diarrhoea or confusion may indicate an infection or complication that requires special treatment.

Hygiene precautions

There has been much misinformation about the risks of HIV infection. The virus is difficult to catch. The risk of becoming infected through the person's blood coming into contact with your skin is very low. In the absence of sores or breaks in the skin, no HIV infections are known to have occurred. Simple precautions can virtually eliminate this already small risk. Ordinary good hygiene is enough to prevent transmission of the virus, even when body fluids are spilled. The virus is easily destroyed with a solution of ordinary household bleach.

An effective disinfecting solution of one part household bleach to ten parts water can be used on floors, sinks, bathrooms, toilets and surfaces. If you have any cuts, sores, or breaks on exposed skin, cover them with a plaster or bandage. You will want to wear gloves to clean up articles soiled with urine, faeces and vomit to avoid all germs. Use disposable hospital-type latex (rubber) gloves to protect against spilled blood and body fluids. These should only be used once and then thrown away. They are readily available from chemists. You might want to wear an apron or smock to prevent your clothing from being soiled.

Medication needles may be present if the person with HIV is diabetic, an injecting drug user, or has haemophilia. Handle needles carefully to avoid sticking yourself. Do not put caps back on needles by hand, and do not remove needles from the syringes because this increases the risk of sticking yourself. Where possible, the person with HIV should dispose of his or her own equipment. If you handle a used needle and syringe, pick it up by the barrel of the

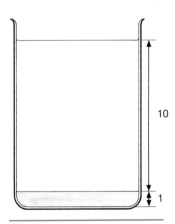

A solution of one part household bleach to ten parts water will make an adequate disinfecting solution

syringe and drop it carefully into a puncture proof container. A doctor or nurse can provide you with a specially made container, a 'sharps box'. Keep the box well out of the reach of children and visitors. Be sure to dispose of the container before it is overflowing with needles.

You can wash clothing and linens used by a person with HIV in hot water (60 °C) and an ordinary detergent, either in an automatic washing machine or by hand. Separate dishes and eating utensils, and special methods of cleaning them are not necessary. People with HIV should not share razors or toothbrushes because these items sometimes draw blood.

Flush all liquid waste containing blood, soluble sanitary pads and tampons down the toilet. Paper towels and other items that are not flushable should be placed in a plastic rubbish bag and sealed securely. Ask the nurse or care providers about further instructions for the removal of sharps boxes and rubbish bags – some local authorities have special arrangements.

Diet and the person with HIV

People with HIV can eat virtually any food that might seem appealing as the healthier the appetite, the better. However, there are some simple precautions to protect them from infections to which they might be susceptible:

- Avoid raw eggs;

- Meat, poultry and fish should be well cooked;

- Scrub fresh vegetables thoroughly;

- Wash your hands before handling any food.

When the person's appetite is poor, small, frequent meals may be more palatable than large, less frequent ones. The diet can be supplemented with high calorie/protein drinks which help maintain weight. Examples are Build-up, Fresubin and Complan, all of which are available from chemists.

Looking after yourself

See Chapter 2, section 6 on Help for the carers and Appendix VII for Addresses of useful organisations and support groups

See also Chapter 7, section 5 on Caring for others and its effects on health

Providing home care can be a stressful and emotionally draining experience. There may come a time when you need someone to talk to, maybe to sort out a particular problem, or for more general advice. If you get to know the avenues of support available to you before there are any major problems, you will have a network to call upon when you need it.

Remember that you are not alone. Others have shared similar experiences and formed self help support groups. It is possibly easier to talk when other people describe experiences that reflect your own.

Be sure to arrange for some back up help so that you can have free time occasionally. When caring for a person with HIV it is important not to ignore your own needs. Unless you take care of yourself, you will reduce dramatically the amount of strength and energy you have left to care for your partner, friend or relative.

Where to get help

It is sometimes difficult to know where to go to for practical help and support, particularly when HIV remains a generally sensitive subject surrounded by hostility, misunderstanding and fear. Many people with HIV and their carers express concern about whether confidentiality will be respected, and who you can trust with information. If you want to talk in confidence to people with training and experience in HIV related issues try an organisation such as the Terrence Higgins Trust or the National AIDS Helpline.

See Appendix VII for Addresses of useful organisations and support groups

Services for people with HIV and their carers vary widely from area to area. There are a number of local organisations which have useful information about the services provided in your locality (see your local phone book). These may include:

- The Citizens' Advice Bureau;

- Public library;

- Community Health Council (which works to improve services to patients in hospitals, surgeries and health centres);

- The Council for Voluntary Services (which co-ordinates voluntary efforts).

Living with HIV is a challenge that has to be faced on an individual basis but, by responding to the needs of the person you are caring for, you help him to meet that challenge and thereby to increase his quality of life.

7.10(n) VIRAL ILLNESS

Viruses are the smallest of all the infectious agents and only reproduce inside living cells. New virus particles are produced because viruses can programme the infected host cells to make a number of virus specific molecules. These molecules are produced and assembled into more virus particles, which are then released to attack new susceptible cells. In this way viruses multiply, invade more and more cells and eventually cause disease.

Any organ of the body may be attacked by some virus or another so that a wide variety of signs and symptoms may be present in a viral infection. However, as viruses are intracellular pathogens there is little in the way of treatment that can be offered. Antibiotics, as already mentioned, are of no use in a viral infection, so the speed and ease with which patients recover depends on their ability to combat disease. Better by far to protect against serious viral illnesses by vaccination.

The earliest classification of viruses was based on the illnesses they caused, for example the viruses that cause generalised diseases such as smallpox, measles, rubella and chicken pox. In these diseases, the virus spreads rapidly via the bloodstream and a number of body organs may be affected including the skin, as rashes occur. Other viruses affect specific body organs. For example, poliomyelitis and rabies affect the nervous system, the common cold and influenza viruses attack the respiratory system while hepatitis A and B viruses affect the liver. Such a classification is not very helpful, however, as some viruses may affect more than one organ. For example, herpes simplex virus (the 'cold sore') affects the skin of the mouth and/or genitals and the nervous system. So nowadays viruses are generally grouped according to their size, shape, structure and method of reproduction.

Treatment and prevention

Although antibiotics have no role to play in treating viruses, there are a few drugs which can be more helpful. Amantadine (Symmetrel) inhibits influenza A viruses by blocking their penetration into the host cells and has been used to prevent individuals with severe heart or lung disease from developing influenza. Acyclovir (Zovirax) inhibits herpes simplex virus and herpes zoster virus and is thus used for patients with cold sores or shingles. To be effective it has to be given as early as possible during the illness, but cannot eradicate the virus totally from the body so recurrence of cold sores is all too common.

Undoubtedly, however, the best way of responding to viruses is to avoid them or to protect ourselves and our children in some other way.

Immunisation or vaccination is one way in which we can prevent certain infections. Our immune system recognises foreign molecules known as antigens and acts to immobilise, neutralise and destroy them. When fully operational, this system protects us from a wide variety of infectious agents as well as from abnormal body cells. If it fails or malfunctions diseases such as cancer, or AIDS may result.

Active immunity can be acquired naturally during bacterial and viral infections but can be produced artificially by the use of vaccines. Most vaccines contain dead or considerably weakened disease producing organisms (pathogens). Such organisms have the ability to produce immunity but not to cause disease. Immunity achieved by vaccination is indistinguishable from the immunity acquired during the course of an infection. However, the individual has not had to suffer all the symptoms of the disease in order to acquire immunity. Vaccines are currently available against the viruses that cause measles, mumps, rubella, influenza, polio and hepatitis as well as some bacterially caused diseases.

The efficiency of the immune system declines slowly but in old age the ability to fight infection is reduced. Indeed, the greater incidence of cancer in the elderly is assumed to be part of this failure of the immune system.

Rhinoviruses

The rhinoviruses cause upper respiratory tract infections including the 'common cold'. The virus enters by the nose, invades the cells of the lining and produces engorgement of the blood vessels, swelling and an increase in secretion hence the 'stuffed up' feeling and the runny nose. Experiments have shown that chilling, including the wearing of wet clothes, does not produce a cold or increase susceptibility to the virus.

The incubation period is short, between two and four days, and the acute illness lasts up to seven days although a non-productive cough may persist for two or three weeks. Usual symptoms include headache, mild cough, malaise and a nasal discharge. Swelling of the nasal linings leads to a decrease in the ability to smell and thus taste may be altered. Tears may overflow as they cannot escape through the blocked passages, leading to the streaming eyes and runny nose of a full blown cold.

A secondary bacterial infection may produce sinusitis, bronchitis or acute otitis media (middle ear infection) especially in children. This will probably respond to antibiotics and your doctor may prescribe some.

The common cold occurs throughout the world and is transmitted through close contact by large droplets. No specific treatment is available and the sufferer should keep warm, drink plenty of fluids, and treat other symptoms appropriately (e.g headache with a mild analgesic such as paracetamol). Paper tissues should be used for nasal discharge and disposed of safely.

Influenza viruses

The orthomyxoviruses cause influenza. They enter the body via the respiratory tract in airborne droplets hence the old adage 'Coughs and sneezes spread diseases'. The incubation period is one or two days. Usual symptoms include fever, chills, muscle pain, and malaise. The fever usually persists for about three days. Complications are not common but pneumonia can occur. Pregnant women and elderly people with chronic illnesses have a higher risk of complications. Children may develop Reye's syndrome which is characterised by nervous system involvement and liver disease.

In the 1940s it seemed that killed influenza vaccine might provide protection. Since then it has become apparent that the virus undergoes periodic 'antigenic shift', a sort of mutation, making existing vaccines useless. However, this should not prevent elderly individuals and those with chronic lung and heart disease from being vaccinated each year. 'Antigenic shift' does explain why serious influenza epidemics can occur suddenly. It is as if we are meeting a 'new' virus and thus have no immunity. Spread is swift and 'flu the result.

No specific treatment exists. The sufferer should go to bed, keep warm and drink plenty of fluids. Aspirin will reduce fever and relieve headache but should not be given to children under 12 years of age because it has been associated with the development of Reye's syndrome. A number of proprietary medicines exist to relieve the symptoms of colds and influenza.

Viruses affecting children

A number of viruses, such as measles, mumps and rubella, can affect adults with quite serious consequences. Far more often, however, they are diseases of childhood and are dealt with accordingly in the appropriate sections. Glandular fever, primarily a disease of teenagers and young adults, is also covered elsewhere.

The herpes viruses

Herpes simplex   Infection with herpes simplex virus may present in several ways. The usual presentation is patches of small blisters (vesicles) on the skin or mucous membranes. Primary infections occur in individuals who have no antibodies and the virus may then reside in the sensory nerves of the host. At times of lowered resistance (e.g. if the person has a cold or 'flu) the lesions recur usually at the junction of the lips with the facial skin. The vesicles rupture leaving a painful ulcer that heals without scarring. Spread is by direct contact with the vesicles. Genital herpes is characterised by similar lesions of the penis in the male or cervix, vulva, vagina or perineum in the female.

Acyclovir can be applied as a cream to the lesions. It will allay the symptoms but not eradicate the virus.

Varicella and herpes zoster   Varicella (chicken pox) is a mild but highly infectious disease, chiefly of children, which has been covered in more detail elsewhere. Herpes zoster (shingles) is a disease of adults that is characterised by an inflammation of sensory nerve roots accompanied by crops of vesicles on the skin supplied by the affected nerves. The illness starts with fever and

See also Chapter 5, section 12 on Common health problems, and Chapter 6, section 6(b) on Infectious diseases

malaise and is soon followed by severe pain in the area of skin supplied by the affected sensory nerves. Within a few days the crops of vesicles appear. The trunk, head and neck are commonly affected, and usually on only one side of the body.

The lesions disappear within three to four weeks. Treatment includes topical applications to the vesicles and analgesia for the pain. Acyclovir may be prescribed. Individuals with herpes zoster can be the source of an outbreak of chicken pox in children, but children with varicella do not cause shingles in adults.

Shingles is an unpleasant disease for the time it lasts, and the sufferer will require careful and sympathetic nursing.

Warts

Warts have an incubation period of up to one year and often disappear with no treatment.

Common skin warts (verrucae)   These can be spread by direct or indirect contact. The sufferer can re-infect herself by scratching. Common warts (verruca vulgaris) are small, flesh coloured raised spots and appear most frequently on the fingers and hand. As they develop they get larger and more pronounced. They sometimes contain black dots.

Plantar warts   Plantar warts occur on the soles of the feet and tend to grow inward, because of weight-bearing, and become uncomfortable. Chiropodists are experts at removing these.

Hepatitis

Viral hepatitis is a disease affecting the liver and is caused by one of five hepatitis viruses the most common of which are the hepatitis A virus and the hepatitis B virus.

Hepatitis A   Hepatitis A virus (HAV) is transmitted via the mouth usually as a result of faecal contamination of food or drink. The incubation period is between two and six weeks. The virus causes inflammation of the liver cells which results in a decreased ability of the liver to function. Thus the patient feels generally unwell, off his food, nauseated and may vomit. His abdomen is tender and he will feel feverish. The skin and whites of the eye become yellow (jaundiced). The urine is dark and the stools pale.

Treatment and care is supportive and symptomatic. Rest in bed or limited activity is recommended until symptoms have subsided. Patients may be unable to tolerate fatty foods and small, high carbohydrate meals may be the answer.

Fatigue is a lingering symptom and convalescence may be prolonged. Alcohol should be forbidden for at least six months while the liver recovers fully. Immune globulin gives temporary passive immunity to HAV and should be given within six weeks of exposure or before travel to an area with epidemic HAV.

Control measures are directed towards the prevention of faecal contamination of water or food. Proper handwashing is essential.

Hepatitis B   Hepatitis B (HBV) is transmitted by blood and other body fluids through breaks in the skin. Needle stick injury, ear piercing, tattooing, sharing syringes and sexual intercourse have all been implicated in the spread of the disease.

Hepatitis B is endemic in South East Asia, Africa, Central and Latin America, Japan, the Soviet Union and parts of Eastern and Southern Europe.

After an incubation period of 15–40 days, 'flu-like symptoms develop in about a third of the patients half of whom will develop jaundice. Ninety per cent of sufferers recover fully but it may take up to six months.

Those patients who do not develop symptoms either become carriers of the disease or develop immunity. The World Health Organisation currently estimates some 200–280 million individuals in the world are carriers, that is to say possible transmitters of the disease.

There is no specific treatment other than rest and alleviation of symptoms. As 10 per cent become chronic carriers who may have chronic persistent hepatitis of a more active form which may lead to liver cirrhosis it is better to avoid the disease.

See also Appendix IV, section ii, for more information about Immunisations

Hepatitis B vaccine is now available and can be prescribed by your family doctor. For immunity to be conferred, three doses over six months must be given. Immunity lasts for around seven years.

Post viral fatigue syndrome (ME)

Post viral fatigue syndrome or myalgic encephalomyelitis (ME) is believed to be caused by one or more viruses. The main features are extraordinary fatigue, headache, muscle pain, and mental disturbances such as mood swings, intolerance of sound and/or light, loss of concentration, and memory lapses.

A particular problem for sufferers of ME is that the disease is difficult to diagnose and, indeed, has been recognised only relatively recently. Individuals may have periods of heightened anxiety while waiting for a diagnosis, and of anger or lowered self-esteem if they feel they are being tacitly accused of malingering. Carers may find they have to be particularly supportive and need to make a special effort to let the patient know that they believe in her symptoms.

The treatment is rest and plenty of it. Extra vitamins such as vitamin B_6, necessary for antibody production, may be beneficial.

Alcohol exacerbates the symptoms. The sufferer should treat her energy reserves as if they were money in the bank and be careful not to overdraw. It is a difficult balancing act – not overdoing things or getting too tired as opposed to resting too much and losing muscle tone. The support of friends and family is essential, for the battle against ME may take many months if not years.

7.11 THE ADULT WITH CANCER

Of all diseases, cancer is one of the most feared, and can give rise to a tremendous amount of anxiety and emotional distress. There are many misunderstandings and myths surrounding cancer which can cause additional problems for patients and their carers at home.

People commonly associate the word 'cancer' with pain, wasting, disfigurement or death. However, it is important to remember that many thousands of patients are cured from cancer while others may live happily for a number of years with their cancer under control. In general, the earlier cancer is diagnosed the better the chances of controlling or curing it. This is the reason for screening programmes and vigilance on the part of the individual (see for example the advice given on breast self-examination, above). The American Cancer Association list a number of early warning signs to look out for, as shown in the box below. This list should be interpreted as a caution, NOT as an aid to self-diagnosis. The appearance of one or more of the signs in no way suggests that you definitely have cancer – but it does mean that you should see your doctor as soon as possible so that the possibility can be eliminated or prompt treatment started.

'Cancer' is a very broad term grouping together several different types of disease. The experience of cancer and its treatment will vary considerably between one patient and another. Therefore,

See section 7.10(a), final paragraphs, for advice on examining your breasts

CAUTION – the early warning signs of a possible cancer (or other serious illness), devised by the American Cancer Society

Change in bowel or bladder habit

A sore that does not heal

Unusual bleeding or discharge

Thickening or lump in the breast or elsewhere

Indigestion or difficulty in swallowing

Obvious change in a wart or mole

Nagging cough or hoarseness

making comparisons with others is not advisable as it can lead to unnecessary worry. It is essential that accurate information and specific advice pertaining to the individual is obtained from the doctor or nurse involved with the overall management.

Undoubtedly, cancer presents unique coping problems for patients and their carers. Support and guidance can be provided from various sources to meet individual needs as far as possible. The variety of options can appear confusing and it is hoped that the remainder of this section will help to clarify what is available to carers, and offer general advice.

7.11(a)   DIAGNOSIS

The experience of being given a diagnosis of cancer can be extremely traumatic for all concerned. Many patients already suspect that the problem is cancer before they are actually told, particularly if they have undergone an extensive series of tests. Even though some degree of mental preparation may have taken place, the official diagnosis can cause immense shock and be difficult to accept initially.

Sometimes the doctor may first approach the carer who is the closest relative in order to discuss the position prior to revealing the diagnosis to the patient. The carer, who knows the patient better than any health professional, can provide useful guidance on how best to deal with the situation. Moral dilemmas can arise, however, where carers feel strongly that the patient should not be told he has cancer. This may stem from the carers' own fears or perhaps from a request by the patient not to be told if he has cancer. There is no easy answer to this difficulty. Each case is highly individual and can only be dealt with as such. It is important that carers share their worries with the health professionals involved and hopefully, after further discussion, a solution can be reached which is satisfactory for all.

See also Chapter 3, section 10 on Bereavement and loss, and section 9 on Sickness and body changes

In response to a diagnosis of cancer, a whole range of different emotions may be experienced by patients and carers alike. As well as shock, there can be grief, anger, a sense of hopelessness and isolation, depression or guilt and many others. There is no set pattern to such reactions. The weeks or months following diagnosis may be a period of time which resembles a bereavement. Some of the confusion at this time can be alleviated if carers understand that these reactions can occur and are therefore able to recognise what is happening. Some will suffer these reactions to a greater extent than others. Everyone is an individual and, as such, will be affected in unique ways by a diagnosis of cancer at all different levels, whether psychologically, socially or spiritually.

See also Chapter 7, section 5 on Caring for others and its effects on health

Carers can do much to help, simply by being there and demonstrating willingness to listen to the patient and sharing in the experience. It is ideal if open, honest communication can be achieved on both sides, if feelings are shared and needs expressed.

Where two-way communication is not present, life can be difficult for everyone following diagnosis. The natural desire to protect loved ones from hurt frequently results in situations where patients and carers try to hide things from each other. There may be a withholding of information or the temptation to pretend that all is well in order to make life more bearable. Although this is done with good intention it does not create an atmosphere of mutual help and support which is often badly needed.

At the same time, a patient ought not to be forced into talking about his cancer or related problems against his will. An advisable approach for carers to adopt would be to encourage patients to share their thoughts and provide plenty of opportunities without using any force.

See also Chapter 7, section 6 on Counselling skills

It is very important that carers seek help in dealing with these sensitive issues. In addition to coping with their own feelings following the diagnosis, carers also take on full responsibility for supporting the patient and this can be extremely difficult. As well as the general practitioner, contact with a nurse can be requested. A specialist nurse such as a Macmillan nurse may be available but first contact is usually with the district nurse who can help co-ordinate the different sources of support. This provides a valuable opportunity for carers to 'offload' any problems and receive the appropriate guidance or counselling.

Following diagnosis, carers may often need to help patients to clarify the facts of the situation. Patients are usually shocked at the time of diagnosis and are unable to take in and remember what the doctor has said. Some doctors are now providing tape-recordings of this initial interview which may be helpful later. It may be that the patient has misunderstood something of great importance or been confused by medical terminology leading to a false perception of the situation. Carers can help by reinforcing the information afterwards providing they themselves are sufficiently well informed. However, it is a useful practice for patients to write down any questions or worries that remain about the cancer itself or impending treatment. This list can then be worked through with the doctor or nurse when they visit at home or else with staff at the hospital where the diagnosis was made.

See Appendix VII for Addresses of useful organisations and support groups

As well as professional help, people with cancer and their carers may wish to make use of the numerous charitable organisations and self-help groups which are in operation. These are available on a local and a national scale and provide excellent information, counselling and support.

7.11(b)   TREATMENT

For some, the fear of treatment outweighs the fear of cancer itself. The methods of treating cancer are frequently misunderstood and confusion surrounding treatment adds to fear and apprehension.

There are three main types of cancer treatment:

- Radiotherapy;

- Chemotherapy;

- Surgery.

The implications of each are discussed later. Patients may receive just one of these forms of treatment or a combination of two or all three. On rare occasions, a choice may be offered to the patient – who then has to decide upon the preferred option following discussion with the consultant in charge.

Usually patients are referred to a cancer treatment specialist but the general practitioner remains in charge of medical care in the home setting. Hospital consultants and general practitioners liaise between each other, transferring information about the patient when necessary.

Treatment may be carried out in a unit of the local hospital, in a regional cancer treatment centre or at home on an outpatient basis when possible. This will vary from one area to another.

Once the diagnosis of cancer has been made, each patient is assessed on an individual basis and a 'tailor-made' programme of treatment is planned. As well as the type and extent of cancer, the patient's age and general state of health will be taken into account when planning the treatment regime. Whichever format of treatment is initiated, it is not unusual for the doctor to introduce changes as the course progresses. This is not a cause to worry and does not mean that plans are going wrong.

Treatment is given for differing reasons. Naturally it is given to cure the disease but where this cannot be guaranteed it may also be used to contain disease, thereby successfully keeping it under control. Where cancer is advanced, treatment can be given to relieve problematic symptoms such as pain.

Usually, the plan of treatment and what to expect will be explained by medical and nursing staff at the unit where it will be given. Once again, there is a great deal of new information for patients and carers to absorb. Writing down the main points can help to some extent but the hospital staff dealing directly with the treatment can provide an excellent source of help.

It is a good idea to keep telephone numbers of useful contacts such as this close at hand. If any problems or uncertainties cause distress, the appropriate help is then readily available.

It is beneficial to approach your general practitioner or district nurse with any queries relating to treatment. Where appropriate they can introduce further support from a Macmillan nurse or a specialist cancer nurse, liaising with the hospital if necessary.

A long course of treatment might have financial implications for carers, especially if the patient is the main 'bread-winner' of the family. Long periods of absence from work or even the loss of a job may result, depending on personal circumstances. Also, carers may be making regular visits to a patient who is hospitalised a long distance away requiring a sizeable cash outlay on travelling costs.

Many people have found benefit from using some other approaches to the treatment of their cancer, in parallel with the orthodox programme of therapy. Such complementary methods include massage, aromatherapy, relaxation techniques, visualisation, hypnotherapy, art therapy and many more. The emphasis in such approaches is on the healing of not only the physical body but also the mind and spirit. It aims to provide a holistic (whole person) angle towards total health revitalisation.

Of those who do find value in the use of these methods, most can successfully incorporate them into their already existing plan of orthodox treatment (such as radiotherapy or chemotherapy). However, it is advisable for patients to discuss the use of complementary therapies with their doctor and express their own viewpoint about the approach to treatment. It should be remembered that patients and their caring relatives are most important members of the treatment team.

One of the reported benefits of using complementary methods is that it gives patients the ability to become directly involved with their own treatment. This can help to increase their feelings of self-worth and encourages a positive outlook which can create a marked improvement for some.

It must be stressed that the use of any complementary therapy must be the choice of the individual patient and must feel right for the patient. Without the willingness and desire to try any one method, the chances of positive benefits are poor.

The wide range of therapies available are either practised privately by individuals or at natural health centres or cancer help centres. Hospitals are also starting to introduce complementary therapies but this will vary from one unit to another. More information can be obtained from your district nurse, Macmillan nurse or other health professionals, the Citizens' Advice Bureau, public library, or the Bristol Cancer Help Centre.

Radiotherapy

Radiotherapy is a method used to damage and destroy cancer cells by means of radiation rays. The treatment is painless and can be described as similar to having an ordinary x-ray picture taken.

See section 7.9 above for more information about the financial implications of long-term illness, and Appendix VI on Benefits

See also Chapter 2, section 3 on Coping with pain

See Appendix VII for Addressses of useful organisations

One of the commonly expressed fears about radiotherapy is that it makes people radioactive. This is NOT the case and there is no cause for alarm. The type of treatment described in this section would never render a patient radioactive at any stage. It is entirely safe for others, including children and pregnant women, to mix with the patient at all times in the home.

In some cases radioactive sources are used to treat cancer by being applied directly onto the affected area of the body. This is always carried out in hospital under conditions of the utmost safety. While differing from the earlier described method of treatment there is still no risk of radioactivity after the treatment has been completed.

As previously indicated, the course of treatment is tailored to the individual's needs. The dosage, length of treatment overall and the body area requiring treatment will vary for each patient. Radiotherapy is usually only given once a day on Mondays to Fridays. Each session of treatment only takes a matter of minutes but the overall period of treatment can vary from several weeks to a few days. For some, a single treatment is all that is needed. Before the treatment is begun, explanations regarding the course and what to expect afterwards will be discussed with patients and carers. Any advice should be sought from the hospital staff as required.

It is important that both patient and carer have been made aware of the potential side-effects of the treatment. The degree to which side-effects appear varies considerably with some patients experiencing none at all. There is no method of predicting how a course of treatment will affect an individual. It is therefore necessary to assess the changing situation on a daily basis.

Side-effects are temporary. They are caused by unavoidable interference to some of the body's normal cells by the radiation. If they do occur, it is usually at least half way through the course and not at the beginning. For some patients, reactions only appear after the treatment has finished. There are some generalised effects of treatment but in the main, reactions are localised. For example, treatment to the scalp can cause hair loss while treatment to the lower abdomen is likely to affect the bowel habit.

Generally speaking, patients may become disillusioned if side-effects to treatment are causing them problems. Carers can help greatly by reassuring them that these problems are temporary and that they will soon get back to normal.

Patients need encouragement to carry on with life as usual following radiotherapy, while allowing for plenty of rest. The vast majority of patients feel more tired than usual during treatment and this can last for up to a few months afterwards. Undergoing a long course of radiotherapy can be every bit as exhausting as having an operation and, frequently, this is not realised.

See also Chapter 6, section 7 on Behavioural and emotional problems in adolescence

See section 7.10(m) below on The adult who is HIV positive

Skin	– Area treated may become pink and sensitive – May become sore, especially in skin folds, such as groins	– Gentle care of skin needed – Avoid scented products such as soap, perfume or talcum powder – Avoid extremes of temperature and exposure to wind or sun – Avoid tight clothing
Head and neck	– Radiotherapy in this area may pose special problems with eating and drinking – Mouth may be sore, with dryness/inflammation of mucous membranes and tongue	– Advice on diet can be obtained from the hospital, district nurse or dietitian – Provide as healthy a diet as possible – Give small frequent meals and try to ensure patient drinks around 3 litres of fluid a day – Food supplements (e.g. Complan, Build-up) may be given – Give mouthwashes every 2 hours – The doctor will prescribe painkillers – Dental check-ups will be required more often than usual and carers may have to remind the patient of appointments
Gastrointestinal system	– Radiotherapy to the abdomen may cause nausea and vomiting – Diarrhoea or constipation may occur	– Make the patient's environment as comfortable as possible – Offer small, regular sips of fluid – Sucking ice cubes or taking fizzy drinks can sometimes help to alleviate the problem – The doctor will prescribe anti-sickness drugs until the problem subsides – The patient should be encouraged to drink plenty and maintain an adequate diet – The doctor will prescribe the appropriate medication

Side-effects of radiotherapy

Should side-effects pose severe problems which cannot be managed adequately at home, the patient will be readmitted to hospital for a short spell for them to be dealt with.

Regular follow-up appointments will be made for the patient to attend hospital so that progress can be monitored.

Chemotherapy

Chemotherapy means 'drug treatment'. In the treatment of cancer, a special group of drugs are used, called 'cytotoxic' agents (i.e. toxic to cells). As this suggests they destroy cancer cells or damage them so that they cannot reproduce. Unlike radiotherapy which is a localised means of treatment, chemotherapy is systemic. This means that by the transport of drugs through the bloodstream it affects the whole body.

This treatment is either given:

- By mouth in tablet form;

- By injection;

- By continuous infusion into a vein (drip).

Patients may be given one drug or a combination of several which is more usual. Specific advice about the selected drugs, how often they are given and how long for, should be obtained from the hospital medical and nursing staff.

All chemotherapy regimes are different but one factor in common with them all is that there is a rest period in between treatments. An example of a treatment plan might be six sessions of chemotherapy given at three weekly intervals. Most patients are admitted to hospital for a short period to receive their treatment and then return home for the rest period until the time comes for the next treatment.

Under some circumstances the treatment itself may take place within the home setting, in one of the following ways:

- The patient, under instructions from the doctor, takes tablets at prescribed intervals;

- The district nurse administers the drug by injection;

- A battery operated pump, pre-programmed by hospital staff to work continuously, delivers the required dosage of drug over a set period. (In this situation a contact number for the hospital ward is given, usually serving as the main link in case of problems.)

The potential side-effects of chemotherapy, as with radiotherapy, vary between individuals and some patients do not find them a problem at all.

If side-effects do occur, again they are temporary and are caused by damage to normal cells by the drugs. Unlike the cancer cells, normal cells recover and regenerate so that no permanent damage is done. The rest periods in between treatments allow the recuperation process to take place.

The many different drugs in use all have a potential for side-effects. Specific advice must be sought in each case. The table overleaf describes some possible generalised effects common to all cytotoxic agents.

It is the psychological aspects of treatment which are often the most difficult for carers to cope with at home. If an unpleasant side-effect has occurred, patients may develop a psychological

A temporary depletion in blood cells makes the person prone to anaemia and bruising and considerably lowers resistance to infection	– Any minor complaint, such as a common cold, can become extremely unpleasant	– While the patient is at home between treatments, reduce contact with crowds and visitors, and keep people carrying colds or other infections away – The patient should keep warm and maintain a good diet and fluid intake – Call the doctor if the patient's temperature rises or his condition is worsening noticeably
Nausea and vomiting	– More likely with some drugs than others	– The doctor will prescribe anti-sickness drugs – The problem is likely to subside quite quickly once the patient is home again
Reduced enjoyment of food	– Chemotherapy can reduce the appetite and change the perception of some tastes	– Give small, frequent meals – Food supplements may be needed
Hair loss	– More likely with some drugs than others	– Reassure patient that hair will grow back once treatment has stopped – Wigs may be available on the NHS – ask your district nurse or at the hospital for details – Encourage the patient to experiment with hats and scarves, and to continue wearing make-up if this is her usual practice when well

Side-effects of chemotherapy

See Appendix VII for Addresses of useful organisations and support groups

barrier affecting subsequent treatments. It appears ironic that it is only when a patient has fully recovered from one treatment, and feels perfectly well again, that he has to go in for the next. The patient may begin to expect the side-effect experienced during the previous treatment making it difficult for him to return for more. Some patients demonstrate physical manifestations of this difficulty in the form of anticipatory vomiting, where just the sight or smell of the hospital can bring on sickness.

These problems can be helped by sharing them with health professionals who will offer advice and help to get the patient through it. Other carers who are going through similar difficulties can also be a good source of support. In addition to all the health professionals mentioned in previous sections, there may be a chemotherapy nurse involved with the situation. In some units it is a chemotherapy nurse whose prime role is to administer the prescribed treatment and provide appropriate advice and emotional support.

Surgery

Unlike radiotherapy and chemotherapy, the surgical removal of cancer tissue is usually very straightforward and is just like having any other form of operation. Surgery is commonly carried out on general hospital wards rather than at specialist cancer treatment units. There are, however, some types of cancer which require operations involving more specialised procedures.

Patients are generally sent home fairly early following surgery so that much of the recovery period takes place at home. Again, good diet is important for the healing of tissues and to regain lost weight. Carers should concentrate on helping the patient to return to his normal activity as soon as possible. Painkillers will have been given to relieve pain from the wound but if this remains a problem the general practitioner should be consulted. The district nurse will perform any wound care that is required, such as removal of stitches or dressings.

The main implications for patients and carers following surgery are dealing with the psychological aspects. If the operation was performed in order to diagnose cancer it can be a great shock to patients afterwards if positive results were found. In other situations, patients may be afraid that not all the cancer has been removed and need reassurance from medical and nursing staff.

See also Chapter 3, section 10 on Bereavement and loss, and section 9 on Sickness and body changes. See Appendix VII for Addresses of useful organisations and support groups

Post-operative shock can be particularly acute where the patient grieves for a lost part of the body. Major operations which commonly cause a lot of psychological distress include the removal of a breast, formation of a colostomy, facial surgery or removal of the womb. Patients may find difficulty in accepting such a loss and the altered body image which results. Sexual problems can develop, as can feelings of low self-esteem. Carers sometimes feel unable to support the patient adequately and may have the added problem of coping with their own feelings of non-acceptance of the surgery.

Specialist help is available. In addition to the health professionals mentioned earlier there are also:

- Breast care counsellors;

- Stomatherapists (dealing with colostomies);

- Many national self-help groups.

7.11(c) ADVANCED CANCER

For some patients, there may come a time when active treatment is no longer of benefit and the main aim of care is to assist the patient to maintain as good a quality of life as possible.

See also Chapter 2, section 5(h), and Chapter 8, section 5 for more information about caring for people who are dying

This stage can be highly stressful for the carers who face an uncertain future and may be observing the deterioration in the health of a loved one. Any unpleasant symptoms experienced by the patient should be discussed with the family doctor so that appropriate medication or gentle form of treatment can be given for their relief. Carers have a useful role in passing on information to the doctor as patients are not always able to do this themselves.

Communication between patient and carer is important and, if possible, the carer can help by focusing on the positive aspects of life. This is not to say that the patient's mental pain should be made light of or that false optimism should be introduced, but the carer can encourage her to concentrate on the good things that she still has in her life. Carers can try to help the patient adapt to a new lifestyle to accommodate the limitations imposed by illness.

Close relatives may need as much support as patients at this stage. Following discussion with the main carer, the district nurse will assist with physical nursing care as required and will also be there to provide emotional support for patient and carer. Others who may be involved include the Macmillan nurse, Marie Curie nursing service and social services.

The hospice facility provides an excellent source of help for carers as well as patients. The philosophy of the hospice movement is to help patients to continue living to their fullest potential, retaining as much independence as possible. The hospice takes account of the wishes of patients and carers when planning admissions. A short respite admission can be arranged, enabling the carer to take a rest which can be badly needed in some cases. The patient is then discharged home as arranged. This service enables patients to remain at home for the most part by providing adequate support for the carer. Hospice admission can be arranged through your family doctor, district nurse or Macmillan nurse.

See Chapter 3, section 10 on Bereavement and loss, and Appendix VII for Addresses of useful organisations and support groups

As well as experiencing the normal process of bereavement when a patient dies, carers are also faced with the loss of their caring role and have to make major adjustments to their own lives. As well as support from family and friends, they can receive help from any of the health professionals already encountered. Support is also offered by various other organisations.

7.12 THE ADULT WITH A PHYSICAL DISABILITY

See also Chapter 2, section 2 on Helping the sick person at home with the activities of living and section 4 on Lifting and transfers

Physical disability in the adult can be due to a congenital abnormality, trauma or disease. Where impairment is due to a congenital abnormality the cause will have been established long before adulthood is reached and both the individual and her family will have had time to make adjustments and revise their expectations of the future during the childhood years. Sudden onset of disability in an adult (for example as a result of a road traffic accident) can, quite literally, turn a whole family's world upside-down as they find themselves having to rethink such basics as where they should be living and how to pay the bills. Disability resulting from disease may give more time for adjustment but can still be most distressing. People whose condition is not readily diagnosed may find themselves becoming extremely frustrated and quite depressed. The effects of long term disability are not limited to physically disabling conditions but may include social and psychological consequences.

The person you are caring for may himself experience many anxieties, for example:

- Fears associated with loss of independence and loss of his role within the family;

- Fears associated with mental, physical and social deterioration;

- Fears about the future;

- A loss of identity and a crisis of sexual confidence;

- Loss of self-esteem;

- Worries about impending adjustments in relationships.

Such anxieties, particularly if occurring together, may result in feelings of anger, denial, helplessness and depression.

You, as a carer may also experience these feelings and may find other difficulties that are frustrating, irritating or that may be extremely distressing. Honest communication is the key aspect when caring for a relative or friend who has a physical disability.

The difficulties that each person experiences are hard to identify individually. The following paragraphs aim, therefore, to give a general overview of principles and advice from which you can pick out the aspects that are specific to people like yourself and those for whom you care.

7.12(a) ENCOURAGING SELF-CARE

People with long term disability may have varying degrees of need. To assist them in preserving their dignity and self-esteem, and to maximise their potential for self-care, you as a carer can help them to adapt to those needs and thereby help yourself.

Allow the sick person to do as much for herself as is possible. Tempting as it may be to save yourself time in the short term by putting on her stockings and shoes for her, encouraging her to do as much as she can for herself can result in a tremendous sense of achievement. Such a positive feeling can only make your relationship easier and more pleasant.

It is essential to allow time for the activities of dressing, washing, bathing, cleaning teeth, toileting and feeding.

Dressing

See also Chapter 2, section 2(n) on Improvising equipment

You may help the person to get up in the morning by himself by tying a rope or sheet to the end of the bed so that he can hold onto it and gradually sit up. Special ropes may be purchased, or you can improvise your own. Other helping aids could include a mechanical back rest or a special electrical bed – this will help you to encourage some form of independence and relieve physical pressure from you. You can use and adapt simple devices to help the person dress himself – for example, using velcro instead of buttons and zips, or making special adaptations to underwear and shoes.

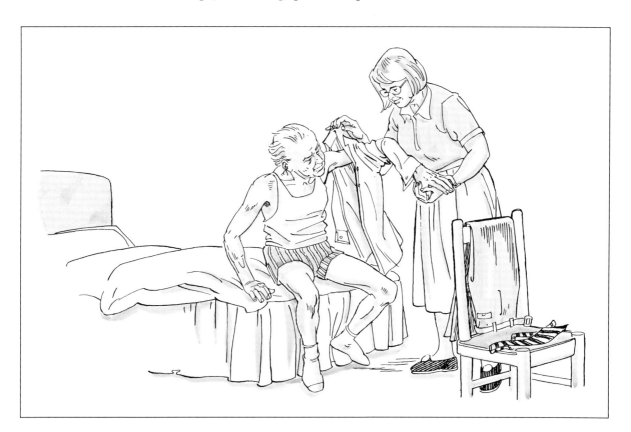

Helping the person to dress

If he is very weak on one side, put his affected arm into the shirt sleeve first

If the person has had a stroke or is very weak on one side you should put his affected arm or leg into the shirt or trouser leg first. Put all the clothes on the upper body first, then all the clothes on the lower body up to the thighs, while the disabled person is sitting or lying on the bed, then helping him to make one standing movement so that you can finish lifting and tucking in clothes and fastening trousers, will prevent undue exhaustion to yourself or your relative.

It is important for the long term disabled person actually to get dressed and not to stay in her night clothes all day. Staying in night clothes only reinforces the idea that the person is ill and can contribute to lowered self-esteem and depression. Getting dressed has the following extra advantages:

- The person is warmer;

- The activity of dressing helps the circulation and muscles;

- The wearing of proper lace-up or strong shoes means that the person is safer when trying to walk.

Washing and bathing

If your relative is unable to get out of bed, you should provide her with an individual bowl, flannel, soap and other personal toiletries. Try to encourage her to perform some small activity herself.

Checking and cleaning the skin on vulnerable pressure points, and turning a bedridden patient regularly, is important to prevent sore areas developing. Talk to your district nurse if this is a possible problem.

You can help your relative by providing a stool or chair in the bathroom. She can sit at the sink to wash, thereby reducing fatigue. Also, a mirror at chair height may enable individuals to

See also Chapter 2, section 2(h), on Keeping clean and well groomed, for more advice on care of the skin

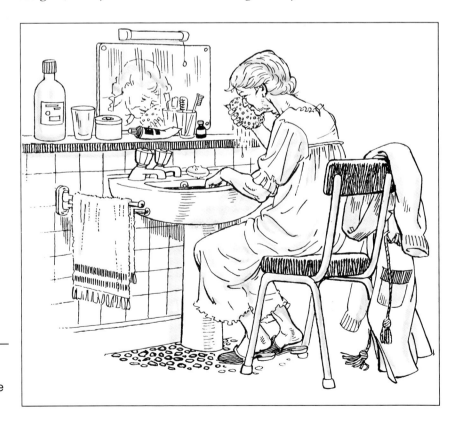

You can help your disabled relative by providing a chair or stool for her to sit on in the bathroom

help themselves put on make-up, shave, brush and comb their hair or clean their teeth. Do not do everything for them if they can do a little to help. If more help than this is needed then bath rails, a bath seat or a hoist will help. Your district nurse or occupational therapist will be able to advise you, after making a full assessment of your home.

Eating and drinking

A sick person with a long term disability may be unable to eat certain foods. Following consultation with your general practitioner you may be able to purchase special foods, or it may be enough to serve puréed or liquidised food.

See Chapter 1, section 1 for more detailed advice on Diet

If you provide regular, small, nourishing meals with plenty of fresh fruit and fibre then the risk of your relative becoming overweight, undernourished or constipated will be reduced.

Some people whose disability affects their hands may need special cutlery or plates to enable them to eat by themselves. The exact design which would be appropriate for any individual will be dictated by the disabling condition and its severity, and to some extent by personal preference. A few of the types of special equipment available are illustrated below but do discuss your relative's individual needs with your district nurse or occupational therapist before you buy any feeding equipment or you may end up with something totally inappropriate.

There are many different types of specially adapted cutlery or crockery available

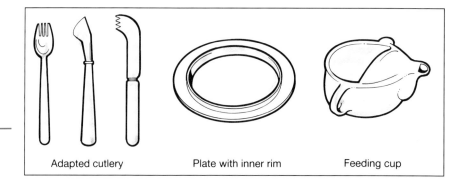

Adapted cutlery   Plate with inner rim   Feeding cup

Elimination

See also Chapter 2, section 2(d) on Eliminating

People with long term disabilities may find toileting a real problem. You, as a carer, may find yourself becoming extremely depressed and frustrated about your ability (or lack of it) to cope. However, there is help available. An occupational therapist will assess your toilet for special hand rails positioned at the right height, and a raised toilet seat. A non-slip floor is essential. Encourage your relative to go to the toilet before he may actually need to. By taking him at certain times, in an unhurried

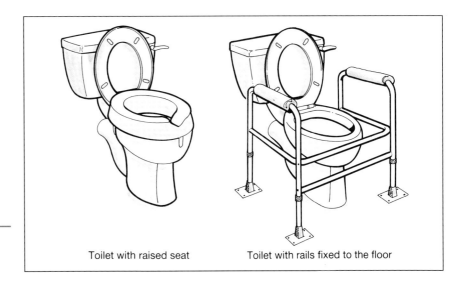

Toilet with raised seat   Toilet with rails fixed to the floor

A raised seat or special handrails may make use of the toilet very much easier

atmosphere, you may prevent problems. Having a toilet, a urine bottle or a portable commode nearby may also be of benefit – however this should be as private as possible.

If the person for whom you care becomes incontinent firstly remember that clothes which are loose and easy to remove may prevent many accidents. People with long term disabilities may feel it is undignified to wear incontinence pads. Ask your general practitioner to refer you to a specialist nurse, a continence adviser, who will be able to suggest ways of dealing with the situation.

7.12(b)   MOBILITY AND EXERCISE

Physical mobility and balance for sick people with a disability may be seriously affected, so prevention of falls is essential.

Your community physiotherapist may be able to advise you about exercises for improving mobility. Severe discomfort and pain may decrease with an exercise programme designed specifically for your relative. Some individuals too may benefit from an exercise programme such as that offered by EXTEND. The benefits of such organised exercise programmes may also include opportunities for social interaction giving the disabled person the chance to make new friendships.

Excess or inappropriate exercise may aggravate some painful conditions so it is important to take advice and strive for a balance between healthy activity and too much exercise.

If you help a relative to walk, check that your garden and the inside of your home are as safe as possible. Remove obstacles such as furniture, slippery mats, the cat or the dog and any trailing wires that may be dangerous. There are a number of walking aids

See appendix VII for Addresses of useful organisations

See also section 7.7 above on Safety at home and outside

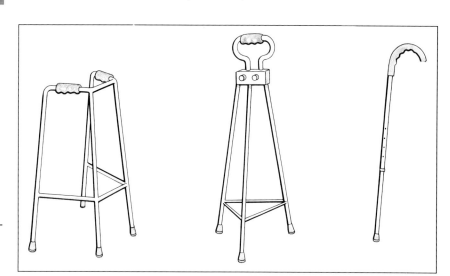

There are a number of
different walking aids
available

available which may make a considerable difference to your relative's ability to get around without help. If a stairlift has been installed in a house where a disabled person lives, it will be useful to have two walking aids – one to be kept at the top of the stairs and the other at the bottom.

To help you and the person you care for to accomplish these activities at home you may need to seek help from an occupational therapist who can be contacted at your local Social Service Department. It is always advisable to seek help from the experts who will make a full assessment before you buy 'over the counter' equipment from high street stores and chemists or from catalogues.

See Appendix VII for Addresses of useful organisations

There are a number of organisations, such as the Disabled Living Foundation, which provide a tremendous source of information and advice about long term disabilities. Such organisations can offer individuals and their carers the benefit of experience with many disability problems; literature, leaflets and catalogues showing helpful equipment; information about specific diseases; and, in some cases, financial or practical help for people with certain long term disabilities.

7.12(c) PSYCHOLOGICAL ASPECTS OF DISABILITY

The needs of the carer

Carers may need time and space to express their feelings and talk to others in a similar situation. Time to pursue a hobby, to go shopping or see friends are all important. Therefore you may find that a plan of specific days or hours set aside for you yourself will benefit you by recharging your batteries. If you wish to leave your relative for a short period, there are voluntary groups that may sit at home while you are out or friends may be willing to help occasionally.

See also Chapter 2, section 6 on Help for the carers and Chapter 7, section 5 on Caring for others and its effects on health

If you feel that the person for whom you care is safe by herself you may wish to provide a hot drink in a thermos flask and a few sandwiches or biscuits within easy reach. Social Services provide a meals on wheels service. In some areas a night-sitting service will make life a little less stressful. It will give you peace of mind if your outings are well planned, and you know that the person for whom you care is safe. The need for respite care is an important one and it is essential for your own health that you recognise this.

The Department of Social Services provides a range of residential homes for disabled people providing long and short term care. If you feel that you need a holiday, or for whatever reason can no longer continue caring for your relative at home, then you should talk to your general practitioner or social worker.

More advice for carers is given elsewhere in this book.

See also Chapter 2, Caring at home, especially sections 1, 2, 4 and 6

The needs of the person with a disability

An individual's sense of self-worth is closely bound up with his body image, and feelings of impotence, dependence and deformity may present real problems for the person you are caring for. At times such feelings may manifest themselves in displays of bad temper or depression. It is important that you realise you are not responsible for such negative feelings and, even though they may appear at times to be directed at you, they do not indicate that you are doing anything wrong. Neither carers nor those they are caring for are necessarily saints but if a good relationship can be fostered and maintained, life will be a great deal easier for both parties. The following suggestions may be helpful:

- Try to keep communicating – as honestly as you are able. Bottled up feelings become even harder to handle.

- Try to ensure that both parties have other, non-involved, people they can talk to (and 'sound off' about the other to, without feeling disloyal).

- Encourage participation in daily life and household chores wherever possible so that not all the help and support is going one way. Someone in a wheelchair may be able to peel vegetables, do the household accounts or even tackle the ironing if the equipment is arranged at an appropriate height.

Self-image can also be improved by helping the person to make himself look as attractive as possible. If financial circumstances allow, a hairdresser can be booked for home visits at regular intervals (many self-employed hairdressers now offer such a service and more cheaply than salon rates) – or ask the district nurse to show you how to wash someone's hair at home. Men should be given the wherewithall (and assistance if necessary) to shave if they so wish and women should be offered the opportunity to wear cosmetics. Even if money is short, clothes can be clean and neat and wherever possible flattering colours should be chosen.

Although traditionally synonymous with lack of attractiveness, disability need not necessarily be so. Sexuality need not be denied either. In many cases, sexual relationships can be continued with affection, good humour and willingness on both sides to make adjustments. An organisation such as SPOD (the Association to aid the Sexual and Personal Relationships of People with a Disability) can provide much helpful advice and reassurance.

If the person with a disability has opportunities for socialising and other outside activities then depression and introspection become less likely.

Both you yourself and the person for whom you care may find it difficult to come to terms with, or feel unable to accept or cope with, long term disability. Support and understanding are needed as adaptations to a change in lifestyle takes place. If you feel that you need extra individual help or advice then do talk to your general practitioner and ask her to refer you to the appropriate professional or organisation.

See Appendix VII for Addresses of useful organisations and support groups

7.12(d)   SOCIAL AND FINANCIAL ASPECTS

Preventing boredom

To prevent boredom and loneliness a rota of visitors could be arranged, although rest periods are important. If however your relative does not want visitors then a chair placed by a window or the use of the television or radio may enhance stimulation and motivation to take interest in the outside world and increase confidence. A daily newspaper or a trip to the corner shop may be the highlight of the day for some individuals, even though this may seem a triviality for you. It is important to try to establish what are the little things which really enhance quality of life.

Information about organisations, clubs and educational facilities will be available from your local library. Financial benefits are always being reviewed and up to date information can be obtained from your local Citizens' Advice Bureau.

Hobbies and other activities

Many pastimes can be continued, or even discovered, after someone has become disabled. The Royal Horticultural Society's garden at Wisley includes among its 'model gardens' one which consists entirely of raised beds at an ideal height for the gardener in a wheelchair. Obviously such major modifications are beyond the

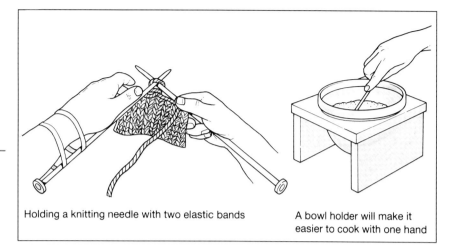

Holding a knitting needle with two elastic bands

A bowl holder will make it easier to cook with one hand

A little help to hold objects – such as a knitting needle or mixing bowl – can enable people to continue hobbies despite reduced function in one hand

See also Chapter 6, section 4 on The child with a physical handicap

scope of many but a hobby such as gardening can still be continued in a modest way with the help of window boxes, terracotta pots on stands and seed trays on tables. Many of the suggestions for participating in card and other games given in Chapter 6 will bring as much pleasure to adults as to children, and the figure above shows ways of continuing hobbies such as cookery and knitting despite impaired function in one hand.

Going out

No one's morale is improved by looking at the same four walls all day and, depending on where you live, it may be possible to get out and about quite a bit. Unfortunately, access to many public places is still not easy for disabled people but if you plan to visit a specific site (such as a National Trust property or other place of interest) it is worth telephoning first to enquire how easy it is to take a wheelchair around, and whether specially adapted toilet facilities are available.

Public transport may be difficult to negotiate but British Rail are usually helpful if you telephone the station in advance and state your needs. Some areas run subsidised taxi services and it is always worth talking to your social worker or local Social Services Department about what is available locally in terms of transport and organised outings for people with a disability.

You may be able to use your own car to take your relative out and if this is the case getting out and about should be a great deal easier. To help a disabled person into the car, you should first open the passenger door as wide as you can and wind the window down. Help the person to stand up in one of the ways shown in Chapter 2, section 4. He can grasp the car door at the bottom of the window frame so that you will not be supporting all his weight (see the figure overleaf). From this position, he should be able to turn himself round to sit down backwards. If necessary, you can help him to

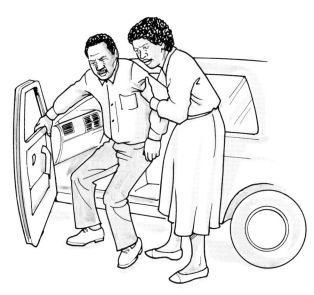

Helping a disabled person into the car

lift his feet into the car. The wheelchair can then be folded and put into the car boot.

When you reach your destination, the procedure can be reversed to help the person out of the car and back into the wheelchair.

If you take your relative out in a wheelchair you may have to negotiate kerbs and even short flights of steps. It is important, when encountering such obstacles, that you retain complete control over the chair. To move off a kerb, hold the chair firmly, with the back wheels on the kerb. Tip the chair back towards you and lower it gently onto the lower level. Transfer some weight back to the front wheels without jerking or jarring the occupant. The procedure should be reversed for getting back up a kerb and you may find it easiest to do this 'backwards' – moving the back wheels onto the kerb first – if traffic allows.

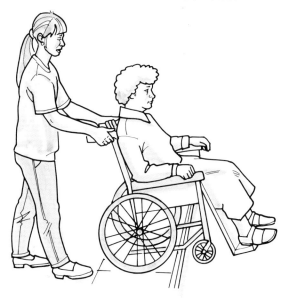

Negotiating the kerb with a wheelchair

Religion

Disability may cause a person to question long held convictions and precipitate some upheaval in her spiritual life. One person who has formerly believed in a God may find that faith shaken, while another – previously agnostic – may find he now needs to search for a deeper spiritual experience. It is important that carers respect the person's spiritual needs as far as possible, even if they are totally different to their own. If someone is going through a religious crisis of some sort, it would be helpful if the appropriate religious leader could be contacted (with the person's permission) and asked to visit.

Disabled people who wish to attend churches or other places of worship to participate in their religion should be helped to do so wherever possible. If you, the carer, do not wish to attend yourself then it may also be a good idea to discuss this with the religious leader as there may well be people in his congregation who can help with transport. Quite apart from the peace of mind that can be fostered by being able to worship as one wishes, regular participation in a religious group will enhance social contact and feelings of self-worth, both of which will have positive effects on the relationship between the individual and his carer.

Where a person is really too ill to leave the house, the religious leader will probably be happy to make home visits. Appropriate religious ceremonies can be performed at home where necessary and this may be a source of great solace and inner strength to the person concerned. Many churches pray for the sick during ordinary services and individuals may derive much comfort from knowing this.

It is equally important, however, that carers who participate in organised worship themselves do not try to force this on an un-willing patient. If you wish to go to church on a Sunday morning, for example, and your relative has no desire to accompany you, then do not press him. Instead, try to persuade a friend or other relative (perhaps on a rota system) to sit with the person for the time during which you will be out of the house. You too have the right to fulfil your own spiritual needs.

Work

A physical disability does not necessarily mean that there is no possibility of paid employment. Indeed, those individuals who do work will find that their financial situation, their social life and their self-esteem are all greatly enhanced. So, what opportunities are open to people with a disability?

Individuals who have been disabled from childhood should have been given thoughtful and sensitive careers advice at school – but where this has not been adequate, the person is advised to contact

See Appendix VII for Addresses of useful organisations and support groups

RADAR (who publish a guide on employment opportunities for disabled people) and the Disabled Living Foundation's Information Service. Those who have become disabled in later life (as a result of an accident or a stroke for example) may also find these sources of help useful but in many cases their situation will differ in that they have been in full time employment up until the onset of the disability. In such cases, a sensible first step is to talk to the personnel manager of the existing employer to see if one can still do one's old job and if not whether transfer to another department can be arranged. A company that has already invested considerable amounts of money in training and nurturing a valued employee may be surprisingly sympathetic and helpful. Some individuals may be able to continue to work on a part time basis – or even from their own home thanks to the wonders of modern technology.

If continuing to work for the same or a similar employer is not a practical proposition, then the local Disablement Resettlement Officer should be contacted. Your social worker or Citizens' Advice Bureau will tell you how to go about this.

If a disabled person intends to work outside the home, thought should be given to such practicalities as transport and the individual's need for rest. Shorter hours, to avoid rush hours and exhaustion, might be the answer for some individuals.

7.13 THE ADULT WITH A LEARNING DISABILITY (MENTAL HANDICAP)

In today's society there are many people who may be classified as having a learning disability. Many of us, indeed, have some learning difficulty or other whether it be manifest in the form of dyslexia, illiteracy or even the lack of computer literacy.

The definition of 'learning disability' will vary from generation to generation and there will also be noticeable differences in definition between cultures and nations. However there are some basic norms against which definitions are made:

- They usually imply that there is a reduction in learning ability or mental functioning;

- Such conditions when they occur are usually permanent and irreversible.

Definitions may also be influenced by an individual's ability to contribute to the workforce of the local area or to the maintenance of community life. Consequently variations in definition may be of little use in understanding the needs of people who present with a variety of learning and support needs.

In the past the definition was made somewhat easier through the application of psychological testing or as they are more commonly known IQ tests. These are rarely used now (except in certain legal situations) because of the lack of useful information they provide. In fact, it may be argued that the application of such criteria restricted the way in which the needs of people with learning disabilities were responded to thereby reducing opportunities for developing their full potential.

The approach now favoured is one that values individuals in their own right and emphasises the abilities and skills of each person, rather than one that focuses on negative aspects of behaviour or skill deficiency. The concept that underpins this approach has been referred to as 'the ordinary life model'.

7.13(a) THE ORDINARY LIFE MODEL

People with learning disabilities are born into ordinary families and usually spend their childhood years at home with their families. They spend these years experiencing opportunities in their local neighbourhoods and meeting friends and neighbours. They participate in family holidays and excursions and many attend local clubs and functions.

This integrated approach compares favourably to the less appropriate approach that removes people with a learning disability from their peers and provides them with segregated activities such as 'handicapped swimming clubs and discos'. This is not to say that many people with learning disabilities do not benefit from such activities with their peers but these should not be provided in isolation from the same activities that are enjoyed by other members of society.

People have the right to live in a home of their own. Dependence on state hospitals and hostels is rapidly becoming a thing of the past and real choices and opportunities are now being afforded to people to live in ordinary houses in their local communities whenever the need or wish to leave the parental home occurs. Some people (no matter how 'severe' their learning disability may be) are sharing accommodation together with two or three others and have tenancy agreements which protect their rights to a secure home of their choice. Other individuals have decided to remain in their parental home with support from care workers and domiciliary workers.

The right to make choices and to participate in decisions affecting their lives is a key aspect of the ordinary life model. This area has been one of the most difficult to achieve but, through the provision of citizen advocacy schemes and by upholding personal rights, unacceptable care practices and living conditions have been challenged and new services have been created.

All people need to feel valued and useful in their day to day lives. A place to work and to spend our leisure is often taken for granted but for a person with a learning disability the reality may be a most impoverished or boring life engaged in routine work or 'self-occupation'. Consequently the design of creative work and daily opportunities should be placed high on the agenda of most service providers.

Similarly, we all need to be valued and have the opportunity to make and maintain friendships. As a prerequisite people will need to meet others and share aspects of daily living. Segregated activities often deny those with learning disabilities the opportunity to meet with different people and to experience a range of life experiences. Through participation in a range of community activities new friendships may be sought and sustained.

Fixing the model in practice

Having considered the philosophy of the ordinary life approach this section now considers some of the ways in which informal carers and parents may assist adults with a learning disability to live fulfilled and meaningful lives. Consideration will be given to these issues under a number of specific headings.

See Chapter 2, section 2 for advice on Helping the sick person at home with the activities of living

Activities of living The majority of people with learning disabilities will require no more assistance in undertaking activities of daily living than the rest of the population. However, a significant number of individuals require considerable assistance in carrying out their daily living functions. Some will require help with dressing, feeding, washing and toilet training and the degree to which assistance will be required will vary from one person to another depending on their actual level of skill acquisition and previous learning opportunities.

This latter point is most important since a number of adults may have been denied the opportunity to learn how to undertake some of these functions for themselves. Busy parents, with little time to engage in training routines, may have found it easier to feed their sons and daughters or to use incontinence aids rather than to spend a number of hours of intensive activity undertaking behavioural programmes. However, a little time spent early on in life undertaking such activities may not only enhance the person's sense of self-worth and independence but may also reduce the workload for parents in the long run.

Let us take an example. An adult with a severe learning disability may require some considerable time investment in the morning and evening in respect of bathing, dressing, feeding and toileting. Carers may prefer to 'speed' the process by using incontinence aids and appliances rather than engaging in time consuming toilet training programmes. However the cost of this 'short-cut' may be high in other ways. Firstly there is the time involved in additional laundry, problems with odour (which may be embarrassing), the cost of replacement linen and clothing (as well as electricity to power the washing machine and tumble dryer) and of course the indignity that the person suffers. Hence it is still possible to find individuals attending day services with clumsy incontinence aids and pads which further restricts their use of swimming pools and leisure activities. Conversely it is now known that the vast majority of people with a learning disability can acquire continence following a relatively simple and cost-effective investment in carer time.

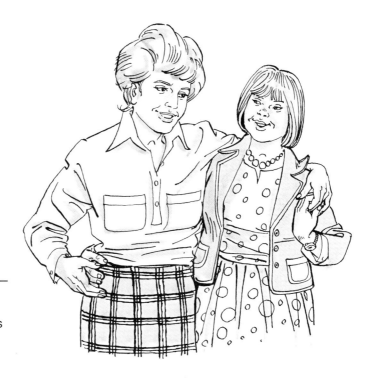

Positive reinforcement – in the form of an appreciative word or a warm embrace – is an important part of any behavioural programme

The application of such behavioural programmes must also be seen to have a positive outcome for the person concerned. These outcomes are not always immediately obvious and must be delivered alongside 'positive reinforcements'. The principle in use here is to ensure that every time a positive response is received that appropriate praise and encouragement is given to 'reinforce' the desired and demonstrated behaviour. This should always be accompanied by using the person's name, and a 'pat on the back' or a warm 'embrace' may also encourage the behaviour to occur again on subsequent occasions. Unfortunately life is rarely as simple as

> - Community mental handicap nurses
> - Specialist social workers
> - Clinical psychologists
> - Consultant psychiatrists for people with a mental handicap
> - Speech therapists
> - Physiotherapists
> - Occupational therapists
> - Parent/consumer representatives

is described here and what reinforces one person's behaviour may not suit another. Hence the search for specific reinforcements must always accompany the design of any programme.

Thus it may be beneficial for carers to seek the advice and support of their local Community Mental Handicap Team (see the box above) to assist them in designing and implementing suitable programmes to encourage independence in areas of daily living. As a result the acquisition of such skills will increase the person's level of competence, enhance her dignity and reduce the longer term burden of care for the family.

Maintaining a safe environment   One of the most commonly discussed areas of need is the requirement of most carers to provide a safe and secure environment for the dependants. This introduces the concepts of *risk* and *responsibility*.

The degree to which people with learning disabilities are able to carry out their lives independently varies greatly between individuals. At a basic level this may be explained by the most common questions raised by parents such as the capacity for their offspring to know 'right from wrong' or when to 'say no'. The answers will of course depend on mental ability on one hand and life experience on the other.

In order to determine the most appropriate degree of support and supervision that people require it will first be necessary to assess the level of personal functioning and ability. This may be achieved by providing opportunities for simulated learning in a controlled situation either at home, college or at work.

Take for example a simple procedure such as learning to pour tea from a teapot. This may appear to be a relatively simple process but in fact it requires that a number of complex senses and behavioural sequences are brought into play. Perhaps the most obvious is the ability to assess the temperature of the tea and to avoid scalding oneself as it is poured. Many people with learning disabilities may be unaware that tea originates in its dried form and is steeped in hot water. They may only receive the finished product as a hot liquid poured by 'mother'. By breaking down the behavioural sequence under controlled conditions it is possible to teach people the exact steps involved in the tea pouring process and by gradually increasing the temperature of the tea the 'trainee' may acquire competence in the procedure – indeed it has been proved that some people with a learning disability learn such routines so thoroughly that the chance of error may be less than that found in the general population.

The lesson from this example is that it is extremely easy to over-protect people from our idea of common danger and yet to deny them the opportunity to acquire new skills under controlled training conditions. This approach is rather like having a swimming pool and never using it in case a perfectly fit and competent swimmer might take cramp one day and die.

Of course such examples are simplistic and very real dilemmas do face parents and carers every day (the independent use of public transport to and from work, and swimming for people with epilepsy for instance). Even in these cases there are procedures that can be followed to calculate and minimise the risks involved. Such decisions are usually shared with members of a number of professional support staff (e.g. nurses, psychologists and consultant psychiatrists for people with learning disabilities). In the final analysis a balance must be struck between asking what the gains and losses are likely to be and thereafter making a decision on balance.

Of course other risks also exist in the environment which may present some degree of danger to some people with learning disabilities. Carers will need to assess their home and garden environments to ensure that adequate precautions have been taken to minimise the risk of unintentional injury. The selective use of safety gates, door catches, fire guards, window fastenings, non-breakable glass, wheelchair harnesses and car seat belts will reduce the risk of accidents at home and in the car. Similarly the effective use of protective headwear for people with severe epilepsy may in fact increase their enjoyment of the community by reducing the risk of head injury and possible containment at home.

Acquiring independence As one grows beyond adolescence a series of emerging needs require attention. Even amongst the more severely disabled members of this group the need to respond appropriately to adulthood is of paramount importance. However for many carers it is hard to reconcile the behaviour and dependency patterns often associated with childhood with a maturing and physically growing body.

The appropriateness of adulthood and its associated life experiences and expectations therefore needs some consideration. Take for example the need for a home of one's own. The majority of people will continue to live with their parents until a choice is made about moving into supported accommodation (this may be a planned move or may occur as the result of a change in coping capacity in the parental home).

Like all adults, people with a learning disability must be offered the opportunity to forge friendships and acquaintances with people outside of their family. This is the first step towards developing the necessary interpersonal skills that will be required when parents decide to share their care with others. Imagine the trauma for all concerned if this decision is taken without preparation and the person with a learning disability is suddenly confronted with the option of moving in to live communally with a group of strangers.

The transition to living outside of the family home must therefore commence at an earlier stage to ensure that positive ties and connections are made before the final move takes place. This can be done positively in most cases and the process begins with the development of a partnership of care between parents and professional carers. Hopefully this will take place close to the family home in a local residential facility and will be phased over a period of time ranging from informal visits for 'tea' through weekend stays to longer spells away from home. The result can be a welcome break for both the person concerned and the family who may choose to use the opportunity 'to charge their batteries' while acknowledging the growth process being undertaken by their relative at the same time. The transition to a change of residence requires sensitive handling and careful planning and consideration for both parties involved in coming to terms with the separation factor involved.

One other example of growing independence and awareness is the right to experience some of the worries and concerns that we all experience during the course of our lives. For example, how do we as carers confront issues relating to the loss of friends who move away from our lives for one reason or another? In the past the simple way to deal with this was to avoid facing up to the truth and to ignore telling the person with a learning disability about the implications or permanency of the loss. Hence the death of a family member may be disguised by saying 'he has gone away for a while' or 'he is in heaven'. The latter may not have any meaning for the person concerned and may be linked to the former statement which implies there will be a return at some stage. One other way was to say nothing.

We now know that no matter how hard it may appear we should face the reality of the situation and share our feelings and experiences with the people we are caring for in order to afford them the dignity of honesty that is required. It is always difficult to assess how successful we have been in delivering news about loss or bereavement – or indeed to assess whether the individual concerned has accepted the news at all. However, loss is a natural part of life and for this reason people (whether or not they have a learning disability) should be enabled to join in the ceremonies that we use to 'say goodbye' and to express our feelings. The following stages of support help us to understand how to respond to the normal loss or grieving process:

- Enable the person to express feelings of loss openly and without reproach;

- Share your own feelings of loss and empathise to give emotional support;

- Provide simple reassurance that the sadness felt will not 'go on forever';

- Involve the support of friends and neighbours and allow others to provide a 'shoulder to lean on';

- Obtain the support of a professional counsellor from the local Community Mental Handicap Team if required.

Feelings of loss are common in the lives of persons with a learning disability and are not only concerned with death. For many people changes in carers and support staff are regular activities and since many people do not have friends who follow them through their lives they become dependent on professional carers who will inevitably move on for career or family reasons. The lack of consistency in friendship networks makes it all the more important to encourage the maintenance of connections within the extended family, with neighbours and with unpaid carers.

Other factors associated with adulthood relate to the need for privacy and 'personal time'. Privacy and opportunities to have some time alone are all important and form an essential part of our lives. How we choose to use our free time is an indication of our independence and permits the expression of personal thoughts and activities.

For people with a learning disability such opportunities may be few and far between since the major part of the waking day is spent in the company of others (often under a watchful eye). Hence time to reflect and to reminisce may be a precious commodity.

Similarly the right to acknowledge sexual needs and to 'explore our bodies' requires similar tact and understanding. This is perhaps one of the most controversial and difficult areas for parents and carers to come to terms with and yet it is one of the most natural of our instinctive behaviours as we mature into adulthood. For the purposes of this chapter it may be helpful to advise on the need to ensure that expression of sexual behaviour is not condemned but is directed appropriately. For example it may be helpful to advise the person that body awareness is a very personal activity and that this must be reserved for specific times in specific (private) places such as the bathroom or the bedroom. Most important of all is the need for parents to consider their own feelings and attitudes and to avoid the temptation to impose their own standards or to censure appropriately expressed behaviours. However, these situations may require advice from a suitably experienced and qualified practitioner and carers should not be afraid to seek advice from their local Community Mental Handicap Team if the need arises.

7.13(b) MAINTAINING OPTIMUM HEALTH

As for other members of the population, adults with a learning disability will need to pay increasing attention to maintaining a healthy lifestyle. However to do so requires that adults in society are able to make important decisions about their lives on the basis of received information and understanding. For people with a learning disability the choices between smoking and overeating may not be so easy to distinguish due to possible lack of comprehension about the consequences of these actions.

Ensuring that a balanced diet is taken is an area of particular concern for those who may be totally dependent on others for selecting, preparing and delivering their meals. In some cases appetite may be poor, while others may have apparently unassuagable intakes at mealtimes. Both require attention since obesity and malnutrition can reduce mental and physical function leading to a deterioration in ability which, when superimposed on an existing disability, can complicate matters tremendously.

Similarly the need for regular health and dental checks with the dentist and general practitioner should not be ignored. Whereas most of us can complain of pain and discomfort (and alert others to seek relief on our behalf) this may not be so obvious for some people with a learning disability. The key question is, how do we know when someone is in pain? In some cases the answer is apparent by changes in gesture, behaviour or posture. In others the cause or symptoms may go unnoticed, and thus reliance on prevention is all the more important. Screening for possible causes *before* pain occurs may reassure carers that everything has and is being done to avoid such problems (for example dental checks before toothache occurs, or regular measurement of blood pressure). Many doctors and dentists offer such checks and carers are recommended to take advantage of them.

*See also Chapter 1,
section 2 on Exercise*

Closely linked to health promotion is the need for regular exercise. For people who have many of their needs met by others, or for whom inactivity is imposed by physical impairment, the need to avoid obesity and to take exercise is all the more important. In such cases, the advice of the community physiotherapist may be very helpful.

In the same way, opportunities should be taken to test regularly for deficiencies in sight or hearing. People who do not engage in well developed forms of verbal communication are particularly dependent on their other senses and so hearing loss and sight difficulties come as a double burden. A significant number of people do require assistance with hearing and vision as they grow older and the provision of spectacles and hearing aids can do much to enable a more stimulating and positive lifestyle.

Finally the importance of following medical advice should be noted. Some people are required to take regular medication to reduce the effects of some physical conditions (such as epilepsy) and in some cases to reduce the effects of emotional distress and anxiety. A well controlled and monitored régime can assist in the promotion of a positive lifestyle and may reduce the effects of underlying handicapping conditions to a minimum.

7.13(c)   SHARING THE CARE

Informal carers are often the most valued and important people in the lives of those with a learning disability. The long term nature of the presenting needs of those individuals requires that consistent, practical advice and support is made available whenever it is called upon during the everyday course of family life.

There are many support groups and services now available to

Examples of the work of the local Community Mental Handicap team

- The provision of advice on self-help skill development e.g. dressing, feeding, toilet training etc.
- Provision of advice on behavioural management
- Provision of advice on the management of specific clinical conditions such as epilepsy, multiple handicap and sensory needs
- Practical assistance with the management and delivery of care
- The promotion of self-help groups
- The provision of parent workshops and training activities
- Advice on aids and adaptations to reduce the effects of handicap
- Facilitation of access to leisure and occupational activities
- The provision and co-ordination of short term (respite) care
- Advice on financial assistance
- The provision of a counselling and advisory service

See Appendix VII for Addresses of useful organisations and support groups

share in the difficulties that may confront carers and these range from self-help groups to professional teams of workers who are employed to provide direct support and advice to families and carers in the community (Community Mental Handicap Teams – see the box featured earlier in this section). For further information about local groups and resources in your area you should contact your local Social Services Department, the Community Health Council or your Citizens' Advice Bureau.

THE LATER YEARS (60 PLUS)

8

8.1   MATURITY AND AGEING

If life begins at 40, then the seventh decade must be one's prime. There are many advantages to ageing, as reported by a variety of older authors. The experiences through which older people have survived and developed can provide young people with a sense of history, of 'where they are coming from'. Hearing about the early life or past experiences of an older friend or family member can greatly enrich the vision of a young person. There are many books available now presenting interviews and reminiscences, featuring people from all walks of life and giving fascinating details of their everyday life and culture – details unlikely to be found in the average history book.

See Appendix VIII for Suggested further reading

Such stories also tell of people's ability to cope with changes. Many older people feel that one advantage of maturity and ageing is that it brings with it an increase in confidence, making them feel able to cope with whatever life throws at them. They have learned to deal with so many complex, distressing, pleasurable, exciting, dull and stressful events that they know that in the event of such situations arising again they will be able to adjust. They are also able to pass on these coping mechanisms to other people, provided they are prepared to listen.

See also section 8.2(d) below on Independence

Another advantage of ageing is having the time to concentrate on learning new subjects and accomplishing good results contrary to expectations and myths. Older people achieve consistently good results with the Open University, GCSEs and other academic courses. The old adage 'you can't teach an old dog new tricks' may have said more about the poor quality of teaching than the inability to learn. Many older people enjoy adult education centres and take up new hobbies and interests for which they have not previously had time.

A wealth of experience, skills and knowledge is accumulated throughout life, and is a valuable resource which should not be lost. One initiative to encourage people to share these skills is the University of the Third Age, a movement discussed in more detail in section 8.2(d) below.

Ageing brings with it numerous other advantages. You may like to consider the advantages which you feel age has given you and reflect on whether or not these outweigh the disadvantages.

- If there is a negative imbalance, what would you like to do about it?

- What ambitions do you have which you have not yet achieved? What will help you achieve these ambitions, and what may hold you back?

- When you have thought about these questions, why not draw up an action plan which will provide you with some deadlines in order to help you realise your ambitions.

If you are not entering these later years yet yourself, but are looking after someone who is, it is hoped that this chapter will help to emphasise for you the positive and life-enhancing aspects of age, at the same time as giving practical and realistic advice.

8.2   LIFE AFTER RETIREMENT

Life after retirement is obviously what you make of it. It can be a time of fulfilment and relaxation after many years of hard work, or it can be a time of loneliness and boredom when life loses its point. Which it is will depend not only on your circumstances but also on your attitude, and a positive approach coupled with some thoughtful and practical preparation will help you to make this period of your life an Indian summer.

8.2(a)   FAMILY LIFE

See also Chapter 3, section 7 on Retirement

Whether you are male or female, married or single, family relationships will now be an important element in your life. Let us take the traditional example of a married couple, the husband having been out at work as the breadwinner while the wife ran the home and cared for her husband and children, perhaps doing a part time job or some voluntary work when the children began to be less dependent on her. Husband and wife will have led separate daily lives, spending time together only in the evenings and at weekends, and when the husband retires and has to spend all his time at home, there will be inevitable stresses and strains between the two unless they have discussed beforehand what pattern their lives should now take, and agreed where their common interests lie and where each should be free to pursue separate activities. Without separate interests, a couple can easily get bored and irritated with each other, the husband missing the status of his job and the involvement with other people, and the wife finding her work doubled and her freedom halved by his constant presence in the house. If they pursue separate hobbies or sports or educational activities, however, they will find life more enjoyable and have more to talk about when they are together, thus enriching their relationship. This, of course, applies to any two people living together, not only to married couples.

A major decision anyone has to take at this point in life is where to live. Is this the time to find your dream cottage in the country or your private castle in Spain where you can lead an idyllic life, or would it be more sensible to stay in the town or city which you know and where your friends are? There are a number of factors to consider. First there is the practical consideration that however fit and active you may be at 65 or even 70, there is bound to come a time in the natural order of things when you will slow down, your joints will stiffen, and you will want a home which is easy to run and to live in, with friends or relatives nearby to turn to in an emergency. If you have children, it will be worth thinking of the possibility of moving to live near them, so that you can see them frequently and enjoy your grandchildren, if you have any. However, it is as well to remember that people's jobs and circumstances alter, sometimes very suddenly: your son or daughter may change jobs and have to move to a different part of the country, or perhaps abroad, leaving you in a district new to you, away from your friends and your familiar territory. So plan carefully for any move, so that you can be sure you won't regret it. A cottage in the country or a luxury seaside flat can become a prison if you are remote from family and friends, and the facilities you need for daily living – shops, library, post office, bank, public transport, doctor's surgery – are not easily accessible. You may find your own home is still the best bet, and that now is the time to spend money on it to make it more comfortable and easy to run.

See also Chapter 3, section 10 on Bereavement and loss

See also Chapter 7, section 2 on Making a will

See Appendix VIII for Suggested further reading

At this time of life, sometimes called the 'third age', there is sadly the likelihood that death will rob you of someone you love, a parent or a marriage partner or perhaps a very close friend. One has to be pragmatic about death, which is the one thing in life that is certain and inevitable, so in deciding where to live after retirement it is important to bear in mind that you may one day lose the person who shares your life, or your partner may lose you, and make sure – both financially and in other ways – that the one who is left will be able to cope alone. Making a will, if you have not already made one, is essential to ensure that shared property goes to the survivor, and that your wishes regarding your estate are carried out.

On a more cheerful note, now that life is more relaxed and you are seeing more of your partner, perhaps going on more frequent holidays together, why not rejuvenate your sex life? Far too many people still regard the act of love between older people as somehow improper or distasteful, but love and affection are just as natural and essential for them as for the young. Changes in the body may affect performance, but your doctor should be able to help and advise you about any problems you may have, and there are several books available which cover the subject in a practical yet sensitive way.

8.2(b) HEALTH

There are many ways in which people of all ages attempt to promote their own health and well-being and, by the time they have reached their later years, many of these will have been tried, tested and found to be relatively successful. A milestone such as one's 60th or 70th birthday can be a good time to take stock of a lifetime's habits and prepare for as fulfilled and healthy a life as possible from that

Strategies for healthy living

- Moderation in the use of alcohol
- Limited use of tobacco
- Obtaining regular medical examinations (with tests appropriate for one's sex)
- Obtaining immunisations and vaccinations as necessary
- Obtaining regular dental examinations
- Using toothpaste, dental floss and/or denture care materials

- Obtaining regular eye examinations
- Performing self-examinations at appropriate intervals (see Chapter 7, section 10(a) for advice on how to examine your breasts)
- Responding to organised health screening programmes
- Seeking information about illness problems and age related health issues

- Monitoring of dietary intake (see Chapter 1, section 1 on Diet)
- Monitoring weight
- Following an appropriate schedule of meals

- Maintaining an adequate sleep pattern (see Chapter 1, section 3 on Sleep)
- Participation in physical activity/exercise on a regular basis

- Informed use of over the counter medications (see section 8.7(a) below on Polymedication)
- Informed use of vitamin supplements
- Not using medications prescribed for other persons

- Getting rid of old or unused medicines and checking expiry dates

- Maintaining an appropriate balance of work and relaxation activities
- Engaging in activities considered to promote a 'positive outlook on life'
- Dressing appropriately for the weather conditions
- Taking proper care of feet and toenails

- Using seat belts when a driver and a passenger (see Chapter 7, section 7 on Safety at home and outside)
- Avoiding settings known to pose environmental hazards of pollution or other contamination
- Staying abreast of new information about health and health care
- Participating in health education activities
- Rearranging furniture and other household items to accommodate physical/sensory changes
- Checking for hazards in the home
- Keeping a First Aid kit and smoke detector in the dwelling (see Appendix II on First Aid)
- Having a repertoire of strategies for the management of stress producing life events (see Chapter 1, section 5 on Stress and Chapter 3 on Normal life crises)

Adapted from the work of William Rakowski

point on. The box on the facing page lists 31 different strategies, developed in America in the 1980s, which older people may undertake to promote their health. Some of these will be discussed in more detail below to enable you to obtain a clearer picture of what they may entail.

Moderation in the use of alcohol

Drinking alcohol is probably the most acceptable and seemingly innocuous of dangerous habits. Alcohol:

See also Chapter 7, section 10(k) on Problems associated with tobacco, alcohol and other drugs

- Prevents the absorption of essential vitamins;

- Can depress your mood despite the expectation that it will have the reverse effect;

- Causes heat loss in cold weather (so the hip flask of brandy to warm you up may in fact make you colder).

People with specific health problems, or those taking certain medicines, should not take alcohol at all. Do talk to your doctor if you are not sure whether this applies to you.

See Chapter 1, section 1 for a discussion of the safe levels of alcohol intake

One of the problems with alcohol intake is that it can be difficult to keep count of exactly how much you are drinking, especially if it is associated with being sociable or hospitable. If you are not sure how much you are drinking, you may find it helpful to keep a diary noting down when you drink and how much (in a similar way to the use of the food diary described in Chapter 1). This may help you to adjust your drinking downwards or to reassure you that you are within safe limits.

If you find that your alcohol intake is over the recommended level, you could try setting aside two or three days when you drink no alcohol at all. If you are going out with friends, you could try sticking to soft drinks (such as tonic water or sparkling mineral water) or low alcohol beer. These are not noticeably 'different' but, anyway, are widely acceptable as alternatives these days.

Limited use of tobacco

Giving up smoking is not very easy, especially if you have been smoking for a long time. Many people need support to help them get over the first few days. If you are trying to give up smoking find out if the nurses at your doctor's surgery are running a 'smokers support group'. If they are then join it, as you will find that sharing your experiences and learning from others will help you.

See also Chapter 7, section 10(k) on Problems associated with tobacco, alcohol and other drugs

Screening checks and preventive measures

Teeth and eyes It is important to obtain dental and vision checks at regular intervals. If you wear dentures, your dentist will ensure that they fit properly. Bone structures change a little with age which may make dentures fit less well creating ulcers and putting you off food and social events.

Ears Hearing may be affected with age and it may be that when you are in a family group, in a pub or adult education class it may seem as though people are mumbling. This could be due to a hearing loss which makes it difficult to hear some but not all sound waves. If you experience difficulties like this, your doctor, having checked for wax in your ears, could refer you to the audiology department of a local hospital where you could have a thorough hearing assessment. If necessary a hearing aid may be provided. This will enable you to hear telephone bells and front door bells ringing and will help you enjoy the company of others without the embarrassment of saying 'pardon' all the time.

Immunisations Immunisations and vaccinations are usually associated with younger people, although some are very important for older people too. It is important to protect yourself against a tetanus infection which is usually associated with injury inflicted in the garden or during a fall. People still die every year from this preventable disease and they are usually people who have let their immunisations lapse. Find out from your doctor whether your tetanus immunisations are up to date.

Another immunisation worth considering is that against influenza which, although not in the same league as tetanus, can nevertheless, be very debilitating. Vaccinations are usually offered to particular groups of people who may be less able to fight the infection and could develop some complications to the disease. These groups of people include those with:

- Chronic lung disease;

- Chronic heart disease;

- Chronic kidney disease;

- Diabetes, and other less common endocrine disorders;

- Conditions involving certain types of treatments.

You will need to check with your doctor to find out whether it is necessary for you to be vaccinated. Vaccinations are usually available from the doctor's surgery late in the year once the particular strain of virus is known and the right immunisation produced by the manufacturers.

Your local health centre

Doctor's surgeries and health centres are changing in their approach to health. At one time people went to the doctor when they were ill

*See Appendix V on
People and resources*

but now people also go because they want advice about how to stay well. In the surgery you may find a number of different nurses who can help you with health issues which are of concern to you. Together with the doctors and associated professionals, they form the primary health care team.

Working together, such teams are now able to provide special services including 'Well Men' and 'Well Women' clinics and various support groups. You could find out more about these services from the notice boards in the surgery, from the receptionists and from other patients and staff.

Some surgeries and health centres have started producing their own booklets telling you about the available staff and the services they offer. Ask your doctor's receptionist whether such literature is available.

Exercise

One of the main reasons for monitoring food intake is to regulate weight which may increase as the opportunities for exercise reduce. Other benefits of exercise include:

- Maintaining or improving mobility;

- Encouraging your heart and lungs to work efficiently;

- Helping to prevent the development of osteoporosis;

- Contributing to a general sense of physical well-being.

If you tend not to be involved in regular exercise at the moment there are ways in which you can gradually introduce exercise into your daily routine without it becoming a chore. If you use the car, to visit friends for example, could you park it a little distance from your destination and walk the rest of the way? This may take a bit of extra time, but 20 minutes of brisk walking every day would improve your general health. Many people say that they feel less lethargic, more energetic and more interested in sex, as well as experiencing fewer aches and pains than they did when they did not exercise.

Some exercise improves suppleness, some increases physical strength and some improve stamina. These three areas – suppleness, strength and stamina – are important to enable participation in an active and independent life. A balanced exercise programme (which should not be embarked upon without advice from your doctor or a trained exercise teacher) will probably include all three types of exercise.

Your local leisure centre may be able to advise you on a fitness programme, or you might find an organisation such as EXTEND, which runs exercise programmes for well elderly people and for disabled individuals very useful.

BREATHING

These exercises help circulation, digestion, and chest problems such as chronic bronchitis and asthma. Clear nasal passages before you start and breath in through your nose and out through your mouth. Make sure you can feel your diaphragm moving.
Starting position: Sitting, posture 2.
Music: Medium waltz.

1. Intercostal – Lateral costal
Place hands over the front of your rib cage just below sternum so that fingertips are touching. Breathe in pushing your hands apart, then breathe out through your mouth allowing hands to come together. Chest should move like a concertina: in and out. Breathe in for 2 and out for 2.
Repeat 3 times.

2. Progressions
Place both hands across top of chest, just below the collar bones. Breathe in pushing hands up away from you, and breathe out, hands coming back. Breathe in for 2 and out for 2.
Repeat 3 times.

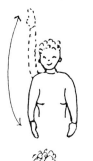

3. Arms at sides. Breathe in and lift right arm out and overhead, count 4; feel the stretch down right side with ribs lifted; breathe out, count 4. Repeat and change to left arm, making four times in all.

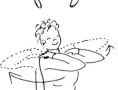

4. Hands on shoulders, elbows forward and at shoulder level. Breathe in for 2 counts, bringing elbows slowly back level with shoulders; feel strong pull across chest. Breathe out, bringing elbows forward, count 2.
Repeat 3 times.

Do these exercises gently at first; if you overbreathe you may feel light-headed or dizzy and must stop at once and have a gentle shake out to use up excess oxygen.
Breathing out should be a relaxation phase.

Breathing exercises from the EXTEND programme

Reproduced by permission of EXTEND

This is a sample page of the EXTEND Booklet, written by Penny Bevan Jones RGN. This is currently under review.
Special note from author: *Anyone having treatment must consult their therapist before proceeding with the described exercises.*

Nutrition

Eating is one of the great pastimes which is more than just to maintain the body. It is about creativity, giving, socialising, sharing and exchanging. Many things can affect the enjoyment of food. Good company, food which is good to look at, to smell and to taste will encourage appetite. Emotional upsets, worry and anxiety, depression and bereavement can have a negative effect on appetite and reduce enjoyment of food.

See also Chapter 1, section 1 for more advice on Diet

Current thinking on nutrition suggests reducing the intake of sugar, fat and salt, while increasing the intake of fibre by half. This is very general advice and the British Diabetic Association (BDA) stresses the importance of looking at each individual's nutritional needs. The BDA recommends that:

- Only elderly people who are overweight or diabetic should reduce sugar and fats;

- Salt should be reduced on medical advice if high blood pressure is a problem;

- Dietary fibre intake should be increased to improve well-being;

- This should be accompanied by an overall increase in fluids.

You may find that with slight adjustments to your present diet taking into account the recommendations of the World Health Organisation (see below), together with an increase in the amount of exercise taken may be enough to help you maintain or reduce your weight, and promote good health. If you have a weight problem you should talk to your doctor who may refer you to a dietitian.

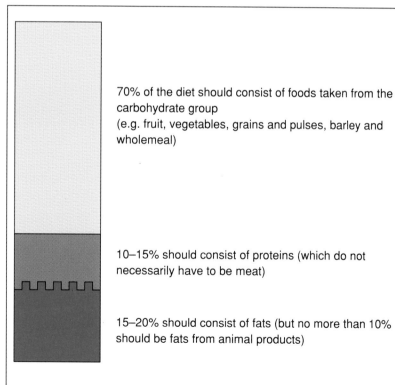

70% of the diet should consist of foods taken from the carbohydrate group
(e.g. fruit, vegetables, grains and pulses, barley and wholemeal)

10–15% should consist of proteins (which do not necessarily have to be meat)

15–20% should consist of fats (but no more than 10% should be fats from animal products)

A healthy diet. The World Health Organisation's recommendations

Adapted from the recommendations given in the World Health Organisation's report *Diet, Nutrition and Chronic Disease*, published in 1990

8.2(c) MONEY

The one thing you don't want to be worried about after retirement is whether you have enough money to live on, and the only way to avoid this is to plan your finances carefully before you retire. Your income after retirement will probably be derived from three main sources:

- A State pension;

- An occupational pension;

- Interest on savings which have been invested.

The sensible thing to do, then, while you are still in employment and earning, is to ensure that these three sources of income will be as ample as possible.

State pensions

See also Appendix VI on Benefits

State retirement pensions are payable to women at the age of 60 and to men at 65, and can be deferred for five years if the individual chooses; deferment will, of course, increase the value. The amount of your State pension will depend on the length of your working life and the number of National Insurance contributions paid by you and your employer. It is possible to find out from the Department of Social Security (DSS) how much your pension is likely to be by completing and sending off a form which is available from DSS offices, where you can also get useful leaflets explaining how your pension is made up, how to claim for it, and what other financial assistance you may be entitled to.

See Appendix VIII for Suggested futher reading

There are a number of useful booklets to help you to understand the details of pensions and financial planning.

Occupational pensions and investments

It is very unlikely that your State pension will be enough to live on, so it is wise to consider joining the occupational pension scheme offered by your employer, or the alternative of joining a private pension scheme. People who are self-employed should certainly provide for the future through a private pension plan. It is worth remembering that you can claim tax relief on all pension contributions. Pension schemes, both occupational and private, vary considerably, so if you are making a choice between the two you should study the conditions very carefully to make sure you get the best benefits, as you should in choosing between private pension plans. The guides listed in Appendix VIII provide useful information, as does the Consumers' Association. The national newspapers, radio and television networks all run regular financial features and programmes offering advice and information on all aspects of handling your financial affairs, including how to invest your savings so as to get the best return on your capital.

Changes in outgoings

In the years before retirement it is a good idea to stock up on expensive items while you can afford them. For instance, buy some good clothes that will last, think about changing your car for a new one, and if you are renting a television set or video recorder, buy these items instead. But don't get depressed at the prospects of having to live on a reduced income: there are a number of financial 'perks' for pensioners, such as:

- Free prescriptions;

- Reduced fares on public transport if you buy a senior citizen's railcard or bus pass;

- Reduced prices for entrance to some places of entertainment.

Also your expenditure will be reduced as you will not have to travel to and from your place of work, and the wear and tear on your clothes and car will be less.

Once you have retired and the pattern of your income has changed, you will want to keep your tax bill down to the minimum. Your State pension will be taxable, but tax will be deducted at source from an occupational pension through the PAYE system, and possibly also from a personal pension. The Inland Revenue increases the personal allowance according to age, first between the ages of 65 and 74, and again at 75 and over, so make sure you claim age allowance on your income tax return. Social security benefits, such as income support, attendance allowance, invalidity pension, and mobility allowance, are tax-free and should be claimed as such. If you take a part time job, however, the income you derive from it will be taxable; and the interest on your investments will also be taxable, except in certain circumstances. The interest on the new TESSA savings accounts is tax free, for example, and people who are not eligible to pay income tax can now receive interest from their savings invested in bank or building society free of tax, after completing an application form. Tax relief can also now be claimed on certain private medical insurance policies for people aged 60 and over. Now that husbands and wives are taxed separately, it is wise to allocate investments between them so as to avoid paying higher rates of tax and to make good use of their separate personal allowances. There are a number of other ways of keeping the income tax you pay to the minimum after retirement, and these are covered in the publications listed in the further reading list at the back of this book. Studying the subject thoroughly could, indeed, give you a new interest in life.

See Appendix VIII for Suggested further reading

8.2(d)   INDEPENDENCE

Now that you are free of the pressures of working life, and of the responsibilities of rearing a family, you will want to enjoy that independence and freedom for as long as possible. However, if you miss the purpose and companionship of work, and if you need to supplement your income, why not look for a part time job? You no longer have to forego part of your pension if you earn more than a certain amount per week; now you can go on receiving your full State pension no matter how much you earn. It is also being recognised that older people are an important part of the work force, that they are more reliable and responsible than the younger generation, and that they can improve a company's business by their helpful attitude towards customers. If you have difficulty in finding a job locally, there are organisations, such as *Success at Sixty* and *Senior Service Bureau* which help older people to find work. If you don't need the money, but would still like to do some useful work, there are many organisations which welcome voluntary workers, such as the British Red Cross Society (BRCS), the Women's Royal Voluntary Service (WRVS), Age Concern, or the League of Friends at your local hospital. Decide first which charitable organisation you would like to join, and contact your local branch, whose address will be in your telephone directory. If you need further help, go to your local Citizens' Advice Bureau – who also, incidentally, employ voluntary workers – or consult your local library.

See Appendix VII for Addresses of useful organisations

Many people find that retirement gives them a golden opportunity to take up a sport or hobby they have not hitherto had time for; adult education classes offer tuition in all sorts of activities, from painting to yoga, and brochures are usually available at public libraries. There may be a Leisure Centre in your locality which also offers a wide range of sporting and other activities. Attending classes at such an institute or centre, or joining the local drama, operatic, music, or literary society, is a good way of meeting people and making new friends, of enjoying some new or favourite recreation, and of keeping mentally alert and physically fit, so that you can relish your independence.

Your interests may lie in the educational field: you may not have had the opportunity to go to college or university after leaving school, and have regretted this all your life. Now you can make up for lost time, not only through your local adult education institute but also through the Open University, the University of the Third Age, or by being accepted as a mature student at university. The Open University offers undergraduate, continuing education, and postgraduate programmes in a wide range of subjects. The system of study is by correspondence, backed up by radio and television programmes and summer schools, and degrees are awarded to successful students. This is an ideal way of studying for a degree if you have

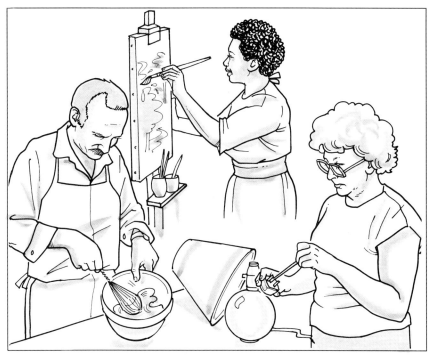

Now may be the time to learn a new skill or discover a hidden talent

– or prefer – to work at home. The University of the Third Age (U3A) originated in France and was established in Britain in 1981; its purpose is to enable older people to extend and share their knowledge, experience, and skills by forming study groups led by a member with knowledge of a particular topic. No qualifications are needed to participate, and none are awarded, so there is no pressure to excel intellectually. If you want to go the whole hog, so to speak, and become a full time university student, you should write to the universities of your choice to find out if they take mature students, and what the pre-entry requirements are. Applications for places have to go through the Universities Central Council on Admissions (UCCA) from whom the necessary form can be obtained. Most universities have a quota of mature students, and value them for their motivation and commitment to learning.

8.2(e) SUPPORTED INDEPENDENCE

We value our independence throughout life, but perhaps never more so than in later life. Most of us dread the thought of becoming so disabled or incapacitated by age or disease that we can no longer manage our own lives, but need the care and support of others; most of us want to end our lives in our homes, not in some kind of institution. Fortunately this is now publicly recognised, and Government policy for community care is to 'enable people affected by ageing or disability to live as independently as possible: the aim is to support people in their own homes or in "homely surroundings" wherever this can be done', according to the Department of Health. To fulfil this aim the health and social services are expected to work closely together with voluntary organisations and the private sector in providing the services needed to maintain a disabled elderly person at home.

The services such a person is most likely to require are:

- Help in the home with housework, shopping, cooking, and other domestic chores;

- Adaptations in the home, such as handrails for stairs, taps that are easy to turn on and off, a raised lavatory seat if the present one is too low;

- Equipment such as walking frames or stair-lifts that enable a disabled person to remain mobile.

There are also day centres where elderly people can go for a meal and for companionship and recreation.

Nursing care in the home is provided by the Community Nursing Service. Another useful service is 'respite care' for a disabled person being looked after by a relative: the elderly person is admitted to a residential home or hospital ward for a short period (usually two weeks) to give the carer a much needed break.

The funds for and availability of such services vary enormously from one district to another, but if you think you need them you should ask your doctor, who will know the extent of the disability which is causing the need, and will be able to advise you of the next step. It is also worth contacting the local branches of the voluntary organisations, such as Age Concern, the Red Cross, and the WRVS, whose work includes running a 'meals on wheels' service, visiting people at home, taking them out in their cars, and organising luncheon and other clubs.

Charges usually have to be made for domiciliary services such as home helps and meals on wheels, and there are social security benefits available to meet the expense of supporting a disabled person at home. These include:

- Community care grants for minor house repairs, bedding, etc.;

- Mobility allowance to help with extra transport;

- Attendance allowance for people who need constant care;

- Invalid care allowance for carers;

- An independent living fund to pay for housework or care.

Your local social services department will also tell you what services the local authority supplies for the elderly and disabled.

See also Chapter 2, section 6 on Help for the carers

See Appendix VII for Addresses of useful organisations and support groups

See also Appendix VI on Benefits

8.3   ACCOMMODATION

8.3(a)   SHELTERED ACCOMMODATION

Sometimes when you get older your housing needs may change. It could be for many reasons, but whatever the reason there are many types of accommodation you can consider. Sheltered accommodation is just one option.

The accommodation

Sheltered accommodation originated several hundred years ago with the introduction of almshouses. Today, almshouses are still in existence, but most sheltered housing is provided by local authorities, private companies and some by housing associations.

The principle of sheltered accommodation is for people of retirement age to maintain their independence with support available when required. It is usually built specifically for the purpose. It can be in the form of bungalows or flats, with accommodation for groups of up to about 40 people.

Different sheltered accommodation complexes vary in the amount of support or assistance provided. A warden is usually based within the group of homes and available 24 hours a day. The warden may visit all the residents each day to check they are not neglecting themselves or developing any illnesses, or whether they have other problems they need help with. Other types of warden-controlled accommodation may operate via an intercom system, where the residents can contact the warden if they need to. The main advantage of this type of housing is an alarm system, which enables the residents to receive help within a few minutes.

Although sheltered accommodation is usually thought of as individual self-contained flats, where the residents cook their own food, do their own laundry and watch their own television sets, there is some sheltered housing where residents have their own room, but share other communal facilities. If you are thinking of moving to sheltered accommodation yourself, you should consider whether you want to live independently, or have your meals prepared for you to eat with other people in the dining room and share the television.

The warden

The role of the warden is to assist with day to day problems and help with any accidents or emergencies. A warden:

- Acts more like a good neighbour than a nurse or home help;
- Does not help with shopping, cooking, cleaning, nor provide assistance with bathing and dressing;
- Will help residents to gain help from other services and relatives;

- May also organise social events, report any repairs and sort out maintenance problems.

Some sheltered accommodation provides more than an on-call warden system, with extra staff. These staff often help the residents with simple nursing duties and housework.

Pros and cons

Sheltered housing provides security and companionship to the frail and people nervous of living alone, in small communities. It is available to rent or buy, but before you decide what to do, consult your local social services department who will be able to give you information and advice about the different types of sheltered housing available in your area. You should find out how much support is available and what is covered by your rent, as you may have to pay extra for special services.

8.3(b) RESIDENTIAL CARE

Most elderly people will see out their lives at home but there are times when, even with all the help a loving family and friends can offer, it is necessary to seek the extra support of residential care. A good residential home will provide the benefits of skilled help always at hand, specialised equipment and companionship. Whether you are looking for residential care from force of circumstances or simply because you are seeking company and comfort, you will want to choose somewhere where the services and way of life suit your needs.

When looking for a place to stay you will need to consider the following points:

- The services offered;
- The atmosphere;
- Cost;
- The environment.

Services offered

Those people who are most severely disabled will need to choose a nursing home which must, by law, have a qualified nurse on duty at all times. Those with less severe disabilities will be able to find a suitable rest home which will have slightly lower staffing levels and so be less expensive. The dividing line between the two types of care is rather vague so, if in doubt, seek guidance from the local home managers.

Different homes will be suited to different types of problem. If you are looking for a placement for somebody else who is confused and liable to wander and get lost, you will need to know how homes deal with that particular situation. Ideally the home will have been designed so that residents can wander about as they wish without coming to any harm. These homes should also use distinctive colours or signs to help the residents to recognise where they are in the home and to find key places such as the toilet. The difference between being continent or incontinent might be as simple as being able to find the right place at the right time. You may hear some homes that specialise in caring for confused people described as EMI units meaning that they are for people who are Elderly Mentally Infirm. It is important to establish that facilities are adequate as homes that are less good at coping with these problems may resort to restricting a confused resident's movements. They may even stop them walking at all by trapping them in their chairs. This can be done by using fixed or heavy tables or by selecting a chair which makes it hard for the resident to get up. In the worst scenario confused people will be controlled by excessive use of sedatives. Other homes may simply tell you that they cannot accept wandering, demented residents.

If your problems are caused by physical handicap you will need to ask about the availability of physiotherapy and whether equipment such as hoists and pressure relieving mattresses are provided. If you are already in residential care, you should find that any sign that a pressure sore (which used to be known as a bedsore) is developing will prompt immediate action. Your nurses will work out what is causing the pressure which is making you sore, and will take steps to eliminate it by suggesting changes of position, or offering you a specially designed cushion or mattress. The choice of equipment will depend on the severity of your problem. In the unlikely case that your sore does not improve it may be that you are not getting the quality of advice you think you are paying for. This is not a matter to be taken lightly.

Incontinence will be competently and cheerfully dealt with by some homes whilst others will prefer not to take people with this problem. If you are only just getting to the toilet on time it might be best to choose a sympathetic home to avoid the upheaval of having to move in the near future. Enormous advances have been made, in recent years, in special pads and sheets designed to improve the lives of people with incontinence. If a home you visit reeks of stale urine the staff have not kept up to date with recent developments. Look elsewhere!

Medical cover is usually provided by general practitioners. This is often the case for NHS as well as private accommodation. In some cases the doctor will have an arrangement to visit regularly.

In others, residents will remain registered with their own general practitioner who will visit on request. Even if the home normally contacts the doctor on your behalf you retain the same rights to approach your doctor that you have always had.

Atmosphere

The most important aspect in any home is the atmosphere. Are staff friendly – do they appear interested in the residents who are already living there? Do the residents seem happy. If you are looking for companionship, find out if the communal sitting rooms are used. Are people reading, chatting, knitting or are they blankly staring into space. Talk to some of them if you can. Only they know what it is really like to live in that home. All homes should smell fresh and be clean but sumptuous furnishings can sometimes disguise a home where care is mediocre. Try to look below the surface.

Whatever the type of residential home it is important to find one that has a way of life that suits you. Different people want different things from their life. While some will choose the order of a highly structured routine, most will want to retain control over their own way of life. Discussion with the manager will reveal how much flexibility there is within the home. Can people get up and go to bed when they like? Can they take a bath when they like, morning or evening?

The most important aspect in any home will be the atmosphere

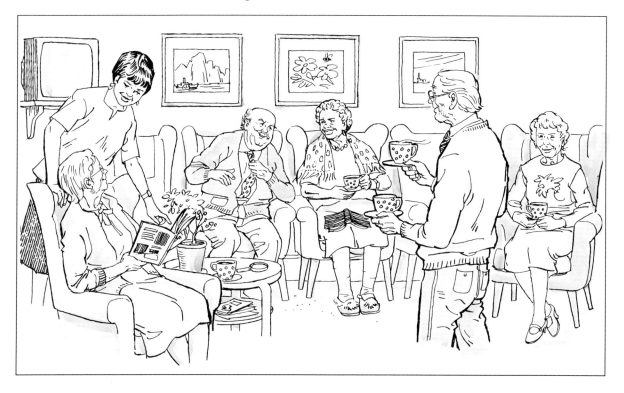

If you enjoy going out ask if you will be given whatever help you need. Some places will organise regular trips to local places of interest or shopping centres but not all residential homes can offer this facility.

Cost

See Appendix VII for Addresses of useful organisations

Cost and facilities can vary enormously making comparison complicated. Nursing home care, in particular, is inevitably expensive. Contact your social services department which may be able to advise you about obtaining financial assistance. If funding is still a problem your local Age Concern group may be able, in some cases, to direct you to organisations which could give you some assistance. Pressure groups make frequent representation to the Government about the financial difficulties that some disabled people suffer. If you are having problems obtaining vital assistance then add your voice by contacting your MP.

Find out exactly what you are getting for your money. Some homes charge extra for laundry and special appliances such as incontinence pads. Physiotherapy and chiropody may be an integral part of care or may be costed separately.

The National Health Service does have some provision for long term care in continuing care wards, in NHS nursing homes and in beds contracted in private nursing homes. To be admitted to any of these beds most health districts require a referral from a consultant geriatrician. Criteria used for assessing potential residents/patients varies from one district to the next but generally places are reserved for the most physically or mentally disabled. Costs are normally covered by the NHS but State pensions are reduced to minimal levels.

In general then, do shop around and do not assume that the cheaper homes are inferior. Many managers work very hard to provide excellent care at a reasonable price.

Environment

Most residential homes provide a good percentage of single rooms. Where there are shared rooms they are usually just for two people. There is often a pay differential between single and shared rooms and larger or more attractive rooms are normally more expensive. Hospital wards, traditionally, still have larger groupings although many now try to place furniture in order to create alcoves which give a greater feeling of privacy.

Policy on furniture varies. Some homes like you to bring your own furniture while others prefer you to use the furnishings they provide. In either case you should check that you will have adequate space for all the clothes, pictures and ornaments that you want to bring with you.

Some homes have resident pets or may be happy for you to bring your own pet in with you. Check if this is important to you.

Unless you are a real country lover, think carefully before deciding to live in a home in an isolated rural position even if the setting is idyllic. You may find you become tired of the beautiful views and long to watch the bustle and crowds on a busy street. You also need to consider the ease with which your friends can visit you. Being in an area well served by public transport might prove useful.

All homes must be inspected and registered so if you are not getting the service you deserve you have recourse to the registering authority. Most homes, however, are run by caring and dedicated people who will work hard to make sure that going into residential care is to start a new and fulfilled life.

8.4 CARING FOR AN ELDERLY PERSON AT HOME

8.4(a) INTRODUCTION

If you are caring for an elderly person at home, then you are one in a million – literally. Contrary to popular belief, we have not abandoned our elderly relatives, friends and neighbours to the mercy of hospitals, homes and other institutions. We do care, often battling against formidable odds to make sure the people who cared for us in the past are cared for in their turn.

Not only are you one in a million as a carer, your financial worth has been estimated, too. If just a small percentage of carers stopped looking after their dependants at home, the cost to the public purse would add up to billions of pounds.

It would be easy to paint a rosy picture of your caring role, to offer you a patronising pat on the back for your sterling work. Perhaps you might then be content to lapse into what has been described as the Florence Nightingale syndrome. When people ask you how you're coping, you will tell them 'Fine, thanks', and carry on in the role of willing martyr. One carer once described how she started baking bread for the first time when her mother came to stay after suffering a stroke. She was determined that her husband and children would have no cause to complain that she wasn't looking after them properly because of mother.

Taking on the responsibility of looking after an elderly person is invariably an open-ended commitment. Unlike children who will, for the most part, eventually leave home to make their own lives, an elderly person could well become more dependent as the years go by. The indignities of immobility, or incontinence, or mental confusion may strike the elderly person you are caring for. The added strain on you and your family could end up by affecting your own health.

Looking after someone with dementia is particularly harrowing. Not to be recognised by your own mother or father is heartrending. Sleepless nights and the worry that your dependant may wander out of the house and come to harm can cause untold stress. Unlike professional carers who can go home at the end of the day, the danger is that you become trapped, your children hesitate before bringing their friends home, your own social life grinds to a halt and the burden becomes too great.

If we lived in an ideal world where money was no object and information and support were readily available the responsibility of caring would be light. We can dream of a house with a self-contained 'granny annexe' attached, of family doctors, district nurses, social workers and health visitors with plenty of time to provide much needed support. Holidays away from home would be no problem because respite care for our elderly dependant would be freely available.

In that ideal world, elderly people would conform to the stereotypical image of apple-cheeked old ladies and jolly old gentlemen, content with their lot and grateful for the care we give them. The reality is somewhat different. None of us, whatever our age, welcomes the thought of journeying down the slippery slope from independence to gratitude when we can no longer look after ourselves.

Campaigning organisations like the Carers' National Association have fought hard to gain recognition for the unpaid work of so-called 'informal' carers. Over the last few years many people, carers and professionals alike, have published books and pamphlets on what it means to be a carer and on what carers need. The professionals are certainly more aware of what is needed in the way of support and services, but provision remains patchy. There are people and organisations, both voluntary and statutory, which can give you help – but you have to know where to look and you have to know the right questions to ask. Despite this age of computerised technology, there is still no single source which pulls together all the available information on everything from benefits to how to get help with bathing the person you care for.

If you have time to read this, probably you have not yet reached crisis point in your life as a carer. You are not yet in a position where your elderly dependant demands every second of your time. You are still able to have quiet moments to yourself. Your family is intact, holidays are still a possibility and not a distant dream. The love that binds you to your elderly charge has not been eaten away by fatigue to be replaced with guilt at your impatience.

See Appendix VII for Addresses of useful organisations and support groups, and Appendix VIII for Suggested further reading

See also Chapter 2, section 6 on Help for the carers

A final word: this introduction has painted a pretty bleak picture of the caring role. It is worth bearing in mind that caring for an elderly person has its rewards, too. There will be moments of great hilarity, of shared excursions, of poignant reminiscence, of your relative, friend or neighbour developing a very special relationship with your children because they have the time to spend together.

The purpose of this section of the manual is to offer you practical advice on coping as a carer so that you never reach crisis point and so that the pleasures of caring balance out the pain and pitfalls.

8.4(b)   PHYSICAL ASPECTS OF CARE

Elderly people are more likely to suffer from physical ailments than their younger counterparts. They are also more likely to have more than one thing wrong with them and to recover from any injury or illness more slowly than someone in their middle years. In addition, it should be remembered that physical illness may send an older person into a temporary state of confusion more easily than a younger one. If you are looking after an elderly person at home, it is important to bear certain principles in mind:

See Chapter 2, section 2 for advice on Helping the sick person at home with the activities of living

- Elderly people must maintain their mobility for as long, and to whatever extent, they can.

- Normal activities of living should be maintained as far as possible and the person's routine disrupted no more than necessary.

See also Chapter 2, section 6 on Help for the carers and Chapter 7, section 5 on Caring for others and its effects on health

- The elderly person's dignity and independence should be respected.

- Looking after a sick elderly person can be tiring and taxing. Don't forget to take care of yourself too.

Mobility

See also Section 8.6(a) below on Problems affecting movement

Joints and muscles stiffen as we grow older and the less they are used the more unlikely they are to revert to their former flexibility. If an elderly person is unable to move, for example through being confined to bed or a chair, it is essential that all joints are helped to retain their normal movements. This is important even if the person is bedridden for a very short time only. The way that this can be achieved is through the use of 'passive' exercises – so termed because the sick person has them done for her. The carer gently moves the patient's limbs through the whole range of movements she would usually perform for herself. This should be done at least twice a day, perhaps in conjunction with washing or dressing. If joints are not 'put through their paces' they may become immobile and 'frozen', which is extremely painful.

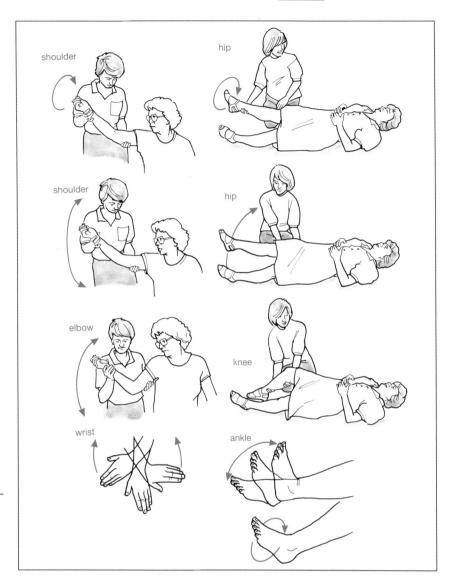

Passive exercises

The carer may have to help the sick person move her joints through all the normal movements so that they do not become stiff and painful

If a joint has not been moved for any length of time it may prove too stiff to move and you then have to be careful not to cause more damage. In such a case, the general practitioner may ask a community physiotherapist to visit. She will assess the patient and plan what care it is best to give. Occupational therapists can provide mobility aids, for example:

- Zimmer frames;

- Bed ladders;

- Walking sticks;

- Raised toilet and bath seats;

- Special cutlery etc.

See also Chapter 7, section 12 on The adult with a physical disability

See also section 8.6(d) below on Problems associated with the feet and legs

They will also assess the home for other needs.

Full mobility needs healthy feet. If feet are painful and shoes don't fit, correct walking is difficult and may lead to falls. Regular visits from a chiropodist are a necessity for most elderly people.

Maintaining a degree of mobility is not only important for keeping a person's joints and muscles in reasonable condition. A number of complications and diseases can result directly from prolonged bedrest, as summarised in the figure below.

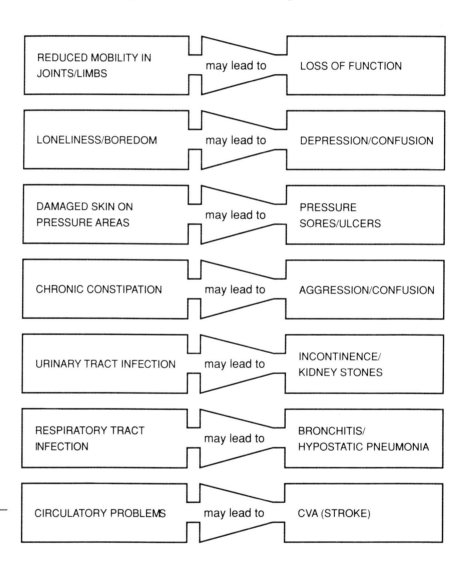

	may lead to	
REDUCED MOBILITY IN JOINTS/LIMBS	may lead to	LOSS OF FUNCTION
LONELINESS/BOREDOM	may lead to	DEPRESSION/CONFUSION
DAMAGED SKIN ON PRESSURE AREAS	may lead to	PRESSURE SORES/ULCERS
CHRONIC CONSTIPATION	may lead to	AGGRESSION/CONFUSION
URINARY TRACT INFECTION	may lead to	INCONTINENCE/ KIDNEY STONES
RESPIRATORY TRACT INFECTION	may lead to	BRONCHITIS/ HYPOSTATIC PNEUMONIA
CIRCULATORY PROBLEMS	may lead to	CVA (STROKE)

Complications associated with long term bedrest

See also Chapter 2, section 2(b) for more information about Breathing

Breathing

Apart from specific chest and throat diseases, there may be other reasons why an elderly person cannot breathe very well. Some of these are considered below.

Hiatus hernia   This is a common problem for people over 50, especially women, and causes pain in the chest leading to breathlessness. Sufferers can be helped by sleeping in a fairly upright position, with a glass of milk or flask of tea and a biscuit by the bedside to be eaten if they wake up in pain in the night.

See also Chapter 7, section 10(f) on Coronary heart disease

Forms of heart disease   If the heart does not pump properly, fluid may gather in the lungs. The doctor may prescribe diuretics ('water tablets') to relieve the congestion, and an elderly person will probably feel safer if she has a commode by the bed. The inability to move quickly and the distress of an 'accident' can cause more breathlessness and maybe broken bones as well.

See the section below on Eating and drinking

Anaemia   Many old people are anaemic and, because the red blood cells carry oxygen, lack of these can cause breathlessness. As old people very often lack iron content in their food, it is necessary to discover what you can about the person's dietary habits.

Obesity   Some people are too stout to move or breathe and losing weight is difficult when you cannot exercise. Diets need to be discussed with care. Why should someone in her eighties be turned into a depressive because she can no longer have sugar in her tea? Sometimes the carer has to accept the inevitable.

Eating and drinking

See also section 8.2(b) above on Health and Chapter 1, section 1 on Diet

Eating habits can change drastically from one generation to another, and you may find that nothing you cook for your elderly relative appears to be appreciated. For example, many younger people now cook green vegetables for a considerably shorter time than used to be the case. The dangers of excess sugar, salt and fats have all contributed to the way we eat today, but someone advanced in years is not going to take kindly to changing the eating habits of a lifetime. If the elderly person is living in your house you may have to try to come to some sort of compromise. Obviously, there will be difficulties if you are cooking for a number of people of different tastes and ages but do take the elderly person's likes and dislikes into account wherever possible. This may include simply keeping quiet instead of voicing your disapproval when the person helps herself to more sugar or salt than you would allow your children, or it may involve providing a weekly treat, such as a favourite dish of her own choosing. You should also be aware that the perception of different tastes declines with age, so other aspects of a meal – presentation, company, familiar rituals etc. – will take on an increasing importance.

Specific diseases may require special diets and your doctor or district nurse will tell you about these. Protein is necessary for good body building and skin care and iron is necessary for healthy red blood cells. The importance of fresh fruit, vegetables and fibre should also be stressed. Try sprinkling a little bran on breakfast cereal or soups to help avoid constipation. Do be careful too to see that the elderly person gets plenty of fluids. This will also help to prevent constipation, as well as making her less prone to bladder infections. For further information, your local health centre, surgery or health advisory council can give you advice on diet, as can the Dairy Council.

Ultimately, however, it is no good providing an elderly person with a healthy meal you know she won't eat. If she's used to bread and butter and jam, she is not going to tuck into a lettuce leaf in order to lose weight. If that is what she is given, her morale will plummet. Part of the value of food comes from the enjoyment surrounding it, so there needs to be discussion about meals. Vitamin supplements and build-up drinks may be necessary, particularly if she is debilitated and her appetite small. Elderly people may also enjoy a pint of beer or a glass of sherry and, in most cases, the pleasure gained thereby will outweigh any adverse effects – particularly if the drink is associated with company and some sense of occasion.

Eliminating

See also the section on Mobility above

Bowel habit   As mentioned above, a common side effect of the reduced mobility and changes in eating habit that may accompany physical illness is constipation. An elderly person's bowel can also become sluggish due to inactivity, decreased elasticity of the bowel wall, incorrect diet, inability to reach the toilet, depression or inadequate knowledge about her own health and body. This can give rise to further problems, including confusion and aggression. Sometimes loose faeces will trickle down on either side of a blockage causing spurious diarrhoea. If this happens it is always best to inform the doctor or district nurse and follow their instructions.

See section 8.6(b) below on Urinary and bowel related problems

Once the bowel has been cleared, it is important to keep it so with correct diet (including plenty of fruit, fibre and fluids) and laxatives if necessary. If you think that laxatives are needed, do discuss their use with your doctor or district nurse as they should not be taken indiscriminately. Some other medications (including ones bought 'over the counter', without a prescription) may cause constipation so make sure that the doctor knows about any medicines or tablets the elderly person is taking.

If there are days of severe constipation alternating with genuine diarrhoea, the doctor should be informed as this can be a sign of bowel disease. Any bleeding from the rectum, vagina or bladder should be reported too. Many elderly people have small bleeding points. Haemorrhoids (piles) are a source of great discomfort and may also cause bleeding. Creams to soothe painful haemorrhoids and reduce swelling can be prescribed by the doctor or bought over the counter after discussion with your pharmacist.

Black faeces may mean that the person is taking iron. If, however, they are black and shiny and smell offensive, then they may well contain blood. The doctor should be informed so that he can send a specimen to the laboratory.

Incontinence of urine The main causes for incontinence of urine – infections, changes in bladder shape and tone, stress incontinence – are discussed in more detail below, as are ways of dealing with them. A related problem is urgency – the need to get to the toilet before the person can manage it.

Helping the elderly person Incontinence of both urine and faeces will make life harder for the carer. There will be more washing and changing to deal with not to speak of floors to clean. It may be very easy to allow exhaustion and frustration to let you forget just how unpleasant and embarrassing incontinence can be for the elderly person herself. If an elderly individual suddenly starts refusing to go out or have visitors, it may well be that continence is becoming a problem. Even a teaspoon of urine can smell unpleasant to others. Inability to perform this most basic and private of bodily functions successfully and independently is extremely upsetting and degrading for the person concerned and anyone in this position deserves every available help.

Some practical suggestions for helping an elderly person to maintain control over elimination are given below.

- Talk to your general practitioner. The problem may be caused by an infection which will respond to treatment or, in other cases, an operation might help. In addition, many practices now have access to a 'Continence Adviser' – a specialist nurse to whom patients can be referred.

- Think about the layout of the house. How far is the toilet from the bedroom? From the living room? Is there somewhere discreet to put a commode nearer to the room where the elderly person spends most of her time? Elderly men can use urine bottles if necessary, and provision should be made for concealing and emptying them.

- Sometimes clothing can be difficult to undo or take off in a hurry, particularly if the person has stiff hands. Large buttons, velcro and easily pulled zips may help. Your continence adviser, or charities such as The Disabled Living Foundation and Age Concern may be able to give advice about modified clothing.

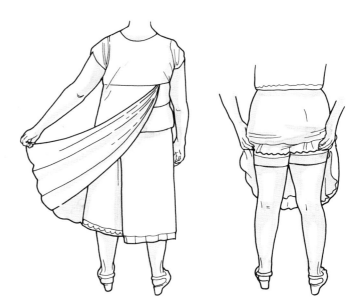

Adapted clothing

A dress that opens down the back and stockings rather than tights will help the person with urgency to get to the toilet on time

- How easy is it for an elderly person to go to the toilet at night time? Is there sufficient light en route? Are there stairs to be negotiated? If a visit to the bathroom in the middle of the night seems like an obstacle course, try discussing alternatives such as a chamber pot, urine bottle or commode in the bedroom.

- During the day, offer to take a disabled elderly person to the toilet at regular intervals (say every half hour). She may be embarrassed to ask you too often or, if she is a little confused, she may forget to ask if not reminded. Helping her down the corridor and into the bathroom at frequent intervals may seem like a waste of time to begin with but it is likely to lead to fewer accidents before very long. This in turn will pay dividends, not only for your workload but also for her self-esteem and your relationship.

- If prevention is not possible, incontinence pads can be worn. Your district nurse or continence adviser can help you choose a suitable brand.

See also section 8.6(f) below on Hypothermia

Keeping warm

It is easy to assume that those elderly people who will suffer from the cold are the ones who live alone, particularly on a very limited income. Certainly such individuals are particularly at risk and a well timed visit from a caring neighbour may save a life. You should be aware, however, that even your own elderly relatives, cared for lovingly at home, may have trouble keeping warm. Elderly people lose their shivering reflex and do not always realise that they are becoming cold. Decreased mobility means that a person will have more difficulty keeping warm than someone who is active. In addition, the person's heat regulation mechanism may become faulty, so that he can suffer undue cold in a very warm room. It is important, therefore, to be alert for the signs of hypothermia and to take certain basic precautions.

- Make sure that the person's environment is as draught free as possible – particularly if he is immobile in bed or a chair.

- Try to ensure that he gets at least one hot meal a day, and several warm drinks – especially in cold weather.

- Pay attention to the patient's hands and feet as these can get particularly cold. Fingerless mittens, thick socks and lined slippers can be worn.

- We lose about one third of our body heat from our heads, so do encourage elderly people to wear a hat out of doors, and indoors too if it is very cold.

- If you are bed-bathing an elderly person or helping her to take a bath or shower in the bathroom, you must be careful to ensure that the room temperature is suitably warm as she may easily become chilled. Let her test the temperature of the bath water herself too before you help her into it.

Cleanliness and grooming

See also Chapter 2, section 2(h) on Keeping clean and well groomed

Skin   Skin needs to be kept clean, washed and dried carefully, especially wherever there are folds of skin such as under the breasts, or between toes and fingers. The navel also needs care, especially if it has not been cleaned properly for some time.

An area which hasn't been touched for ages must be handled very carefully as the skin underneath may be quite sore. Vigorous attempts to clean encrusted dirt, dried skin and exudate will certainly cause pain. It is best to treat the area first with warm oil (arachis or olive oil), and gradually the dirt will loosen and come away of its own accord. If necessary, use a little healing cream (such as Sudocrem) or one of the baby barrier creams (such as Drapolene or zinc and castor oil cream) which prevent water or excretions from damaging the skin. Cream should never be applied too thickly and the area underneath should be kept clean, washed and dried, with old cream removed and fresh applied if necessary. Never use talcum powder and cream together as this clogs the pores.

If the skin is infected, keep the area clean and dry and ask the doctor to advise you about appropriate use of topical preparations (creams, lotions etc.).

If limbs are permanently bent, skin will become excoriated as it is very difficult to wash and dry between the surfaces. Even small areas, such as fingers, must not be neglected. Following a stroke,

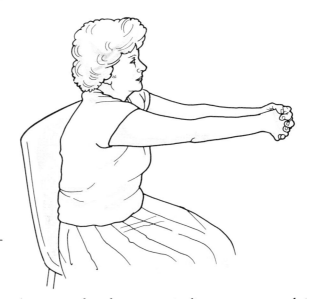

Encourage your relative to straighten her affected arm with her strong one

for example, the person's fingers may curl inwards towards the palm. Encourage her to straighten these fingers with her other hand, and to straighten this arm with her strong arm. (Never call an affected limb a 'bad' limb; 'good' and 'bad' do not equate with illness and can cause physically disabled people to feel negative about the afflicted parts of themselves to the extent of deliberately neglecting them. We are not speaking here of the neglect which comes through loss of contact with the affected side.) Make sure nails are cut short so that they do not dig into the palm. If you do put talcum powder between skin surfaces, make sure that there is not enough to clog or mask the skin underneath.

Old people's skin may be very dry. This may be due to poor nutrition or lack of fluid intake, in which case these problems need to be rectified. A good, gentle body lotion is preferable to the use of talcum powder which tends to dry the skin. Hard rubbing should be avoided as it may cause damage. Baby lotions and oils in the bath water are useful as moisturisers and should not cause an allergic reaction.

Areas needing particular attention are anywhere where there may be body pressure (e.g. heels, elbows, buttocks) or wherever there are skin folds (e.g. between the buttock cheeks, groins, armpits, underneath the breasts for women). These latter are often neglected because they are not noticed until they become very sore. They may become infected and start to smell offensive. If this happens, you should inform your doctor who can prescribe an anti-fungal ointment. The affected areas will need to be washed and dried with special care, perhaps two or three times a day, until they are healed. The towels and flannels used should be kept specifically for this area.

The genitals are another area needing careful attention, and should be washed and dried thoroughly twice a day. Any sign of infection should be reported immediately to the doctor. Again, it is useful to keep a towel and flannel specially for this area.

Some patients develop pressure sores from lying or sitting too long in one place. Certain areas of the body are particularly at risk. Try to change a person's position at least every four hours, and every two hours if at all possible as old people's skin is particularly fragile. This may be difficult if you are the only carer and the patient is heavy. Ask for help, and keep on asking if necessary.

Keep sheets and pillow cases dry and free from crumbs and wrinkles. Bedclothes should be reasonably loose over the body – and sometimes a bed cradle will help to alleviate pressure. Sheepskins under buttocks or as chair covers, as bootees for heels and as elbow protectors, help to prevent skin chafing. A pillow between the knees may also help when the person is lying in bed. Correct lifting techniques are dealt with elsewhere in this book and dragging a person up the bed can cause friction and soreness.

See also Chapter 2, section 4 on Lifting and transfers

Hair   A person feels very different if she is well groomed. There may be local hairdressers willing to visit the housebound and some of these are very inventive. If this is not possible, you may be able to wash the patient's hair yourself. Make sure that ears are dry and that they are not injured by rough pillow handling when the head is being moved.

See also section 8.6(c) below on Problems with hearing and sight

Ears   These need careful cleaning. Nothing should ever be pushed down them 'to clean the wax'. A certain amount of wax provides necessary protection for the ears. If it is causing deafness, the doctor will decide what to do.

See also section 8.7(c) below on Diabetes in the elderly

Nails   Nails should be kept short. Toenails should be cut straight across, fingernails should be rounded and the cuticles pushed down with a towel after the hands have been washed. People with diabetes are more prone to infection, therefore it is advisable for a chiropodist to care for the feet of a person with this disease. You may be able to arrange a home visit through your general practitioner but it is more likely that you will have to pay for a private visit. If you make the arrangements yourself, do check that the chiropodist is a state registered practitioner.

Teeth   Old people's gums tend to shrink causing dental problems. Teeth need cleaning at least twice daily. If they are false, they should be soaked overnight in a special cleaning solution such as Steradent. Dentures should be well fitting if the wearer is to be able to eat properly.

A clean denture does not necessarily mean a clean mouth. Offer mouthwashes after meals, and check that gums, tongue and throat are clean and healthy looking. Any white spots should be reported to the doctor as they may indicate an infection. If this is suspected, it is best that the individual uses his own cutlery, plate and cup unless you have an efficient means of sterilisation available.

Dental appointments should continue regularly and the dentist may be able to make home visits if necessary.

Clothing   Clothing should be warm, loose but well fitting, and attractive. It is not good for anyone's morale to stay in nightwear and dressing gown all day and, as mentioned above, elderly people can easily become hypothermic.

See the section above on Keeping warm

When helping an elderly person to dress, let him do as much as he can for himself. After all, he has probably got plenty of time on his hands, so it doesn't matter if he's slow. Zips or velcro fastenings, easy to reach, lessen frustration and enhance the sense of achievement. With repetition and patience, even a confused person can learn to dress himself at least partially, even if he does sometimes need a little prompting.

Avoiding danger

See also Chapter 2, section 2(i) on Avoiding danger and Chapter 7 section 7 on Safety at home and outside

Apart from the dangers of malnutrition and hypothermia, discussed above, elderly people may be at particular risk from falls and other similar accidents. This is especially worrying at a time when the bones are increasingly brittle and when immobility following an accident can bring a host of other complications in its wake. The dangers caused by confusion and memory loss (when, for example, a person forgets to turn the oven off) will be considered elsewhere. This section will concentrate simply on ways of avoiding accidents and minimising the effects of falls.

See also section 8.6(c) below on Problems with hearing and sight

Eyesight   Vision deteriorates with age – and this is especially true of night vision. An elderly person is more likely to fall when moving around at night simply because she cannot see where she is going. The section on 'Eliminating' above looks at ways of avoiding hazardous journeys to the bathroom at night. It is also important that the elderly person can reach a night light or bedside lamp with ease, and lights in passageways or over stairwells should be left on at night if at all possible, if there is any likelihood of the elderly person walking along that way.

Eyesight should be tested regularly and spectacles need to be kept clean. Many elderly people are operated on successfully for cataract and glasses can help them to see and read again. In such cases, it is important to remind the person to turn the whole head when looking at something. Spectacles cannot cover the whole field of vision that eyes do, even though they are attempting to do the job of the lens of the eye. In severe cases, it may be appropriate to discuss with your general practitioner whether you should apply to be registered blind or partially sighted.

See section 8.3 above on Accommodation

The home environment   Sometimes an elderly person's home environment will need to be radically altered – for example, he may need to go into a nursing home or sheltered accommodation. On occasions, just moving his room to the ground floor so that he no longer has to negotiate stairs may make a great deal of difference (providing that there is still access to toilet and washing facilities). Other basic safety precautions include the following.

- Make sure that any stairway the elderly person will be using is fitted with sturdy handrails.

- Floors should be uncluttered (you may have to watch other members of the family carefully over this), and free from ridges in the carpet, loose rugs or slippery surfaces.

- If the person has his own facilities for boiling a kettle, make sure that he has a model that turns itself off.

- A smoke alarm should be fitted in the house of an elderly person living alone – if she is deaf, this should flash a light as well as make a noise.

The house can hold many hazards for elderly people – inadequate handrails on stairs, loose rugs, toys and other clutter on the floor, kettles and other appliances that can't turn themselves off

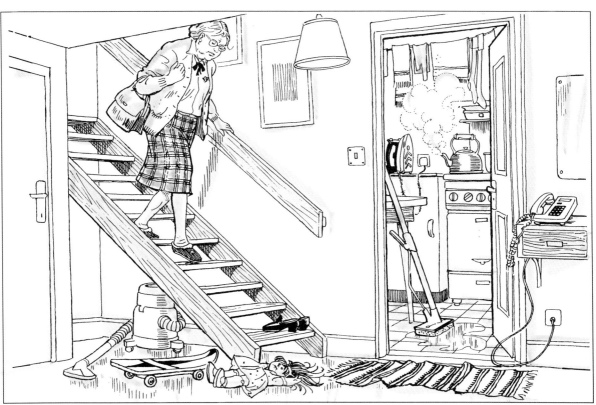

See also Chapter 2, section 2(i) on Avoiding danger and section 2(j) on Communicating and expressing needs

Communication   If accidents do happen, it is important that help can be summoned quickly. The following suggestions may perhaps be useful:

- If your relative lives in a self-contained part of the house, fix up an ordinary doorbell with a push button in her room and a bell which rings in your quarters. Make sure that the push button is easily accessible for her and that batteries are checked and changed regularly.

- If she is bedridden or immobilised in a chair, an ordinary domestic intercom, such as those used as baby alarms, will enable her to tell you if she needs you.

- If she is going to be in the house alone for any length of time, make sure that the telephone is within easy reach.

- Write the number of your doctor, district nurse, and local hospital up above the telephone and ensure that anyone who deputises for you if you are absent knows they are there.

See Appendix II on First Aid, for advice on what to do while waiting for the doctor to arrive

If the person you are caring for does have a fall, call the doctor immediately even if she does not seem very damaged. With an elderly person, you cannot be too careful.

8.4(c)   THE CONFUSED ELDERLY PERSON

Many people look after elderly confused relatives in their own home. This role can be both rewarding and demanding. The rewards obviously come from looking after someone you love and have lived and shared your life with for some time. Your relative will probably look well cared for, be dressed in her own clothes and live in her own home. Some people think that this kind of quality care is achieved relatively easily, but anyone who is involved in caring for an elderly confused person is well aware of the tremendous amount of work involved and the stress that can be caused as a result of taking on this caring role.

It is useful to identify the ways in which carers can maximise the patient's independence and assist her to carry out her activities of living, because in this way carers will enable elderly people to do as much as possible for themselves.

Physical causes of confusion

See also section 8.7(g) below on Severe confusion and dementia

The previous section deals largely with the physical care of elderly people and for that reason it is not discussed in any detail here. However, there are some physical causes of confusion which need to be understood. The most frequent causes of confusion in elderly people, are the dementing illnesses or Alzheimer's disease. These illnesses can result in either the loss of brain tissue or, as a result of insufficient blood supply to the brain, a lack of the oxygen so necessary for people to function effectively. Sometimes these problems can be helped by medical intervention, but more frequently they are long term and difficult to reverse. This does not mean, however, that carers cannot enhance the lifestyle of the person for whom they care, and assist to some extent in achieving a reduction in confusion. The following list indicates some of the causes that may be reversible from the carer's perspective:

- Dehydration;

- Malnutrition;

- Short term infection (for example, a cold or influenza);

- Constipation;

- Pain.

Methods of reducing physical causes of confusion

Fluid and roughage intake   There is an interrelationship between dehydration, constipation and some infections, in that if a person has insufficient fluid to drink, this causes confusion and can result in both constipation and problems like urinary tract and chest infections. A regular intake of *at least 2 litres of fluid* a day will ensure that the person has enough fluid passing through his body to reduce the chances of infection and constipation. Most cups contain about 150 mls of fluid and water glasses about 200 mls, while some fluid will be given in the form of soups, as milk on cereal, or as sauces including custard. Therefore most people need between ten and twelve drinks a day, in the form of cups of tea or coffee and glasses of water or squash. There are of course other causes of constipation, including inadequate roughage in the diet, and it is important to see that elderly people do have sufficient vegetables, fruit and bran in their diet.

See also the section on Eliminating in 8.4(b) above

The elderly person should have 10 – 12 drinks a day to avoid becoming dehydrated

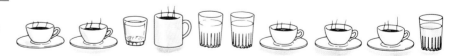

See also Chapter 2, section 3 on Coping with pain

Reducing pain and treating infections   Pain can be missed when people are confused, and it is often assumed as with very young children that they do not feel pain. However, elderly people are of course subject to long term chronic complaints such as arthritis, which can be very painful, or they may simply have a headache or a stomach ache like anybody else. Initially, aspirin or paracetamol are the ideal things to give to elderly people as long as your doctor is happy with such medication and has assured you that this will not interact with anything else that the person is taking.

If it is clear that this kind of pain relief is insufficient to reduce the person's pain completely, then advice should be sought from your general practitioner who may be able to prescribe something stronger.

When people have short term illnesses such as 'flu, this can sometimes cause an increase in confusion which may be difficult to deal with. However, as long as people have sufficient fluid intake, pain relief medication and where appropriate, are given antibiotics, this should pass relatively quickly.

See the section on Eating and drinking in 8.4(b) above

See also Chapter 1, section 1 on Diet

See also section 8.7(b) on Short term memory loss and living in the past, and section 8.7(g) on Severe confusion and dementia

Diet   For a variety of reasons, many elderly people may not eat as wisely as they should. This is often related to income and the effort it takes to prepare an adequate diet. Malnutrition occurs when people have not had enough of the right foods and it can lead to severe confusion, which is why it is important that all elderly people have balanced diets. This does not mean that they have to eat things they do not like, but rather that they should have enough dairy food, meat, plenty of vegetables and enough sugar in the form of cakes and biscuits to give them a balanced and nourishing diet.

Mental deterioration and confusion

Having checked that you have done everything possible to overcome the physical causes of confusion, it is important to turn to the most common causes of confusion which are those of mental deterioration as a result of either Alzheimer's disease or other forms of dementing illness. The term 'dementia' is used to describe progressive loss in mental functions caused by the destruction of brain cells. This results in a gradual decline in the ability to remember, to learn, to think and to reason. This condition is far more common in people over 65, but does sometimes strike people in their forties. Symptoms vary from person to person and initially they can be difficult to distinguish from the ordinary forgetfulness that most of us suffer when we are under stress, anxious or gradually ageing. The most striking problems associated with the confusion caused by mental deterioration are:

- Forgetfulness – short term memory loss;

- Disorientation in time and place;

- Wandering – with the risk of getting lost;

- Difficulty in recognising friends and relatives;

- Mood changes.

These problems naturally cause much anxiety to carers but there are ways of reducing them in the earlier stages of the diseases. They will be discussed one at a time, although inevitably some of the methods for coping with each problem, apply to them all.

Short term memory loss   It can be a source of frustration to carers that an elderly person with confusion can remember very clearly the date that he was married and describe the wedding, or the day his child was born in graphic detail, but is unable to remember whether or not he has had his breakfast. This is not the elderly person's fault but part of the disease. It may be useful to think of it in terms of a field with a gate. Any information that has already gone through the gate and into the field stays there, but nothing new can get through the gate. In this way, the person can remember what is already in the field, in other words what is already in his memory, but can no longer add new information. This accounts for the fact that he can remember the past but not the immediate past. This symptom is not curable, but there are ways of reducing the stress to both the person and the carer. This can be done by accepting initially that it is not the person's fault – he is not forgetting on purpose.

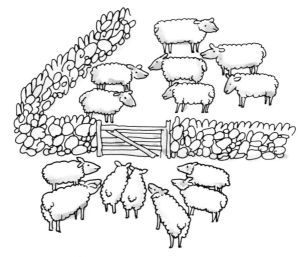

Think of the memory as a field with a gate. Once the gate has been shut no more information can get through

See also Chapter 2, section 6 on Help for the carers

Having accepted this, it may be useful just to remind him gently that, yes he has had his breakfast, for example, without saying 'can't you remember?' If you say 'can't you remember?' to somebody who clearly cannot, he is likely to become increasingly distressed. It can also be quite distressing for the carer, of course, when someone keeps saying every five minutes. 'Have I had my breakfast? When am I going to have my breakfast?' when they actually had it two hours ago. Carers in this stressful situation should feel able to seek out and ask for support.

Similarly, it can be useful to label things so that the elderly person can remember what was what, for example putting a label on the television may help her to remember the name of it, or at least reduce the amount of times that she asks you what that piece of machinery is called. In addition, it is very important to try and leave furniture and other items arranged in the same or a similar way to help her to remember. For example, if you were suddenly to change all the bedcovers, she might start to get into the wrong bed because she cannot remember which one is hers. If, however, you leave an old counterpane on her bed that she remembers very clearly as the counterpane that has been on her bed in the past, this can help her to remember which is her bed.

Disorientation in time and place   You may find that the person for whom you care cannot remember the time of the day, the date, the month or even the year in which he is living. In such case, you may help to orientate him by having a large clock in the room where he sits, so that at least he will be aware of the time. Some people find 'tear-off' calendars where you leave just 'today's' date, useful for the same reason. People who have made regular use of a clock or calendar in the past, certainly do seem to find these objects help to make them aware of the time. It is important to have items that are big enough for the person to see, because a tiny watchface that is difficult to read may not actually help an elderly person with poor eyesight to orientate himself at all.

Suggestions to help orientate a confused person in time and place

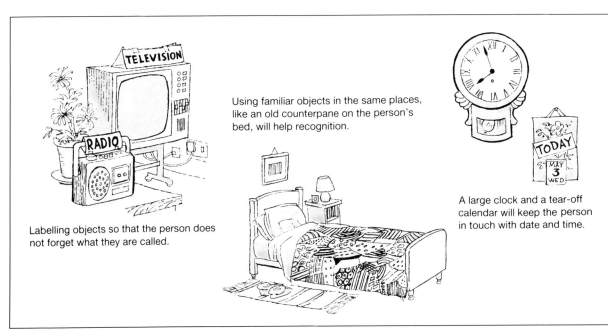

Using familiar objects in the same places, like an old counterpane on the person's bed, will help recognition.

Labelling objects so that the person does not forget what they are called.

A large clock and a tear-off calendar will keep the person in touch with date and time.

Having lights on during the day and off at night may also help, although it may be necessary to keep some lights on at night so that people can see their way around to the toilet for example.

Reading the newspaper with elderly people, and pointing out current events, may help to keep them aware of what is happening in the present.

One way of orientating elderly confused people to the place where they are is to use signs such as 'this is the bedroom', 'this is the bathroom'. However, if they are in their own homes, they often are less confused about exactly where they are. If your relative or friend goes into hospital or local authority care for respite, it may be necessary to take some of her own belongings with her to orientate her towards the area in which she is to sleep. You may find other little tips that help you and the person for whom you care to remember the time and place in which they are, and if so do use them.

Wandering   It can be extremely difficult to stop people wandering if they are so inclined. In some instances, it is necessary to ensure that they cannot get out of the house by locking the door. Although this initially may seem unkind, it is certainly less so than allowing people to wander the streets, not knowing where they are. It is neither useful nor humane, however, to tie elderly people down in a chair or a bed, so that they do not wander. Basic human rights dictate that they should at least be allowed to move within their own room or within their flat or house. This can, of course, cause concern to the carer, particularly if he thinks that the

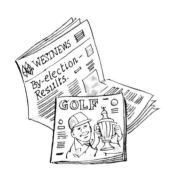

Seeing a daily newspaper is delivered, and making time to look at it with the person, will help to keep him in touch with the outside world.

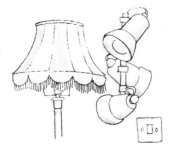

Turning lights off at night and putting them on in the darker hours of daytime will help to give a sense of different periods of time.

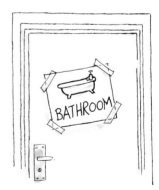

Using signs to label rooms will help the person to know where she is.

person being cared for is a danger to herself in terms of forgetfulness and may leave a gas ring on for example. It is always difficult to weigh up the risks of giving independence to an elderly, confused person against their rights. The only guidance that can be really useful, is to say that the carer should discuss the individual situation with his family and, where appropriate, health professionals such as the district nurse and family doctor.

Where wandering has become a severe problem and the person is clearly a danger to herself, it may be time to seek long term outside help. Many carers are reluctant to have the person who they love and have cared for over a long period, admitted to long term care but, although this should be seen as a last resort, it will sometimes be necessary for the health and safety of the person herself and indeed her carer.

Difficulty in recognising friends and relatives It is always distressing when elderly confused individuals do not recognise their friends or relatives, and there are only a few ways of improving this situation. One may be to start a conversation by reminding the person who you are, by saying 'it is Mary, or Susan or Joseph – your daughter, your wife, your son'. Sometimes, this initial orientation statement does help the elderly person to remember. If it does not, however, you may find it useful to take the person back into the past and say, 'Do you remember when we got married, when I was born, when I went to school?' This helps the elderly person to think back to a time when he can remember you, even though he may remember you, if you are his child, as a child rather than as the 45 year old adult you really are. Where this problem occurs, it is important to remember that it is not through any fault of yours that the person cannot quite remember who you are, or place you, and that the more distressed about it you become, the more it is likely to cause him distress also. Whenever possible, therefore, try to treat this lightly and go on to have as sensible a conversation as you can. You will reduce both your own anxiety and the other person's by not making a big issue out of it.

Mood changes Unfortunately, mood changes do occur with the dementing illnesses. These can range from bursting into tears, or suddenly being physically or verbally aggressive. These mood changes can be distressing to carers, particularly if the person for whom they are caring has never been moody in the past. The best way of dealing with this situation is to try to identify the cause of the sudden mood change. If you can do this, and avoid repetition of the cause in the future, you may well reduce sudden changes of mood. For example, it may be that giving an elderly person rice pudding can result in her suddenly turning and screaming, 'You know I have never liked rice pudding. Why have you given it to me?' It may be that in the past she has really liked rice pudding but has suddenly taken an aversion to it, so to argue and try to get her to eat will only cause further distress. It is better simply to dismiss the matter and ask her what she would like instead. Another situation that can suddenly cause mood change, is violent noise or too much stimulation in a room at any one time. Therefore, do try and reduce loud or sudden noise and conversation going on between several members of the family while the elderly confused person is present.

Independence

At the beginning of this section, it was suggested that wherever possible, carers should maximise the patient's independence. In particular, this involves giving the individual choices about simple things in her everyday life, such as what she would like to eat or what she would like to wear. By encouraging this kind of choice, you will be helping the person to remain as independent as she possibly can for the period that the disabling illness allows. The more that choice is reduced, the more likely it is that the person becomes dependent on you, doing less and less for herself.

The main test that you must always consider when allowing people who are confused to do things for themselves is *'Can they do it safely'?* If the answer is 'Yes', then, even if they are irritatingly slow, do try to allow them to do it for themselves. In this way, you are allowing them the dignity of independence even if it can be a little frustrating for you. If, however, the answer to the question is, 'No, they are not able to carry out the activity of living, whether it be cooking or having a bath, in safety', then it is important that you provide assistance.

Respite care

See also Chapter 2, section 6 on Help for the carers

It is not selfish to ask for assistance, or for your relative or friend to be admitted for short term respite care, if you are getting close to the end of your tether. This is because while caring at home is always difficult, caring for a confused person who sometimes is unable to let you know how much she appreciates your help, can be doubly stressful. Talk to your general practitioner or district nurse if you feel you need respite from caring for a week or two. Your own health, and your relationship with the elderly person, can only benefit from the break.

8.5 DYING AND DEATH

*See also Chapter 2,
section 5(h) The dying,
Chapter 3, section 10
Bereavement and loss
and Chapter 7, section 6
on Counselling skills*

Bereavement, chronic illness and the special needs of people who are dying are considered in some detail elsewhere in this book. Certain aspects of death and dying are particularly likely to be encountered by the very elderly person (for whom, after all, death is a natural 'next step') and her carers. This section looks at such aspects and also covers other, more practical and general information which may not have been covered elsewhere.

8.5(a) THE REALITY OF DEATH

Death comes in many guises. It can be a cruel shock or a blessed release from pain. It can be lingering and distressing, sudden and violent or quiet and peaceful. Surely most of us would wish, for ourselves and for those we care about, a gentle death in familiar surroundings with loved ones in attendance.

Like their younger counterparts, elderly people can die in road traffic accidents, intensive care units or hospital wards. They are more likely than young people, though, to die at home in bed or in their favourite armchair. Certainly frail people living at home or with relatives, needing a high level of physical care and not expected to recover, are more likely to be elderly than from one of the younger age groups. Caring for such a person, and knowing that he will never be fit again, can be distressing and draining for the carer. This will probably be even more true if the person being cared for is much loved. Changes, deterioration and suffering are most difficult to bear when they affect someone who has been very important to us.

In some cases, the person you are caring for may be admitted to hospital, subsequently dying there. This is particularly likely if she:

- Has an accident;

- Develops a sudden illness;

- Has a long standing illness which becomes complicated.

Whether a person dies at home or in hospital cannot always be her decision (or that of her carers). If there is a choice, then planning with health professionals should help to avoid pitfalls and regrets that the step taken may not, after all, have been for the best.

8.5(b) HELPING YOURSELF AS A CARER

Whether the realisation of death comes as a short sharp shock through information received, or as a gradual dawning awareness

See also Chapter 2, section 6 on Help for the carers and Chapter 7, section 5 on Caring for others and its effects on health

that health can only deteriorate, there will be a period of numbness, of denial, before one can begin to accept the reality of the situation. This will be equally true for you as a carer, facing the prospect of bereavement, and for the sick person himself.

Once the numbness starts to wear off, both you and the person you care for will start to feel pain, anger and bitterness. If you are the primary carer, you will probably have to support the sick person through this difficult phase, and quite apart from the distress that his physical and psychological pain will cause, you may find yourself on the receiving end of his rage as he struggles to come to terms with what is happening to him.

It is very important that you do not try to cope alone. Do you have a good friend to whom you can turn who can offer you the support you will need? Such a friend need not necessarily be in a position to do anything, but if she will listen, non-judgmentally, allowing you to mirror your thoughts and clarify your feelings you will probably find that you feel better for talking.

Other resources are available to you too and it is important that you use all the professional help available. Don't be ashamed to ask for information about borrowing mobility aids, incontinence laundry aids or extra financial help such as Night Attendance Allowance. Your general practitioner will contact a social worker for you if you ask her to, and may also refer you to a Macmillan nurse or a bereavement counsellor. You can also consult the district nurse or your local Citizens' Advice Bureau.

• General practitioner	• Bereavement counsellor
• District nurse	• Social worker
• Macmillan nurse	• CAB counsellor
• Marie Curie nurse	

People available to help you

Marie Curie nurses are available in some areas and can provide 'sitters' when you need to go out or take time off, or sometimes during the night.

It is not always easy to assess the length of a person's illness, or the form it will take. You must include yourself in your forward planning and not ask too much of yourself. If you try to do everything yourself, 24 hours a day, you will either:

• Become ill yourself, in which case someone else will have to look after you; or

• 'Burn out' and withdraw, because you cannot cope, causing feelings of guilt in yourself and of rejection in the person for whom you are caring. You will become short tempered and say things you may regret afterwards.

Most patients don't expect too much, but there has to be a contract, even if it is unspoken, an acknowledgement of the expectations of each for the other and the limits to which both can go. Don't try to do what is beyond you.

8.5(c)   PRACTICAL CARE

See also section 8.4(b) above on Physical aspects of care, and Chapter 2 on Caring at home

If the elderly person you are caring for suffers from deteriorating health or a specific illness you will need to follow the advice for practical physical care given in the previous section and in Chapter 2 of this manual. The details of caring for a person who is dying will not be very different from those of caring for someone who is ill but who may recover but they may, sometimes, be perceived rather differently. In particular, if the duration of a person's life is expected to be limited, then the quality of what life remains becomes especially important.

Life is for living

As long as there is breath in the body, there is hope. If someone is told, tentatively, that she has three months to live, then those three months become the most important time of her life. If she goes on to live for a year, every day beyond the three month deadline could be seen as a gift. For as long or as short a time as it lasts, life should be as full as possible and, if it can be so arranged, the sick person should be able to make choices and have her day arranged around her, as she wants it, rather than being pushed into someone else's routine. For example, she may not always want a morning wash. If she has had a bad night and been unable to get to sleep until 5 am, she will probably not appreciate being woken up for a wash two hours later.

Little things can be very important. Find out what really makes your patient's day. If he is very weak, in the terminal stages of illness, these won't be big things. Rather, they may include a hot cup of tea, served in a clean china cup and not slopped in the saucer, a daily newspaper arriving on time or a favourite radio programme. A book rest to help him read more easily and large print books, or cassette tapes, or hearing someone he cares for reading aloud to him, these may all give enormous pleasure. Other people may enjoy the sight and fragrance of cut flowers or a pot plant, may gain great comfort from holding, stroking and talking to a loved family pet or take great pride in looking at photographs of grandchildren or great-grandchildren and hearing about their exploits.

Comfort and dignity

A sick room needs to be clean, tidy and uncluttered, but not clinical. The dying person should have his most precious belongings around

See the section on pressure sores in Chapter 2, section 2(h), on Keeping clean and well groomed

See also Chapter 2, section 4(e) on Turning the patient who cannot move himself

him, within reach. For as long as he is able, he should be up – even if he has to be wheeled into another room to be with the rest of the family. His bed should be clean and his sheets smooth but not too tightly drawn across his feet. Prevention of pressure sores and general physical care have been dealt with earlier in this book but the more the person does for himself the better. It is hard to come to terms with increasing dependence and this should be avoided for as long as possible. On the whole, however, you will find that when a person can no longer help himself, he will accept the necessary help from others rather than just flounder. When he can no longer move himself, he will need to be turned regularly, to avoid soreness and skin damage. Your district nurse should be able to help with this.

A person in the terminal stages of illness who cannot care for himself will need regular attention to his mouth, nose and eyes. He may be able to use a mouthwash but if not you can clean his mouth with swabs of cotton wool dipped in this. Use a different swab for each side, top and bottom and make sure that the patient doesn't 'gag' on it. False teeth must be cleaned daily.

The nose can be cleaned with warm water, and a little vaseline or white petroleum jelly will prevent nostrils becoming cracked and sore. Vaseline or lip salve can be applied to the lips, especially if the sick person can only breathe through his mouth or is being prescribed oxygen (as shown in the illustration below).

A person who is unconscious may have his eyes incompletely closed. If he has no blinking reflex his eyes will become dry and he will be in danger of becoming blind. Make sure that his eyes are

Some patients may be given oxygen at home

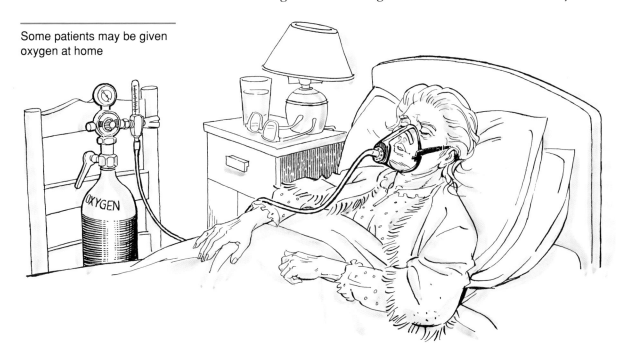

bathed regularly, with cooled boiled water or a prepared saline solution and cotton wool swabs. The district nurse will show you how to insert eyedrops if these are needed. She will also teach you how to manage any tubes (for example, a urinary catheter or a feeding tube).

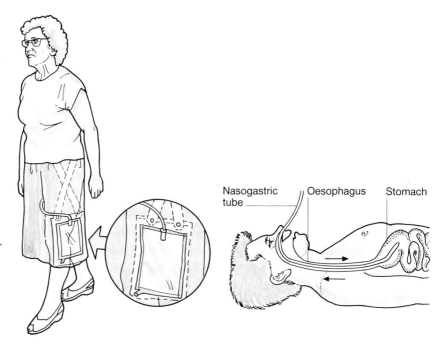

Tubes and related equipment

The person you are caring for may have a tube and catheter bag to collect her urine, or may need to be given nutrients through a naso-gastric feeding tube

Nasogastric tube | Oesophagus | Stomach

All these procedures are artificial and degrading, and it is important to preserve the person's dignity as far as possible. The following suggestions may help.

- Make sure that the sick person has clean and attractive nightwear. Natural fabrics such as cotton are more comfortable, and unsuitable colours, such as orange for a person with jaundice, should be avoided.

- Sick people should not be uncovered unnecessarily when they are washed. Hair should be clean and nicely styled, men should be shaved (unless of course they prefer not to be) and women should be encouraged to apply make up if they so wish.

- Dirty plates and other utensils should never be left by the bedside.

- Plants and cut flowers should be fresh and well watered.

See Chapter 2, section 6 on Help for the carers

If you are feeling tired and under stress yourself, it can be tempting sometimes to cut corners with physical care on the assumption that, if someone is going to die next week anyway it will not matter too much if his mouth is not cleaned. This temptation should be resisted at all costs. Tell your doctor or district nurse that you need more support, co-opt help from friends or relatives, but do try not to let the standard of care the sick person is receiving drop. You will feel guilty and regretful later and his last days may not be as comfortable as they should be.

Pain

See also Chapter 2, section 3 on Coping with pain

No one should have to suffer continual pain. While it is the doctor's right to prescribe pain-relieving drugs, the carer has an important role to play in reporting the effect of medication and seeing that it is taken regularly. If the patient cannot swallow tablets, the drug may have to be given in another form. Tablets should not be crushed without first consulting the doctor as certain ones may irritate the stomach if prepared in this way.

People vary in their reaction to drugs; what helps one may not help another. Certain combinations may cancel each other out and it may take the doctor a little time to get the dose right for a particular patient. You can help by giving the doctor as much information as you can about effects of the medication and by supporting and encouraging the patient.

It is particularly important to remember the following.

- Addiction to a drug should not be a cause for concern when a person is terminally ill and should never be a reason for decreasing pain relief.

- It is a mistaken kindness to omit a dose of pain-relieving medicine because the person is sleeping. She needs regular doses to keep the pain under control and if one is omitted she may wake in pain. Analgesia should be given before pain surfaces; no one should ever have to beg for it.

- Pain is not necessarily caused by the disease. There may be another very simple explanation such as constipation. Don't always look for the worst reason first.

Chronic pain can be helped by a number of measures such as massage, relaxation techniques or the distraction of hobbies, music and company. Drugs are only one line of response in pain relief.

8.5(d) SOCIAL AND EMOTIONAL NEEDS

It is important to help the dying person not to become bored. Ideally, too, he should be able to see as much of his friends and other relatives as he wishes, without getting overtired. There is a fine line to be walked between overloading a sick person and isolating him but, in general, visits from outside the home are nearly always welcome.

They provide topics for conversation and the dying person may be able to say things to an outsider that he feels he cannot say to someone too close for fear of hurting her.

Some people may be embarrassed about visiting a dying person, or afraid that they will not know how to behave. They may need some encouragement, or even more active persuasion, and reassurance that they need only be themselves might be in order.

Occasionally, situations arise where either the dying person or the carer (or even both) tries to believe or act as though the other does not know that the situation is terminal. In most cases, however, such behaviour is unrealistic or even insulting. You don't have to use the word 'death' to each other, you certainly don't have to be brutal, as long as you both accept that you know the important things can be discussed and old misunderstandings set right. Without mutual respect and openness, dying may become a restless and lonely business and bereavement full of regrets.

In old age or at time of crisis many people return again to religious practices which they may have let lapse over the years. For others, of course, religion will always have had a major part to play. Even if carers are not believers themselves they should respect such needs and encourage visits from the appropriate religious leader and members of the local group. Whatever rituals are part of the patient's religion should be administered as and when they are desired. If the sick person has not practised his religion for some years he may fear the reaction of religious leaders and church members but few believers in a loving God will add to his burdens of grief and guilt. He is more likely to find recognition of his fear and anger, with support to help him work through these negative feelings. After all, he too is being bereaved, of life, and unless he can come to terms with this in his own way he may become depressed.

8.5(e)   MIXED FEELINGS

There are times when death is positively longed for, perhaps because the elderly person has suffered so much or is the last of his peer group to be left alive. This is not necessarily sad for relatives. It is sometimes consoling to feel that 'Dad only wanted to be with Mum, and now he has got his wish'.

Some relatives, however, get very upset at hearing an elderly person express his desire to die. This may be due, in part, to a desire not to let the person go, not to accept the fact of the situation. Alternatively it may be that such a wish is seen as a slur on themselves as carers, suggesting that they have not been able to keep their parent or loved one happy at home.

It is extremely unlikely that any expressed desire for death on the part of an elderly person should really indicate dissatisfaction with care received. It is more likely to be indicative of a desire to face up to the fact that goodbyes are imminent and that the person feels physically and spiritually ready to 'move on'. To want to hold on to a well loved parent and to keep him with us is natural, but it also shows a selfishness that is crying out for more time. The old person's attitude in such circumstances is sensible, healthy, and usually the outcome of a fulfilled and satisfied life.

More distressing perhaps are those situations where the relatives, worn out by continual care and the pain of seeing a loved one suffering, recognise in themselves a desire for the old person to die. Such carers may suffer pangs of irrational guilt, not realising that their feelings are perfectly natural. They are not trying to kill their relative nor wishing her life away. Like her they are suffering the limitations and frailties of this human condition. Carers need to acknowledge to themselves just how far they are able to cope and where their boundaries lie. An honest acceptance by each individual of his own limits is the key to inner peace and psychological balance. Such an awareness will make for a more healthy pattern of grieving when the inevitable bereavement comes.

8.5(f) DEATH AND AFTERWARDS

The death itself

People who have been ill for a long time or who are very elderly may die so quietly that you hardly notice that last breath. Others may breathe deeply, or with difficulty. A 'rattle' may be distressing for relatives. It is not causing added suffering however; the secretions which cause it can be alleviated by medication. Facial muscles may twitch and causes grimaces – again, these do not necessarily indicate pain but can be upsetting for those who see them.

Don't be afraid to hold the dying person's hand and to talk to him, even if he cannot reply. Hearing is the last of our senses to go so your voice will comfort and reassure him. Do be careful, too, what you say to others in his presence.

It may be that a doctor or nurse is present if the patient dies at home. If not, get a neighbour to phone your doctor – and stay with you too if you do not want to be alone. It is hard to think coherently when you are numb with shock and grief.

Practicalities

The doctor must come to certify death before the person's body can be removed from the house. You need the doctor's certificate to register the death at your local registry office – get someone to come

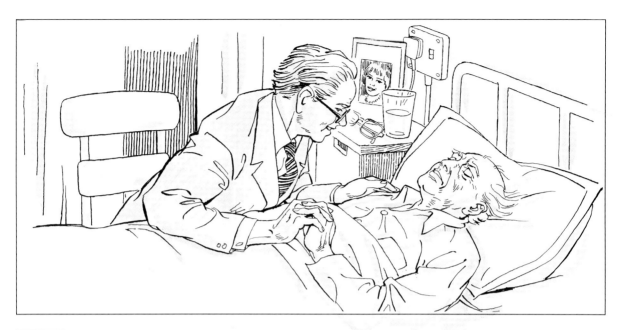

You may be able to give great comfort to a dying person by holding his hand and talking to him – even if he is unable to respond

with you when you go to do this if you can as you may find you need the support. The death is registered in the locality where the person dies, even if this is not her home town.

The funeral cannot take place until after the death has been registered, but this does not mean that you cannot contact the funeral director first. He will be able to take the situation in hand for you and relieve you of much of the mundane work. Your main task will be to grieve and if you have too much to attend to you will not be able to do so. The funeral director will be able to arrange the kind of funeral you want, the service, flowers, newspaper notices, refreshments, thank yous and so forth. It is his job to see that everything runs as smoothly as possible for you. He will also tell you what financial assistance you can claim from the DSS and how you should go about this.

If the death takes place in hospital, you will be informed by the ward staff where to obtain the death certificate and told which part of this certificate the funeral director needs in order to remove the body from the hospital mortuary. You may need copies of the certificate for insurance purposes and these can be obtained for a small fee when you register the death.

After the funeral

You are entitled to compassionate leave from work when a close relative dies. This is usually three days but can be six at the employer's discretion. Bereavement is as bad as an illness. If you are not fit to return to work straight away go to your doctor – you are not malingering. To push your feelings into the background is to hoard up problems for later.

Life will never be quite the same again but you will pick up the threads. Ignore people who tell you, 'It's time you pulled yourself together' after a few weeks. A bereavement of two years or more is considered 'recent' by psychologists.

To an extent, the speed with which you recover will depend on what has gone before. You may have done much of the grieving over months of seeing someone you love suffering. The finality of death may hit you in waves – you may suddenly cry for no reason at all, you may feel unable to function properly, may be forgetful or feel as though life is passing before your eyes in slow motion. All of these responses are normal and will pass eventually. Don't push yourself too hard though, this is a time to be gentle with yourself.

Above all, don't make major decisions – either for yourself or for an elderly relative left alone. It is unwise to make big changes at times of great emotional trauma. It is tempting, for example, when an old lady dies leaving her husband alone, for her daughter living in another part of the country to say, 'Come and live with us Dad, it will be so much better than living alone.' If the widower has spent a great deal of time with his daughter previously this arrangement may work but such a move could prove very unwise. The old gentleman is leaving a place he knows, a place of memories that he can share with friends. He is going to live with a younger family who may all be out for most of the day. It will take time to meet neighbours of his own age group and they won't have known his wife. It would be better by far to wait and see how he manages at his own home alone and let him reach a decision himself over the following months.

8.6 ## COMMON HEALTH PROBLEMS

The mere fact of chronological age is no reason for life to become less dignified or less worth living. In society at large and, it must be said, even within the caring professions, certain conditions, or symptoms such as incontinence, confusion and even depression can wrongly be seen as an inevitable part of the ageing process. Because of this many older people and their carers might be led to the view that their troubles are a normal consequence of old age, and nothing particular can be done about them. These factors can sometimes combine to add feelings of shame and resentment to problems that are already difficult enough. It should always be borne in mind that even if the conditions you, or those you are caring for, suffer from are such that they cannot be cured, there is help available to make them at least a little easier to cope with. Problems of pain can almost always be relieved, problems relating to continence can often be cured or contained, problems relating to mobility can be helped by sometimes simple and sometimes ingenious appliances and changes in furniture.

Inclusion in this chapter does not mean that the problems described are inevitable, nor does exclusion of any problems that you or those you care for may suffer from mean that they are beyond assistance.

8.6(a) PROBLEMS AFFECTING MOVEMENT

So much else about our lives depends on our ability to be able to get around. People living alone will find that they need not actually feel lonely if they are able to go to the shops or visit friends. Other problems can be worsened by immobility, for example physical difficulty with getting to the toilet can lead on to problems relating to incontinence. Being isolated in one room can make one feel totally dependent on others making time pass very slowly and allowing only inward thinking.

Of the problems relating to lack of mobility probably the most common is arthritis. This is potentially a very painful condition which involves the joints. The commonest types are rheumatoid and osteoarthritis, both of which can be extremely distressing to sufferers themselves and to their carers.

Osteoarthritis

See also Chapter 7, section 10(i) on Orthopaedic problems

The development of osteoarthritis is slow and progressive, being due to a degeneration of cartilage between the joints. Most commonly affected are the joints that bear weight, such as the knees, hips and hands. Osteoarthritis is rarely found in the wrists, elbows or feet. It is worth noting that the disease is not likely to spread and that involvement of one side of the body does not necessarily mean that the other side will be affected. At first the affected joint will feel stiff, but tends eventually to become painful especially on movement. Because of this the joint will not be used if it can be avoided which can lead to further stiffening, and the limb around the joint may look twisted.

Treatment of osteoarthritis depends on which part of the body is affected and the extent to which the joint is deformed. In many cases the only drugs that need to be prescribed will be those that provide pain relief and have anti-inflammatory properties. Aspirin is commonly used. Do remember though that all drugs can have side effects so be sure that you ask what they are and take proper advice before setting out on any long term treatment.

Along with pain relief, will go a mixture of rest and mild exercise for the affected part of the body.

The amount of weightbearing on the joint should be reduced. It is an idea for those who are heavier than they should be to try to reduce their weight, so the joints in the lower part of the body do not have quite so much work to do. It is estimated that the use of a simple appliance such as a walking stick can reduce the force of weightbearing by as much as 50 per cent. Any of these appliances should be prescribed for use by a qualified person, such as your doctor or physiotherapist, after he has made an assessment of what is actually required.

A gentle exercise programme will help ensure that the muscles maintain their strength and that joints do not further waste through lack of use. This sort of exercise, along with gentle warming and massage, can often provide relief. Your district nurse or physiotherapist should show you how these methods work before you try them for yourself. This is especially important with heat treatments some of which will only be carried out by the physiotherapist because, if they are used incorrectly, they could be harmful.

If, after a proper assessment, all of the above fails to relieve the symptoms of osteoarthritis of the hips or knees, your doctor might suggest that surgery may be required. This will be for an operation called an *arthroplasty*, or total joint replacement. These operations have a high success rate and patients often describe how they feel they have been given a new lease of life. Of course the doctors will want to be sure that the risks involved in the surgery itself do not place potential patients at greater risk than the condition that they are trying to cure so such procedures will follow a full examination and detailed tests.

The operation itself will entail a stay of two to three weeks in hospital and a lot of physiotherapy to ensure that the new replacement joint is functioning fully.

Total joint replacement

The diagram shows how a 'prosthesis' or artificial joint replaces an arthritic hip

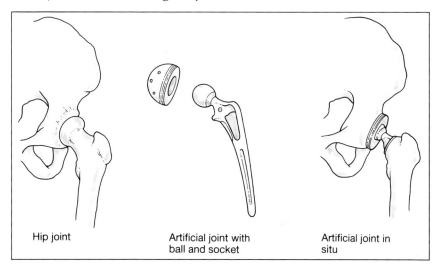

Hip joint   Artificial joint with   Artificial joint in
                   ball and socket   situ

See also Chapter 2, section 2(n) on Improvising equipment

Rheumatoid arthritis

Although the cause is different, rheumatoid arthritis shares many of the characteristics of osteoarthritis. Perhaps the biggest difference is that it tends to affect the smaller joints of the hands, wrist, knee, ankle, elbow and shoulder. These joints also tend to be affected 'symmetrically', i.e. the joints on both sides of the body, both hands, both wrists, etc. will often be affected. Treatment for rheumatoid arthritis, as for osteoarthritis, aims to control pain and reduce the inflammation. Drugs will be given for this and, in addition, there is a carefully worked out routine of rest and support for the affected joints while the muscles are gently exercised. An additional problem however, is that because of the parts of the body that are affected, particularly the fingers, hands and wrists, there may be a need to adapt many basic household objects in order that they can be used. For example, consider how difficult it would be to open a tin, or to hold a knife and fork if your fingers were twisted. Such aids may be available from the community occupational therapist, or can be bought privately, or improvised. Ensure that any appliances are exactly right for you by taking advice.

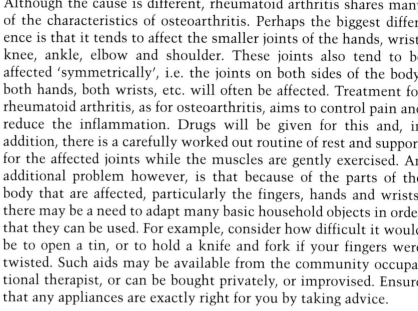

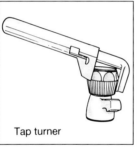
Tap turner

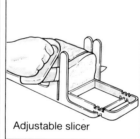
Adjustable slicer

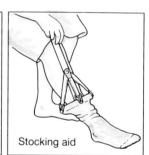
Stocking aid

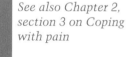
Aids for people with arthritis

Quality of life

See also Chapter 2, section 3 on Coping with pain

Arthritis that is unrecognised and untreated can cause a great deal of pain and distress. It must never be underestimated how unpleasant pain is, and how pain can inhibit actions. Pain control is an important aspect of the treatment of arthritis. Also of importance is the need to adapt to some of the constraints imposed by the condition. An adapted toilet downstairs, chairs which make standing and sitting easier and the use of special knives and forks could make the difference between dependence and independence. As long as the problem is recognised and advice and help is sought it should be possible for life to be a great deal more liveable.

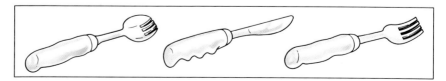

Special thick-handled cutlery will be easier to grip

Fractures

See also Chapter 7, especially sections 8(c) on Women in mid-life, and section 10(i) on Orthopaedic problems

Elderly people are at greater risk than their younger counterparts of breaking their bones, in the event of even a minor fall. This is because the bones become thinner and more brittle with age. The main cause of this thinning of the bone is the condition osteoporosis (which also causes compression of the spinal joints). This condition is particularly likely to affect women after the menopause. More information about osteoporosis is given elsewhere in this book.

8.6(b) URINARY AND BOWEL RELATED PROBLEMS

See also Chapter 2, section 2(d) on Eliminating and vomiting

Problems with elimination among elderly people are usually concerned with infections, continence or changes in bowel habit. Infections may contribute directly to incontinence, and also to the person's general health and well-being.

Urinary tract infection

The urinary tract provides an ideal breeding ground for many different types of micro-organisms. Sometimes the first sign of a urinary tract infection will be that the urine smells different from normal – perhaps stronger, or 'fishy'. The urine may also be dark in colour, cloudy or even bloodstained.

A person suffering from a urinary tract infection may feel pain across the bladder or in the lower or mid back. He may need to pass urine often and this may burn or be painful. He may have a raised temperature and feel generally unwell. The doctor will want a specimen of urine and will probably prescribe a course of antibiotics.

Plenty to drink A common contributing factor to urinary tract infection is that some elderly people may not drink enough, especially if they are concerned about night time bedwetting.

It is vital that the older person drinks about 10–12 cups or glasses of fluid a day, to prevent him becoming dehydrated. As well as increasing the likelihood of urinary tract infection, dehydration can also contribute to confusion and constipation.

Incontinence – a problem to be tackled

Unfortunately, many people (including some professionals) regard difficulties with continence as synonymous with old age. This is a total misconception. Most elderly people have no problems controlling elimination and many of the problems that do occur are temporary and reversible.

Incontinence may be defined as 'the passing of urine or faeces in a socially unacceptable place'. Although a distressing problem, particularly for the sufferer, incontinence should never be regarded as an illness in itself. Rather, it indicates an underlying problem. This is likely to be something relatively minor and easily treated but, on rare occasions, it may be a more serious condition.

An awareness that incontinence is merely a symptom of something else means that the carer, or the sufferer herself, is likely to contact the family doctor sooner rather than later. The importance of taking this step cannot be overstressed. In addition to being able to diagnose and treat underlying infections and other conditions, the doctor may be able to refer the person to a continence adviser. Continence advisers are specially trained nurses who will work with individuals to help them to overcome the problem in what ever way is most appropriate. If your general practitioner cannot put you or your relative in touch with such a person, The Association for Continence Advice will be able to help.

See Appendix VII for Addresses of useful organisations

Incontinence of urine

Incontinence of urine is far more common than incontinence of faeces. Many people (of all ages) find that they have the occasional urinary 'accident'. Stress incontinence is not uncommon among women who have had children, due to weakening of the pelvic floor muscles, while men in middle and later life may experience problems due to enlargement of the prostate gland.

The main causes of urinary incontinence, in order of prevalence, are listed below.

See Chapter 4, section 6(c) and Chapter 2, section 2(d) for more information on pelvic floor exercises

- 'Stress incontinence' is caused by weak muscles in the bladder outlet and pelvic floor. A small amount of urine may leak if the person coughs, sneezes or otherwise exerts herself. Stress incontinence may be treated by pelvic floor exercises. Hormone replacement therapy may be prescribed for some women and, very occasionally, surgery may be needed.

- 'Urge incontinence' describes a sudden, urgent need to pass urine – which may mean that the person doesn't quite make it to the toilet on time. This is caused by an 'overactive' or unstable bladder trying to squeeze out urine before it is really necessary. This condition can be treated by a 'bladder training programme' (which the district nurse or continence adviser will draw up) enabling the person to go to the toilet at gradually longer intervals. Drugs to calm down bladder muscle may sometimes be prescribed to be taken in addition to such a programme.

- In 'obstructed outflow', the bladder outlet is partially obstructed, usually by constipation or an enlarged prostate gland. The urine cannot be passed normally so the bladder overfills and overflows causing 'dribbling incontinence'. Removal of the obstruction should cure the problem.

- An 'underactive bladder' fails to empty completely resulting in overflow. This is often caused by nerve damage resulting from an underlying condition such as diabetes, multiple sclerosis, Parkinson's disease or stroke. The problem may be helped by widening the bladder outlet, or by teaching the person how to empty the bladder using a small plastic tube or catheter.

- Indirect causes include psychological and emotional factors and environmental factors, all of which are considered below. The person's diet and any drugs being taken may also have a bearing on the problem, as may the amount of fluids drunk and any urinary tract infection.

With so many possible causes for urinary incontinence, it is imperative that the reason for the problem is established as soon as possible. Incontinence in older people often has several contributory factors so a careful individual assessment by a professional is crucial. Sufferers should be urged not to delay contacting their general practitioner or the Association for Continence Advice.

Once the cause (or causes) has been established, treatment can begin. With appropriate help, some 50 per cent of sufferers can become completely dry again, while symptoms can be improved for most of the remainder.

Normal life need not grind to a halt even if incontinence persists. There is a wide range of appliances (usually available from your district nurse or general practitioner). These range from special pads and pants which are discreet to wear to protective covering for the mattress. In a few cases, the individual may need to have an indwelling urinary catheter fitted to drain the urine from the bladder directly into a sealed bag. If this happens the person or his carer (or both) will be given detailed instructions on how to care for the catheter and change the bag as well as on how to avoid introducing infection.

Incontinence of faeces

There are a number of possible causes of faecal incontinence, and the major ones are listed below.

See also section 8.4(b) on Physical aspects of care

- Constipation – with impaction of faeces and overflow (which looks like diarrhoea) – is by far the most common cause. This is because, even if the normal stool passage is blocked by hard faeces, liquid faeces can get past the obstruction ('spurious diarrhoea' as described in 8.4(b) above). Impaction can usually be assumed to be the cause for people who have been immobile for any length of time.

See Chapter 2, section 2(d) for pelvic floor exercises

- Muscle ring weakness and weakness of the muscles of the pelvic floor may make control of bowel movements difficult. This may be improved by exercises – talk to your district nurse or continence adviser.

- 'Neurogenic' (nerve damage) causes may include stroke, multiple sclerosis or dementia.

- Severe diarrhoea from any of many causes, with a frequent, urgent need to go to the toilet, may result in distressing 'accidents'. The general practitioner should always be consulted in cases of severe diarrhoea as the cause will need treating. In the meantime, the sufferer should be encouraged to drink plenty of fluid as dehydration is a real possibility.

See also section 8.6(a) above on Problems affecting mobility

- Certain physical conditions (for example arthritis) may be indirect causes of faecal incontinence because of their effects on the person's mobility.

The person's diet and level of hydration will also affect his bowel function, as indeed may some drugs. Certain types of pain killers, antacids and iron supplements may have a constipating effect while some antibiotics may cause diarrhoea. You should talk to your doctor about any side-effects of prescribed or over the counter medicines you or the person for whom you are caring are taking.

Environmental factors and incontinence

See also Chapter 2, section 2(d) on Eliminating, and section 8.4(b) above on Physical aspects of care

Problems with continence may be due solely or partially to the person being unable to get to the toilet on time. Ways of countering this problem are considered in more detail in Chapter 2 of this manual as well as in 8.4(b) above.

Emotional and psychological factors

These can be many and varied. The three major causes tend to be anxiety, depression and confusion.

- **Peristalsis**
  The muscular action of the bowel which moves food and other matter along it

Anxiety   This has the effect of stimulating peristalsis (which may contribute to faecal incontinence), also of stimulating the desire to empty the bladder more frequently.

See also Chapter 7, section 10(b) on Depression and anxiety

Depression   Depressive states can remove the sufferers' willpower, with the effect that they do not bother to go to the toilet before it is too late. The resultant 'accident' may lower self-esteem even further thus compounding the problem.

See also section 8.4(c) on The confused elderly person

Confusion A person who is confused may quite simply forget to visit the toilet at regular intervals, or she may forget where the toilet is. This may mean that the carer has to anticipate her needs and remember for her.

Psychological help If the person you are caring for suffers from any of the above problems, it is very important that you seek professional advice. Your general practitioner will be able to refer you to an appropriate specialist. All three problems may be temporary or treatable and, if they are resolved, the person's normal pattern of eliminating should resume.

Management of incontinence

- The underlying cause of incontinence must be found before any treatment can be started.

- Good skin care is essential after any episode of urinary or faecal incontinence. Both contain substances which can damage the skin if left. Urine in particular contains ammonia which becomes extremely smelly below body temperature.

- Inform your doctor of any episodes of incontinence; there may be a physical cause which will respond to a simple remedy.

- Make a mental note of the times of any episodes of incontinence and watch to see if a pattern emerges. Give the doctor as much information as you can about the person's normal bowel habit as well as any factors that appear to predispose him towards incontinence. These may include, for example, activity, any medication being taken, dietary and fluid intake and previous medical history.

- For faecal incontinence, the doctor may perform a rectal examination and may prescribe a course of tablets, suppositories or enemas.

- If infection is suspected as a contributory factor to urinary incontinence, the doctor may ask the patient to supply a specimen of urine. If infection is found, the problem may be treated with a course of antibiotics.

- The patient's level of activity and usual diet should be looked at carefully as they may need to be modified – especially if constipation is a contributory cause of faecal incontinence.

- Your doctor may refer the patient to a continence adviser, a specially qualified nurse who will give advice and may draw up a bladder or bowel training programme.

- Remember that incontinence is not normal just because somebody has reached a certain age. It can often be treated or controlled, usually relatively easily. It should never be allowed to become a terrible secret that a family keeps to itself, away from the very people who might be able to help.

8.6(c) PROBLEMS WITH HEARING AND SIGHT

See also Chapter 7, section 10(l) on Visual and hearing problems

Our senses of hearing and sight are the two most important ways we have of getting information about the world around us. Unfortunately, as we grow older, there tends to be a diminution of both senses falling short of the extremes of deafness and blindness, but nevertheless adding at least some measure of difficulty to our ability to remain in full, independent contact with all that is going on around us. There are quite severe legal tests to register as either blind or partially sighted, and most older people will not fall into these categories, However, if you feel that sight is a problem, your general practitioner may be able to help.

Hearing problems

Hearing problems are notoriously difficult to detect because of the popular misapprehension equating deafness with mental retardation. People are generally either too shy to admit that they have a problem, or may be working so hard at trying to compensate for the deficiency that they may genuinely not realise that there is one. The easiest method of detection is during conversation. You should be aware that a problem may exist when you are asked repeatedly to speak up, or repeat yourself. Equally, replies such as obviously uncomprehending smiles, inappropriate 'yes' or 'no' answers or obvious attempts at lip reading might indicate hearing difficulties. A sure sign is to say something while standing outside the line of vision. This should not be carried out in an attempt to 'catch' somebody out, but rather in an attempt to prove that perhaps the time has come to seek help.

It is estimated that it is normally the higher range of hearing that is affected in older people, so making it difficult to recognise people by voice alone, or to be able to understand fully what is being said in a large group.

A real problem for people suffering from hearing difficulties is that because their disability cannot be seen, it can be considered to be in some way not real.

Unfortunately, studies suggest that there is an association between deafness in old age and depression. This may be in part due to the person with hearing difficulties feeling that it is too hard to try to maintain contact with the outside world, fear of going out of doors and becoming more dependent on others for information.

Types of hearing loss   Hearing loss can be described as being:

- Conductive or

- Sensorineural.

In conductive hearing loss the problem has been caused by something, perhaps injury or certain diseases, actually preventing sound waves being conducted to the inner ear. A common example of this is a build up of ear wax, which can be easily remedied in your local surgery by a doctor or nurse who will syringe the ear. The build up of ear wax is very common and in no way reflects on the hygiene of the person involved.

It is very dangerous to try to poke about in your ears, or anyone else's, with cotton tips or any other small objects, as there is a risk of perforating the eardrum. A basic rule of thumb is that you should never put anything smaller than your elbow into the ear.

Sensorineural hearing loss is caused by problems within the ear and the hearing centres, so a hearing aid is of only limited use in such cases.

Whichever type of hearing loss is present, the problem should be referred in the first instance to your family doctor.

Resources available Your doctor should be able to arrange a hearing test which will let you know which type of hearing aid is suitable. These range from models available under the NHS to expensive commercial models. Again it is important that the model selected is suitable for the person who will actually be wearing it. Unfortunately what a hearing aid does is to amplify all sound, so people need help with using one. Remember a hearing aid is of no use on the table, nor if its batteries are defective, nor if it is not cleaned regularly.

It might be possible to have some of the many aids and adaptations available fitted at home. These include lights on telephones as well as the traditional bell, and attachments for television sets to ensure that the volume does not upset the neighbours. An organisation such as the Royal National Institute for the Deaf will be able to give more detailed information and advice.

See Appendix VII for Addresses of useful organisations and support groups

Helping the hearing disabled Bear in mind the following points when you are talking to somebody who is suffering from a problem with hearing.

- Ensure that your whole face, and particularly your lips, can be seen.

- Do not shout. This will actually distort your mouth.

- Without laughing at the person, try to have a sense of humour when mistakes are made.

- Encourage the person to ensure that her eye sight is maximised, by the use of glasses if necessary, in order that she can make the most of visual cues.

- Try to be sympathetic. The tone of your voice may be all the person hears and this also can convey very important messages.

Problems with vision

Fading sight can be a problem that affects people of all ages. However, as we get older it can become more pronounced. For the majority of people this may mean only that they need to wear spectacles to be able to read, or it might mean real difficulty in perception of colours or depth of vision which could cause problems, for example, in climbing stairs.

It is estimated that the older person's vision is not acute to changes in light, so it is better to have a generally brightly lit room, rather than the room lit just by one or two lamps. There are obvious implications too for night driving.

The effect this can have on a person's confidence can be shattering. Fortunately, people can become very resourceful in learning where objects are in a room, can switch from small print books to large print or even talking books. However restricted sight can reduce the quality of life.

Two common conditions affecting the ageing eye are cataracts and glaucoma.

Cataracts   A cataract is a clouding in the lens of the eye, caused by a densening in the cells that make up the lens. Surgery is often recommended and recovery of sight can lead to a dramatic improvement in the quality of life.

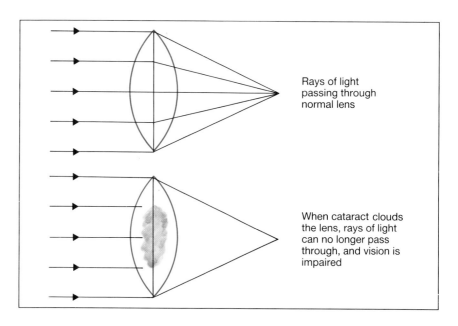

Rays of light passing through normal lens

When cataract clouds the lens, rays of light can no longer pass through, and vision is impaired

What happens if you develop a cataract

See Appendix VII for Addresses of support groups and useful organisations

Glaucoma   This condition is caused by increasing pressure within the eye if fluid is not able to be drained away. Again surgery or medication can often relieve this condition.

The idea of surgery on the eye can be potentially daunting, but these operations are now quite routine and have helped many people to regain the use of one of their most important senses.

A whole range of aids are available for those with impaired sight. Advice should be sought from your doctor, health visitor, optician, or from one of the relevant societies.

Helping the visually disabled Some ways of helping people with visual handicap are given below.

- Try to ensure that the room is well lit, allowing available sight to be maximised.

- Do not walk up on somebody unannounced. Say 'hello' before touching him to let him know you are there.

- Encourage the person to keep in touch by use of resources such as large print books and talking newspapers.

- Don't automatically do everything, but rather help and encourage him to do things for himself wherever possible.

8.6(d) PROBLEMS ASSOCIATED WITH THE FEET AND LEGS

Foot care

As we get older, our circulatory system has to work harder to ensure that we get the oxygen-providing blood supply we need to all parts of the body. Because the body tends to be very efficient, it ensures that those parts of the body that need this supply most in order to maintain vital functions, such as the heart and brain, are well supplied. If the heart has to work too hard, it selects these essential organs as being of top priority while the extremities (e.g. fingers and toes) have to make do with what can be provided.

Because of this, foot care becomes more important as we get older. If it is ignored a cut can lead to an infection or even, in extreme cases, to gangrene. The reduced blood supply means that the antibodies that help to fight infection are not present in sufficient numbers to be effective and the reduced oxygen to these parts means that tissue damage is not repaired as quickly.

What you can do You should inspect your feet regularly, looking for signs of sores, cracks, blisters or infection or irritation. Ingrowing toenails and overlapping toes are a source of irritation and infection.

Feet should be soaked in warm water at least once a week and should be dried thoroughly, including between the toes. Nails should be cut carefully so as to avoid leaving sharp points which can snag or cut.

The choice of footwear is important, socks or stockings should not be tight enough to restrict blood flow. You might find it helpful to have your shoe size checked to ensure a proper fit.

This simple routine should be enough to ensure that you do not have any serious problems with your feet. However, if you have any particular difficulties, or are diabetic, you should seek advice from your doctor, district nurse or chiropodist.

- **Chiropodist**
A health care professional specialising in foot care

Varicose veins

As mentioned above, the circulatory system of an older person might find that it is being expected to work harder than it is able, and blood pressure increases. Congestion may follow. Blood in the veins can pool, putting increasing pressure on the small valves within the veins and causing them to become varicosed. The veins of the legs are the most susceptible to this.

Often the only treatment required is the use of elasticated stockings which will give support to the muscles and aid the return of blood. Leg exercises as described in Chapter 7, section 10, might also help. In severe cases, the veins themselves can be stripped.

Varicose ulcers

These can be caused by the inability of the veins to drain blood due to varicose veins, immobility, or heart conditions such as congestive cardiac failure. The legs become swollen, interfering with the distribution of nutrients to the skin. This can produce a localised skin reaction made worse by scratching or even, in some cases, by ointments put on to reduce the discomfort. Also, importantly, the tissue dies. This sequence of events can cause infection and skin breakdown resulting in an ulcer.

Varicose ulcers are notoriously slow to heal and so it is important that the sufferer complies with the doctor or nurse's advice about taking antibiotics to fight the infection, wearing the stockings to help with the swelling and sitting with the legs raised in order to help with the return of blood from the limbs.

As mentioned above, the risk of infection in the lower limbs is potentially very high and leg ulcers, unless cared for scrupulously, could be both prolonged and dangerous.

See also Chapter 7, section 10(h) for more information about the causes, incidence and treatments of Varicose veins

Key pointers to avoiding foot and leg problems

> - Make sure your feet and legs are clean and dried thoroughly after washing
> - Ensure toenails are kept short and cut without snags
> - Look out for any cuts and abrasions and notify your doctor or district nurse if this happens
> - Don't wear socks, stockings or shoes that interfere with the blood supply to your feet

8.6(e)   DEPRESSION

It is common, especially for younger people, to think of old people as being depressed anyway. The reasoning goes that the old may have lost either a spouse, or near friends. They are not able, physically, to do the things they once did, and they are in many ways close to the end of their life.

See also Chapter 7, section 4 on Mental health and section 10(b) on Depression and anxiety

It is normal for any of us to be sad when we think of loved ones we have lost or of other types of loss we may have sustained, but depression is different to sadness in many ways even though there are some similarities.

Depression can be seen as being both persistent and exaggerated sadness. It can probably be best recognised by those closest to the person involved. It can change a person from somebody able to cope with life into somebody who is constantly in a state of anxiety, unable to cope with any setback, unable to make decisions, unable to take any pleasure from former hobbies, constantly tired but unable to sleep. Such a person may also take to drinking to excess. When the condition gets worse the person may feel unable or unwilling to eat, lose normal self respect if formerly very neat and tidy, and might even think of or plan suicide. Plainly this is a condition far removed from just ordinary, understandable sadness.

Unfortunately, as with several other topics considered in this section, such signs could be put down to 'just normal old age' and so be missed until a real crisis intervention is called for.

What can you do to help?

Detailed advice on helping and supporting a depressed person is given elsewhere but a few key points are given below.

See also Chapter 2, section 5(c) on caring for The emotionally ill, Chapter 7, section 6 on Counselling skills and Chapter 7, section 10(b) on Depression and anxiety

- If you are concerned that the person you are caring for may be depressed, have a word with your doctor or district nurse telling them what worries you about the person's behaviour. Let the doctor know how long it has been going on.

- Try to be supportive.

- If it gets too much, remember that it is an illness and that it can be cured.

- Maintain your friendship with the person you are caring for.

- Look after yourself.

8.6(f) HYPOTHERMIA

Winter months tend to be greeted by children with great expectations. Free from worries about heating and other bills, they can look forward to the darker, colder months bringing with them the excitement of bonfires, ghost stories, snowballs and, best of all, Christmas. It would be wrong to think that these aspects of family life are not enjoyed by very many elderly people, after all they may well be the grandparents who are able to provide the treats and tell the stories so eagerly looked forward to. However, for many elderly people, especially those living on fixed incomes, the colder weather can also bring with it fear of a condition that seems to catch society unprepared each year – hypothermia.

It is a terrible pity that this condition should find itself in a chapter on common health problems, but each winter's grim statistics, coupled with the relative ease with which the condition could be avoided, perhaps make it an important inclusion.

Hypothermia is said to exist when the body temperature falls below 35°C (95°F). This becomes particularly serious if the temperature reduction is prolonged and even more so if the victim is not physically well and nourished.

Although hypothermia is associated in the public imagination with severe, almost arctic, conditions, it should be stressed that the physical and mental condition of the victim are of great relevance. Hypothermia can occur even after exposure to relatively mild cold, especially in the already infirm.

Physical effects of hypothermia

In its normal response to cold, the body responds initially by increases in pulse rate, an increase in the metabolic rate by which it uses up the body's stores of fuel and by shivering. All of this produces extra heat which hopefully should see us through until there is a rise in temperature. However, with prolonged exposure to cold, the internal temperature lowers, resulting in depression of the heat regulating centre in the brain. Eventually there is depression of metabolism, and a slowing of both muscular and mental ability. If left untreated, the victim will eventually fall into a coma before suffering circulatory and respiratory failure.

Symptoms of approaching hypothermia can be detected by simple observation, easily carried out on a visit by either a family member or friend. These include noticing:

- If the temperature in the room feels cold;

- Whether the person's skin appears pale and 'waxy';

- Whether the skin is cold to the touch, even though the person is not shivering;

- Whether speech is slurred and the person appears more drowsy than normal.

Any of these should prompt further investigation. A health check may further reveal signs of slower than normal pulse, and lower than normal blood pressure.

Who is at risk?

As has been stated, given the right set of unfortunate circumstances, anybody of any age could become prone to hypothermia.

Classically, however, victims tend to be older people already suffering from a combination of medical and social problems. Unfortunately in terms of self-diagnosis, because of a generally slower metabolic rate, the older person will often feel reasonably warm even although her body may be cold.

The many elderly people living alone, especially those with chronic ailments that hinder mobility, are considered to be a high risk group, classically the symptoms of hypothermia might not be recognised and it may be many days before anybody realises that the person has not been seen for some time and raises the alarm. Again, the symptoms, especially of slurred speech and drowsiness or lessened mental faculties, might be mistaken by the lay person as being down to 'old age'.

Certain medicines may accelerate the loss of body heat. These include certain antidepressants or even aspirin. Others still may interfere with the ability of blood vessels to constrict or dilate in response to temperature changes. These factors should be taken into account when somebody is taking a great deal of tablets for different conditions and talked over with the doctor.

First aid

Hypothermia is a medical emergency and should be treated as such. Intervention is based around the need to help the victim to regain normal body temperature. The first rule is that under no circumstances must the patient be rewarmed too quickly and that direct heat, for example a hot water bottle, must never be applied. This at first may seem strange, and has often been a temptation to well meaning helpers. This is because there will have been quite severe vasoconstriction by which the body is trying to conserve heat. Any rapid or direct external heat, such as a hot drink, or bringing the electric fire closer, will quickly cause the vessels to dilate with the result that the patient will be in great danger of

- **Vasoconstriction**
  Narrowing of the blood vessels reducing blood flow

Key pointers to preventing hypothermia

- Keep warm. See if you can discuss with your fuel company the most economical way to warm your house
- Try to wear several layers of clothes during the colder months of the year. Extra layers trap warm air
- Wear a hat. Around 60–70 per cent of body heat escapes through the head
- Eat your meals. If you do not eat enough your body cannot build up enough energy to provide you with heat when you need it
- Put a thermometer on the wall so you can check the temperature
- If you live alone, try to ensure that you keep in touch with somebody regularly, at least by telephone
- See if you are entitled to any extra benefits. They are yours by right
- Try to keep an emergency stock of food, just in case you can't get out

being sent into shock. A general rule of thumb is that the temperature should not be allowed to rise by more than 1°C per hour. If possible the victim's pulse rate, respiratory rate and temperature should be checked so the ambulance can be informed.

Ideally the victim should be rewarmed by means of a blanket and other covers. Hands, feet and especially the head should be kept covered, as it has been estimated that most of the body's heat escapes from this route.

Prevention is better than cure

Ideally, hypothermia would never occur. Given adequate diet, a visit from a relative or neighbour and an awareness of the need to keep warm during the colder months, this problem could be largely prevented. It is important that those in the 'at risk' groups realise that they are able to get advice and assistance from health professionals as well as from social service departments. The fuel companies have to a large extent responded well to suggestions on how they can help those on low incomes to pay bills at an affordable rate, and are loathe to use their ultimate weapon of cutting off supplies during the winter months. It is the very avoidability of hypothermia that makes death because of it such a tragedy.

8.7 LESS COMMON HEALTH PROBLEMS

8.7(a) POLYMEDICATION

Older people tend, on the whole, to be of a generation that respects those in authority. The idea of questioning what is said, especially by a doctor, will not come easily. Therefore, if an older person, with a multitude of ailments is seen on different occasions by different general practitioners and hospital doctors and is prescribed something from each of them, it is not surprising that quite a sizable collection of pills and tablets may soon be amassed. This situation is unfortunately not uncommon, and potentially it could lead to several dangerous consequences.

- Each of the medicines that you are given by your doctor will have a number of side-effects. In themselves they may not be particularly dangerous, but in combination with other tablets they could produce unwanted reactions.

- If several different doctors have prescribed tablets, it is possible that they each do not know that the others are involved. While singly they have prescribed the correct safe dose, too many similar tablets could lead to an overdose.

- When faced with a mountain of tablets, it is possible that you will decide not to take them because it seems too much bother, or they are too difficult to swallow. This could lead to essential medications being omitted.

- When you have too many tablets in front of you, they could look confusing and so you may end up taking the wrong tablets, in the wrong quantity, at the wrong time.

Each of these examples is the result of what is known as polymedication (*poly* meaning many).

This is accepted as not being in the best interest of any patient and so many doctors, along with pharmacists, are trying to ensure that such mistakes are not made.

The best way of ensuring that polymedication does not happen is to tell your doctor which medicines you are already on, or better still take them with you. You might well find that this will prompt him into reviewing your need for tablets and you could end up with significantly fewer, but the ones you will be left with will be specific to your needs and much safer.

You should include any medicines that you have bought for yourself from the chemists and any remedies that you may be trying out.

Signs of polymedication

There are a number of signs suggesting that a person is taking too many medicines.

- Confusion can result if somebody is taking too much medicine, as the chemical balance in the body is disturbed.

- Several different medicine and tablet containers – it might be the case that you have many pills to take; this should be safe so long as your doctor knows and has agreed that you need them all.

- Different pills in the same container – each set of tablets should be in its own container. If you mix them up, you run the risk of taking the wrong ones at the wrong time.

- Nausea, giddiness, headaches, blurred vision and abdominal pains are some of the most common drug side effects. You should see your doctor if you experience any of these.

If you are unsure about the medicines that you are taking, or feel that one or more are making you feel worse, get advice from your doctor or your pharmacist. You should only ever take medicines as you have been advised to by somebody properly qualified. Do not, for example, think that because one pill works well two will work better. Under no circumstances should you ever take any tablets that are not meant specifically for you. Do not for example, take a heart pill from somebody else, even if it seemed to do him the world of good.

Another problem involving medicines concerns diuretics, the so called 'water pills'. Every now and again magazines make use of the fact that our bodies are composed of a very high percentage of water. It is not uncommon for slimmers to take diuretics in the hope that this will help them shed weight quicker. THIS IS DANGEROUS AND COULD KILL.

Return any medication that you are no longer using to the pharmacist for disposal. All medicine has an expiry date and it could actually do a lot more harm than good to take medicines that are past this date.

8.7(b) SHORT TERM MEMORY LOSS AND LIVING IN THE PAST

Memory and forgetting

There are many theories about memory and forgetting. Many experts believe that the memory is divided into two sections, long term memory and short term memory. It is thought that the short term memory can only hold so many 'items' at any one time, but while they are there they are available for recall at any time.

Into the long term memory go those items from the short term, for storage until some event sparks off our need to recall them.

It is thought that in the long term memory are our recollections of everything that ever happened to us, down to the smallest detail and that we never really ever forget anything, a bit like the elephant. The trouble is that because we tend to have too much going on, having to live life at the time, we are unable always to find where abouts in the long term memory we have stored items and so cannot bring information back to short term memory where we could use it.

It is thought that as we get older, we tend to use our short term memory less and begin to 'sort through' the items that we hold in the long term. This, in essence, is the basis of several theories concerning what it actually means to grow older.

It was noticed by American researchers in the 1960s that older people tended to withdraw from their roles in society as they got older. They worried less about ambition and became more content with things in the home. They stopped being members of clubs and associations that would be good for their careers and instead tended to pursue activities that gave them more personal pleasure. From this work was drawn the theory of 'Disengagement' which held a great deal of sway over the way policy makers and professionals made their decisions.

Another American, Robert Butler, saw these events in a slightly different way, which he used as the basis for a body of work called 'Life Review'. Butler argued that in old age we need to take some time to take stock of our life and the things we have achieved, they need to be evaluated and it is this process that makes it possible to gain satisfaction or even to make amends for our past wrongs. This is obviously a huge task, to review one's whole life. So possibly this is a reason as to why, as we get older less of our short term memory is available to us.

We still, however, have to live in the present. To help us do this, it is generally found that the best memory aids are those that we have always used – such as the diary which was such an invaluable tool in the days before retirement.

Habit, or usual routine, remains a good way of remembering just where you put things. If you always keep the keys in a certain place you will always know to look there, and even if the worst happens you will at least know that they are missing. Similarly, there is nothing wrong in writing yourself a note to remind you of things that you must do, or people who have arranged to call, and placing this in a prominent place in the house, say next to the clock.

Declining memory can be a worrying aspect of growing older, it should not be confused with mental illness or dementia. Although these conditions may include short term memory loss they are at a very different end of the spectrum from that normally associated with ageing.

Living in the past

This is an accusation thrown at older people, usually by those young enough to know no better. In fact to an extent we all live in the past, or rather the past is a place we go to when we want to compare how things are now to how things were then. This is an activity that is by no means exclusively confined to older people.

Many writers point out that reminiscence is a universal experience. It is something that we all do at various times and is not necessarily entered into consciously. Rather, it can be brought about by a whole range of stimuli including smells, tastes, moods and music which in turn can trigger daydreams and reveries. Indeed it can be one of life's great pleasures, a reason for us to attempt to keep in touch with people and to go to extreme lengths to get in contact with family and friends at special times like birthdays, weddings, Christmas and other anniversaries. Equally there will be few of us who have not, on occasion, dwelt on the way things were.

If we take the point made by Robert Butler, that as we get older we need to review our life, it can be seen why so much thought and time is spent on the past. However, like all interests it can become a problem. If the living in the past entails the person thinking she is talking to people who are long dead, or trying to buy goods with old money, the help of a psychiatrist might be called for. Except in such extreme cases, the person's interest in the past should be respected. However, as with anybody who becomes obsessed with just one topic of conversation, it might need to be pointed out tactfully that she is in danger of becoming boring.

If the reason why an older person is dwelling on the past is that there is nothing significant or interesting happening for her at present or in the future, then it could be that she might be helped or encouraged to use her memories to shine some light on the present. Older people are witnesses to some of the most major changes that have happened in this century. They might be persuaded to help local historians or schools to make a record of the changes that have occurred locally.

8.7(c) DIABETES IN THE ELDERLY

Diabetes is a condition that affects people of all ages. Unfortunately, the incidence of non-insulin dependent diabetes increases with age. The main causes are thought to be heredity, obesity, stress and certain drugs, but there is no certain answer.

See also Chapter 7, section 10(c) for more information about Diabetes

As we get older there appears to be less likelihood of diabetes being caused by heredity alone.

The effects of diabetes

The condition prevents the body from using glucose, which it needs in order to obtain energy. The first sign that an older person has diabetes may be seen as the result of a routine urine examination either in hospital or at a visit to the doctor for some unrelated problem. The signs of diabetes which may alert the doctor are complaints of weight loss, thirst, passing a lot of urine, or itching as a result of the presence of sugar in the urine. If mature onset diabetes is diagnosed, there will be a full medical examination to assess whether the condition has caused any complications – these can range from ulcerations on the legs and feet to eye problems.

Treatment

Diabetes in older people is treated by reducing blood sugar levels and ensuring that complications do not arise. Few older people who develop diabetes in later life need injections of insulin; the vast majority can be controlled through adjustments to the diet and by tablets. Skilled dietary advice is needed, and this can be obtained through your health visitor or community dietitian.

Many hospitals and health centres have a diabetic clinic where urine and blood sugar levels can be monitored on a regular basis. You will be shown how to do this yourself and also how to calculate which foods have which values in order to ensure that you can prepare your own diet.

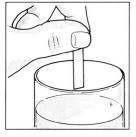
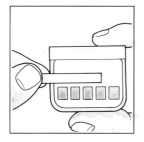
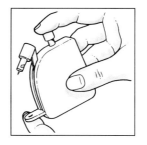
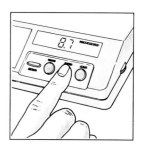

Testing urine for glucose levels

Testing blood for glucose levels

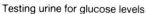

You will probably be taught how to test your own urine and blood for glucose levels

Unfortunately, diabetes is not curable at present and you need to take care of yourself to ensure that it does not get out of control. One aspect of this is that you should be extra vigilant about any cuts, especially on the feet and legs, and should let your doctor know quickly about any infections you may pick up.

It is a good idea to carry a card identifying that you have diabetes in case of any accidents, in order that you can get the right sort of help if required.

So long as people with diabetes stick to the diet as they are advised, take the proper medication and enjoy the right balance of rest and exercise, there is no reason why this condition should get out of control.

Hypoglycaemia

Hypoglycaemia means low blood sugar which, if untreated, could be very dangerous. The causes are either too much insulin, too much oral antidiabetic medication, too little food or too much exercise. Signs are:

- Loss of temper;
- Hunger;
- Impairment, or even loss, of consciousness;
- Sweating;
- Rapid pulse.

Treatment is needed urgently and will consist of oral glucose (if the person is conscious and able to swallow) or injection. It is a good idea to carry glucose with you; ask at the clinic which preparations are the most convenient.

8.7(d)   HEART AND CIRCULATION PROBLEMS

See also Chapter 7, section 10(f) on Coronary heart disease and Appendix I, section viii on Blood and the circulatory system

The body depends on its blood supply for many reasons. Blood carries oxygen to all parts in order that each organ can carry out its work. It also transports white cells to sites of cuts or other breaches of the body's integrity in order that they can start to resist any resulting infection. Blood carries nutrients to all cells to enable them to function and carries away waste products so that they can be expelled and so not build up and become toxic.

In order to circulate around the body the blood needs to be pumped by the heart. The blood is carried away from the heart, while rich in oxygen, to all parts of the body by arteries and back from the body towards the lungs and heart by the veins.

There is some debate as to whether or not any actual age-related changes occur normally in the heart as the body grows older. Certainly it would seem that heart and circulatory problems increase as people get older, but this may be only because of other factors such as stress, the effects of prolonged smoking, drugs, lack of exercise and other factors including diet. It is worth noting that not all cardiac problems are fatal, but they have the capacity to be if not treated properly. Anybody with a heart-related problem is potentially very ill and will need to take life a lot more easily than before. If you are caring for a person with a heart problem, you should be aware of the indications of pain, understand that because the heart is not working properly, the patient is likely to be tired or lethargic, and also that he is likely to be quite frightened.

Congestive cardiac failure (CCF)

Congestive cardiac failure is one of the more common heart conditions that older people suffer from. It occurs when the efficiency of the heart is compromised, because of a failure of the heart to work effectively as a pump thus causing congestion in the circulatory system. There could be many reasons for this, including:

- Other heart related problems;

- Chronic lung problems;

- A blockage in the circulatory system.

The typical signs of this are sudden breathlessness, often on exertion, coughing up clear frothy sputum, weight gain and difficulty in breathing while lying down (commonly in bed at night) which may cause insomnia. The lower parts of the body, especially the legs, may look swollen due to fluid being unable to return to the circulation and be redistributed.

Treatment consists of trying to determine and correcting the underlying problem that has caused the CCF. The symptoms will be treated as they present, so for the breathlessness the patient will be advised to sleep upright, perhaps in a chair rather than in bed, as this will relieve some of the congestion on the lungs. Activity levels will have to be assessed as this will need to be kept down to the level that does not cause breathlessness.

The fluid retention will be cured by diuretic medicines – 'water tablets' – which will cause the patient to pass a great deal of urine. If such medicines are prescribed, access to the toilet should be made as easy as possible.

The heart itself may be encouraged to work more slowly, but harder by the use of a tablet known as digoxin. There is a danger that this drug can build up in the bloodstream as it is not always passed out in the urine. In order to check for this you might be asked to have blood taken at intervals. However a rule of thumb is to check your pulse before you are due to take the tablet. If the pulse is below sixty beats per minute do not take it but instead tell the doctor immediately.

Once the cardiac failure has been controlled, a gradual programme of rehabilitation can be introduced. This will entail careful monitoring of fluid in and out, advice over the use of salt in the diet and gentle exercise. The question of salt in the diet is one that needs to be discussed with your doctor because salt retains water in the body, which we want to get rid of, but it is possible that the diuretic tablets may contain salt. This is soon clarified when your tablets are decided upon. You may be aware of feeling extra tired or breathless and should let your doctor know if this happens.

Angina

Angina is chest pain caused by a temporary insufficient supply of blood to the muscles of the heart itself. It most often happens under times of stress or on exertion. The sensation is described as being like a gripping pain with crushing or as a heavy feeling under the chest bone. The pain can travel down the left arm or to the neck, throat or jaw.

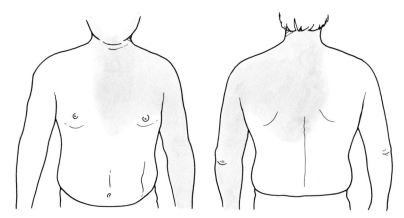

Possible sites for angina pain

Treatment is by a type of medication called glyceryl trinitrate, designed to allow blood quickly to the heart muscle. This is given either as tablets which, instead of being swallowed, are placed under the tongue or in the form of a patch, rather like a sticking plaster, which is placed on the chest.

You may need to review your lifestyle following a diagnosis of angina. This would include giving up smoking, and avoiding those activities which bring about an attack.

Arteriosclerosis and atherosclerosis

Arteriosclerosis is more commonly known as 'hardening of the arteries'. Usually affected will be the larger and medium sized arteries supplying, in particular, the heart or the brain.

In atherosclerosis there is also the build-up of lesions known as plaques which consists of fatty deposits within the lining of the artery. As they collect more fatty deposit they can reduce the size of the space available for blood to pass through. The main causes of atherosclerosis are:

* High blood pressure;

* Smoking;

* High levels of blood fat.

Hypertension (high blood pressure)

This is the most common circulatory condition in older people, and is a common cause of heart failure and stroke. If the high pressure is sustained over a long period of time it can make the heart work harder with the potential of it failing, or can seriously damage the effectiveness of the kidneys, brain and eyes.

Hypertension is referred to as being either *primary* or *secondary*.

Primary hypertension is also known as idiopathic or, more commonly, essential hypertension.

Secondary hypertension is so called because there is a reason for its occurrence. This can be:

* Heart problems;

* Problems in the central nervous system;

* Endocrine disturbance;

* Problems in the kidney;

* Other causes which make the heart work harder than it is able, including smoking and obesity.

Treatment This is based on treating the underlying problem. The aim of treatment obviously is to reduce the blood pressure in order

See also Chapter 7, section 10(e) for more information on Blood pressure problems

to prevent serious problems and to have the person adjust her lifestyle in order to reduce the demands placed on the heart and circulatory system.

The treatment will depend on the height and consistency of the blood pressure and evidence of any existing damage. For those with mild hypertension all that is required may be advice on the need to reduce weight, avoid over excitement and cut down the intake of salt. Those who have higher hypertension may have to take medication to lower the blood pressure and the restrictions on work and diet may be more severe.

Your doctor will want to monitor your blood pressure at regular intervals to ensure that whichever course of treatment you are following is succeeding.

Anaemia

Anaemia means literally 'without blood'. The condition itself is not quite as dramatic as it sounds, but is still potentially serious as it implies a reduction in the blood's oxygen carrying capacity.

The most common forms of anaemia are:

• Iron deficiency anaemia;

• Vitamin B_{12} or pernicious anaemia;

Iron deficiency anaemia The most common cause of this is persistent mild blood loss, perhaps from an ulcer. Also, older people tend not to include as much iron in their diets to prevent the deficiency occurring.

The patient will complain of increasing fatigue, especially after effort and at the end of the day. Skin will look pale and the patient might complain of feeling cold. The pulse will rise as the heart tries to maintain the supply of blood around the body.

Treatment is with iron supplements, either as tablets or by injection. In severe cases, blood transfusion will be necessary. Obviously any bleeding will have to be stopped, and this may necessitate admission into hospital.

Vitamin B_{12} or pernicious anaemia In this condition there is a lack of a substance in the stomach known as intrinsic factor. This prevents the absorption of vitamin B_{12}. It can result in damage to the nervous system (known as subacute combined degeneration of the spine) which usually shows itself some time after the condition has actually set in, once the liver has depleted its stocks of vitamin B_{12}. The patient's skin will look pale with a tint of yellow; the tongue in particular will be sore.

Because vitamin B_{12} is needed for the nervous system, nerve endings might become affected. This results commonly in the hands and feet losing their full sensation, often described as feeling as though one is wearing gloves and stockings.

Treatment consists of blood transfusion, injections of vitamin B_{12} and iron tablets.

8.7(e) CHEST PROBLEMS

Respiratory conditions, that is problems relating to breathing in one way and another, tend to be far more common in older people than younger people. In most recognised respiratory conditions, this is a result of prolonged exposure to irritants ranging from pollutants in the environment (such as chemicals or dust resulting from work place activity prior to clean air legislation) to possibly the most common cause of illness in adults, smoking.

See also Chapter 7, section 10(g) on Chest diseases

It is difficult for a non-smoker to understand either the addictive nature of tobacco or the difficulty in overcoming what appears to be a habit that costs a great deal of money, is so unpleasant to others and leaves those in its grasp so open to infections and is potentially lethal.

However, in the generation of older people who are now suffering the consequences of their habit, smoking was seen as

Some suggestions for controlling chest disorders

- The main cause of all breathing related illness is smoking

- It is important to ensure that the person suffering with these conditions drinks plenty of fluid; this can mean between 3–4 pints of fluid (10–12 cups or glasses) every day

- The person suffering from these conditions is likely to feel very frightened; it is important that you should remain calm and know the best ways to help

- If the condition causes sputum to be produced this should be treated as if it were infected, handle paper tissues carefully and ask about disposal in your area

- Be sure about the correct use of oxygen equipment

- Keep items that the patient may need within easy reach

- Remember that the breathing will be helped if the person can remain upright; prop him up with plenty of cushions or pillows. He will feel more comfortable like this anyway

- Ask about help which might allow you to get some time to yourself

- Encourage children and others not to smoke

- Try to give up yourself if you have not done so already

being not only a smart thing to do but even as some form of badge representing their admittance into adulthood.

It is without doubt that for many smokers in the early, or acute phases of respiratory illness, stopping smoking will be of benefit. But for those whose conditions are very far advanced, for example those with very long standing chronic bronchitis, a strict regime of smoking cessation might produce few benefits and actually make what quality of life is left feel like misery imposed by the very person who is trying to help most. Therefore, it might be advisable to try to get the smoker, rather than feel like a martyr, to agree only to smoke within agreed limits and in agreed conditions.

In some cases difficulty in breathing may require some form of home use of oxygen breathed in through a mask. This would be a prime time to impose an absolute smoking ban as the potential risk of explosion is great.

Three respiratory conditions, perhaps more commonly associated with older people than with any other age group, are:

- Pneumonia;

- Chronic bronchitis;

- Pulmonary tuberculosis (TB).

Pneumonia

The common symptoms of pneumonia in an older person are those for many other infections, namely a high temperature, an increase in heart rate which can be measured by taking the pulse, general feelings of being unwell, and loss of appetite for both food and drink. As well as these the person affected will have a cough and almost certainly produce sputum after coughing. This will look infected to even the most untrained eye, being green or yellow in colour, and there may also appear to be traces of blood. On investigation by the doctor, an x-ray will be requested and a course of antibiotics prescribed. All being well, the condition can respond within a few days. It is important, however, that the course of antibiotics is completed even after the symptoms have gone.

During the time that the condition is being treated, it is vital that the person affected drinks plenty of fluids, in order to replace fluids lost, the amount most commonly quoted is 1500 ml, which roughly amounts to around three pints of fluid per day. It is also important that the patient should remain as well nourished as possible, within what appetite she has, and that further complications are prevented. These can include ensuring that seats or the bed are as comfortable as possible and that the parts of the body that touch the seat or bed are moved in order to prevent pressure sores developing.

See also section 8.4(b) above on Physical aspects of care

Chronic bronchitis

This is the respiratory disease that seems to affect smokers most. It is thought that the reason for the condition being more common in men than in women is reflected by the prevalence in the past of male over female smokers but it is possibly due also to the conditions in places of work more traditionally associated with male rather than female employment.

The features of chronic bronchitis are coughing and subsequent production of sputum all through the year. This becomes worse at certain periods, commonly the winter months.

The affected person may suffer from bouts of pneumonia but generally the sputum that is produced is thick in appearance rather than being infected.

Apart from treating any infection with courses of antibiotics generally little else can be done to stave off the recurrence of this condition. There are medications, known as bronchodilators, which will help with breathing by widening for a period the tubes through which air goes in and out of the lungs.

If oxygen therapy is prescribed for home use, the danger of explosion as indicated above must be considered. As well as this, it must be remembered that the concentration of oxygen to be taken must be that ordered by the doctor and delivered through the correct mask due to the risk of giving too much and driving out the levels of carbon dioxide which stimulates the body to go through the physical task of breathing. For this reason, it is advisable that explanation is obtained from either your doctor or district nurse.

A common result of respiratory conditions of the severity of chronic bronchitis is the distress caused to the person affected of feeling unable to get enough air to breathe. There are various methods available to assist, including keeping a window open if

The importance of giving the correct concentration of oxygen to a patient requiring oxygen therapy (O_2 = oxygen; CO_2 = carbon dioxide)

In the healthy person	⇨	CO_2 and O_2 exchanged in respiration
In the person with chronic bronchitis	⇨	Respiration inadequate: CO_2 retained in the body
Chronic bronchitis with controlled oxygen therapy	⇨	Enables efficient exchange of CO_2 and O_2
Chronic bronchitis treated with too high a concentration of O_2	⇨	Suppresses O_2 intake, ultimately leading to CO_2 poisoning

feasible, and putting a table in front of the patient's chair or bed so he can stretch out over it in order to maximise his lung capacity.

If the condition has developed to such an extent, the patient may well act as if he is unable to think of, or concentrate upon, anything else. This is understandable, but can lead to him becoming a 'respiratory cripple'. This can place a great deal of strain upon carers as it is difficult to leave such an individual alone without provoking great anxiety, which in turn can lead to an outbreak of respiratory distress.

Advice from the district nurse will go some way towards helping by ensuring that objects needed can be placed within easy reach, that a plentiful supply of tissues and sputum cartons is at hand and that both the carer and patient are aware of the correct use of any medication. It might be the case that the chronic bronchitic at home is able to obtain some help from the local council or other agency in order to adapt the home circumstances to be more suited to his restricted lifestyle.

See Appendix VII for Addresses of useful organisations

Pulmonary tuberculosis (TB)

This once very common condition is now most commonly associated with older adults. Many of those who suffer from it will have actually contracted it at some time in the past, but the disease will have lain dormant for many years until a change in the body's resistance precipitates the onset.

The symptoms are similar to those of chronic bronchitis, the difference being shown after x-ray examination and a microscopic investigation of the sputum. The condition itself is contagious and unfortunately can come to light after other people have been infected – which bears out the importance of chest x-ray investigations of older people suffering with persistent coughs.

There is a well established routine of drug therapy for those suffering from TB which consists of doses of medication being given for up to a year. Most patients will recover although in some cases the infections can be overwhelming. Those who have been in contact with the sufferer should be traced in order that they can be screened for the disease.

8.7(f)   CANCER

Although 'cancer' is a word which is synonymous in the imagination of many people with death, it becomes less common as a cause in older people, especially those who reach the age of around 80. This is due in part to the fact that as we get older, the rate at which the cells in our body divide becomes ever slower and

See also Chapter 7, section 11 on The adult with cancer

so the chances of a malignant condition advancing to fatal proportions are reduced as the time taken for these malignant changes to take effect are considerably slower.

A more detailed description of the treatments for cancer is given elsewhere in this book. In older people, however, especially those whose condition is advanced, radical surgery and intensive chemotherapy may well be more upsetting and demand too high a price in terms of life expectation and the quality of that life to be of great value. This does not for one moment mean that such treatment is never of benefit, but that the price demanded in terms of side-effects and their own related dangers to life need to be carefully discussed and evaluated between the older person and his advisers both family and medical.

Only if the condition is producing pain, or is likely to result in pain are treatments such as radiotherapy of value to control the growth of malignancy in those whose health is otherwise unlikely to be restored. Equally, depending on where the tumour is located, it might be more realistic to take alternative action in order to allow the quality of life to remain as high as possible.

In considering the alternatives to radical treatment, it is important to understand that there should be no reason for the person suffering with cancer to fall into a position where she is in pain as a result of the condition. Most hospitals now have a pain control team, often led by a specialist nurse, which can advise doctors (including general practitioners) about the various types of medication and other treatments available. The work of the Macmillan nurses is well known as is that of other charitable foundations specialising in terminal care and support.

See Appendix VII for Addresses of useful organisations

If, following discussion, it is felt that on balance radical treatment is inappropriate, the way is open for planning the control of symptoms that are likely to emerge as a result of the main condition. The prime concern is to ensure that life is as comfortable and, within the limits imposed by the condition, as normal as possible. Depending on the site of the main tumour or any subsequent spread certain difficulties may present. These can include the following.

- Difficulties in swallowing – which are commonly associated with tumours in or around the upper digestive tract. Softer foods such as stews or casseroles may be more palatable, or meals can be liquidised. There are now several brands of commercially available meals in liquidised form.

- It is important that nausea, should it occur, is treated – with medication if required. Nausea can lead to the patient feeling weak and unable to maintain sufficient nutrients to perform many tasks.

- Jaundice is a side-effect of tumours in or around the pancreas and liver. The skin may take on a yellowish tinge as a result of the bile salts being released. These can result in the skin becoming itchy. Bathing, either in the bath or by means of a form of blanket bath, followed by soothing lotion will make your patient feel fresher and less itchy.

- Urinary and faecal dysfunction may occur as a result of localised tumours. Specialist advice is essential. The symptoms may be controlled by the use of medication, catheterisation, pads or even the formation of a stoma to by-pass the problem.

- Mental confusion and mood changes may occur. Advice should be sought from your general practitioner or district nurse. Admission to hospital or a nursing home might be advisable.

- Pain – this is possibly the biggest single fear that comes with the pronouncement of the diagnosis of cancer. Pain relief and control techniques are now well advanced and with the help of the general practitioner, district nurse or specialist team, there should be no reason for pain to become unbearable.

8.7(g) SEVERE CONFUSION AND DEMENTIA

There is a fear that dementia is the natural state to which all older people return. Many people who know no better talk about second childhood as if there is no escape from this harrowing condition.

See also section 8.4(c) above on The confused elderly person

Statistically the chances of dementia grow as we age, reaching its highest percentage at and over the age of 80, when 20 per cent of individuals suffer from some form of dementia. Looking at it more optimistically that means that 80 per cent of all people of that age and over will *never* suffer from the syndrome in any way.

The word 'senile' in relation to dementia is actually of little use. The word itself merely means 'old', but is often used as if to describe more fully what is actually going on. This confusion is rife – even among the ranks of some professionals who may themselves be susceptible to the common illusion that older people will inevitably be prone to a decline in mental function.

In fact a great many causes might be responsible for the mental confusion that is often presented as dementia and it is a tragedy if all of these causes are not first ruled out before the diagnosis of dementia is arrived at – if for no other reason than the despair that meets the pronouncement of dementia, an irreversible condition that cannot be cured. Once the diagnosis is reached, therefore, treatment (in terms of medically attempting to reverse the condition) is almost inevitably withdrawn.

Common disorders that can produce confusion which may be mistaken for dementia include the following:

- Constipation – it is relatively common for the relief of constipation to produce a sudden reversal of confused behaviour.

- Polymedication – the effects of a huge array of drugs prescribed for many different ailments can mix together to cause confusion. Once the problem of over-prescribing has been dealt with, the body has a chance to rid itself of the build up of poisons.

- Infections – particularly urinary tract infections – can produce toxins that affect one's mental state. Judicious use of antibiotics can clear up more than the infection alone.

- Migraine.

- Tinnitus.

- Deafness and the sense of social withdrawal that comes with being unable to participate in one's surroundings, can lead to inappropriate behaviour. Correct use of hearing aids might solve the problem.

As can be seen from the above list, which is by no means exhaustive, confusion can be the result of such a large range of factors that it simply is not good enough to arrive at a conclusion of dementia without excluding all other possible factors.

If after excluding all of the other possibilities the diagnosis is dementia, how can one then go about organising one's life in order to 'stand by' the dementing loved one?

See section 8.4(c) above for more detailed advice on The confused elderly person

It is important to realise that not everybody will be able to cope with all of the demands that a dementing person has the potential to make. You should feel able to discuss the possibility of looking for hospital or nursing home support, even if only on a short term or respite basis, in order that your own mental and physical health is not compromised.

If after weighing up all of the alternatives, care outside the home environment is decided on, this in no way should reflect on the relationship between the people involved, nor should the remaining partner feel guilt about the decision. However, this is easier said than done and such decisions are obviously so personal that they can only be taken by the people involved directly.

APPENDICES

PART
III

APPENDICES

HOW THE BODY WORKS

I.i INTRODUCTION

The human body is a highly complex network of different systems – like a computer – interacting to maintain equilibrium in the body (the process of homeostasis). The smallest organised unit of the body is the cell, which uses nutrients and oxygen to produce energy. This in turn is used by the cell for general purposes (such as growth and repair) or specialised needs (e.g. enzymes to digest food in the gut or transmitters to send messages in the brain). Groups of similar cells make up tissues, which are then combined as organs with one special purpose (for instance the heart or liver). Organs which interact closely are grouped together as systems, and although all systems of the body act interdependently, it is easier to consider each separately.

I.ii THE SKIN

The skin consists of an outer layer or epidermis and an underlying dermis. The skin has four main roles:

- **Protection** against bacteria and viruses, chemicals and some types of radiation, for instance ultraviolet radiation in sunlight, and loss or entry of too much water.

- **Sensation**, which enables us to interact with the environment by means of touch and response to heat and cold.

- **Temperature regulation** – heat can be lost when blood vessels in the skin dilate (widen) and saved when they constrict (narrow). Cooling is also achieved by sweating. Some insulation is provided by the hairs standing on end and trapping air, and by a layer of fat below the skin.

- **Production of vitamin D** (needed for healthy bones and teeth) when sunlight falls on the skin, although most vitamin D comes from food.

I.iii BONES AND JOINTS

There are over 200 bones in the body making up its supporting framework, the skeleton. These bones are composed of a cartilage framework hardened by calcium, and are constantly being remodelled in response to outside forces working via muscles and tendons. Bones have a tough outer cortex and a spongier internal area, the marrow, which helps to lighten them. It is in the marrow of some bones (e.g. the ribs and upper ends of the humerus), that blood cells are produced.

The skeleton protects delicate internal organs and also acts as a site of attachment for muscles.

The sites at which bones meet are known as joints. Some of these, such as the sutures which are found between the bones of the skull, are fixed, preventing movement. A different type of joint – a synovial joint – is found where movement is to occur. Ball and socket joints such as the shoulder and hip allow most freedom, whereas hinge joints such as the knee and elbow allow movement in one plane only. The joint is strengthened by a capsule surrounded by tough ligaments, which, if they are injured, make the joint unstable.

Between the bones of the spinal column, the vertebrae, lie spongy intervertebral discs which act as shock absorbers.

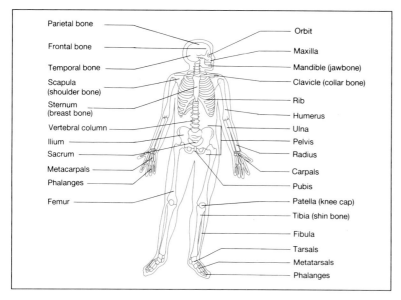

Parietal bone
Frontal bone
Temporal bone
Scapula (shoulder bone)
Sternum (breast bone)
Vertebral column
Ilium
Sacrum
Metacarpals
Phalanges
Femur

Orbit
Maxilla
Mandible (jawbone)
Clavicle (collar bone)
Rib
Humerus
Ulna
Pelvis
Radius
Carpals
Pubis
Patella (knee cap)
Tibia (shin bone)
Fibula
Tarsals
Metatarsals
Phalanges

The skeleton

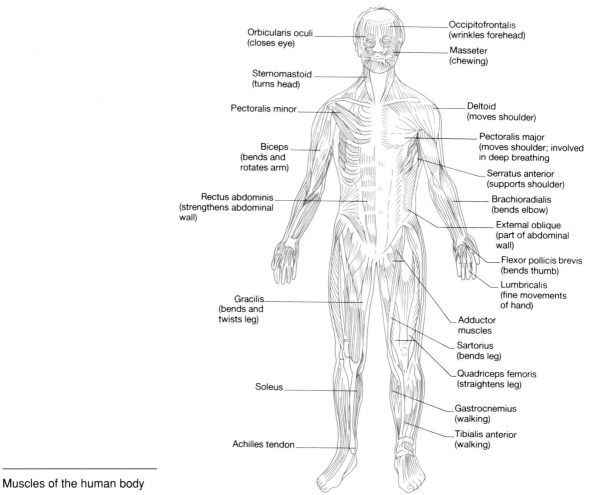

Orbicularis oculi (closes eye)
Sternomastoid (turns head)
Pectoralis minor
Biceps (bends and rotates arm)
Rectus abdominis (strengthens abdominal wall)
Gracilis (bends and twists leg)
Soleus
Achilles tendon

Occipitofrontalis (wrinkles forehead)
Masseter (chewing)
Deltoid (moves shoulder)
Pectoralis major (moves shoulder; involved in deep breathing
Serratus anterior (supports shoulder)
Brachioradialis (bends elbow)
External oblique (part of abdominal wall)
Flexor pollicis brevis (bends thumb)
Lumbricalis (fine movements of hand)
Adductor muscles
Sartorius (bends leg)
Quadriceps femoris (straightens leg)
Gastrocnemius (walking)
Tibialis anterior (walking)

Muscles of the human body

I.iv MUSCLES AND TENDONS

Nearly half the body's weight is accounted for by the muscles attached to the skeleton (striated or voluntary muscles) of which there are more than 400. They are mainly under conscious control and act to maintain posture, generate movement and, by means of shivering, keep the body warm.

Striated muscles are made up of individual cells or fibres containing proteins called actin and myosin which can slide into spaces between each other and shorten the muscle. The ends of the muscle are attached either directly or indirectly, via tendons, to bone, although some muscles in the face attach directly to the skin.

A second class of muscle – smooth or involuntary muscle – is found in the internal organs, for example the gut, and is not under conscious control.

The third class of muscle, heart muscle, is peculiar to that organ.

I.v THE NERVOUS SYSTEM

The nervous system is the main control system of the body. It has two parts, the peripheral and the central nervous systems.

The basic functioning unit is the neurone, a cell with many projections like tree branches, which interact (synapse) with other nerve cells, to stimulate or inhibit them and to pass or receive messages by means of chemicals called neurotransmitters.

The peripheral nervous system has two main types of neurone:

- **Sensory neurones** carry messages into the central nervous system from sensory receptors in the skin or organs;

- **Motor neurones** relay commands from the central nervous system outwards, e.g. to a gland or muscle.

Thirty-one pairs of spinal nerves (to supply the body) and twelve pairs of cranial nerves (to the

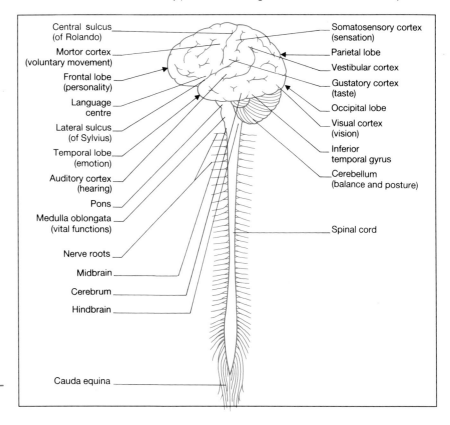

Central sulcus (of Rolando)
Mortor cortex (voluntary movement)
Frontal lobe (personality)
Language centre
Lateral sulcus (of Sylvius)
Temporal lobe (emotion)
Auditory cortex (hearing)
Pons
Medulla oblongata (vital functions)
Nerve roots
Midbrain
Cerebrum
Hindbrain
Cauda equina

Somatosensory cortex (sensation)
Parietal lobe
Vestibular cortex
Gustatory cortex (taste)
Occipital lobe
Visual cortex (vision)
Inferior temporal gyrus
Cerebellum (balance and posture)
Spinal cord

The nervous system

head and neck) are the start of the peripheral nervous system, joining directly to the central nervous system. These then divide to finer and finer nerves throughout the body.

The autonomic nervous system (ANS) is a specific part of the peripheral system which sends subconscious, involuntary commands to the glands and organs. The sympathetic division of the ANS prepares the body for action, while the parasympathetic division is concerned with functions that take place largely at rest, e.g. digestion.

The central nervous system is made up of the brain and spinal cord. The spinal cord is a transmission system, carrying messages up to and down from the brain. Integration and interpretation of information take place in the brain and commands are sent to the body so that it can respond to changing needs.

There are three main functional, but inter-relating, divisions of the brain.

- The cerebral hemispheres, which make up 90 per cent of the brain tissue, control higher functions such as memory, speech and intelligence.

- The cerebellum is involved in posture, muscle tone and co-ordination of movement.

- The brain stem controls basic vital functions such as respiration, circulation and consciousness.

Some tasks can be located specifically to certain areas of the brain, e.g. vision to the occipital lobe, whereas others are more diffuse. In general, one side of the brain controls the *opposite* side of the body.

The brain and spinal cord are covered by three protective tissue layers, the meninges. Between two of these lies the cerebrospinal fluid (CSF), which acts as a protective cushion. CSF is also found in a central channel running through the spinal cord. This channel expands into larger chambers called ventricles within the brain.

I.vi THE ENDOCRINE SYSTEM

The second control system is the endocrine system. Endocrine glands release substances called hormones, directly into the bloodstream. Hormones act as messengers affecting specific target organs. The response is slower than communication via nerves, but the system is better for longer term control.

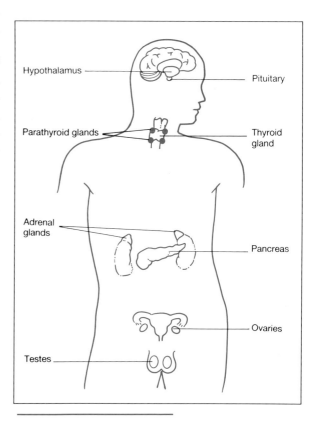

The endocrine system

An area of the brain called the hypothalamus controls the main endocrine gland, the pituitary, and thus provides a link between the nervous and endocrine systems. The hypothalamus also has a direct effect on the adrenal (otherwise known as supra-renal) glands.

The pituitary glands release a number of hormones:

- Growth hormones, for new muscle, bone etc.;

- Prolactin, which affects milk production in the breasts;

- Oxytocin, which stimulates the uterus and breasts;

- Antidiuretic hormone, which causes more water to be reabsorbed in the kidney when the water level in the body is low;

- Four other hormones, targeting the adrenal glands, the thyroid, the testes and ovaries, and the skin (to increase pigmentation).

The outer layer (cortex) of the adrenal glands produces small amounts of sex hormones (androgens and oestrogen) and hormones which affect carbohydrate metabolism and sodium and water balance. The adrenal gland's inner medulla forms adrenaline and nor-adrenaline. These prepare the body for action-when threatened – the so-called fright, fight or flight response.

The thyroid gland influences metabolic rate, growth and development, by the release of the hormone thyroxine, and also produces calcitonin which decreases the blood level of calcium, important in bone formation, blood clotting and normal cell function. Calcitonin is antagonised (opposed) by parathyroid hormone from the parathyroid glands which increases blood calcium levels.

The pancreas, as well as producing digestive enzymes, makes the hormones insulin and glucagon. Insulin decreases blood glucose concentration and glucagon increases it. Between them, these hormones affect the amounts of stored or available energy in the body.

The ovaries and testes are also endocrine glands, but are described in section xi below.

I.vii THE RESPIRATORY SYSTEM

The respiratory system acts to exchange oxygen and waste carbon dioxide. Air enters through the mouth and nose, the latter having cells specialised for the sense of smell. Here it is warmed and humidified before passing to the pharynx and larynx, where harmful substances can be trapped in sticky mucus. The mucus (phlegm) is then propelled to the outside by fine hairs (cilia). Coughing and sneezing reflexes also help to remove

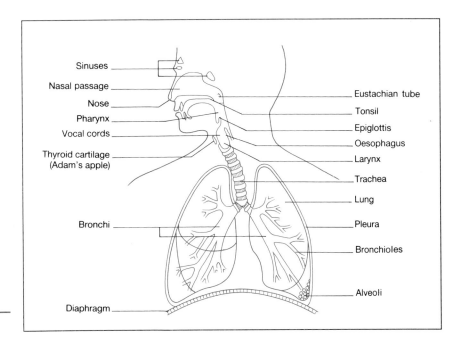

The respiratory system

unwanted particles. A flap of tissue, the epiglottis, covers the top of the trachea (windpipe) during swallowing to prevent food and liquid entering the lungs.

The larynx houses the vocal cords which vibrate as air passes over them to form the basis of the voice.

The trachea divides into two main branches, one to each lung, which divide into smaller bronchi and bronchioles. Finally they lead to alveoli, shaped like bunches of hollow grapes and covered in blood vessels, where the gas exchange takes place.

Covering the lungs and lining the chest wall are two fine membranes, the pleurae, with a thin layer of fluid between them. The membranes stick together by capillary action so, when the chest expands and the diaphragm flattens in inspiration, the lungs are pulled open and air sucked in. During expiration the muscles relax and the lungs recoil to their original shape, pushing the air out.

I.viii   BLOOD AND THE CIRCULATORY SYSTEM

All nutrients and oxygen reach the body cells via the blood, which also removes all the waste products and carries heat round the body. Blood is manufactured in the marrow of certain bones and is made up of:

- **Red blood cells** (red corpuscles or erythrocytes) whose red pigment haemoglobin binds to oxygen;

- **White blood cells** (white corpuscles or leucocytes) which help to defend the body against bacteria, cancer cells etc., by either directly attacking them or producing antibodies to neutralise them;

- **Platelets** (thrombocytes) which act in conjunction with clotting factors in the plasma to stop bleeding;

- **Plasma** – the fluid containing these cells, along with, for example, minerals, gases, hormones, vitamins, nutrients and waste products, as well as clotting factors. If clotting factors are removed from plasma it is known as **serum**.

The right side of the heart pumps blood via the pulmonary artery (the only artery in the body carrying deoxygenated blood) to the lungs, where carbon dioxide is given off and oxygen taken up. The blood then returns to the left side of the heart which pumps it into the aorta, the major artery, and then to the rest of the body. The arteries divide to give progressively smaller vessels – arterioles – which sub-

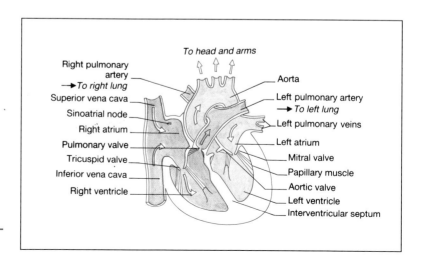

The heart

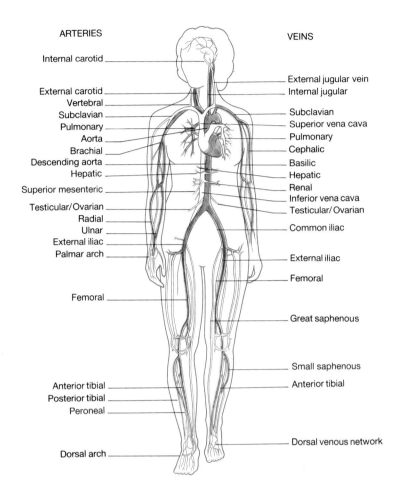

ARTERIES

- Internal carotid
- External carotid
- Vertebral
- Subclavian
- Pulmonary
- Aorta
- Brachial
- Descending aorta
- Hepatic
- Superior mesenteric
- Testicular/Ovarian
- Radial
- Ulnar
- External iliac
- Palmar arch
- Femoral
- Anterior tibial
- Posterior tibial
- Peroneal
- Dorsal arch

VEINS

- External jugular vein
- Internal jugular
- Subclavian
- Superior vena cava
- Pulmonary
- Cephalic
- Basilic
- Hepatic
- Renal
- Inferior vena cava
- Testicular/Ovarian
- Common iliac
- External iliac
- Femoral
- Great saphenous
- Small saphenous
- Anterior tibial
- Dorsal venous network

Major arteries and veins of the human body

divide to very fine capillaries, where nutrients and oxygen are given up to the tissues and waste products collected. The capillaries join to form venules and then veins, and blood is returned to the heart by the two major veins, the venae cavae. Thus the circulation is a double loop.

The heart has its own pacemaker, the sino-atrial node. This controls the heart contraction by generating electrical impulses which spread throughout the muscle. It is these that are registered on an ECG (electrocardiogram). Characteristic abnormalities of the ECG are produced by different heart conditions.

I.ix THE LYMPHATIC SYSTEM

This is a specialised system, part of its function being to collect fluid and small proteins that leak from blood vessels, and to return them to the circulation via a chamber in the neck known as the thoracic duct.

At certain points along the lymphatic vessels lie lymph nodes or glands which detect and combat antigens in the fluid by stimulating defensive cells (lymphocytes) to attack them directly or with antibodies. Lymphocytes are also present in the blood stream.

This process is normally directed against outside invaders or cancer cells, but some-

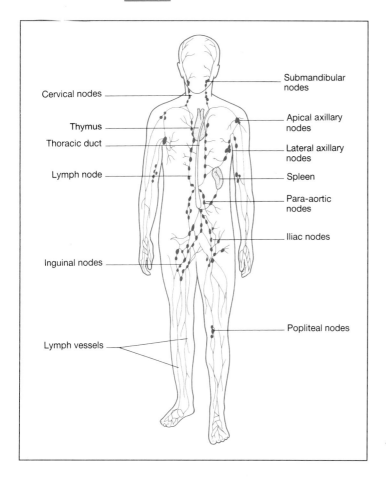

Cervical nodes

Thymus

Thoracic duct

Lymph node

Inguinal nodes

Lymph vessels

Submandibular nodes

Apical axillary nodes

Lateral axillary nodes

Spleen

Para-aortic nodes

Iliac nodes

Popliteal nodes

The lymphatic system

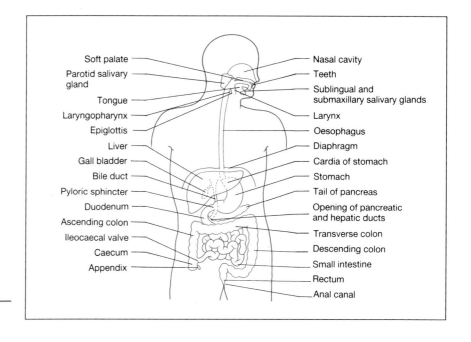

Soft palate

Parotid salivary gland

Tongue

Laryngopharynx

Epiglottis

Liver

Gall bladder

Bile duct

Pyloric sphincter

Duodenum

Ascending colon

Ileocaecal valve

Caecum

Appendix

Nasal cavity

Teeth

Sublingual and submaxillary salivary glands

Larynx

Oesophagus

Diaphragm

Cardia of stomach

Stomach

Tail of pancreas

Opening of pancreatic and hepatic ducts

Transverse colon

Descending colon

Small intestine

Rectum

Anal canal

The digestive system

times mistakenly targets the body's own cells, leading to autoimmune disease.

The spleen is the main site of destruction of old red blood cells and is also involved in immune responses, while the thymus activates lymphocytes.

I.x   THE DIGESTIVE SYSTEM

Food and drink must be digested to release vital nutrients. The body needs:

- **Proteins** for growth and repair;

- **Carbohydrates** for energy;

- **Fats** for energy and hormone and cell membrane production (vitamins A, D, E and K are also found in fat);

- **Vitamins** B and C;

- **Mineral salts** and **trace elements**;

- **Roughage** and **water**.

Digestion starts in the mouth where the teeth (20 deciduous or milk teeth in the child and 32 permanent teeth in the adult) cut and grind the food into manageable pieces. Saliva from three pairs of salivary glands lubricates the food and begins digestion of some of the carbohydrate present. The tongue, besides being vital for clear speech, carries about 10,000 taste buds.

From the mouth, food travels to the stomach, where churning splits it up further. Food is stored here to be released to the intestines in easily handled amounts. The stomach produces:

- **Acid** to curdle milk, kill bacteria and activate digestive enzymes;

- **Pepsin** to digest proteins;

- **Intrinsic factor**, vital for the absorption of vitamin B_{12}, used for nerve function and red blood cell formation.

From the stomach, food enters the small intestine where digestion continues:

- **Pancreatic enzymes** digest carbohydrates, fats and proteins;

- **Bile salts** from the gall bladder emulsify fats.

The structure of the small intestine provides a large surface area to absorb the broken down nutrients etc. These enter the blood and are passed to the liver, which recombines them to form energy stores and new substances suitable for the body to use. The liver also:

- Produces bile;

- Inactivates hormones;

- Destroys some poisons and drugs;

- Helps the system break down red blood cells.

A large amount of roughage, water and surplus nutrients has been left in the gut, and now enters the large intestine. Here, water and salts are absorbed, and the remaining debris (faeces) is stored until defaecation.

I.xi   THE GENITOURINARY SYSTEM

The kidneys maintain the volume and composition of the body's fluids and are major regulators of the internal environment. They have five main functions:

- **Removal** of nitrogenous waste, e.g. urea;

- **Regulation** of the level of acid or alkalinity in the body (acid-base balance) and of chemicals (electrolytes) influencing it, e.g. sodium and potassium;

- **Control** of water levels;

- **Production** of the hormone erythropoietin which stimulates the production of red blood cells;

- **Activation** of vitamin D.

Each kidney is made up of more than a million units called nephrons which continuously

The final product of the kidney's action is urine, which is stored in the bladder before being voided through the urethra. In men this passage is also shared with the reproductive system, whereas in women it is separate.

In men, sperm are manufactured in the testes, along with the hormone testosterone which is responsible for male characteristics such as beard growth and for maintaining the reproductive system. The sperm mature and are stored for up to 70 days in the hugely coiled epididymis before ejaculation. Secretions from the prostate gland and seminal vesicles supply energy and help to mobilise the sperm.

In women between puberty and the menopause, an ovum (egg) from the ovary is released approximately every month into a fallopian tube. Fertilisation usually takes place here and the egg then implants into the prepared wall of the uterus (womb). If there is no implantation, the blood-filled lining of the uterus breaks down and is lost during menstruation. The ovary also produces the hormones oestrogen and progesterone which control the menstrual cycle, cause ovulation and prepare tissues for possible pregnancy.

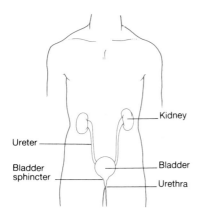

The basic urinary system

filter the blood and remove vast quantities of water and dissolved substances. Some of these (e.g. vitamins and glucose) are returned to the body, as is 99 per cent of the water, whereas urea, for example, is eliminated. The amount of other substances reabsorbed varies according to the needs of the body. In control of acid-base balance, the kidney works very closely with the lungs: any build-up of carbon dioxide makes the blood more acid and the kidney can compensate for this.

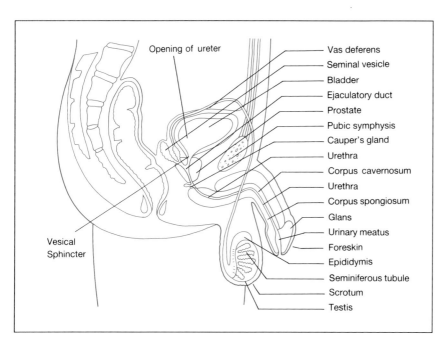

The male reproductive system

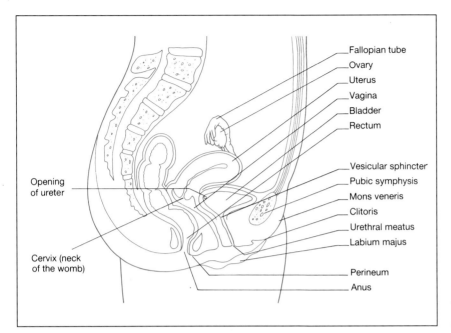

Fallopian tube
Ovary
Uterus
Vagina
Bladder
Rectum

Vesicular sphincter
Pubic symphysis
Mons veneris
Clitoris
Urethral meatus
Labium majus

Opening
of ureter

Cervix (neck
of the womb)

Perineum
Anus

The female reproductive
system

I.xii   THE EYE AND EAR

The special senses of sight and hearing are
vital for interaction with the environment.

The eye
The eyeball is protected by the bony orbit and
washed by tears from the lacrimal ducts at the
upper outer edge of the eye. In blinking, the
eyelids act like windscreen wipers.

Two types of light-sensitive cell, rods and
cones, are found in the retina. Rods are sensitive to low levels of light and are used for night
vision. Cones are specialised for colour vision
and for seeing in bright light. Cones are concentrated at the macula, where the image from
the lens is most accurately focused.

The lens changes shape when the ciliary
muscles contract or relax. Further muscles in
the iris (the coloured part of the eye) control
the amount of light entering the eye through
the pupil.

Information from the retina passes into the
optic nerve to travel to the brain, the two optic
nerves joining *en route*.

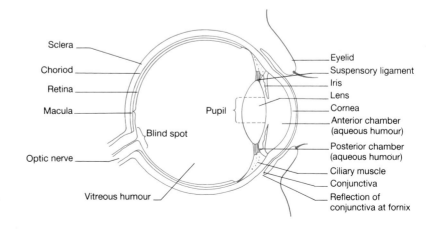

Sclera
Choriod
Retina
Macula
Optic nerve

Blind spot

Vitreous humour

Pupil

Eyelid
Suspensory ligament
Iris
Lens
Cornea
Anterior chamber
(aqueous humour)
Posterior chamber
(aqueous humour)
Ciliary muscle
Conjunctiva
Reflection of
conjunctiva at fornix

The eye in cross-section

The ear

The pinna (outer ear) and auditory canal funnel sound in the form of air vibration towards the eardrum. The eardrum's movements relay the vibration to the three tiny bones of the middle ear, the malleus (hammer), incus (anvil) and stapes (stirrup). These act as a system of levers transmitting the sound with increased force to the inner ear (cochlea) where specialised cells are stimulated. The impulses generated are transmitted along the auditory nerve to the brain.

The Eustachian tube is a passage from the middle ear to the pharynx ('voice box'), allowing pressure to be equalised across the eardrum so that it can move more freely.

The three semicircular canals, lying at right angles to one another, are involved in balance and orientation, checking the position and movement of the head relative to gravity.

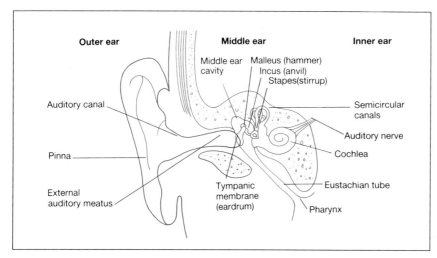

The ear in cross-section

FIRST AID

This section aims to provide easy-to-find advice on dealing with accidents at home. Basic first aid measures will be outlined and indications given as to when medical help should be sought. The major life-saving skills of external cardiac (heart) compression and mouth-to-mouth breathing will be mentioned but not described in detail since these techniques should be taught by and learned from a trained instructor. Supervised practice is essential to ensure their correct performance. Short courses in these and other First Aid skills are available through local branches of the British Red Cross Society and St John Ambulance and readers are advised to undertake such a course.

All possible measures should be taken to PREVENT accidents in the home and the need for appropriate use of gates, guards and locks cannot be overstressed, particularly where there are young children. Accidents do happen, however, despite all preventive measures.

II.i BASIC FIRST AID MEASURES

The aims of First Aid are threefold:

- To save life;
- To prevent deterioration;
- To aid recovery.

BRUISES

A bruise occurs when there is bleeding into the tissues under the skin and may occur following any blunt injury.

Aims

- Stop the bleeding;
- Reduce swelling and discomfort.

Actions

- Apply a cold compress to the injured area using a flannel or ice cubes/packs wrapped in a cloth. This will stop the bleeding, limit the size of the bruise and reduce swelling.

- Position the limb comfortably. If the bruise is large, the limb should be elevated if possible to help reduce swelling.

CUTS AND GRAZES

A cut will result in bleeding from an area of the body surface.

Aims

- Arrest bleeding;
- Prevent infection.

Actions

- Wash hands if possible to minimise risk of infection;

- If bleeding is not profuse, clean the wound using soap and water;

- Apply pressure directly on the wound using a clean cloth until the bleeding stops;

- Cover with an appropriate dressing – an adhesive plaster or gauze and bandage.

If bleeding is severe, raise the limb and apply firm pressure for 2–3 minutes.

If blood is spurting out in jets, press firmly and summon help.

A large wound may need stitching so seek medical advice once it is clean and covered.

If there is a foreign body or bodies (gravel or wood for example) remove it if possible using tweezers. Large foreign bodies should be left in place, a dressing applied around them and medical help sought.

N.B. Head wounds usually bleed profusely and the cut may be difficult to find.

NOSEBLEED (EPISTAXIS)

This occurs when a tiny blood vessel in the nose is broken. There may be no apparent cause.

Aims

- Maintain a clear airway so that the subject can breathe;

- Stop the bleeding.

Actions

- Sit subject down with head leaning forward, as shown in the figure;

- Loosen any tight clothing around the neck;

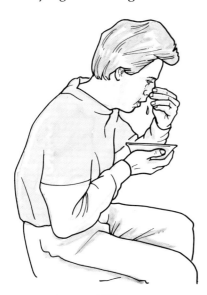

Stopping a nosebleed

- Ask subject to breathe through his mouth whilst pinching the soft part of his nose for 10 minutes (do this for him if necessary);

- Provide a vessel or towels to catch dribble and blood;

- Repeat the above is bleeding persists after 10 minutes;

- Clean up once bleeding has ceased.

If bleeding persists, seek medical advice.
Do not plug the nose.
Do not allow the subject to blow his nose or exert himself for 2–4 hours.

INSECT BITES AND STINGS

Bees, wasps and hornets can cause painful stings and some insects can inflict painful, irritating bites. Occasionally individuals are allergic to insect stings, in which case medical help should be sought at once and resuscitation may be necessary (see page 631).

Aims

- Remove sting if still in skin;

- Reduce swelling;

- Relieve pain.

Actions

- If the sting is visible use tweezers to remove it. Hold it close to the skin and take care not to squeeze the poison sac.

- Apply a cold compress to help reduce pain and swelling.

- Apply proprietary creams (e.g. Anthisan) to reduce local inflammation.

If stings are in the mouth, rinse with cold water or give the sufferer ice cubes to suck.

If breathing is affected, place the casualty in recovery position (see page 630) and telephone for an ambulance.

ANIMAL BITES

Animal mouths (including human mouths) contain many germs which can infect bite wounds. Many animals have sharp, pointed teeth which cause deep puncture wounds through which tetanus may be introduced.

Aims

• Clean wound thoroughly;

• Prevent further infection.

Actions

• Wash the wound thoroughly with warm, soapy water for 5 minutes;

• Cover with a clean, preferably sterile, dressing;

• Seek medical advice if anti-tetanus injections are not up to date.

If the wound is large or bleeding severely, seek medical aid.

N.B.   Dog bites should be reported to the police.

SPRAINS AND STRAINS

A *sprain* occurs when tissues and ligaments around a joint are pulled or torn. Some sprains cause only very minor damage, others are much more serious.

Aims

• Reduce pain and swelling;

• Prevent further damage.

Actions

• Expose the area and apply ice packs to reduce swelling;

• Elevate the affected limb and immobilise with cushions in the most comfortable position;

• Pad with cotton wool and apply a crêpe bandage to provide support.

If swelling or pain is severe, seek medical advice.

A *strain* occurs when muscles are over-stretched or torn by violent movement such as sport or lifting. There will be acute pain at the injury site and swelling may also occur.

Aims

• Make subject comfortable;

• Seek medical aid.

Actions

• Elevate the limb if possible;

• Support with pillows in the most comfortable position;

• Apply cold compress for about 30 minutes to reduce swelling;

• Apply crêpe bandage to help support the injured area;

• Seek medical help.

BURNS AND SCALDS

A burn is an injury to the skin and underlying tissues. It may be caused by extreme heat or cold, chemicals, electricity or radiation. A scald is a burn caused by wet heat (e.g. steam, water, hot oils or fat). The management of the injury is the same for dry or wet burns.

Aims

• Stop further burning;

• Relieve pain which can be extreme;

• Reduce swelling;

• Prevent infection.

N.B.   MANY BURNS REQUIRE MEDICAL ATTENTION. These include all burns larger than 3–4 cm $(1-1\frac{1}{2}$ in.) in diameter, burns involving more than just the surface of the skin and burns caused by chemicals or electricity. If in any doubt, seek medical advice.

Actions

- Stop further burning by dousing flames with water or wrapping burning area in towels or other cloths (do not use nylon or plastic);

- Remove any hot items from the skin (e.g. clothes, hot objects);

- Run cold water over the affected area for 10 minutes to stop burning and relieve pain (see figure). If the area cannot be put under a tap, apply cloths or towels soaked in cold water and change these every few minutes.

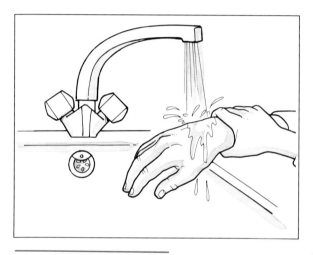

Cooling a burn

- Remove constricting articles such as rings and watches from the surrounding area before swelling begins.

- Cover burn lightly with a clean (sterile if possible) dry dressing.

- Keep casualty warm while seeking advice or assistance.

If the burn is extensive, call an ambulance for emergency transfer to hospital.

DO NOT break blisters over burns.

DO NOT apply butter, lotions or creams to burned areas.

DO NOT use adhesive plaster on any burned area.

POISONING

Poisoning occurs when a substance enters the body in sufficient quantity to damage it. Poisons may enter the body through the mouth (e.g. tablets, plants or fluids), through the skin (e.g. insecticides and other poisonous sprays) or via the lungs (e.g. noxious fumes and vapours). In some instances, poison may enter by injection as in poisonous bites or stings or by intentional hypodermic needle injection.

Children almost always poison themselves by accident (not so adults) and it is vital that all possible measures are taken in the home to avoid such an event. Substances commonly ingested include household cleaning products such as bleach, medicines and tablets (particularly brightly coloured ones which look like sweets), garden insecticides and poisonous plants and seeds. Children are often totally unaware of the dangers of swallowing or inhaling these substances and every effort should be made to ensure their safe storage out of the reach of children.

Poisons act on the body in many different ways and may cause temporary or permanent damage. The first aid measures remain the same, whatever the cause of poisoning and whatever symptoms the casualty has.

N.B.   MEDICAL AID OR ADVICE SHOULD ALWAYS BE SOUGHT, WHATEVER THE CAUSE OF POISONING.

Aims

- Ensure that subject can breathe adequately;

- Seek medical advice or transfer to hospital at once.

Actions

- Try to find out what has been taken, how much and when;

- Ensure that the casualty is able to breathe properly;

- Place in recovery position (see page 630) if vomiting, drowsy or unconscious;

- Be prepared to resuscitate if necessary (see page 631);

- Call medical help at once – if in any doubt, arrange urgent transfer to hospital (dial the emergency services).

DO NOT make the subject vomit unless told to do so – it may make things worse.

Food poisoning occurs when food containing bacteria is cooked or stored incorrectly. The very young, the very old and those who are already ill are most at risk from this type of poisoning.

Nausea, vomiting, diarrhoea, fever and headache are common indications of food poisoning and may occur from 2–48 hours after eating the affected food.

Aims

- Avoid dehydration;

- Seek medical aid if necessary.

Actions

- Give plenty of fluids to drink;

- Withhold food until vomiting and diarrhoea subside;

- Encourage to rest until symptoms abate;

- Seek medical help if symptoms are severe or persist beyond 24–48 hours.

CHOKING

Choking occurs when food or other matter taken into the mouth goes 'down the wrong way' and causes the windpipe to be partly or totally blocked. Children are most at risk, especially very young children who tend to put things into their mouth as part of normal investigation.

The person who is choking will be extremely frightened and unable to breathe or speak. He may or may not cough and will become blue around the mouth and lips as oxygen in the blood is used up. He will become unconscious and die if the matter is not expelled from the windpipe.

Aims

- Ensure adequate air enters the lungs;

- Arrange emergency transfer to hospital if necessary.

Actions

- Remove any obstruction in the mouth by hooking it out with a finger (e.g. large pieces of food, false teeth). This method of clearing the airway is described in more detail on page 631.

- Encourage the subject to cough in order to dislodge the obstruction.

- If choking persists, lie the **child** face down across your lap or knee and support his chest with one hand. With the other hand slap the child between the shoulder blades (see the figure below). The force required in this manoeuvre will vary with the size of the child but a sharp blow is needed. Repeat this three or four times if necessary.

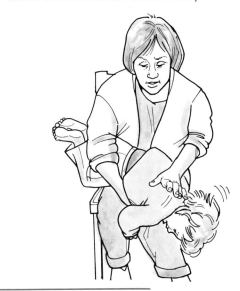

Slapping a choking child

Adult subjects should be helped to bend over so that the head is lower than the lungs and given a sharp slap between the shoulder blades, again repeated two or three times if necessary.

- If choking still persists, an attempt must be made to force air out of the lungs at speed in an effort to blow the obstruction out.

This technique, known as the abdominal thrust, may cause damage to the abdominal organs and **should only be used when all other methods have failed**. Sit the **child** on your lap, facing forward, and place one arm across his tummy while supporting his back with the other. Clench the fist of the front arm (as shown in the figure) with the thumb inwards and place it below the ribs, at the top and centre of the abdomen. Press the clenched fist inwards and upwards in a quick movement which should be hard enough to dislodge the obstruction. Repeat two or three times if necessary.

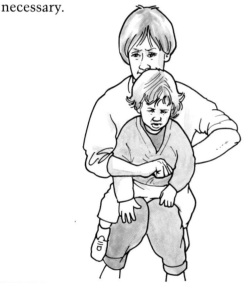

Abdominal thrust for child

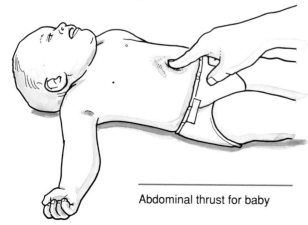

Abdominal thrust for baby

Babies should be laid on their backs on a firm surface and the abdominal thrust performed using two fingers, as shown in the figure.

Adults will require a much more powerful thrust to push air from their lungs and two grasped hands should be used from a position standing or kneeling behind the subject.

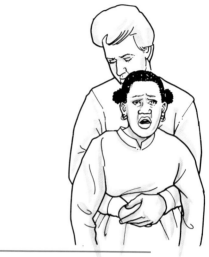

Abdominal thrust for adult

IF SUBJECT BECOMES UNCONSCIOUS the back slap and abdominal thrust may still be performed with the casualty on the floor. Once choking has stopped, the casualty should be transferred to hospital.

IF BREATHING STOPS, dial the emergency services for an ambulance and perform artificial ventilation (mouth-to-mouth breathing) until help arrives (see page 631).

N.B. Breathing may restart at any time if the obstruction is dislodged and the subject should be encouraged to sit or lie quietly until he recovers fully. He may be given sips of cold water to drink as long as he is fully conscious.

UNCONSCIOUSNESS

A person may become unconscious or semi-conscious if there is an interruption in the normal activity of the brain. A semiconscious

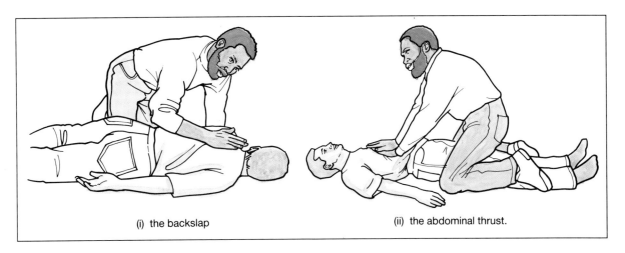

(i) the backslap   (ii) the abdominal thrust.

The unconscious casualty

person will appear drowsy or vague and be unable to answer questions properly, whilst one who is fully unconscious will not respond at all and will collapse. Causes of unconsciousness are varied and include injury to the head, poisoning, fainting, stroke, diabetes, epilepsy and infantile convulsions.

WHATEVER THE CAUSE, THE TREATMENT REMAINS THE SAME.

Aims

- Ensure the patient can breathe adequately;

- Arrange emergency medical assistance.

Actions

- Open the mouth and clear out any debris such as false teeth or food with your fingers (see page 631);

- Check that the patient is breathing adequately;

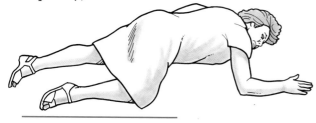

Recovery position

- Turn the subject into the recovery position (shown in the figure). See page 630 for details of how to achieve this;

- Keep subject warm but ensure that there is a good air supply;

- Dial the emergency services to arrange transfer to hospital;

- Stay with subject until help arrives.

Do not attempt to give anything to eat or drink. There is one exception to this rule – someone who is a known diabetic and who is only semiconscious may be given sugar lumps, glucose tablets or a sweet drink if you think it safe to do so.

DISLOCATIONS

When one or more bones move out of position at a joint, they are said to have dislocated. The cause may be a direct blow to the joint or elsewhere along the bones causing the bones to slide out of position at their weakest point. The thumb, finger, shoulder and jaw joints are the ones most usually dislocated. Dislocations may occur at the same time as fractures and if there is any doubt about the nature of the injury it should be treated as a fracture. The subject will feel great pain at the site of the dislocation and will be unable to move the affected joint. The area will look deformed.

Aims

- Make as comfortable as possible;

- Arrange transfer to hospital.

Actions

- Sit or lie the casualty down – she will probably feel faint;

- Avoid any movement of the affected area by immobilising it as appropriate with bandages, slings, pillows or cushions;

- Arrange for casualty to be taken to hospital.

DO NOT allow the subject to eat or drink as an anaesthetic may be necessary and would be delayed by this.

DO NOT attempt to put the bones back into place as this may cause more damage to the delicate structures surrounding the joint.

FRACTURES

A fracture is a break or a crack in a bone and may be caused by direct force to the area as in a fall or blow or by indirect force to the bone such as twisting or wrenching. Young bones do not break easily and tend to crack (known as greenstick fractures); older bones are more brittle and snap relatively easily sometimes as the result of a fairly minor injury.

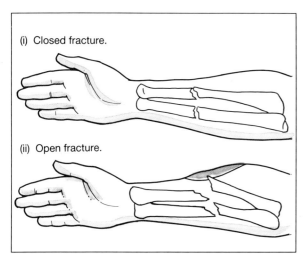

(i) Closed fracture.

(ii) Open fracture.

There are two main types of fracture – open and closed. A closed fracture occurs when the skin surface around the broken bones remains intact, though there may be a lot of damage to the tissues around the bones. In an open fracture, the skin is broken and the bones are in direct contact with the air – they may indeed be sticking right out and be clearly visible. There is a great danger with open wounds that infection may enter from the outside environment and care must be taken to avoid this right from the beginning.

Fractures are usually extremely painful and the area may look deformed. The casualty may have heard the bone crack and will be unable to move the affected area properly. There is often a lot of bleeding around a fractured bone – it may be obvious in an open fracture but not in a closed one. Severe bleeding can make the casualty shocked and very ill so urgent medical help must be sought.

Aims

- Prevent any further damage by immobilising the fracture site;

- Remove casualty to hospital for medical attention.

Actions

- Check the casualty is breathing properly and is conscious – any problems with either must be dealt with first as they could threaten life. (See page 630 for guidelines on restoring adequate breathing and page 626 for treatment of the unconscious casualty.)

- Stop any severe bleeding by pressing firmly on the bleeding point for 5 minutes. This should be done before the fracture is dealt with.

- Steady the fractured limb above and below the injury;

- Immobilise by bandaging to a firm structure which will act as a splint. The body may be used as a splint for a fractured arm; the other leg for a fracture of the lower limb. If possible move the uninjured part, not the injured, whilst doing this. Ideally some soft padding should be placed between bony joints such as knees or in obvious hollows. Bandages may be improvised from any soft cloth and should be applied firmly but not tightly.

- If the fracture is open, cover the wound first with a sterile or clean dressing. If necessary, place padding (sterile if possible) around any bones that protrude through the skin and put a dressing over the top.

- Check that blood flow to the limb is getting past the fracture site – the skin should look pink and feel warm and a pulse should be detectable below the injury.

- Remove any tight articles, especially rings and watches, from the broken limb. It is important to do this as soon as possible before swelling begins.

- Arrange for casualty to be taken to hospital at once – call an ambulance if in any doubt and for any lower limb fracture.

DO NOT try to move someone with a fracture unless they are in danger.

DO NOT allow him to eat or drink anything since this may mean a delay in his hospital treatment.

DO NOT allow the person to become cold – cover with a coat or blanket if possible.

BACK AND NECK INJURIES

The spine is made up of 33 irregularly shaped bones called vertebrae. The bones support the back and head and provide protection for the spinal cord which runs from top to bottom through the bones. The spinal cord is a bundle of nerve fibres which run from the brain to all parts of the body; damage to it can result in paralysis or loss of sensation to parts of the body. Between the vertebral bones are pads of cartilage, the intervertebral discs, which allow the spine to bend and twist.

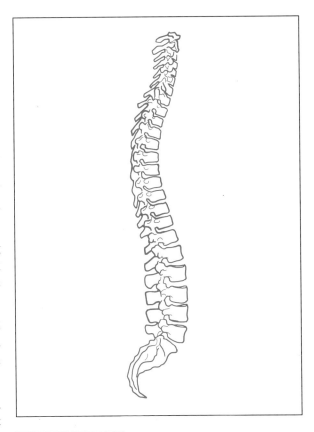

The spine

It is possible to injure the spine in a number of ways; it may be strained or sprained, the intervertebral discs may come out of place or the spine may be fractured. Of these, fractured spine is by far the most serious as the spinal cord may be involved resulting in permanent damage to part of the body. If there is any doubt at all about the nature of a back or neck injury, always err on the side of caution and treat it as a fracture.

Aims

- Prevent further damage to the spine and spinal cord;

- Arrange transport to hospital if necessary.

Actions

- DO NOT MOVE THE CASUALTY UNLESS IT IS ESSENTIAL.

- Check that the casualty is conscious and breathing properly (deal with these problems first).

- Steady and support the head without moving it. Do not pull or twist. Pad around head and neck with cushions, pillows or pads to keep it still.

- If the casualty must be turned (vomiting or unconscious), try to roll the body in a straight line with the head and neck supported in their natural position.

- Stay with the casualty until medical help arrives – call doctor or emergency ambulance according to severity of injury. Medical advice should be sought in all but the most minor injuries.

II.ii IMPORTANT FIRST AID TECHNIQUES

A person must be able to breathe properly and have an adequately working heart in order to function normally. There is a real danger of death in the following situations:

- Unconsciousness or vomiting resulting in a blocked airway;

- Breathing or heartbeat stopping;

- Severe blood loss, which means oxygen cannot be carried to body tissues.

The techniques outlined in this section will help to maintain life in these situations until help arrives.

Mouth-to-mouth breathing and external heart compression cannot be taught in a book and will be dealt with only briefly. Readers are advised to learn these techniques properly and practise them under supervision by attending a short course organised by local Red Cross or St John Ambulance groups. To find the address of your local group, contact the head office at the address given in Appendix VII, or consult your local telephone directory.

THE RECOVERY POSITION

This position is the one of choice for all unconscious casualties, providing they are breathing adequately and their heart is beating properly. Placing a person in this position will ensure that his tongue cannot fall to the back of the mouth and block the passage of air to the lungs. It also allows any secretions or vomit to drain freely out of the mouth, again avoiding the danger of airway blockage.

The position is also of use for those casualties who need to lie down and who are likely to vomit as it reduces the amount of movement needed to keep the air passages clear.

Once in the recovery position, the patient will be kept still because of the position of his limbs. Further movement should only be necessary in extreme situations such as the heartbeat stopping. The casualty can normally be kept in this position until help arrives.

The nature of the injuries will determine to some extent how the casualty is turned to the recovery position and the utmost care must be taken with those with injuries to the neck or spine (see page 629).

The casualty should be straightened out with limbs close to the body. Kneel on the floor beside him and roll him gently towards you as shown in the figure. Position the limbs as shown on page 627 for maximum safety.

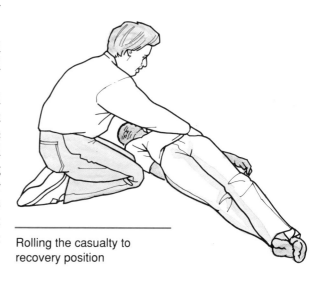

Rolling the casualty to recovery position

CLEARING THE AIRWAY

A casualty, whether conscious or unconscious, needs a clear airway in order to breathe adequately. The airway may be blocked by vomit or food particles, by objects put into the mouth such as false teeth or small toys, or by the tongue falling to the back of the mouth if the casualty is unconscious.

The airway may be cleared as follows:

- Turn the casualty's head to side and open the mouth (kneel beside her).

- Hook your first two fingers (only one for a child) and sweep all around the mouth quickly, hooking out any debris. Take care not to push objects further down, especially when the casualty is a child.

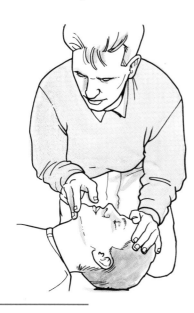

Opening the airway

- Now open up the air passages at the back of the throat by lifting the jaw forward with your fingers under the casualty's chin and pressing the head backwards with your other hand on her forehead as shown in the figure above.

- If breathing does not commence, begin mouth-to-mouth breathing at once.

MOUTH-TO-MOUTH BREATHING

This technique should be learned from a recognised instructor and practised under supervision.

Mouth-to-mouth breathing is a means of breathing for the casualty until his own breathing resumes or he can be mechanically ventilated. After clearing and opening the airway, check for signs of breathing by watching the chest for signs of movement, and by listening and feeling for breaths with your face held close to his mouth and nose. If there is no sign of breathing, proceed as follows.

- Turn the casualty onto his back if possible.

- Kneel beside the casualty's head and open his airway as described above.

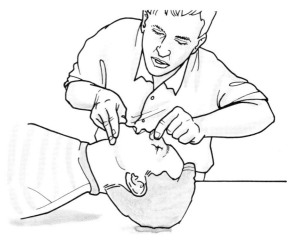

Mouth-to-mouth breathing

- Take a deep breath in, pinch the casualty's nostrils with your finger tips, and seal your mouth around his (see the figure above). With small children there is no need to pinch the nose as your mouth will be able to seal a child's mouth and nose.

- Blow steadily into the casualty's mouth; watch his chest to see it rise.

- Remove your mouth and allow air to be exhaled (casualty's chest will fall).

- Repeat inflation as long as necessary.

- When breathing resumes, turn the casualty to recovery position.

If the casualty's heartbeat stops, commence external chest compression.

EXTERNAL CHEST COMPRESSION

This technique should be learned from a recognised instructor and practised under supervision.

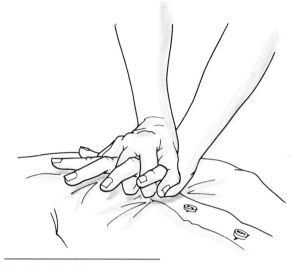

Hand position for external chest compression

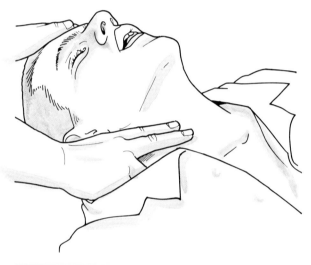

Feeling the carotid pulse

External chest compression is a means of pumping someone's heart for them when their heartbeat has stopped. If the heart does not beat, oxygen will not reach the brain and the person will die. External chest compression is always performed in conjunction with mouth-to-mouth breathing.

Before beginning external chest compression, make sure there is no circulation by feeling for the carotid pulse in the neck.

If there is no carotid pulse, proceed as follows:

- Lay casualty flat on his back on a firm surface and kneel beside his chest;

- Locate the bottom of the breastbone, at the lower end of the ribs and measure two finger breadths up from this point;

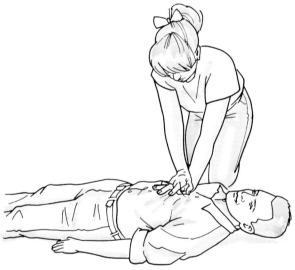

External chest compression

- Place the heel of one hand on the breastbone immediately above the two fingers and the heel of the other hand on top of this – the fingers should be clear of the ribs.

- Keep your arms straight and lean down on them so that the chest is depressed 4–5 cm ($1\frac{1}{2}$ –2 inches). Repeat at a rate of 80 compressions per minute.

- After 15 compressions, move to the head and give two breaths by mouth-to-mouth ventilation.

- Check the circulation every 3 minutes or so and stop compressions as soon as you can feel a pulse.

For children much less pressure is needed; use ONE HAND only at a faster rate, about 100 compressions per minute. Depress the chest 2.5–3.5 cm (1–1½ inches) and give one ventilation after every five compressions.

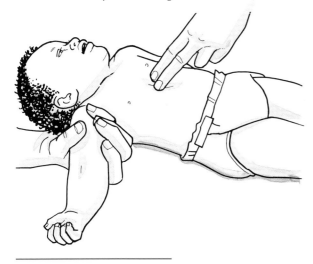

External chest compression
for babies

For babies and children under two support the head and neck with one hand under the back and use TWO FINGERS only to press the chest 1.5–2.5 cm (½–1 inch) at a rate of 100 per minute.

IF ANY OF THE TECHNIQUES IN THIS SECTION ARE NECESSARY THE CASUALTY REQUIRES URGENT MEDICAL ATTENTION – DIAL THE EMERGENCY SERVICES.

II.iii THE FIRST AID KIT

It is a good idea to have a first aid kit to hand at home or in the car when travelling. Any clean, dry, preferably airtight, container will do as a receptacle for your stocks. It should be clearly labelled and easily accessible; if it contains medicines of any sort it should be stored out of reach of children. A number of proprietary brands of kits are available but you may prefer to make up your own which is tailored to your likely requirements.

Suggested contents for a first aid box are as follows:

- Cotton wool – small packs are better than large for this purpose;

- Adhesive plasters – waterproof or fabric according to your preference – individually wrapped ones are best and you will need a variety of sizes;

- Sterile gauze dressings – small, medium and large;

- Triangular bandage (sling) – a large silk or cotton headsquare or cut sheeting will do;

- Safety pins for fastening bandages;

- Cotton gauze bandages;

- Crêpe bandages – several widths if possible (2 and 3 inch are most useful);

- Scissors and tweezers.

You may also wish to keep a small selection of your favourite topical lotions and creams, for example a soothing cream for bites and stings (Waspeze or Anthisan), calamine lotion for rashes and sunburn, arnica ointment for bruising to name but a few. In general, the more selective you can be with the contents of your box, the better. It is not recommended that you keep tablets and linctuses in a first aid kit – these should be securely stored elsewhere in the house.

PUTTING ON A BANDAGE

There are a few simple rules which, if followed, will make bandaging easy and effective. Here they are:

- Choose a bandage of appropriate size – a small bandage for a small limb, a large for a large;

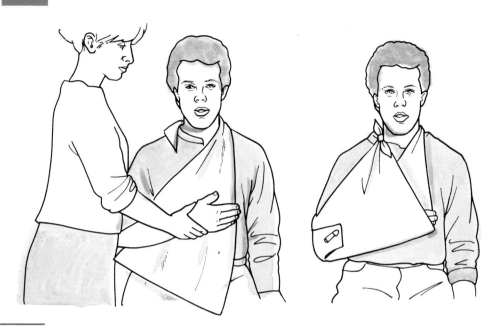

Applying a sling

• Choose the correct type of bandage – cotton for holding a dressing in place, crêpe if you need to provide support to the joint or limb;

• Ask the casualty to sit or lie down;

• Try to stand or sit in front of the injured part;

• Apply the bandage evenly covering about half of the previous turn with each new turn;

• Leave fingers or toes exposed whenever possible;

• Bandage firmly but not so tightly that circulation is cut off (check from time to time that swelling has not made the bandage tight).

PUTTING ON A SLING

Triangular bandages or slings have many uses but are most commonly used to support an injured arm which may or may not be bandaged. They are easy to put on if you follow these guidelines:

• Support the injured arm while sliding the sling behind it so that the point of the sling is at the elbow side (this is best done with the casualty sitting down) – see the figure above;

• Bring the lower part of the sling up over the hand and forearm and to the shoulder on the injured side;

• Bring the other end round the back of the neck and tie with a reef knot, on the shoulder of the injured side;

• The hand should be slightly higher than the elbow when you have finished and the fingertips must be left exposed, as shown in the figure;

• Neaten the elbow end with a safety pin.

DRUGS AND MEDICINES

A wide variety of different drugs are available for medicinal use. Some of these can be bought 'over the counter' at your local chemist but the majority will need to be prescribed by a doctor who will check that a drug is suitable for you.

Huge volumes have been devoted to the listing and description of drugs, their uses, benefits, side-effects and the circumstances under which they should not be used. Some books are aimed specifically at the concerned general reader and give considerable detail about all the drugs with which you are likely to come into contact. The 'Suggested further reading' list (Appendix VIII) gives more information about these.

The data given in this Appendix is necessarily selective; in a book of this nature it is really only appropriate to consider some of the most common types of drug and, in particular, those which may have been mentioned in earlier chapters. The intention is to give enough information to answer everyday queries while at the same time providing readers with signposts for amassing more detailed knowledge.

Drugs and medicines: safety first

- If your doctor is writing a prescription for you, be sure to remind her if any of the following apply:

  - you are taking any other medicines already;
  - you have reacted badly to the drug in question on a previous occasion;
  - you are pregnant or breast feeding;

- When buying over the counter medicines, always ask the advice of the pharmacist. If the medicine is for a child, tell the pharmacist the child's age.

- Keep all medicines in a locked cabinet, out of reach of any children.

- Always complete the course of medication, as advised by your doctor – unless you develop a reaction to the drug while taking the course in which case you should contact your doctor immediately for advice.

- Take only medicines that have been prescribed for you and don't let anyone else take your medicines.

- Return all unused or out of date medicines and tablets to the pharmacist to be disposed of safely.

III.i ANTIBIOTICS (DRUGS TO COMBAT BACTERIAL INFECTION)

Group name	Examples	Notes
Penicillins	Ampicillin Amoxycillin Flucloxacillin Penicillin V	Some individuals are allergic to penicillins. If you know this to be true in your case you should make sure your doctor knows.
Cephalosporins	Cephalexin Cephradine	Some people who are allergic to penicillins are also allergic to cephalosporins. If you are allergic to penicillins, make sure your doctor knows.
Sulphonamides and trimethoprim	Co-trimoxazole (Septrin)	Not suitable for pregnant women or babies under six weeks old. Make sure your doctor knows if you are breast feeding as these drugs should be used with caution.
Tetracyclines	Doxycycline Minocycline Oxytetracycline Tetracycline	Not suitable for pregnant women, nor for children under the age of 12. Make sure your doctor knows if you are breast feeding, as these drugs should be used with caution.
Other antibiotics	Erythromycin Metronidazole	 Around 25% of people will experience adverse effects including nausea, vomiting and headache if they drink alcohol while taking metronidazole.

III.ii DRUGS TO COMBAT PAIN

Group name	Examples	Notes
Non-narcotic analgesics	Aspirin Paracetamol	Aspirin should not be given to children under the age of 12.
Combinations of narcotic and non-narcotic analgesics	Co-proxamol Co-dydramol	These may make you drowsy. If they do, you should not drive or operate machinery.
Narcotics (opioids)	Codeine Morphine Diamorphine Pethidine	To be taken only under medical supervision as uncontrolled use could lead to addiction. They may cause drowsiness (see above), but if you need to take them regularly, the drowsiness usually wears off. They cause constipation. Your doctor will probably prescribe a laxative if you need to take a narcotic for any length of time.
Anti-inflammatory analgesics (NSAIDs)	Ibuprofen Naproxen Diclofenac Indomethacin	These irritate the stomach so should be taken with or just after food or a glass of milk. Not suitable for use during the last three months of pregnancy. Check with your doctor before taking them if you are breast feeding.
Local anaesthetics	Benzocaine Bupivacaine Lignocaine	Some patients may be particularly sensitive to certain drugs applied to the skin, so any adverse reactions should be reported to your doctor.

III.iii DRUGS TO REDUCE ACID SECRETIONS IN THE TREATMENT OF STOMACH OR DUODENAL ULCERS

Group name	Examples	Notes
H_2-receptor blockers	Cimetidine Ranitidine	If you are pregnant or breast feeding, tell your doctor before taking these drugs.

III.iv DRUGS PRESCRIBED FOR PEOPLE WITH CARDIOVASCULAR PROBLEMS (e.g. HIGH BLOOD PRESSURE, ANGINA)

Group name	Examples	Notes
Beta blockers	Atenolol Propranolol	Should not be taken during late pregnancy. Make sure your doctor knows if you are breast feeding. Not used in patients with asthma.
Diuretics	Amiloride Bendrofluazide Frusemide Hydrochlorothiazide	These increase the amount of urine you produce. Your doctor may not want you to take them if you are pregnant.
ACE inhibitors	Captopril Endopril Lisinopril	Should not be taken during pregnancy.
Nitrates	Glyceryl trinitrate (GTN) Isosorbide dinitrate Isosorbide mononitrate	Glyceryl trinitrate tablets deteriorate quickly once the bottle has been opened. A bottle should be discarded eight weeks after opening and a new supply obtained. GTN can be bought without a prescription. Nitrates sometimes cause headaches initially but this usually diminishes rapidly. Tell your doctor if the problem continues.
Calcium antagonists	Nifedipine Diltiazem Verapamil Amlodipine	Generally, these are not used during pregnancy. Some of these drugs should be used with caution during breast feeding, so make sure your doctor knows if you are.

III.v DRUGS PRESCRIBED FOR PEOPLE WITH RESPIRATORY PROBLEMS (e.g. ASTHMA)

Group name	Examples	Notes
Bronchodilators	Salbutamol Terbutaline	Correct use of inhalers is important. If you are not sure that your technique is correct, read the accompanying leaflet (if there is one) or ask your doctor or pharmacist.
Corticosteroids	Beclomethasone	Correct use of inhalers is important (see above). Corticosteroids need to be used regularly as their effect is to prevent asthma attacks rather than to produce immediate bronchodilation. Rinsing your mouth with water after using a steroid inhaler will reduce the risk of mouth infections due to yeast (Candida).

III.vi ANTIDEPRESSANTS AND SEDATIVES

Most of these drugs can cause drowsiness, and hypnotics taken at night can cause hang-over drowsiness the next day. Drinking alcohol will make drowsiness worse. If you are affected, you should not drive or operate machinery.

Group name	Examples	Notes
Hypnotics	Nitrazepam Temazepam	For treatment of insomnia on a short term basis only. The drugs lose their effectiveness quickly and there is risk of dependence (addiction) if they are used for more than a few weeks. If they are used for long periods, withdrawal may lead to insomnia and anxiety.
Anti-anxiety drugs	Diazepam Lorazepam	For short term use only – there is risk of dependence and problems with withdrawal (as with hypnotics, see above). Unsuitable for use in pregnancy.
Tricyclic antidepressants	Amitriptyline Dothiepin Lofepramine	Generally not recommended in late pregnancy. Some drugs are more sedative than others. Improvement in depression is not immediate; it usually takes 2–4 weeks and may take longer (e.g. 6 weeks). Improvement in sleep (sedative drugs only) should be immediate.
Monoamine oxidase inhibitors (MAOIs)	Phenelzine Tranylcypromine Isocarboxazid	MAOIs can react adversely with a number of common foods and over the counter medicines. Ask your doctor for detailed advice and check with your pharmacist before taking any other medicine.

III.vii CONTRACEPTIVE PREPARATIONS

Group name	Examples	Available as	Notes
Combined (oestrogen/ progestogen) pill	Eugynon Microgynon Ovran Ovranette	Tablets (usually 21 in pack for 28 day cycle)	Not suitable for all women – discuss with your doctor and read the leaflet in the pack.
Mini (progestogen only) pill	Microval Noriday	Tablets (28 in pack for 28 day cycle)	Not as reliable as the combined pill. Must be taken at the same time every day. Read the leaflet in the pack.
Spermicides	C-film Duragel Ortho-Creme Orthoforms	Film Gel Cream Pessaries	Should only be used in conjunction with a barrier method (condoms or diaphragm)

IMMUNISATIONS

IV.i IMMUNISATION SCHEDULE FOR INFANTS, CHILDREN AND YOUNG PEOPLE

Age	Immunisations given
Two months	First triple vaccine (diphtheria, pertussis, tetanus) Polio
Three months	Second triple vaccine (diphtheria, pertussis, tetanus) Polio
Four months	Third triple vaccine (diphtheria, pertussis, tetanus) Polio
12–18 months	MMR (measles, mumps, rubella)
School entry (4–5 years)	Diphtheria/tetanus booster Polio booster
10–14 years	BCG (tuberculosis) (Girls only) rubella * There should be an interval of at least 3 weeks between the BCG and rubella immunisations
15–18 years	Tetanus booster Polio booster

IV.ii IMMUNISATION FOR ADULTS

Tetanus

A booster dose 10 years after the primary course and again 10 years later maintains a satisfactory level of protection which will probably last throughout your lifetime. However, if you have a tetanus-prone wound such as a puncture wound or a cut that has been in contact with soil or manure, the doctor may consider a booster dose.

Rubella (German measles)

Vaccination is available to women of child-bearing age provided they are not pregnant. Any woman vaccinated against rubella is advised not to conceive for at least one month after the vaccination.

Influenza

Vaccination should be considered for elderly people and for children living in long stay hospitals and residential homes. Individual protection should be considered for those at special risk, for example individuals who suffer from any of the following conditions:

- Chronic lung disease;

- Chronic heart disease;

- Chronic renal disease;

- Diabetes mellitus;

- Conditions involving immunosuppressive therapies.

BCG (for tuberculosis)

It is recommended that the following groups be vaccinated with BCG provided they have not had a successful BCG vaccination previously and that a tuberculin skin test is negative:

- Health care personnel who are likely to come into contact with infectious patients;

- Veterinary and other staff who handle animal species known to be susceptible to tuberculosis;

- Contacts and close relatives of people known to be suffering from tuberculosis;

- Immigrants from countries where tuberculosis is prevalent;

- Those intending to stay in Africa, Asia, Central or South America for more than one month.

Hepatitis B

Vaccination against hepatitis B should be considered for the following groups of individuals:

- Family contacts of people with hepatitis B;

- Health care personnel;

- Police and members of the emergency services;

- Individuals visiting countries where hepatitis B is endemic;

- Haemophiliacs and others receiving regular blood transfusions or blood products.

Immunisation for travellers

For those travelling abroad immunisation against the following diseases may be recommended:

- Cholera;

- Malaria;

- Typhoid fever;

- Yellow fever.

Consult your doctor or travel agent if you think this could apply to you.

This information has been compiled from the Department of Health's *Immunisation Against Infectious Diseases*, 1990 edition.

PEOPLE AND RESOURCES

If you are caring for family members or friends in the community, or if you have health or other problems yourself, there are a number of sources from which you will be able to obtain help. These sources can be broadly grouped under three main headings:

- Health services;

- Social services;

- The voluntary sector.

Your main contacts with the health services will be through your local general practitioner and health centre, or perhaps directly with a hospital. Community health services will be co-ordinated from the health centre, as shown in the table (on the right), while more complex problems will be dealt with in hospital. The ways in which contact with

The health centre/doctors' surgery

Community health services are co-ordinated from here. The staff are likely to include the following:
- Receptionist
- General practitioner
- Practice nurse
- District nurse
- Community psychiatric nurse
- Specialist nurse (e.g. diabetic specialist nurse, continence adviser)
- Health visitor
- Community midwife
Some health centres also include a dentist and dental assistant.

hospital are initiated and maintained are illustrated (below).

GOING TO HOSPITAL

First point of contact	Referred on to
Outpatient department (referred by general practitioner)	Departments where investigations are undertaken (e.g. x-ray)
	Medical wards
Accident and emergency department/casualty (self-referral or ambulance)	Surgical wards
	Treatments
	Operating theatre
	Discharge into community
Obstetric/midwifery services (usually in partnership with general practitioner and community midwife – see Chapter 4)	Antenatal clinic/ward
	Labour ward
	Postnatal wards
	Special care baby unit (SCBU)
	Discharge into community

SOCIAL SERVICES

Your local Department of Social Services is responsible for many services including the following:

- Social workers;

- Home helps;

- Meals on wheels;

- Arranging residential care;

- Laundry services.

Readers should be aware, however, that availability of these services is likely to vary from one area to another.

THE VOLUNTARY SECTOR

Resources offered by the voluntary sector include:

- Citizens' Advice Bureaux;

- Charitable organisations and agencies (see Appendix VII for a list of useful addresses);

- The Macmillan Nursing Service;

- The Women's Royal Voluntary Service (WRVS).

If you feel you need some sort of help but are not quite sure where to begin, it might be best to start by talking to your family doctor and paying a visit (between 10 am and 2 pm) to your local Citizens' Advice Bureau.

BENEFITS

There are a number of different benefits to which you may be entitled, depending on your situation. Sorting out exactly what is due to you may be quite complicated and it is always worth starting with a visit to your local Citizens' Advice Bureau. The staff at these bureaux are well versed in all the Welfare Benefits likely to be appropriate and they are usually very helpful about pointing you in a direction which enables you to find out the information you need. Another useful source of information is DSS Leaflet FB2 Which Benefit, (available in a number of different languages as FB22) which you can pick up from your Post Office, local Social Security Office or Citizens' Advice Bureau.

The chart below gives brief information about the benefits, loans and allowances to which you may be entitled. It must be stressed that such information serves as an introduction only, but it is to be hoped that it will enable you to find out more.

If you are . . .	You may be entitled to . . .	For further information . . .
On a low income	Income Support Cash help while working Housing Benefit Help with your Community Charge A loan or grant from the Social Fund Family Credit	See DSS Leaflet IS1 See DSS Leaflet FB4 See DSS Leaflet RR1 See DSS Leaflet CCB1 See DSS Leaflets SB16 and SFL2 See DSS Leaflet FC10 and Claim Pack FC1

Pregnant	Statutory Maternity Pay
	Maternity Allowance
	A Maternity Payment from the Social
	    Fund if on Income Support or Family
	    Credit
		See DSS Leaflets FB8 and NI17A
		
		See DSS Leaflets SB16 and SFL2

Looking after one or more children
 	
– as a single
   parent
 	
– as a guardian
 	
– looking after
   a disabled child
	Child Benefit
	
	One Parent Benefit
	Widowed Mother's Allowance
	
	Guardian's Allowance
	
	Attendance Allowance
	Mobility Allowance
	Severe Disablement Allowance
		See DSS Leaflet CH1
		
		See DSS Leaflet CH11
		See DSS Leaflet NP45
		
		See DSS Leaflet NI14
		
		See Claim Pack OS2
		See DSS Leaflet NI211
		See DSS Leaflet NI252
		
		See also DSS Leaflets FB8 (Babies
		   and Benefits) and FB27 (Bringing
		   up Children?)

Looking after a sick or disabled adult at home	Invalid Care Allowance A loan or grant from the Social Fund if on Income Support	See DSS Leaflet DS700 See DSS Leaflets SB16 and SFL2

continued next page

If you are . . .	You may be entitled to . . .	For further information . . .
Sick, disabled or injured yourself	Statutory Sick Pay	See DSS Leaflet NI244
	Sickness Benefit	See DSS Leaflet NI16
	Invalidity Benefit	See DSS Leaflet NI16A
	Mobility Allowance	See DSS Leaflet NI211
	Severe Disablement Allowance	See DSS Leaflet NI252
	Attendance Allowance	See Claim Pack OS2
	Constant Attendance Allowance	See DSS Leaflet NI205
	Industrial Injuries Disablement Benefit	See DSS Leaflet NI6
		See also DSS Leaflet FB28 (Sick or Disabled?)
Elderly	Retirement Pension or	See DSS Leaflet NP46
	Over 80 Pension	See DSS Leaflet NI184
	Income Support	See DSS Leaflet IS1
	Housing Benefit	See DSS Leaflet RR1
	Help with your Community Charge	See DSS Leaflet CCB1
	A Cold Weather Payment from the Social Fund if on Income Support	See DSS Leaflet CWP1
		See also DSS Leaflet FB6 (Retiring?)
Widowed or recently bereaved	Widow's Pension	
	Widow's Payment	See DSS Leaflet NP45
	Widowed Mother's Allowance	
	A one-off payment from the Social Fund to help you pay for the funeral if on Income Support or Family Credit	See Form SF200
		See also DSS Leaflet D49

You may also find one or more of the following leaflets helpful.

DSS Leaflet No.	Title
IS26	Income Support if you are under 18
FB23	Young People's Guide to Social Security (16–18)
FB30	Self-Employed?
N12	Industrial Disease
FB8	Unemployed?
NI12	Unemployment Benefit
IS50	Income Support for People in Residential Care/Nursing Homes
CCB2	Community Charge in Different Languages
AB11	Help with NHS Costs
D11	Dental Treatment NHS
G11	NHS Sight Tests and Glasses
H11	NHS Hospital Travel Costs
P11	NHS Prescriptions
NI246	How to Appeal

ADDRESSES OF USEFUL ORGANISATIONS AND SUPPORT GROUPS

Accept Clinic (advice centre for people with drinking/tranquillizer problems)
724 Fulham Road, London SW6 5SE;
Tel 071-371 7477

Action Against Allergy
24–26 High Street, Hampton Hill, Middlesex
TW12 1PD

Action for Dysphasic Adults
Canterbury House, 1 Royal Street,
London SE1 7LN;
Tel 071-261 9572

Action for Victims of Medical Accidents
24 Southwick Street, London SE1 1TY;
Tel 081-291 2793

Action on Smoking and Health (ASH)
109 Gloucester Place, London W1H 3PH;
Tel 071-935 3519

Advice and Rights Centre for the Handicapped (ARCH)
90 Upper Street, London N1;
Tel 071-359 6535

Age Concern
Astral House, 1268 London Road,
London SW16 4ER;
Tel 081-679 8000
• *Many local groups – see your phone book*

Al-Anon (for relatives)
61 Great Dover Street, London SE1 4YF;
Tel 071-403 0888

Alcohol Concern
305 Grays Inn Road, London WC1X 8QF;
Tel 071-833 3471

Alcoholics Anonymous (General Services Office)
PO Box 1 Stonebow House, York YO1 2NJ;
Tel 0904 644026
• *Many local groups – see your phone book*

Alzheimer's Disease Society
158–160 Balham High Road, London
SW12 9BN;
Tel 081-675 6550/7/8/9

Amarant Trust (clinic/advice centre for HRT and menopause)
80 Lambeth Road, London SE1 7PP;
Tel 071-401 3855

Anorexia and Bulimia Nervosa Association
Annexe C, Tottenham Town Hall,
Town Hall Road, London N15 4RX;
Tel 081-885 3936

Anthony Nolan Bone Marrow Trust
The Royal Free Hospital, Pond Street,
London NW3 2QG;
Tel 071-431 5306

Arthritis and Rheumatism Council
41 Eagle Street, London WC1R 4AR;
Tel 071-405 8575

Arthritis Care
5 Grosvenor Crescent, London SW1X 7EE;
Tel 071-235 0902

Association for all Speech-Impaired Children (AFASIC)
347 Central Market, Smithfield,
London EC1A 9NH;
Tel 071-236 3632

Association for Continence Advice
c/o Disabled Living Foundation,
380 Harrow Road, London W9 2HU;
Tel 071-266 2059

Association for Improvements in the Maternity Services (AIMS)
21 Iver Lane, Iver, Bucks SL0 9LH;
Tel 0753 652781

Association for Postnatal Illness
25 Jerdan Place, London SW6 1BE;
Tel 071-386 0868

Association for Spina Bifida and Hydrocephalus (ASBAH)
22 Upper Woburn Place, London WC2H 0EP;
Tel 071-388 1382
• *Many local groups – see your phone book*

Association for the Prevention of Addiction
37–39 Great Guildford Street,
London SE1 0ES;
Tel 071-620 1919

Association of Breast Feeding Mothers
10 Herschell Road, London SE23 1EG;
Tel 081-778 4769

Association of Community Health Councils for England and Wales
30 Drayton Park, London N5 1PB;
Tel 071-609 8405
• *See under 'Health Authority' in your local phone book for the address of your Community Health Council*

Association of Hypnotists and Psychotherapists
12 Cross Street, Nelson, Lancashire BB9 7EN;
Tel 0282 699378

Association of Radical Midwives
8A The Drive, Wimbledon, London SW20;
Tel 081-540 2040

Asthma Society
300 Upper Street, London N1 2XX;
Tel 071-226 2260

Back Pain Association
31–33 Park Lane, Teddington, Middlesex TW11 0AB;
Tel 081-977 5474

Baby Life Support Systems (BLISS)
17–21 Emerald Street, London WC1N 3QL;
Tel 071-831 8996
• *Ask your SCBU/health visitor if there is a local group*

Barnardos
Tanners Lane, Ilford, Essex IG6 1QG;
Tel 081-550 8822

Body Positive (HIV self-help group)
51b Philbeach Gardens, London SW5 9EB;
Tel 071-835 1045

BREAK (Holidays for the elderly)
20 Hooks Hill Road, Sheringham, Norfolk NR26 8NL;
Tel 0263 823170

Breast Care and Mastectomy Association
15–19 Britten Street, London SW3 3TZ;
Tel 071-867 8275 (admin);
071-867 1103 (helpline)

Bristol Cancer Help Centre
Grove House, Cornwallis Grove, Clifton, Bristol BS8 4PG;
Tel 0272 743216

British Acupuncture Association
34 Alderney Street, London SW1V 4EU;
Tel 071-834 1012

British Agencies for Adoption and Fostering
11 Southwark Street, London SE1 1RQ;
Tel 071-407 8800

British Association for Cancer United Patients (BACUP)
121 Charterhouse Street,
London EC1M 6AA;
Tel 071-608 1785 (admin);
071-608 1038 (counselling service)

British Association for Counselling
1 Regent Place, Rugby, Warwickshire
CV21 3BX;
Tel 0788 578328

British Chiropractic Association
Premier House, 10 Greycoat Place,
London SW1P 1SB;
Tel 071-222 8866

British Colostomy Association
15 Station Road, Reading RG1 1LG;
Tel 0734 391537

British Council for the Rehabilitation of the Disabled
25 Mortimer Street, London W1;
Tel 071-637 5400

British Deaf Association
38 Victoria Place, Carlisle, Cumbria
CA1 1HU;
Tel 0288 28719

British Diabetic Association
10 Queen Anne Street, London W1M 0BD;
Tel 071-323 1531

British Dietetic Association
Daimler House, Paradise Circus, Queensway,
Birmingham B1 2BJ;
Tel 021-643 5483

British Epilepsy Association
Anstey House, 40 Hanover Square,
Leeds LS3 1BE;
Tel 0532 439393

British Heart Foundation
41 Fitzhardinge Street, London W1 4DH;
Tel 071-935 0185
• *Many local groups – see your phone book*

British Holistic Medical Association
179 Gloucester Place, London NW1 6DX;
Tel 071-262 5299

British Institute of Mental Handicap
Wolverhampton Road, Kidderminster,
Worcester DY10 3PP;
Tel 0562 850251

British Kidney Patients' Association
Bordon, Hampshire;
Tel 0420 472021

British Medical Acupuncture Society
77–79 Chancery Lane, London WC2

British Migraine Association
178A High Road, Byfleet, Weybridge, Surrey
KT14 7ED;
Tel 0932 52468

British Nutrition Foundation
15 Belgrave Square, London SW1X 8PS;
Tel 071-235 4904

British Polio Fellowship
Bell Close, West End Road, Ruislip,
Middlesex HA4 5LP;
Tel 0895 75515

British Pregnancy Advisory Service (BPAS)
Ansty Manor, Wooten Warren, Solihull,
West Midlands B95 6DA;
Tel 0564 793225
• *Many local centres – see your phone book*

British Psychological Society
St Andrew's House, 48 Princess Road East,
Leicester LE1 7DR;
Tel 0533 549568

British Red Cross Society
9 Grosvenor Crescent, London SW1X 7EJ;
Tel 071-235 5454
• *Many local groups – see your phone book*

British Sports Association for the Disabled (BSAD)
Hayward House, Barnard Crescent,
Aylesbury, Bucks HP21 9PP;
Tel 0296 27889

The Brittle Bone Society
c/o Mrs MTJ Grant, Ward 8,
Strathmartin Hospital, Strathmartin,
Dundee DD3 0PG;
Tel 0382 817771

Brook Advisory Centre
153a East Street, London SE17 2SD;
Tel 071-708 1234
• *Many local centres – see your phone book*

**Cancer Aftercare and Rehabilitation Society
(CARE)**
21 Zetland Road, Bristol BS6 7AH;
Tel 0272 427419

Cancer Care Marie Curie
28 Belgrave Square, London SW1X 8QG;
Tel 071-235 3325

Cancer Link
17 Britannia Street, London WC1X 9JN;
Tel 071-833 2451

Cancer Relief Macmillan Fund
15–19 Britten Street, London SW3 3TZ;
Tel 071-351 7811

Cancer Research Campaign
2 Carlton House Terrace, London SW1Y 5AF;
Tel 071-930 8972

Carers' National Association
29 Chilworth Mews, London W2 3RG;
Tel 071-724 7776

Charity Search
25 Portview Road, Avonmouth,
Bristol BS11 9LD;
Tel 0272 824060 (10am–2pm)

Chartered Society of Physiotherapy
14 Bedford Row, London WC1R 4ED;
Tel 071-242 1941

Chest, Heart and Stroke Association
CHSA House, 123–127 Whitecross Street,
London EC1Y 8JJ;
Tel 071-490 7999

Child Development Research Unit
University of Nottingham,
University Park Road,
Nottingham NG7 2RD

Childline
2nd Floor, Royal Mail Building, Studd Street,
London N1 0QR;
Tel 071-359 9090 (admin);
0800 1111 (helpline)

Child Poverty Action Group
1–5 Bath Street, London EC1V 9PY;
Tel 071-253 3406

Children's Society
Edward Rudolph House, Margery Street,
London WC1X 0JL;
Tel 071-837 4299

Cleft Lip and Palate Association
Dental Department, The Hospital for Sick
Children, Great Ormond Street,
London WC1N 3HJ;
Tel 071-405 9200

Coeliac Society
PO Box 220, High Wycombe,
Buckinghamshire HP11 2HY;
Tel 0494 37278

Colostomy Welfare Group
2nd Floor, 38–39 Eccleston Square,
London SW1V 1PB;
Tel 071-825 9244

Combat Care Home
Theydon Road, Theydon Bois, Epping,
Essex CM16 4DY;
Tel 0378 77588

Commission for Equal Opportunities
Overseas House, Quay Street,
Manchester M3 3HN;
Tel 061-833 9244

Commission for Racial Equality
Elliot House, 10–12 Allington Street,
London SW1E 5EH;
Tel 071-828 7022

**Community Health Councils (advice and
help for users of the NHS)**
• *See under 'Health Authority' in your local phone
book for the address of your Community Health
Council*

Compassionate Friends (support group for bereaved parents)
6 Denmark Street, Bristol BS1 5DG;
Tel 0272 292778

Consumers' Association
2 Marylebone Road, London NW1 4DX;
Tel 071-486 5544

Counsel and Care (advice and help for older people)
Twyman House, 16 Bonny Street,
London NW1 7PG;
Tel 071-485 1550

Coronary Artery Disease Association
Tavistock House North, Tavistock Square,
London WC1H 9TH;
Tel 071-387 9779

Coronary Prevention Group
Central Middlesex Hospital, Acton Lane,
London NW10;
Tel 081-965 5733

Crossroads Care
10 Regent Place, Rugby, Warwickshire
CV21 2PN;
Tel 0788 73653
• *Many local groups – see your phone book*

Crusaid (hardship fund for people with AIDS)
21 Upper Tachbrook Street,
London SW1V 1SN;
Tel 071-834 7566

CRUSE (national association for the widowed and their children)
Cruse House, 126 Sheen Road, Richmond,
Surrey TW9 1UR;
Tel 081-940 4818

CRY-SIS (support group for parents of crying babies)
BM CRY-SIS, London WC1N 3XX;
Tel 071-404 5011
• *Ask your health visitor if there is a local group*

Cystic Fibrosis Research Trust
5 Blyth Road, Bromley, Kent BR1 3RS;
Tel 081-464 7211

Department of Health
Richmond House, 79 Whitehall,
London SW1;
Tel 071-210 5983/3000

Depressives Associated
PO Box 5, Castle Town, Portland, Dorset
DT5 1BQ

Disability Alliance
Universal House, 88 Wentworth Street,
London E1 7SA;
Tel 071-247 8776

Disability Now
12 Park Crescent, London W1N 4EQ;
Tel 071-636 5020

Disabled Living Foundation (information service for the disabled)
380–384 Harrow Road, London W9 2HU;
Tel 071-289 6111

Disfigurement Guidance Centre
PO Box 7, Cupar, Fife KY15 4PF

Divorce Conciliation and Advisory Service
Shaftesbury Centre, Percy Street,
Swindon SN2 2AZ;
Tel 0793 514055

Down's Babies Association
Quinbourne Community Centre,
Ridgeacre Road, Quinton,
Birmingham BR3 2TU;
Tel 021-428 1003

Down's Syndrome Association
153 Mitcham Road, Tooting, London
SW17 9PG;
Tel 081-682 4001

Drink Crisis Centre
124 Brook Drive, London SE11 4TQ;
Tel 071-820 9947

Duke of Edinburgh Award Scheme
5 Prince of Wales Terrace, London W8 5PG;
Tel 071-937 5205

Eating Disorders Association
Sackville Place, 44–48 Magdalen Street,
Norwich, Norfolk NR3 1JE;
Tel 0603 621414

Emergency Bed Service
28 London Bridge Street, London SE1 9SG;
Tel 071-407 7181

Endometriosis Society
245a Coldharbour Lane, Brixton,
London SW9 8RR;
Tel 071-737 0380

EXTEND (movement to music for the over 60s and handicapped people of all ages)
1A North Street, Sheringham,
Norfolk NR26 8LJ;
Tel 0263 822479

Families Anonymous (friends and relatives of people who misuse drugs)
310 Finchley Road, London NW3 7AG;
Tel 071-431 3537

Family Planning Association (FPA)
Margaret Pyke House,
27–35 Mortimer Street,
London W1N 7RJ;
Tel 071-636 7866

Family Rights Group
The Print House, 18 Ashwin Street,
London E8 3DL;
Tel 071-923 2628

Family Welfare Association
501 Kingsland Road, Dalston,
London E8 4AU;
Tel 071-254 6251

Foresight (association for the promotion of preconceptual care)
The Old Vicarage, Church Lane, Witley,
Godalming, Surrey;
Tel 0428 684500

Foundation for the Study of Infant Deaths (cot death research and support)
35 Belgrave Square, London SW1X 8QB;
Tel 071-235 1721

Friedreich's Ataxia Group
The Common, Cranleigh, Surrey GU6 8SB;
Tel 0483 272741

Frontliners (help for people with AIDS)
c/o Mildmay Mission Hospital,
Hackney Road, London E2 7NA;
Tel 071-256 0407

Gamblers Anonymous
PO Box 88, London SW10 0EU;
Tel 081-741 4181

Gay Bereavement Project
The Vaughan M Williams Centre,
Colindale Hospital, Colindale Avenue,
London NW9 5GH;
Tel 081-200 0511

Gay and Lesbian Switchboard
Tel 071-837 7324

General Council and Register of Osteopaths
56 London Street, Reading, Berkshire;
Tel 0734 576585

General Medical Council
44 Hallam Street, London W1N 6AE;
Tel 071-580 7642

Gingerbread (association for one parent families)
35 Wellington Street, London WC2E 7BN;
Tel 071-240 0953

GRACE (Mrs Gould's residential advisory centre for the elderly)
PO Box 71, Cobham, Surrey KT11 2JR;
Tel 0923 62928

Haemophilia Society
123 Westminster Bridge Road,
London SE1 7HR;
Tel 071-928 2020

Handicapped Adventure Playground Association (HAPA)
HAPA Office, Fulham Palace,
Bishops Avenue, London SW6 6EA;
Tel 071-736 4443

HEADWAY (national head injuries association)
7 King Edward Court, King Edward Street,
Nottingham NG1 1EW;
Tel 0602 240800

Health and Safety Executive
Baynards House, 1 Chepstow Place,
Westbourne Grove, London W2 4TF;
Tel 071-221 0870

Health Education Authority
Hamilton House, Mabledon Place,
London WC1 9BD;
Tel 071-276 3000

Health Visitors' Association
50 Southwark Street, London SE1 1UN;
Tel 071-378 7255

Help for Health (patient care information service)
Wessex Regional Library Unit,
South Academic Block,
Southampton General Hospital,
Southampton SO9 1XY;
Tel 0703 777222

Help the Aged
16–18 St James's Walk, London EC1R 0BE;
Tel 071-253 0253
• *Many local groups – see your phone book*

Holiday Care Service
2 Old Bank Chambers, Station Road, Horley,
Surrey RH6 9HW;
Tel 0293 774535

Hospice Information Service
St Christopher's Hospice,
51–59 Lawrie Park Road, Sydenham,
London SE26 6DZ;
Tel 081-778 9252

Hyperactive Children's Support Group
c/o Sally Bundy, 59 Meadowside, Angmering,
West Sussex BN16 4BW

Hysterectomy Support Group
c/o Anne Webb, 11 Henryson Road, Brockley,
London SE4 1HL;
Tel 081-690 5987

Ileostomy Association
79 Blackscotch Lane, Mansfield,
Nottinghamshire NG18 4PF;
Tel 0623 28099

Imperial Cancer Research Fund
PO Box 123, Lincolns Inn Fields,
London WC2A 3PX;
Tel 071-242 0200
• *Many local groups – see your phone book*

Incest Crisis Line
Tel 071-890 4732/01; 071-422 5100

Institute of Complementary Medicine
21 Portland Place, London W1N 3AF;
Tel 071-636 9543

Institute for the Study of Drug Dependency
1 Hatton Place, London EC1N 8ND;
Tel 071-430 1991

Institute of Child Health
30 Guildford Street, London WC1N 1EH;
Tel 071-242 9789

Institute of Medical Ethics
Tavistock House North, Tavistock Square,
London WC1;
Tel 071-387 8132

Institute of Neurology
The National Hospital, Queen Square,
London WC1N 3BG;
Tel 071-837 3611

Institute of Policy Research
8 Wilfred Street, London SW1E 6PL;
Tel 071-828 1540

Institute of Psychiatry
The Maudsley Hospital, De Crespigny Park,
London SE5;
Tel 071-703 5411

Invalid Children Aid Nationwide (ICAN)
10 Bowling Green Lane, London EC1R 0BD;
Tel 071-253 9111

Invalids at Home
23 Farm Avenue, London NW2 2BJ

Jewish Care
221 Golders Green Road,
London NW11 9DZ;
Tel 081-458 3282

Keep Able – The Catalogue
Fleming Close, Park Farm, Wellingborough,
Northants NN8 3UF;
Tel 0993 679426

**Kielder Adventure Centre (special provision
for children with a physical disability)**
Low Craneclough, Kielder Water, Falstone,
Hexham, Northumberland;
Tel 0660 50232

King George's Fund for Sailors
1 Chesham Street, London SW1H 9BZ;
Tel 071-235 2884

**Lady Hoare Trust for Physically Disabled
Children (associated with arthritis care)**
Mitre House, 44–6 Fleet Street,
London EC4Y 1BN;
Tel 071-583 1951

**La Leche League (information, support and
counselling for breast feeding mothers)**
B M 3424, London WC1N 3XX;
Tel 071-242 1278
• *Ask your health visitor if there is a local group*

**Let's Face It (support group for people who
have had disfiguring facial surgery)**
10 Wood End, Crowthorn,
Berkshire RG11 6DQ;
Tel 0344 774405

Leonard Cheshire Foundation
26 Maunsel Street, London SW1P 2QN;
Tel 071-828 1822

Leukaemia Care Society
14 Kingfisher Court, Vennybridge,
Pinhoe, Exeter EX4 8JN;
Tel 0392 64848

Liberty (national council for civil liberties)
Tabard Street, London SE1 4LA;
Tel 071-403 3888

Macmillan Cancer Relief
Anchor House, 15–19 Britten Street,
London SW3 3TY;
Tel 071-351 7811
• *Ask at your health centre for details of local
branches*

Malcolm Sargent Cancer Fund for Children
14 Abingdon Road, London W8 6AF;
Tel 071-937 4548

**Marcé Society (an international society for
the understanding, prevention and treatment
of mental illness related to childbirth)**
Secretary: Dr Trevor Friedman,
Leicester General Hospital,
Gwendolen Road, Leicester, LE5 4PW;
Tel 0533 490490

Marie Stopes House (Well Woman Centre)
108 Whitfield Street, London W1P 6BE;
Tel 071-388 0662

Mastectomy Association
15–19 Britten Street, London SW3 3TZ;
Tel 071-867 8275; 071-867 1103 (helpline)

Maternity Alliance
15 Britannia Street, London WC1;
Tel 071-837 1265

Medic-Alert Foundation
12/15b Caledonian Road, London N1 9UU;
Tel 071-833 3034

**MENCAP (national society for children and
adults with a mental handicap)**
123 Golden Lane, London EC1Y 0RT;
Tel 071-454 0454
• *Many local branches – see your phone book*

Mental After Care Association
Bainbridge House, Bainbridge Street,
London WC1A 1HP;
Tel 071-436 6194

Mental Health Act Commission
Hepburn House, Marsham Street,
London SW1;
Tel 071-217 6016

Mental Patients' Union (for patients detained against their will)
12 Kings Court, Barry Road,
London SE22 0JB

Migraine Trust
45 Great Ormond Street,
London WC1N 3HZ;
Tel 071-278 2676

MIND (national association for mental health)
22 Harley Street, London W1N 2ED;
Tel 071-637 0741
- *Many local branches – see your phone book*

Miscarriage Association
c/o Clayton Hospital, Northgate, Wakefield,
West Yorkshire WF1 3JS;
Tel 0924 830515
- *Many local branches – see your phone book*

Motor Neurone Disease Association
PO Box 246, Northampton NN1 2PR;
Tel 0604 250505;
Linkline/helpline 0800 626262

Multiple Births Foundation
c/o Dr Elizabeth Bryan, Queen Charlotte's
and Chelsea Hospital, Goldhawk Road,
London W6 0XJ;
Tel 071-748 4666

Multiple Sclerosis Society
25 Effie Road, Fulham, London SW6 1EE;
Tel 071-736 6267
- *Many local groups – see your phone book*

Muscular Dystrophy Group
Nattrass House, 35 Macaulay Road,
London SW4 0QP;
Tel 071-720 8055

Myalgic Encephalitis Society
PO Box 8, Stanford-le-Hope, Essex SS17 8EX;
Tel 0375 642466

Narcotics Society
PO Box 246, London SW1

National Advisory Centre on the Battered Child
Denver House, The Drive,
Bounds Green Road, London N11

National AIDS Trust
286 Euston Road, London NW1 3DN;
Tel 071-383 4246

National Ankylosing Spondylitis Society
5 Grosvenor Crescent, London SW1X 7EE;
Tel 071-235 9585

National Association for Gifted Children
1 South Audley Street, London W1Y 5DG;
Tel 071-499 1188

National Association for Maternal and Child Welfare
46 Osnaburgh Street, London NW1 3ND;
Tel 071-383 4115

National Association for the Childless
318 Summer Lane, Birmingham BR19 3RL;
Tel 021-388 2153

National Association for the Welfare of Children in Hospital
Argyle House, 29–31 Euston Road,
London NW1 2SD;
Tel 071-833 2041

National Association of Bereavement Services
68 Chalton Street, London NW1 1JR;
Tel 071-388 2153

National Association of Citizens' Advice Bureaux (NACAB)
Myddleton House, 115 Pentonville Road,
London N1 9LZ;
Tel 071-833 2181
- *See your phone book, under 'Citizens' Advice Bureaux' for the address of your local CAB*

National Association of Disablement Information and Advice Services (DIAL UK)
Victoria Buildings, 117 High Street,
Clay Cross, Derbyshire S45 9DZ;
Tel 0246 864498

National Association of Laryngectomy Clubs
11 Elvaston Place, London SW7 5QG;
Tel 071-581 3023

National Association of Victim Support Schemes
Cranmer House, 39 Brixton Road,
London SW9 6DZ;
Tel 071-735 9166

National Asthma Campaign
300 Upper Street, London N1 2XX;
Tel 071-226 2260

National Autistic Society
276 Willesden Lane, London NW2 5RB;
Tel 081-451 1114

National Blood Transfusion Service
Tel 0800 300 333

National Caesarean Support Campaign
c/o Sue Johnson, 11 Duke Street, Astley,
Manchester M29 7BG

National Care Homes Association
5 Bloomsbury Place, London WC1 2QA;
Tel 071-436 1871

National Childbirth Trust (NCT)
Alexandra House, Oldham Terrace,
London W3 6NH;
Tel 081-992 8637
• *Many local branches – see your phone book*

National Council for the Divorced and Separated
41 Summit Avenue, London NW9 0TH;
Tel 081-205 8316

National Council for One Parent Families
255 Kentish Town Road, London NW5 2LX;
Tel 081-267 1361

National Deaf-Blind and Rubella Association (SENSE)
311 Grays Inn Road, London WC1X 8PT;
Tel 071-278 1005

National Deaf Children's Society
45 Hereford Road, London W2 5AH;
Tel 071-229 9272

National Eczema Society
Tavistock House East, Tavistock Square,
London WC1H 9SR;
Tel 071-388 4097

National Federation of Kidney Patients' Associations
Acorn Lodge, Woodsets, Nr Worksop, Notts
S81 8AT; Tel 0909 487795

National Institute of Medical Herbalists
41 Hatherley Road, Winchester,
Hants SO22 6RR; Tel 0962 68776

National Kidney Research Fund
42 Lower Marsh, London SE1 7RG;
Tel 071-928 5058

National Osteoporosis Society
1 Riverside, PO Box 10, Radstock,
Bath BA3 3YB; Tel 0761 431472

National Schizophrenia Fellowship
28 Castle Street, Kingston upon Thames
KT1 1SS; Tel 081-547 3937
• *Many local groups – see your phone book*

National Society for Epilepsy
Chalfont Centre for Epilepsy,
Chalfont St Peter, Gerrards Cross,
Bucks SL9 0RJ;
Tel 0240 73991

National Society for PKU and Allied Disorders
26 Towngate Grove, Mirfield, West Yorkshire

National Society for the Prevention of Cruelty to Children (NSPCC)
67 Saffron Hill, London EC1N 8RS;
Tel 071-242 1626/071-404 4447
• *Many local groups – see your phone book*

National Toy Libraries Association
68 Churchway, London NW1 1LT;
Tel 071-387 9592

National Family Planning Centre
Queen Elizabeth Medical Centre, Edgbaston,
Birmingham B15 2TG
Tel 021-472 1311

Nippers (information and support for parents of premature and sick newborns)
c/o Sue Lawley, 12A Beatty Road,
London N16 8EB;
Tel 081-241 0398
- *Ask your SCBU/health visitor if there is a local group*

Nutrition Society
Grosvenor Gardens House,
35–37 Grosvenor Gardens, London SW1 0BS

Open University
Milton Keynes, Buckinghamshire MK7 6AA;
Tel 0908 27066

Parents Anonymous (for parents who fear they may batter their children)
6 Manor Gardens, London N7
Tel 071-263 8918

Parents for Safe Food
102 Gloucester Place, London W1H 3DA;
Tel 071-981 5676

Parents of Murdered Children Support Group (part of Compassionate Friends)
c/o 10 Eastern Avenue, Prittlewell, Southend,
Essex SS2 5QU;
Tel 0702 68510

Parkinson's Disease Society
22 Upper Woburn Place, London WC1H 0RA;
Tel 071-383 3513

Partially Sighted Society
Queens Road, Doncaster, South Yorkshire
DN1 2NX

Patients' Association
18 Victoria Square, London E2 9PF;
Tel 081-981 5676

PETS (Pre-eclamptic toxaemia society)
c/o Dawn James, Ty Iago, High Street,
Llanbers, Gwynedd LL5B 4HB;
Tel 0286 872477

Phobic Society
4 Cheltenham Road, Chorlton-cum-Hardy,
Manchester M21 1QN;
Tel 061-881 1937

Phoenix House (drug dependency)
1 Eliot Bank, London SE23 3XE;
Tel 081-407 2789

Physically Handicapped and Able-Bodied (PHAB)
Tavistock House North, Tavistock Square,
London WC1H 9HX;
Tel 071-338 1963

Positively Women (for women with HIV)
5 Sebastian Street, London EC1V 0HE;
Tel 071-407 5501

Pregnancy Advisory Service (PAS)
11–13 Charlotte Street, London W1P 1HD;
Tel 071-637 8962

Pre-School Playgroups Association
61–63 Kings Cross Road, London WC1X 9LL;
Tel 071-833 0991

Psoriasis Association
7 Milton Street, Northampton NN2 7JG;
Tel 0604 711129

Psychiatric Rehabilitation Association
1 Bayford Mews, Bayford Street, London E8;
Tel 081-985 3570

Rape Crisis Cente
PO Box 69, London WC1X 9NJ;
Tel 071-837 1600
- *Many local centres – see your phone book*

Raynauds and Scleroderma Association
112 Crewe Road, Alsager, Cheshire ST7 2JA;
Tel 0270 872776

RELATE (national marriage guidance council)
Herbert Gray College, Little Church Street,
Rugby, Warwickshire;
Tel 0788 573241
- *Many local centres – see your phone book*

Release (for people addicted to drugs)
388 Old Street, London EC1V 9LT;
Tel 071-729 9904/603 8654

Renal Society
64 South Hill Park, London NW3 2SJ

Retirement and Nursing Home Advisory Service
Cain and Paton, 4 Ives Close, Aldersey Road, Guildford, Surrey GU1 2ET;
Tel 0483 578160

Royal Association for Disability and Rehabilitation (RADAR)
25 Mortimer Street, London W1N 8AB;
Tel 071-637 5400

Royal Association in Aid of the Deaf and Dumb
27 Old Oak Road, London W3 7SL;
Tel 081-743 6187

Royal College of Midwives
15 Mansfield Street, London W1M 0BE;
Tel 071-580 6523

Royal College of Nursing
20 Cavendish Square, London W1M 0AB;
Tel 071-409 3333

Royal National Institute for the Blind (RNIB)
22 Great Portland Street, London W1A 4XX;
Tel 071-388 1266
• *Many local groups – see your phone book*

Royal National Institute for the Deaf (RNID)
105 Gower Street, London WC1E 6AH;
Tel 071-387 8033

Royal Scottish Society for the Prevention of Cruelty to Children
Melville House, 41 Polwarth Terrace, Edinburgh EH11 1NU;
Tel 031-337 8539

Royal Society for the Prevention of Accidents (RoSPA)
Cannon House, The Priory, Queensway, Birmingham B4 6BS;
Tel 021-200 2641

St John Ambulance Association
1 Grosvenor Crescent, London SW1X 7EE;
Tel 071-235 5231
• *Many local groups – see your phone book*

Salvation Army
101 Queen Victoria Street, London EC4;
Tel 071-236 5222
• *Many local centres – see your phone book*

Samaritans Incorporated
10 The Grove, Slough, Berkshire SL1 1QP; Tel 0753 532713
• *Many local groups – see your phone book*

Schizophrenia Association
Bryn Hyfryd, The Crescent, Bangor, Gwynedd LL57 2AG;
Tel 0248 354048

Scoliosis Association
380–84 Harrow Road, London W9 2HU;
Tel 071-289 5652

Sickle Cell Society
54 Station Road, London NW10 4UA;
Tel 081-961 4006

Society of Compassionate Friends (parents who have lost a child)
6 Denmark Street, Bristol, BS1 5DQ;
Tel 0272 292778

Spastics Society
12 Park Crescent, London W1N 4EQ;
Tel 071-387 9571
• *Many local groups – see your phone book*

Spinal Injuries Association
76 St James' Lane, London N10;
Tel 081-444 2121

Spinal Muscular Atrophy (Jennifer Macaulay Trust for SMA)
11 Ashtree Close, Wellesbourne, Warwick;
Tel 0789 842377

SPOD (society to aid personal and sexual relationships of disabled people)
286 Camden Road, London N7 0BJ;
Tel 071-607 8851

SSAFA (soldiers, sailors and airmen's families association)
27 Queen's Gate, London SW1H 9BZ;
Tel 071-222 9221

Stillbirth and Neonatal Death Society (SANDS)
28 Portland Place, London W1 4DE;
Tel 071-436 5881

Stress Syndrome Foundation
Cedar House, Yalding, Kent ME18 6JD

Sue Ryder Foundation
Cavendish, Sudbury, Suffolk CO10 8AY;
Tel 0787 280252

Support After Termination for Fetal Abnormality (SAFTA)
29–30 Soho Square, London W1V 6JB;
Tel 071-439 6124

TAG – The Arthogryposis Group
Witts End, Ghyll Road, Scotby, Carlisle CA4 8BT;
Tel 0228 72553

Terrence Higgins Trust (for AIDS patients and their families)
52–54 Grays Inn Road, London WC1X 8JU;
Tel 071-831 0330

Thalassaemia Society
107 Nightingale Lane, London N8 7QY;
Tel 081-348 0437

Tranquillizer Withdrawal Advice and Support
1 Mosley Street, Heaton, Newcastle-upon-Tyne, NE1 1YE;
Tel 091-261 6338

Turning Point (drug-related problems)
New Loom House, 101 Backchurch Lane, London E1 1LU;
Tel 071-702 2300

Twins and Multiple Births Association (TAMBA)
59 Sunnyside, Worksop,
North Notts S81 7LN;
Tel 0909 479250
• *Many local groups – ask your midwife or health visitor for details*

University Central Council on Admissions (UCCA)
PO Box 28, Cheltenham, Gloucester GL50 1HY

Urostomy Association
Buckland, Beaumont Park, Danbury, Essex CM4 4DE;
Tel 0245 414294

Vegan Society
7 Battle Road, St Leonards on Sea,
East Sussex TN37 7AA;
Tel 0424 427393

Vegetarian Society
Parkdale, Denham Road, Altrincham,
Cheshire; Tel 061-928 0793

Vitiligo Group
PO Box 919, London SE21 8AW;
Tel 081-776 7022

Ways and Means (Nottingham Rehabilitation)
Ludlow Hill Road, West Bridgford,
Nottingham, NG2 6HD;
Tel 0602 452345

Wireless for the Bedridden
816 Corbets Tey Road, Upminster, Essex RM14 2AJ;
Tel 0402 250051

Women's Environmental Network
287 City Road, London EC1V 1LA;
Tel 071-490 2511

Women's Health Concern (WHC)
Ground Floor, 17 Earl's Terrace,
London W8 6LP;

Women's Health and Reproduction Rights Information Centre
52 Featherstone Street, London EC1Y 8RT;
Tel 071-251 6332

Women's Royal Voluntary Service (WRVS)
234–44 Stockwell Road, London SW9 9SP;
Tel 071-416 0146

Write Away (pen-pals for handicapped and able-bodied children)
c/o Nichole Levine and Hilary Wainer,
PO Box 175, New Ash Green,
Dartford DA3 8PQ;
Tel 081-452 3330

SUGGESTED FURTHER READING

This Appendix lists some suggestions for further reading on the various topics covered in this book. You are recommended to look through additional sections of the Appendix as some titles are undoubtedly relevant to more than one section of the book – so, for example, if you are interested in reading more about the very young child, it would be well worth your while looking at the booklists under the headings 'Pregnancy and parenthood' and 'The older child and adolescent'. Similarly, all readers may benefit from looking at the list under the heading 'I Health and Caring'.

I HEALTH AND CARING

British Medical Association (1990) *Complete Family Health Encyclopedia*. Dorling Kindersley.

Borbely, A. (1986) *The Secrets of Sleep*. Penguin.

British Red Cross (1984) *Practical Nursing*. Dorling Kindersley.

Chartered Society of Physiotherapy (1988) *Handling the Handicapped*. Woodhead Faulkner.

Copperman, Harriet (1983) *Dying at Home*. Scutari Press.

Davies, S. and A. Stewart (1987) *Nutritional Medicine*. Pan.

Faulder, Caroline (1985) *Whose Body is It?* Virago Press.

Hodgkinson, P.E. and M. Stewart (1991) *Coping with Catastrophe*. Routledge.

Holford, P. (1981) *The Whole Health Manual*. Thorsons.

Kohner, Nancy (1988) *Caring at Home*. Health Education Authority/The Kings Fund.

Lake, Tony (1984) *Living With Grief*. Sheldon Press.

Melzack, K. and P. Wall (1982) *The Challenge of Pain*. Penguin.

Ministry of Agriculture, Food and Fisheries. (1985) *Manual of Nutrition*. HMSO.

Murray, Michael and Joseph Pizzorno (1990) *Encyclopaedia of Natural Medicine*. Optima.

NAGE (1989) *Eating a Way Into the '90s*. British Diabetic Association.

Nicholson, J. and M. Lucas (1984) *All in the Mind*. Thames Methuen.

Orton, C. (1989) *Care For The Carer*. Thorsons.

Rodmell, S. and A. Watt (1986) *The Politics of Health Education*. Routledge.

Schiff, Harriet (1979) *The Bereaved Parent*. Souvenir Press.

Smith, Tony (1987) *The New Macmillan Guide to Family Health*. Macmillan.

St John's Ambulance (1988) *Caring for the Sick*, 2nd ed. Dorling Kindersley.

Skynner, Robin and John Cleese (1983) *Families and How to Survive Them*. Mandarin.

Trevelyan, Joanna, David Dowson and Ruth West (1989) *Thorsons Guide to Medical Tests*. Thorsons.

Truswell, A. S. (1986) *ABC of Nutrition*. British Medical Association.

Whitfield, Clive (1990) *People Who Help*. Profile Productions.

Winn, Denise (1987) *The Hospice Way*. Optima.

World Health Organisation (1990) *Diet, Nutrition and Chronic Disease*. HMSO.

The Family File. (A format devised by a group of mothers for keeping personal and health details for all the family.) Septima.

II THE STAGES OF LIFE

PREGNANCY AND PARENTHOOD

Billings, A. and A. Westland (1980) *Natural Family Planning*. Allen Lane.

Blackie, Penny (1986) *Becoming a Mother After Thirty*. Blackwell.

Bryan, Elizabeth (1984) *Twins in the Family*. Constable.

Bryan, Elizabeth (1992) *Twins, Triplets and More*. Penguin.

Campbell, R. and A. Macfarlane (1987) *Where to be Born? The debate and the evidence*. National Perinatal Epidemiology Unit.

de Crespigny, Lachlan and Rhonda Dredge (1991) *Which Tests for My Unborn Baby?* Oxford University Press.

Fenwick, Elizabeth (1990) *The Johnson & Johnson Complete Book of Mother and Baby Care: a practical parents' handbook from conception to three years*. Dorling Kindersley.

Fletcher, Gillian (1991) *The National Childbirth Trust: Get into Shape after Childbirth*. Ebury Press.

Guillebaud, John (1985) *Contraception: your questions answered*. Pitman.

Hart, Graham (1989) *The First Time Father*. Corgi.

Inch, Sally (1989) *Birthrights: a parents' guide to modern childbirth*. Green Press.

Junor, V. and M. Monaco (1984) *The Home-birth Handbook*. Souvenir Press.

Kitzinger, Sheila (1987) *Freedom and Choice in Childbirth*. Viking.

Kitzinger, Sheila (1989) *Pregnancy and Childbirth*. Michael Joseph.

Kohner, Nancy (1988) *Pregnancy Book*. Health Education Authority.

Lewis, Charlie (1986) *Becoming a Father*. Open University Press.

Macfarlane, Aidan (1977) *The Psychology of Childbirth*. Fontana.

McConville, Brigid (1990) *The Parent's Green Guide*. Pandora.

McIntyre, A. (1988) *Herbs for Pregnancy and Childbirth*. Sheldon Press.

Marshall, Fiona (1992) *Coping Successfully with Your Second Baby*. Sheldon Press.

Maternity Alliance. *Getting Fit For Pregnancy*. Available from The Maternity Alliance, London.

Oakley, A., A. McPherson and H. Roberts (1984) *Miscarriage*. Fontana.

Pearce, J. C. (1979) *Magical Child*. Paladin/Granada.

Rosambeau, M. (1987) *How Twins Grow Up*. The Bodley Head.

SANDS *A Little Lifetime: a booklet for parents whose babies have died at or around the time of birth*. Health Education Bureau (Ireland) and SANDS.

Sapstead, Anne Marie (1990) *Banish Post-Baby Blues*. Thorsons.

Szarewski, Anne (1991) *Hormonal Contra-ception*. Optima.

Ward, Jane (1989) *One Parent Plus: a handbook for single parents*. Optima.

Warner, Jennifer (1991) *Helping the Handicapped Child with Early Feeding*. Winslow Press.

Wesson, Nicky (1989) *Alternative Maternity*. Optima.

Wesson, Nicky (1989) *Home Birth: a practical guide*. Optima.

Winston, Robert (1987) *Infertility: a sympathetic approach*. Optima.

THE FIRST FIVE YEARS

Bunker, Caroline (1990) *Feed your Child Safely*. Ebury Press.

Green, Christopher (1990) *Toddler Taming: a parents' guide to the first four years*, Revised edition. Century.

Jolly, Hugh (1985) *Book of Childcare*, 4th ed. Allen & Unwin.

Jones, Maggie (1990) *The Mothercare Guide to Safety and Your Child*. Mothercare/The Child Accident Prevention Trust.

Karmel, Annabel (1991) *The Complete Baby and Toddler Meal Planner*. Ebury Press.

Kitzinger, Sheila (1991) *Breastfeeding your Baby*. Dorling Kindersley.

Kohner, Nancy (1989) *Birth to 5*. Health Education Authority/Harper & Row.

Leach, Penelope (1989) *Baby and Child: from birth to age five*, 2nd ed. Penguin.

Messenger Davies, Maire (1991) *The Breastfeeding Book*, 2nd ed. Frances Lincoln.

Royal College of Midwives (1988) *Successful Breastfeeding*. Available from The Royal College of Midwives, 15 Mansfield Street, London W1M 0BE

West, Richard (1983) *Family Guide to Children's Ailments*. Hamlyn.

THE OLDER CHILD AND ADOLESCENT

Aarons, Maureen and Tessa Gittens (1992) *A Handbook of Autism*. Routledge.

Brooks, Sue and Richard Newton (1991) *Down's Syndrome*. Optima.

Chadwick, David and Sue Usiskin (1991) *Living with Epilepsy*, Revised ed. Optima.

Coleman, J. (1989) *Teenagers in the Family* (Booklet and cassette tape for parents) and *Teenagers under Stress* (Booklet and cassette tape for parents). Both available from The Trust for the Study of Adolescence, 23 New Road, Brighton, East Sussex.

Department of Transport (1990) *Keep on the Safe Side: a handbook for young cyclists*. HMSO.

Disabled Living Foundation (1978). *The Garden and the Handicapped Child*. Haigh and Hochland.

Elliot, Michelle (1986) *The Willow Street Kids*. True stories told by children to whom they have happened – for children. Piccola.

Elliot, Michelle (1990) *Feeling Happy, Feeling Safe: a safety guide for young children*. Piccola.

Harpin, Phillippa *With a Little Help* (series). Available from the Muscular Dystrophy Group of Great Britain.

Hillson, Rowan (1988) *Diabetes: a young person's guide*. Optima.

Lansdown, Richard and Marjorie Walker (1991) *Your Child's Development: from birth to adolescence*. Frances Lincoln.

Lintner, Brenda (1991) *Living With Teenagers*. Optima.

Markham, Ursula (1990) *Helping Children Cope with Stress*. Sheldon Press.

Millard, Diana (1984) *Daily Living with the Handicapped Child*. Croom Helm.

Open University (1988) *Health Choices*. Available from The Open University, PO Box 188, Milton Keynes, MK7 6DH

Stanton, Marion (1992) *Cerebral Palsy*. Optima.

Whiteside, Mike (1990) *Childhood Asthma: a doctor's complete treatment plan.* Thorsons.

THE ADULT YEARS

Ashton, David (1991) *The 12-Week Executive Health Plan.* Kogan Page.

Baum, Michael (1988) *Breast Cancer: the facts.* Oxford University Press.

BBC Radio 4 (1986) *The In Touch Handbook: a guide to services for visually handicapped people.* Available from Broadcasting Support Services, PO Box 7, London W3 6XJ.

Beard, M. (1984) *Understanding Premenstrual Tension.* Pan.

Benz, Cynthia (1988) *Coping with Multiple Sclerosis.* Optima.

British Medical Association (1987) *Living With Risk.* John Wiley.

British Medical Association (1989) *Infection Control.* Edward Arnold.

Comfort, Alex (1991) *The New Joy of Sex.* Mitchell Beazley.

Clyne, Rachael (1989) *Cancer – Your Life Your Choice,* 2nd ed. Thorsons.

Consumers' Association (1988) *Which? Wills and Probate.*

Connor, S. and S. Kingman (1989) *AIDS: the search for the virus.* Penguin.

Dalton, Katharina (1969) *The Menstrual Cycle.* Pelican.

Darnbrough, Ann and Derek Kinade (1991) *Directory for Disabled People.* 6th ed. Woodhead Faulkner.

Davies, Paul and F. Clifford Rose (1987) *Answers to Migraine.* Optima.

Disability Alliance (1990) *The Disability Rights Handbook.* Available from The Disability Alliance, 25 Denmark Street, London WC2H 8NJ.

Dixon, Allan and Anthony Woolf (1989) *Avoiding Osteoporosis.* Optima.

Evans, P. (1979) *Cystitis and How to Cope With It.* Granada.

Farrell, Elaine (1991) *The Mental Health Survival Guide.* Optima.

Feneley, R. C. L. and J. P. Blannin (1984) *Incontinence: help for an unmentionable problem.* Patient Handbook No. 18. Churchill Livingstone.

Ford, Janet and Philippa Merriman (1990) *The Gentle Art of Listening.* Bedford Square Press.

Glasspool, Michael (1984) *Eyes.* Optima.

Greenwood, Sadja (1991) *Menopause the Natural Way: looking forward to the future.* Optima.

Hart, Frank Dudley (1981) *Overcoming Arthritis.* Optima.

Hawkridge, Caroline (1989) *Understanding Endometriosis.* Optima.

Hillson, Rowan (1988) *Diabetes Beyond 40.* Optima.

Hillson, Rowan (1991) *Thyroid Disorders.* Optima.

Hillson, Rowan (1992) *Diabetes: a new guide.* Optima.

Jay, Peggy (1985) *Help Yourselves,* 4th ed. Ian Henry Press.

Julian, Desmond and Clare Marley (1991) *Coronary Heart Disease: the facts,* 3rd ed. Oxford University Press.

Lane, Donald and Anthony Storr (1992) *Asthma: the facts,* 3rd ed. Oxford University Press.

Martin, Michael and Brian Grover (1986) *Hearing Loss: causes, treatment, and advice.* Churchill Livingstone.

Martin, Michael and Brian Grover (1990) *Ears and Hearing.* Optima.

McKenzie, Robin (1983) *Treat Your Own Neck.* Spinal Publications, Waikanae, NZ.

McKenzie, Robin (1985) *Treat Your Own Back*, 2nd ed. Spinal Publications, Waikanae, NZ.

Miller, David (1988) *Living With AIDS and HIV.* Macmillan.

Mulcahy, Risteard (1990) *Beat Heart Disease*, Revised ed. Optima.

Nichols, Philip (1981) *Disabled: an illustrated manual of help and self-help.* David & Charles.

Phillips, Angela and Jill Rakuson (1990) *The New Our Bodies, Ourselves.* Penguin.

Priest, Robert (1988) *Anxiety and Depression.* Optima.

Sagar, Harvey (1991) *Parkinson's Disease.* Optima.

Smith, Tom (1991) *Living with High Blood Pressure.* Sheldon Press.

Swaffield, Laura (1960) *Stroke: the complete guide to recovery and rehabilitation.* Thorsons.

Symes, David (1990) *Cholesterol – Reducing Your Risk.* Optima.

Webb, Ann (1989) *Experiences of Hysterectomy.* Optima.

THE LATER YEARS (60 PLUS)

Age Concern (1990) *Your Rights: a guide to money benefits for older people.* Age Concern England.

Age Concern (1990) *Your Taxes and Savings: a guide for older people.* Age Concern England.

Bennett, Gerry (1989) *Alzheimer's Disease and Other Confusional States.* Optima.

Consumers' Association *Which? Way to Save and Invest.*

Consumers' Association (1990) *Which? Way to Save Tax.*

Fenely, R. C. L. and J. P. Blannin (1984) *Incontinence: help for an unmentionable problem.* Patient Handbook No. 18. Churchill Livingstone.

Forgey, William (1991) *The Basic Essentials of Hypothermia.* ICS Books.

Franks, Helen (1987) *What Every Woman Should Know About Retirement.* Age Concern England.

Greengross, Sally (1985) *Ageing: an adventure in living.* Human Horizon Series.

Greengross, Wendy and Sally Greengross (1989) *Living, Loving and Ageing.* Age Concern England.

Help the Aged (1991) *Take Care of Yourself: a health handbook for older people.* Winslow Press.

Hemmings, S. (1985) *A Wealth of Experience: the lives of older women.* Pandora.

Leach, Robert (1989) *Financial Planning for the over 50s.* Longman for Allied Dunbar Financial Services Ltd.

Letts, Penny (1991) *Managing Other People's Money.* Age Concern England.

Manthorpe, Jill (1990) *Elderly People – Rights and Opportunities.* In association with Age Concern. Self-help guides. Longman.

Mares, Penny (1991) *In Control: help with incontinence.* Age Concern England.

Micklewood, Paulette (1991) *Caring for Confusion.* Scutari Press.

Muir Gray, J. A. and Heather McKenzie (1980) *Caring for Older People.* Penguin.

Muir Gray, J. A. and Heather McKenzie (1986) *Take Care of Your Elderly Relative.* Beaconsfield.

Shapiro, J. (1989) *Ourselves. Growing Older. Women Ageing with Knowledge and Power*. Fontana/Collins.

Skeet, Muriel (1982) *The Third Age: a guide for elderly people, their families and friends*. Darton, Longman & Todd.

Whitlock, Ralph (1984) *Three-score-years-and-ten*. Ian Henry Publications.

III ADDITIONAL INFORMATION

HOW THE BODY WORKS

Ross, J. W. R and K. Marks (1986) *Baillière's Anatomy Illustrated*. Baillière Tindall.

Vannini, V. and G. Pogliani (1980) *The New Atlas of the Human Body*. Corgi.

FIRST AID

Playfair, A. S. (1986) *First Aid*. Made Simple Books, Heinemann.

St John's Ambulance Brigade/St Andrew's Ambulance Brigade/British Red Cross Society (Latest Edition) *First Aid Manual*. Dorling Kindersley.

DRUGS AND MEDICINES

British Medical Association (1988) *BMA Guide to Medicines and Drugs*. Dorling Kindersley.

British Medical Association/Royal Pharmaceutical Association (Updated six-monthly) *British National Formulary*. BMA/The Pharmaceutical Press.

Bold type indicates main entry